Melvin A. Shiffman (Editor)

Breast Augmentation

Melvin A. Shiffman (Editor)

Breast Augmentation

Principles and Practice

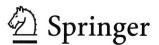 Springer

Melvin A. Shiffman, MD, JD
Chairman, Surgery Section
Tustin Hospital and Medical Center
17501 Chatham Drive
Tustin, CA 92780-2302
USA

ISBN 978-3-540-78947-5   e-ISBN 978-3-540-78948-2

DOI 10.1007/978-3-540-78948-2

Library of Congress Control Number: 2008925097

Cover design: Frido Steinen-Broo, eStudio Calamar, Spain
Reproduction, typesetting and production: le-tex publishing services oHG, Leipzig, Germany

Printed on acid-free paper

9 8 7 6 5 4 3 2 1

springer.com

Foreword

It is a great pleasure and privilege to recommend this book on breast augmentation, having spent over 25 years of my life dealing with and operating on breasts. It is still fascinating to understand why breast augmentation has become one of the most common cosmetic operations in the world. The psychology and body image that influence a woman's decision to have this operation are still a mystery. Many books and articles have been written about various techniques; however, you will find all of this condensed in this book, with the latest information and research to help you understand this relatively simple operation. Varying approaches and different implants have puzzled many surgeons and patients alike, and this book provides enlightenment.

Implants and materials used in this operation are discussed and argued in this book and settle the score on which implant should be used in the 21st century. The positioning of the implants either above or below the muscle is discussed in detail, and the reasons behind the authors' preferences are well demonstrated. Capsule formation has been considered as a sequela of the operation, and many speculations have been put forward as to the likely cause. However, to date, no surgeon or theory has convinced me that the answer has been found as to the likely cause of this condition, and that is why the treatment has been toward symptomatic management rather than prevention and cure.

The size of the implants and the final result have depended mostly on the surgeon's experience and the patient's psychological state. There is no precise way to accurately determine the size; however, my measurements and ideas have been put forward to help both novice and experienced surgeons alike. New ideas and measurements have also been put forward. Indications and information on where to draw the line between augmentation and mastopexy and when to combine the two operations are discussed.

The purpose of this book is to discuss the current thoughts and trends in breast augmentation and to detail the current techniques used, as well as to discuss various common complications of this procedure, how to deal with these problems, and how to treat these conditions using the current thoughts and tried and tested methods.

A unique contribution to the gratification of these human needs has been the development of surgical techniques that are safe, reasonable, and available. These are described in this book and seem to answer many questions, based on scientific and sound anatomical bases.

Anthony Erian

Preface

Breast augmentation is one of the most common cosmetic procedures performed. Women who are concerned about the size of their breasts will seek an improved appearance with augmentation to conform to their own body image. Despite the prolonged litigation and settlement of lawsuits concerning silicone breast implants and their possible association with autoimmune disease, there has been a resurgence in the frequency of breast augmentation. It has ultimately been shown that silicone is not the cause of the claimed autoimmune disease. Additionally, introduction of a cohesive gel implant that does not contain silicone gel fluid that can "bleed" into the pocket has contributed to a decrease in capsule contracture.

Surgeons performing breast augmentation have to be well informed, not only about the variety of techniques that are available but also about the possible risks and complications of the procedure. The surgeon should be capable of deciding which procedure to use to correct any defect or deformity and of avoiding or treating the variety of possible complications of the surgery. The patient should understand that the possibility exists for a second or even third procedure on the breast after augmentation.

This book is an attempt to bring together, as much as possible, augmentation surgery techniques, the possible complications of each one, and the means of correcting breast imperfections. It also includes chapters on embryology, anatomy, benign and malignant breast diseases, mammograms, body dysmorphic disorder, implant choice, breast augmentation principles, the various pockets and incisions, and medical-legal aspects. The international contributors are experts in the field of breast augmentation and have helped put together a much needed textbook to cover the varieties of breast problems and their solutions.

Melvin A. Shiffman

Contents

List of Contributors

Adrien Aiache, MD
9884 Santa Monica Blvd., Apt BH310
Beverly Hills, California 90212-1622
USA
E-mail: aaiachemd@sbcglobal.net

Robert W. Alexander, MD, DMD, FICS
Assistant Professor (Clinical), University of Texas, Health Science Center
at San Antonio, Department of Surgery
Affiliate Associate Professor, University of Washington, Department of Surgery
3500 188th St. SW, Suite 670
Lynnwood, Washington 98037
USA
E-mail: rwamd@cybernet1.com

Robert J. Allen, MD
Medical University of South Carolina
125 Doughty Street, Suite 480
Charleston, South Carolina 29403
USA
E-mail: boballen@diepaslap.com

Antonino Araco, MD
Attending Surgeon
Dolan Park Hospital
Stoney Lane
Tardebigge, Bromsgrove B60 1LY
UK
E-mail: araco@libero.it

Andre Auersvald, MD
Clinica Auersvald
Alameda Presidente Taunay 1765
Curitiba, Parana 80430-000
Brazil
E-mail: andreauersvald@uol.com.br

Luiz Augusto Auersvald, MD
Clinica Auersvald
Alameda Presidente Taunay 1765
Curitiba, Parana 80430-000
Brazil
E-mail: andreauersvald@uol.com.br

Richard A. Baxter, MD, FACS
Clinical Instructor
University of Washington School of Medicine, Seattle
6100 219th Street, SW, Suite 290
Mountlake Terrace, Washington 98043
USA
E-mail: drbaxter@baxterplasticsurgery.com

Joel Beck, MD, FACS
66 Bovet Road
San Mateo, California 94402-3125
USA
E-mail: jbeck@baysurgery.com

Hilton Becker, MD
5458 Town Center Road, Suite 101
Boca Raton, Florida 33486
USA
E-mail: hbeckermd@msn.com

George John Bitar, MD
Medical Director, Bitar Cosmetic Surgery Institute
Visiting Lecturer, Department of Plastic Surgery, University of Virginia
8650 Sudley Road, #203
Manassas, Virginia 20110
USA
E-mail: georgebitar@drbitar.com

Pierangelo Bosio, MD
Department of General Surgery
University of Modena Medical School
Policlinico Di Modena, via Del Pozzo 71
41100, Modena
Italy
E-mail: pierangelo.bosio@libero.it

R. James Brenner, MD, JD, FACR, FCLM
Chief of Breast Imaging, Professor of Radiology
University of California
UCSF-Mt. Zion Hospital, Radiology H2804
1600 Divisadero Street
San Francisco, California 94115-1667
Bay Imaging Consultants
Walnut Creek, CA 94598
USA
E-mail: james.brenner@radiology.ucsf.edu

Robert R. Brink, MD
66 Bovet Road
San Mateo, California 94402-3125
USA
E-mail: moonsheyn@yahoo.com

Valerio Cervelli, MD, PhD
Professor of Plastic Surgery
University of Tor Vergata
Via Montpellier
00133 Rome
Italy

Greg Chernoff, BSc, MD, FRCSC
9002 N. Meridian Street, Suite 205
Indianapolis, Indiana 46260
USA
E-mail: greg@drchernoff.com

Nicholas V. Chugay, DO
4210 Atlantic Avenue
Long Beach, California 90807
USA

Mark W. Clemens, MD
Resident, Department of Plastic Surgery
Georgetown University Medical Center
3800 Reservoir Road NW
Washington, DC 20007
USA
E-mail: clemensmd@gmail.com

Andre Ricardo Dall'Oglio Tolazzi, MD
Volunteer Assistant Plastic Surgeon
Federal University of Parana
Rua Brigadeiro Franco, 2507, Ap.102
Curitiba-PR, 80250-030
Brazil
E-mail: artolazzi@yahoo.com.br

Amal Dass, MD, MBChB, BAO (Ire), LRCP & SI, MRCS (Edin)
Fellow in Cosmetic Surgery
Blk 10B, Braddell View, #02-06, S
579721 Singapore
E-mail: amaldass_2000@yahoo.com

Steven P. Davison, DDS, MD, FACS
Associate Professor of Surgery
Department of Plastic Surgery
Georgetown University Medical Center
3800 Reservoir Road, NW
Washington, DC 20007
USA
E-mail: spd2@georgetown.edu

Danielle M. Deluca-Pytell, MD
400 E. Main Street, 2nd Floor North Building
Mount Kiscoe, New York 10549
USA
E-mail: delucapytell@verizon.net

Christine Anne Diedwardo, MD
Lahey Clinic, 41 Mall Road
Burlington, Massachusetts 01805-0002
USA
E-mail: christine.a.diedwardo@lahey.org

Alexandre Dionyssopoulos, MD
Assistant Professor
Aristotle University of Tessaloniki
Tessaloniki
Greece

Anthony Erian, MD, MBBCH, Bs (Lon), LRCP, FRCS (Eng) FRCS (Edin)
Orwell Grange, 43 Cambridge Road
Wimpole, Cambridge
UK
E-mail: erian@erian.demon.co.uk

Gaetano Esposito, MD
Professor of Plastic Surgery, University of Tor Vergata, Rome
Centro Ustioni Ospedale
S.Eugenio Piazzale Umanesimo, n.10
00143 Roma
Italy
E-mail: gaetanoesposito@fastwebnet.it

Renato Da Silva Freitas, MD
Assistant Professor of Plastic Surgery, Federal University of Parana
Plastic and Reconstructive Surgery Unit
Hospital de Clinicas of Federal University of Parana
R. General Carneiro, 181, 9° andar
Curitibas-PR 80060-900
Brazil
E-mail: dr.renato.freitas@gmail.com

Felix-Rüdiger G. Giebler, MD
Vincemus-Klinik
Brückenstrasse 1-A
25840 Friedrichstadt/Eider
Germany
E-mail: info@vincemus-klinik.de

Caroline Glicksman, MD
Jersey Shore University Medical Center, Neptune, New Jersey
Center for Special Surgery, Wall, New Jersey
Ocean County Medical Center, Brick, New Jersey
2164 Highway 35
Sea Girt, New Jersey 08750-1013
USA
E-mail: docglicksman@aol.com

Ruth M. Graf, MD, PhD
Professor of Plastic Surgery, Federal University of Paraná
Rua Solimões, 1175
Mercês, Curitiba – Paraná
Cep: 80810-070
Brazil
E-mail: ruthgraf@bighost.com.br, ruthgraf@bsi.com.br

Gianpiero Gravante, MD, PhD
Clinical Fellow in Hepatobiliary and Pancreatic Surgery
University Hospitals of Leicester
Research Fellow of Physiology, University of Tor Vergata, Rome
Via Umberto Maddalena 40/a
00043 Ciampino, Roma
Italy
E-mail: ggravante@hotmail.com

Daniel P. Greenwald, MD
1208 East Kennedy Boulevard, Suite 221
Tampa, Florida 33606
USA
E-mail: docdan@bs-ps.com

Darryl J. Hodgkinson, MD, MBBS (Hons), FRCS (C), FACS FACCS
The Cosmetic and Restorative Surgery Clinic
20 Manning Road
Double Bay, New South Wales 2028
Australia
E-mail: dr_hodgkinson@bigpond.com

Julie C. Holding, MD
6.124 McCullough Building, 301 University Boulevard
Galveston, Texas 77555-0724
USA
E-mail: jcholdin@utmb.edu

Lisa M. Hunsicker, MD
Revalla Plastic Surgery
7720 S Broadway, Suite 380
Littleton, Colorado 80122
USA

Ali Infield, BA
Department of Psychiatry
Research Assistant, Center for Weight and Eating Disorders
University of Pennsylvania School of Medicine
3535 Market Street
Philadelphia, Pennsylvania 19104
USA
E-mail: infieldl@mail.med.upenn.edu

J. Arthur Jensen, MD, FACS
Assistant Professor of Plastic Surgery, Geffen School of Medicine at UCLA
Adjunct Assistant Professor, John Wayne Cancer Center
2001 Santa Monica Boulevard, Suite 790W
Santa Monica, California 90404
USA
E-mail: Dr.J.Jensen@gmail.com
JAJCA@aol.com

Lin Jinde, MD
Hangzhou Municipal Plastic Surgery Hospital
168, Shangtang Road
Hangzhou, Zhejiang Province, 310014
China
E-mail: hzljd@sohu.com

José Juri, MD
Clínica Juri Cirugía Plástica
Cerviño 3252
1425 Capital Federal, Buenos Aires
Argentina
E-mail: info@clinicajuri.com.ar, clinicajuri@bcnsite.com

Bobby Arun Kumar, MD, MB BS (UNSW) BSc (UNSW)
P.O. Box 155
Pyrmont, New South Wales 2009
Australia
E-mail: getbare@hotmail.com

Franck Landat, MD
2, rue Glesener, L.
1630 Luxembourg
Luxembourg
E-mail: drlandat@pt.lu

Mary E. Lester, MD
Medical University of South Carolina
96 Jonathan Lucas Street, 426 CSB
Charleston, South Carolina 29425
USA
E-mail: lesterma@musc.edu

Susana Létiz, MD
Juramento 4462
1430 Capital Federal, Buenos Aires
Argentina
E-mail: suletiz@hotmail.com

Apostolos D. Mandrekas, MD, PhD
Director, Artion Plastic Surgery Centre
11 D. Vassilious Sreet, N. Psyhiko
Athens 15451
Greece
E-mail: amandrekas@artion-plasticsurgery.com

James W. May, Jr., MD
Chair, Division of Plastic & Reconstructive Surgery
Massachusetts General Hospital,
15 Parkman Street, WACC 435
Boston, Massachusetts 02114
USA
E-mail: jwmay@partners.org

W. Thomas McClellan, MD
Department of Plastic & Reconstructive Surgery
Lahey Clinic, Burlington, Massachusetts
Morgantown Plastic Surgery Associates
1085 Van Voorhis Road, Suite 350
Morgantown, West Virginia 26505
USA
E-mail: wtmcclellan@gmail.com

John McCurdy, Jr., MD
Formerly Assistant Clinical Professor of Surgery
University of Hawaii John A. Burns School of Medicine
1188 Bishop Street, Suite 2402
Honolulu, Hawaii 96813
USA
E-mail: johnmccurdy@hotmail.com

Sid J. Mirrafati, MD
Mira Aesthetics
1101 Bryan Avenue, Suite G
Tustin, California 92780-4401
USA
E-mail: drmirrafati@youngerlook.com

Richard Moufarrège, MD, FRCS(C)
Assistant Professor
University of Montreal
Private practice: 1111, rue St-Urbain, Suite 106
Montreal (Quebec), H2Z 1Y6
Canada
E-mail: plasticsurg_moufar@hotmail.com

Toma T. Mugea, MD, PhD
Professor, Plastic and Aesthetic Surgery
Oradea Medical University
Director Medestet Clinic
9/7 Cipariu Square
Cluj-Napoca
Romania
E-mail: drmugea@medestet.ro

Robert X. Murphy, Jr., MD, MS
Department of Surgery, Division of Plastic Surgery
Lehigh Valley Hospital
Cedar Crest & I-78, P.O. Box 689
Allentown, Pennsylvania 18105-1556
USA
E-mail: sally.lutz@lvh.com, robert.murphy@lvh.com

David T. Netscher, MD
Clinical Professor, Division of Plastic Surgery
Baylor College of Medicine
Adjunct Professor of Surgery, Cornell University, Houston, Texas
Chief of Plastic Surgery, Veterans Affairs Medical Center, Houston, Texas
Private practice: 6624 Fannin Street, Suite 2730
Houston, Texas 77030-2339
USA
E-mail: netscher@bcm.tmc.edu

Gilvani Azor De Oliveira e Cruz, MD
Chief Professor, Plastic Surgery Unit
Federal University of Parana
Rua Saint´ Hilaire, 717, Aptº 2002, Agua Verde
CEP: 80254-140
Curitiba, PR
Brazil
E-mail: gilvani@ufpr.br

Daniele Pace, MD, MsC
Rua Solimões, 1175 Mercês, Curitiba, Paraná Brasil
Cep 80810-070
Brazil
E-mail: danielepace@hotmail.com

Beniamino Palmieri, MD
Department of Surgery
University of Modena Medical School and Reggio Emilia
Policlinico IV floor
Via del Pozzo, 71
41100 Modena
Italy
E-mail: palmieri@unimo.it

Edward A. Pechter, MD, FACS
Assistant Clinical Professor of Plastic Surgery
University of California, Los Angeles
25880 Tournament Road, Suite 217
Valencia, California 91355-2844
USA
E-mail: drpechter@aol.com

Myron M. Persoff, MD
3659 South Miami Avenue
Miami, Florida 33133-4227
USA
E-mail: drpersoff@drpersoff.com

Linda G. Phillips, MD
Distinguished Truman G. Blocker, Jr., MD, Professor
Chief, Division of Plastic Surgery
Program Director, Plastic Surgery Residency Program
University of Texas Medical Branch, Galveston
6.124 McCullough Bldg., 301 University Boulevard
Galveston, Texas 77555-0724
USA
E-mail: lphillip@utmb.edu

Rocco C. Piazza, MD
53 Campau Circle, NW
Grand Rapids, Michigan 49503
USA
E-mail: rpiazzamd@gmail.com

Luis A. Picard-Ami, Jr., MD
PTY 8016, 1601 N.W. 97th Avenue
Miami, Florida 33102
USA
Consultorios Médicos Paitilla #513
Panamá City
Panamá
E-mail: picardami@psi.net.pa

Lukas Prantl, MD, PhD
Director, Department of Plastic Surgery
University of Regensburg
Franz-Josef-Strauss-Allee 11
93042 Regensburg
Germany
E-mail: lukas.prantl@klinik.uni-regensburg.de

Mark A. Randolph, MS
Massachusetts General Hospital
Division of Plastic Surgery Research Lab
15 Parkman Street, WACC 457
Boston, Massachusetts 02114
USA
E-mail: marandolph@partners.org

Angelo Rebelo, MD
Clinica Milenio
Rua Manual Silva Leal, 7A, 11C
1600-166 Lisboa
Portugal
E-mail: clinicamilenio@netcabo.pt

Robert S. Reiffel, MD
12 Greenridge Avenue, Suite 203
White Plains, New York 10605-1238
USA
E-mail: r.reiffel@verizon.net

Anileda Ribeiro Dos Santos, MD
Volunteer Assistant Plastic Surgeon
Federal University of Parana
Rua Pe. Anchieta, 640, Aptº 501, Champagnat
CEP: 80430-060, Curitiba, PR
Brazil
E-mail: aniledaribeiro@yahoo.com.br

Asaad Samra, MD
Former Resident, Division of Plastic Surgery, Baylor College of Medicine
The Samra Group
733 North Beers Street, Suite U1
Holmdel, New Jersey 07733
USA
E-mail: asamramd@aol.com

David B. Sarwer, PhD
Departments of Psychiatry and Surgery
The Edwin and Fannie Gray Hall Center for Human Appearance
Center for Weight and Eating Disorders
University of Pennsylvania School of Medicine
10 Penn Tower
3400 Spruce Street
Philadelphia, Pennsylvania 19104
USA
E-mail: dsarwer@mail.med.upenn.edu

Shawkat A. Sati, MD
Clinical Instructor, Tufts University
Lahey Clinic, Department of Plastic & Reconstructive Surgery
41 Mall Road
Burlington, Massachusetts 01805
USA
E-mail: shawkat.sati@lahey.org

Ingrid Schlenz, MD
Consultant, Department of Plastic and Reconstructive Surgery
Wilhelminenspital
Montleartstrasse 37
1160 Vienna
Austria
E-mail: ingrid.schlenz@wienkav.at

Brooke R. Seckel, MD
Lahey Clinic, Department of Plastic & Reconstructive Surgery, Burlington,
Massachusetts
Boston Plastic Surgery Associates
Emerson Hospital
John Cuming Building, Suite 700, 131 ORNAC
Concord, Massachusetts 01742
USA
E-mail: drseckel@gmail.com

Asuman Sevin, MD
Plastic and Reconstructive Surgery Department
Ankara Numune Training and Research Hospital
Zirvekent 2. Etap Sitesi C-1/43
Cankaya, 06550 Ankara
Turkey
E-mail: basevin@gmail.com

Kutlu Sevin, MD
Professor, Plastic and Reconstructive Surgery Department
Ankara University Faculty of Medicine
Zirvekent 2. Etap Sitesi C-1/43
Cankaya, 06550 Ankara
Turkey

Melvin A. Shiffman, MD, JD
Chairman, Section of Surgery
Tustin Hospital and Medical Center
17501 Chatham Drive
Tustin, California 92780-2302
USA
E-mail: shiffmanmdjd@yahoo.com

Tetsuo Shu, MD
Daikanyama Clinic
4F, 1-10-2 Ebisu-Minami, Shibuya-ku
Tokyo, 150-0022
Japan
E-mail: shu@mpint.co.jp

John E. Skandalakis, MD, PhD
Chris Carlos Distinguished Professor of Surgical Anatomy and Technique
Director, Centers for Surgical Anatomy & Technique
Professor of Surgery, Department of Surgery
Emory University School of Medicine
Clinical Professor of Surgery, The Medical College of Georgia, Augusta, Georgia
Clinical Professor of Surgery, Mercer University School of Medicine, Macon, Georgia
1462 Clifton Road, NE, Suite 303
Atlanta, Georgia 30322
USA
E-mail: cfroman@emory.edu, cpainte@emory.edu

Ned Snyder IV, MD
901 W. 38th Street, Suite 410
Austin, Texas 78705
USA

Colin Song, MD, MBBCh, FRCS, FAMS
Head and Senior Consultant
Department of Plastic Reconstructive and Aesthetic Surgery
Director, Post Graduate Medical Institute
Singapore General Hospital
Outram Road
169608 Singapore
E-mail: colin.song@sgh.com.sg

Katsuya Takasu, MD, PhD
Takasu Clinic Building 8F
16-23 Tuabaki-cho, Nakamura-ku
Nagoya, 453-0015
Japan
E-mail: tomoko@takasu.co.jp, info@takasu.co.jp

Shizu Takasu, MD
Takasu Clinic Building 8F
16-23 Tuabaki-cho, Nakamura-ku
Nagoya, 453-0015
Japan
E-mail: tomoko@takasu.co.jp, info@takasu.co.jp

Bien-Keem Tan, MD, MBBS, FRCS, FAMS
Senior Consultant, Department of Plastic Reconstructive and Aesthetic Surgery
Singapore General Hospital
Outram Road
169608 Singapore
E-mail: bienkeem@singnet.com.sg

Maria Fernanda Valotta, MD
3 de Febrero 986
1426 Capital Federal, Buenos Aires
Argentina
E-mail: cplastica@doctoravalotta.com.ar

Melvyn Westreich, MD
Department of Plastic Surgery
Assaf HaRofeh Medical Center
Tzrifin, 70-33
Israel
E-mail: mwestreich@hotmail.com

Chin-Ho Wong, MBBS, MRCS (Ed), M Med (Surgery)
Chief Resident, Department of Plastic, Reconstructive and Aesthetic Surgery
Singapore General Hospital
Outram Road
169608 Singapore
E-mail: wchinho@hotmail.com

Elisabeth Würinger, MD
Department of Plastic and Reconstructive Surgery
Wilhelminenspital
Montleartstrasse 37
1160 Vienna
Austria
E-mail: dr.elisabeth.wueringer@utanet.at

Robert Yoho, MD
797 S. Arroyo Parkway
Pasadena, California 91105
USA
E-mail: ryrobert@pacbell.net

George J. Zambacos, MD
Associate
University of Athens
27 Skoufa Street
Kolonaki, Athens 10673
Greece
E-mail: gzambacos@aestheticsurgery.gr

Part I
Anatomy, Benign Breast Disease, Malignant Breast Disease, Mammograms

Chapter 1

Embryology and Anatomy of the Breast

John E. Skandalakis

1.1
Introduction

In the middle and fore-part of each side of the Chest, there rise two fleshy Eminences, called the Breasts, which are a good deal larger in Women than in Men. The Breasts of Women are composed of Glandular Bodies, interspersed with an infinite Number of Vessels, which serve for the Secretion of Milk. Those of Men are only composed of Skin, Flesh, and Fat … In general, the Breasts of Men ought to be small, and a little plain. Those of Women ought to be round, high, and have the Figure of two Hemispheres, separated from one another by a middle Interstice.

Nicolas Andry de Bois-Regard, Orthopaedia (1743) [1]

1.2
Embryogenesis

The ectoderm and the mesenchyme are responsible for the genesis of the male and female breast. The ectoderm is responsible for the formation of the ducts and alveoli, and the mesenchyme is responsible for the connective tissue and its vessels.

In the ventral area of the body, the milk line (ridge) develops (Fig. 1.1). Usually, it extends from the axilla to the inguinal area. However, occasionally the milk ridge extends down into the triangle of Scarpa. The pectoral part of the milk ridge produces the right and left mammary primordia. The proximal and distal part of the extrapectoral ridge disappears.

Kopans [2] stated that the breasts have the same ectodermal origin as skin glands (Fig. 1.2). The ectodermal thickening of the mammary primordium grows into the dermis [3]. This produces 16–24 solid cords of ectodermal cells growing within the underlying mesoderm (dermis). Later, these buds will become canalized and form the lactiferous ducts and alveoli. The epidermal surface of the future nipple is at first a shallow depression during the final trimester; near term it becomes everted and ready to accept the lactiferous ducts.

Howard and Gusterson [4] stated that very little is known about the molecular mechanisms that initiate breast formation. A small part of the ridges remains in the pectoral area, which is responsible for the genesis of the right and left breasts as well as for the embryological mammary anomalies. The typical developmental harmony between ectoderm (epithelial ductal lining and acini) and mesenchyme (the skin and the supporting elements) occasionally goes awry, producing congenital anomalies of the breast.

Each mammary lobe has one lactiferous duct, which terminates at the nipple of the mammary gland. The pathway of the lobes is from the nipple to the connective and fatty tissue of the superficial fascia. Thus, the breast can be conceptualized as a grouping of large glands that originate from the epidermis. Langebartel [5] termed

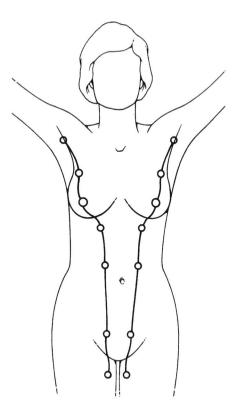

Fig. 1.1 The milk line. Mammary glands usually develop in humans from the pectoral portion of the line. Supernumerary mammary structures may develop from other positions along the line (From Skandalakis et al. [58], with permission)

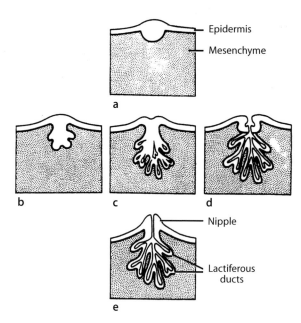

Fig. 1.2 Development of the breast. **a–d** Stages in the formation of the duct system and potential glandular tissue from the epidermis. Connective tissue septa are derived from mesenchyme of the dermis. **e** Eversion of the nipple near birth. (From Skandalakis et al. [58], with permission)

the female breast "mostly a mound of fat, with fascias and fibrous strands and the mammary gland (active or inactive)."

Kopans [2] analyzed breast development: "The breast develops in the superficial layer of fascia that lies just beneath the skin. It is not clear whether the superficial layer splits into a deep and superficial layer to form an incomplete envelope around the gland, or whether the elongating ducts invaginate the fascia, which then ends up enveloping the gland" (Fig 1.3).

The chronology of breast development is presented in Table 1.1.

The breast characteristically presents changes when still in utero as well as during the extrauterine period. Russo and Russo [6] divide these changes into two phases:

- Developmental phase: Early stages of gland morphogenesis from nipple epithelium to lobule formation
- Differentiation phase: Differentiation of mammary epithelium

Remember: The ridges disappear early, but a small portion remains in the pectoral region. This is responsible for the genesis of "a single pair of glands," according to Bland and Romrell [7].

Neville et al. [8, 9] have summarized the stages of human mammary development (Table 1.2), noting the role of the mammary fat pad in the development of the mammary epithelium. The fat pad provides signals that mediate ductal morphogenesis and alveolar differentiation.

The genesis of the breast is an enigma. Sakakura [10] and Robinson et al. [11] have discussed mesenchymal interactions.

1.3
Congenital Anomalies

The axilla is the most common area in which accessory breast tissue can be found [2]. The multiple but rare congenital anomalies of the breast may be associated with various other syndromes. It is not within the scope of this chapter to study these syndromes or their associated anomalies.

1.3.1
Amastia

By definition, amastia is the absence of one or both breasts. This congenital phenomenon is very rare. The first reports of unilateral amastia [12], bilateral amastia

Table 1.1 Timeline of breast development

4th–6th fetal week	Development of milk lines or mammary (ectodermal) ridges
10th fetal week	Atrophy of the proximal and distal part of the milk lines; the middle (pectoral) part is responsible for the genesis of the breast
5th fetal month	Development of the areola and 15–20 solid cords
Later	Lactiferous ducts; mammary glands develop from the milk lines
After birth	Nipple is visible
Puberty	Ducts develop acini at their ends

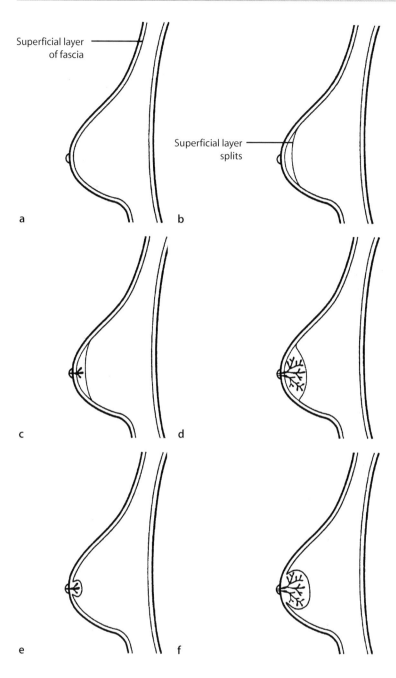

Fig. 1.3 It is unclear how the breast develops with respect to the superficial fascia, which runs just under the skin. **a** The fascia may split, forming a deep and superficial layer with the breast in between (insinuation). **b–d** The other possibility is that as the ducts elongate and grow back into the soft tissues, they may be enveloped by the fascia (invagination; **e, f**). (From Kopans [2], with permission)

[13], and amastia (with or without athelia) associated with Poland syndrome [14] were all published in the 1800s. In 1917, Deaver and McFarland [15] reported other congenital anomalies in association with amastia.

In females, unilateral breast absence is the most common form of amastia. Bilateral amastia has been reported in male and female patients [16].

Trier [17] divided his presentation of 43 cases of amastia into three categories:

- Bilateral amastia
- Unilateral amastia
- Bilateral amastia with congenital ectodermal defects

According to Merlob [18], 40% of all cases of amastia are associated with other congenital malformations (skeletal, facial, renal, genital). Several syndromes are associated with this condition [19–22]. Familial occurrence has been observed by various investigators

Table 1.2 Stages of mammary development (*GH* growth hormone, *IGF-1* insulin-like growth factor-1, *HGF* human growth factor, *TGF-ß* transforming growth factor-ß, *PRL* prolactin, HER heregulin, FIL feedback inhibitor of lactation)

Developmental stage	Hormonal regulation	Local factors	Description
Embryogenesis	???	Fat pad necessary for ductal extension	Epithelial bud develops in 18–19-week fetus, extending a short distance into mammary fat pad with blind ducts that become canalized; some milk secretion may be present at birth
Pubertal development	—	—	—
Before onset of menses	Estrogen, GH	IGF-1, HGF, TGF-ß, ???	Ductal extension into the mammary fat pad; branching morphogenesis
After onset of menses	Estrogen, progesterone, PRL?	—	Lobular development with formation of terminal duct lobular unit
Development in pregnancy	Progesterone, PRL, placental lactogen	HER, ???	Alveolus formation; partial cellular differentiation
Transition: lactogenesis	Progesterone withdrawal, PRL, glucocorticoid	Unknown	Onset of milk secretion: Stage I: midpregnancy Stage II: parturition
Lactation	PRL, oxytocin	FIL, stretch	Ongoing milk secretion, milk ejection
Involution	Withdrawal of prolactin	Milk stasis (FIL??)	Alveolar epithelium undergoes apoptosis and remodeling; gland reverts to prepregnant state

From Neville [8], with permission

[23–24], and complete absence of a breast in siblings has been reported [25].

Greydanus and colleagues [26] state that amastia is the result of "complete mammary ridge involution, including the pectoral ridge on the affected side."

1.3.2
Athelia

Athelia, from the Greek word ΘΗΛΗ, is the congenital absence of one or both nipples and areolas of the breast. Athelia, which may be the rarest of all breast anomalies [27], may result from a developmental failure of the lower cervical and upper thoracic somites [28]. The fatty stroma is the precursor of the mammary fat pad [29], and without a good stroma, the overlying breast tissue cannot grow.

Ishida et al. [29] reported that athelia "is always associated with other anomalies… but [is] usually associated with amastia." These authors stated that "individuals generally present absence of the nipple–areola complex inside a constellation of other alteration. So, athelia cannot be classified in distinct groups." Latham et al. [30] cautioned that athelia, which is "uniformly described in the literature as being associated with a syndrome or a cluster of syndromes," should be differentiated from amastia (absence of breast tissue and nipple–areolar complex) and amazia (absence of breast tissue).

The inverted nipple is not an athelic phenomenon. According to Lawrence and Lawrence [28], it is the result of the persistence of fibers from the original invagination of the mammary pit (dimple).

1.3.3
Polythelia

More than two nipples, each with an areola, are present in polythelia. Schmidt [31] stated, "Not every supernumerary areola has a nipple, but every supernumerary nipple has an areola. The term 'polythelia' means a developed areola with a nipple." Supernumerary nipples may be found anywhere along the embryonic milk line [32]. Merlob [18] reported the prevalence of supernumerary nipples in various ethnic population studies as ranging from 0.22% to 11–16%. He stated that polythelia may be sporadic, familial, or syndromic.

Table 1.3 presents congenital malformations and diseases associated with polythelia.

1.3.4
Polymastia

The presence of more than two breasts, which are usually located at the mammary ridge, is called polymastia. The terms "ectopic breast" and "supernumerary breast" also appear in the literature. Darwin [33] viewed both polymastia and polythelia as atavistic traits, representing human phylogeny.

Supernumerary breasts and nipples have a 1–2% incidence of all live births [7, 34].

What embryogenetic explanation can be found for the reported cases of supernumerary mammary organs on the vulva, legs, or dorsal trunk? Dixon and Mansel [35] stated that the cause is unknown. Ectopic and normally located breasts may be equally subject to pathology (mastitis, cancer, etc.).

Polymastia is associated with other anomalies, both obvious and more hidden. Mehes and colleagues [36–38] and Goeminne [39] advise complete evaluation of the patient with ectopic breast(s) to rule out other problems, such as renal anomalies.

1.3.5
Breast Asymmetry

Araco et al. [40] defined breast asymmetry as "an asymmetric morphology of the shape, volume, or position of the breast, the nipple–areola complex, or both." Tuberous breast deformity (an aberration of breast shape) includes a spectrum of symmetrical and asymmetrical defects, both unilateral and bilateral [41].

In megalomastia, the breast is extremely enlarged. Unilateral megalomastia is extremely rare [42].

Micromastia is a congenital condition in which the breast fails to develop beyond its prepubertal state, despite the presence of mammary gland tissue [27]. The condition may be unilateral or bilateral. The etiology of micromastia (hypoplasia, aplasia) is unknown; however, unilateral hypoplasia may be associated with several syndromes, such as congenital renal hyperplasia and other autosomal dominant inherited conditions.

1.3.6
Gynecomastia

Gynecomastia refers to enlargement of the male breast. The development and then spontaneous regression of mild gynecomastia is common and usually asymptomatic in young men. Gynecomastia is also relatively common in older men; it is usually idiopathic and commonly regresses spontaneously [3].

1.4
Anatomy

The female breast is practically enveloped by the superficial fascia of the anterior chest wall (Fig 1.4). The superficial fascia is continuous with the superficial abdominal fascia of Camper below and the superficial fascia of the neck above, merging anteriorly with the dermis of the skin.

The base of the breast has the following extensions:
- From the 2nd rib (above) to the 6th or 7th rib (below)
- From the sternal border (medial) to the midaxillary line (lateral)

Table 1.3 Polythelia and associated conditions

Urinary tract abnormalities	Cardiac abnormalities	Miscellaneous abnormalities
Renal agenesis	Cardiac conduction disturbances	Pyloric stenosis
Renal cell carcinoma	(especially left bundle branch block)	Epilepsy
Obstructive disease	Hypertension	Ear abnormalities
Supernumerary kidney(s)	Congenital heart anomalies	Arthrogryposis multiplex congenita

From Pellegrini and Wagner [32], with permission

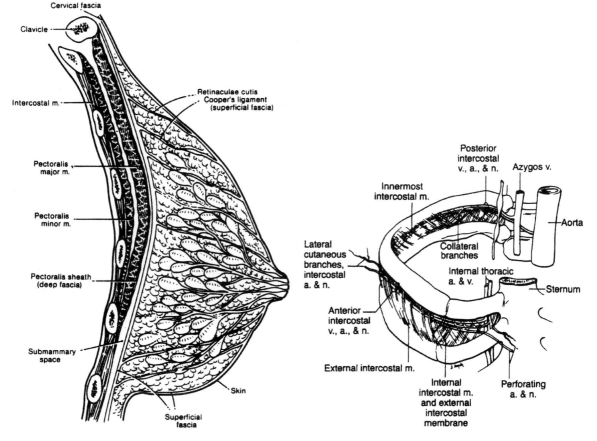

Fig. 1.4 Diagramatic sagittal section through the nonlactating female breast and anterior thoracic wall. (From Skandalakis et al. [58], with permission)

1.4.1
Superficial Fascia

The superficial fascia of the anterior chest wall is the home of the breast. The fascia completely envelops the lobes of this organ; each breast is formed by 15–20 lobes of glandular tissue. The lobes and lobules are separated by connective tissue, the septa. The subcutaneous tissue is thin or thick and travels deeply, forming the septa. Adipose tissue is also present between the lobes [43].

Two muscles are closely related to the breast: the pectoralis major and the serratus anterior. Two-thirds of the base of the breast rests anteriorly on the pectoralis major muscle. The other one-third of the breast is located anterior to the serratus anterior muscle. A small amount of breast tissue may lie over the aponeurosis of the external oblique muscle [44].

Fig. 1.5 A segment of the body wall illustrating the relationship of structures to the ribs. Two ribs are shown as they extend from the vertebrae to attach to the sternum. The orientation of muscle and connective tissue fibers is shown. The external intercostal muscle extends downward and forward. The muscle layer extends forward from the rib tubercle to the costochondral junction, where the muscle is replaced by the aponeurosis, called the external intercostal membrane. The internal intercostal muscle fibers with the opposite orientation can be seen through this layer. The innermost intercostal muscle fibers are present along the lateral half of the intercostal space. The intercostal nerve and vessels pass through the intercostal space in the plane between the internal and innermost intercostal muscle layers. Anterior intercostal arteries arise from the internal thoracic artery; anterior intercostal veins join the internal thoracic vein. Posterior intercostal arteries arise from the aorta; posterior intercostal veins join the azygos venous system on the right and the hemiazygos system on the left. Lymphatics follow the path of the blood vessels. Anteriorly, lymphatics pass to parasternal (internal mammary) nodes that are located along the internal mammary vessels; posteriorly, they pass to intercostal nodes located in the intercostal space near the vertebral bodies. (From Romrell and Bland [59], with permission)

A small amount of breast tissue travels toward the axilla in the majority of women. The surgeon in the operating room should remember that this breast tissue is the only part beneath the deep fascia. It is well known as the tail of Spence, and it enters the axilla through an opening of the deep fascia of the medial axillary wall. This opening is the well-known hiatus of Langer.

1.4.2
Deep Fascia

The deep fascia, known as the deep pectoral fascia, envelops the pectoralis major muscle and travels below with the deep abdominal fascia. The deep fascia also attaches medially to the sternum, and laterally and above to the clavicle and axillary fascia (Fig. 1.5). Along the lateral border of the pectoralis major muscle, the anterior lamina of the deep pectoral fascia unites with the fascia of the pectoralis minor muscle and, more inferiorly, with the fascia of the serratus anterior. A posterior extension of this fascia is continuous with the fascia of the latissimus dorsi and forms the so-called suspensory ligament of the axilla.

Deep to the pectoralis major muscle, the clavipectoral fascia envelops the pectoralis minor muscle and part of the subclavius muscle and attaches to the inferior aspect of the clavicle, dividing into two laminas that are anterior and posterior to the subclavius (Fig. 1.6). The posterior layer is fused with the fascial anchor of the midportion of the omohyoid muscle and is connected deeply with the axillary sheath. It extends between the axillary fascia, the clavicle, and the coracoid process. Laterally it unites with the anterior layer of the pectoralis major fascia.

The axillary fascia lying across the base of the axillary pyramidal space is an extension of the pectoralis major fascia and continues as the fascia of the latissimus dorsi. It forms the dome of the axilla (Fig. 1.7). As noted earlier, the lamina of muscle fascia that interconnects the pectoral musculature and the anterior border of the latissimus dorsi is referred to as the suspensory ligament of the axilla. Occasionally, there is a muscular interconnection within this fascia, which is called the suspensory muscle of the axilla. The suspensory muscle of the axilla can confuse the unwary surgeon, particularly when he or she performs axillary surgery on a patient who is not having a total mastectomy.

The prevertebral fascia gives off a sheet that covers the floor of the posterior triangle of the neck. The axillary vessels and the nerves to the arm pass through the sheet and floor, and take with them a tubular fascial sleeve, the axillary sheath.

The clavipectoral fascia (Fig. 1.7a) can be thought of as consisting of five parts:

- The attachment to the clavicle and the envelope of the subclavius muscle
- That part between the subclavius and pectoralis minor muscles, referred to by some as the "costocoracoid membrane"
- The thickened lateral band between the 1st rib and the coracoid process, the costocoracoid ligament
- The pectoralis minor envelope
- The suspensory ligament of the axilla attaching to the axillary fascia

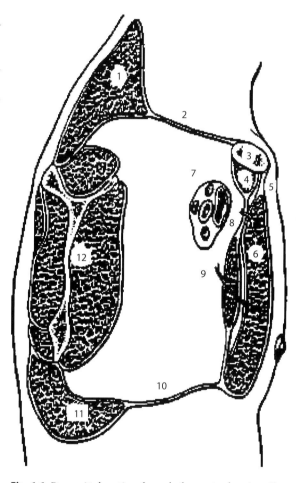

Fig. 1.6 Parasagittal section through the pectoral region. Trapezius muscle (*1*), cervical investing fascia (*2*), clavicle (*3*), subclavius muscle (*4*), pectoral fascia (*5*), pectoralis major (*6*), axillary sheath (*7*), lateral pectoral nerve, piercing the clavipectoral fascia (*8*), medial pectoral nerve, entering pectoralis minor muscle (*9*), suspensory ligament of axilla (*10*), latissumus dorsi muscle (*11*), blade of scapula (*12*). (From Colborn and Skandalakis [60], with permission)

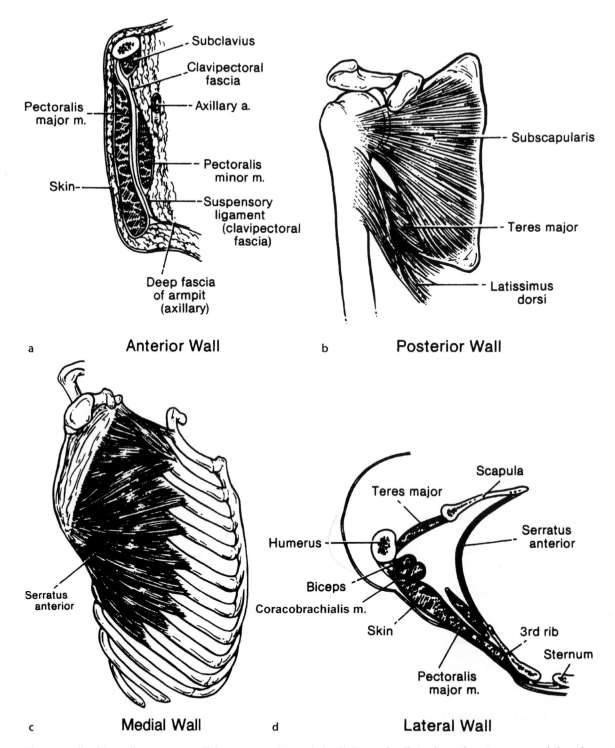

Fig. 1.7 Walls of the axilla. **a** Anterior wall. **b** Posterior wall. **c** Medial wall. **d** Lateral wall. (Redrawn from Basmajian and Slonecker [61])

1.4.3
Axilla

Despite the fact that textbooks almost always present the axilla in any discussion of the breast, it should be remembered that the axilla is the home of the nerves and vessels of the upper extremity. These are enveloped by a fascia, the axillary sheath, which is a continuation of the prevertebral fascia of the route of the neck. The axilla also contains lymph nodes, adipose tissue, the tendons of the long and short heads of the biceps, and various fasciae (e.g., pectoral, clavipectoral).

The axilla is located between the upper extremity and the thoracic wall. By definition, it is pyramidal, with an apex, a base, and four walls. The apex is a triangular space that extends into the posterior triangle of the neck by an opening (the cervicoaxillary canal). The space is bounded by the clavicle anteriorly, the scapula posteriorly, and the 1st rib medially. The base is formed by the axillary fascia.

The four walls of the axilla are formed as follows (Fig. 1.7):

- The anterior wall is formed by the pectoralis major and minor muscles, the subclavius muscle, and the clavipectoral fascia.
- The posterior wall is formed by the scapula and three muscles (subscapularis, teres major, and latissimus dorsi).
- The medial wall is formed by the serratus anterior muscle.
- The lateral wall is formed by the bicipital groove of the humerus.

Table 1.4 presents the muscles and nerves with which the surgeon must be familiar.

Table 1.4 Muscles of the breast and their nerve supply

Muscle	Origin	Insertion	Nerve supply
Pectoralis major	Medial half of clavicle, lateral half of sternum, 2nd–6th costal cartilages, aponeurosis of external oblique muscle	Lateral lip, bicipital groove	Lateral and medial pectoral nerves
Pectoralis minor	2nd–5th ribs	Coracoid process of scapula	Lateral and medial pectoral nerves
Deltoid	Lateral half of clavicle, lateral border of acromion process, spine of scapula	Deltoid tuberosity of humerus	Axillary nerve
Serratus anterior (three parts)	1. 1st and 2nd ribs 2. 2nd–4th ribs 3. 4th–8th ribs	Costal surface of scapula at superior angle Vertebral border of scapula Costal surface of scapula at inferior angle	Long thoracic nerve
Latissimus dorsi	Back, to crest of illium	Crest of lesser tubercle and intertubercular groove of humerus	Thoracodorsal nerve
Subclavius	Junction of 1st rib and its cartilage	Groove of lower surface of clavicle	Subclavian nerve
Subscapularis	Costal surface of scapula	Lesser tubercle of humerus	Upper and lower subscapular nerve
External oblique aponeurosis	External oblique muscle	Rectus sheath and linea alba, crest of ilium	—
Rectus abdominis	Ventral surface of 5th–7th costal cartilages and xiphoid process	Crest and superior ramus of pubis	Branches of 7th–12th thoracic nerves

Adapted from Skandalakis [67], with permission

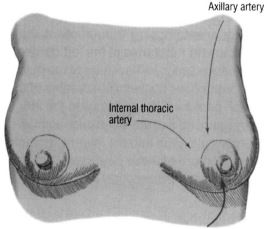

a **18%**

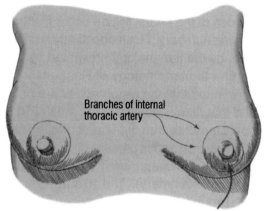

b **30%**

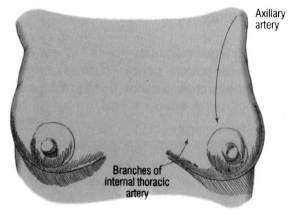

c **50%**

Fig. 1.8 a The breast may be supplied with blood from the internal thoracic, the axillary, and the intercostal arteries in 18% of individuals. **b** In 30%, the contribution from the axillary artery is negligible. **c** In 50%, the intercostal arteries contribute little or no blood to the breast. In the remaining 2%, other variations may be found. (From Skandalakis et al. [58], with permission)

1.4.4
Vascular Supply

1.4.4.1
Arterial Supply

The arterial supply of the breast forms a rich anastomotic plexus. With considerable variation, the breast is supplied with blood from three sources (Fig. 1.8): the internal thoracic artery, the branches of the axillary artery, and the intercostal arteries.

1.4.4.1.1
Internal Thoracic Artery

The internal thoracic artery produces the largest vessels supplying the breast, and the internal thoracic branches supply most of the blood to the breast. The internal thoracic (or internal mammary) artery is a branch of the subclavian artery; it courses parallel with the lateral border of the sternum behind the transversus thoracis muscles. From the internal thoracic artery, perforating branches pass through the intercostal muscles of the first six interspaces and the pectoralis major muscle to supply the medial half of the breast and surrounding skin (Fig. 1.9). Perforating arteries pierce the thoracic wall adjacent to the sternal edge in the 1st–4th intercostal spaces. The mammary rami of the first two of these perforating branches are the largest, although in some cases the 1st and 3rd or 2nd and 4th are the largest. About 2 cm lateral to the main perforating vessel, a second perforating branch is usually found. Typically these arteries descend laterally toward the nipple–areolar complex so that most of the arterial supply arises above the level of the nipple (Fig. 1.10). Therefore, radial incisions in the upper half of the breast are less likely to injure the major arterial supply than are transverse incisions. Morehead [45] stated that the inferior parts of the breast below the level of the nipple are almost free of major vessels.

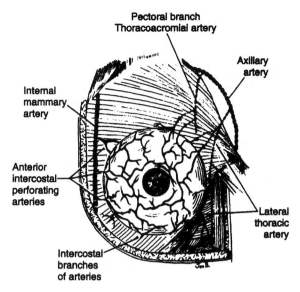

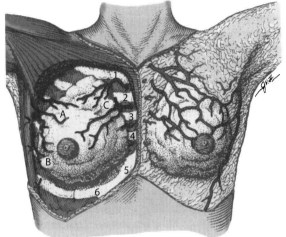

Fig. 1.9 Arterial distribution of blood to the breast, axilla, and chest wall. The breast receives its blood supply via three major arterial routes: 1) medially from anterior perforating intercostal branches arising from the internal thoracic artery, 2) laterally from either pectoral branches of the thoracoacromial trunk or branches of the lateral thoracic artery (the thoracoacromial trunk and the lateral thoracic arteries are branches of the axillary artery), and 3) from lateral cutaneous branches of the intercostal arteries that are associated with the overlying breast. The arteries indicated with a *dashed line* lie deep to the muscles of the thoracic wall and axilla. Many of the arteries must pass through these muscles before reaching the breast. (From Romrell and Bland [59], with permission)

Fig. 1.10 Blood supply of the breast. Arteries are shown on the right breast. The arterial supply is derived chiefly from (*A*) direct mammary branches of the axillary artery, (*B*) branches of the lateral thoracic artery, and (*C*) perforating branches of the internal thoracic artery. Veins are shown on the left breast; the venous drainage is comparable. The rib levels are indicated by numbers. (From Colborn and Skandalakis [60], with permission)

1.4.4.1.2
Branches of the Axillary Artery

The axillary vasculature supplies the lateral portion of the breast. Branches from the axillary artery to the breast include the small supreme thoracic artery, the pectoral branches of the thoracoacromial artery, the lateral thoracic artery, and the subscapular artery, which gives twigs of supply to the lateral aspect of the breast. The lateral thoracic artery is the most important of these vessels.

1.4.4.1.3
Intercostal Arteries

In addition to the vasculature described above, the lateral half of the breast may also receive branches of the 3rd, 4th, and 5th intercostal arteries. Small branches of the intercostal arteries in the 2nd, 3rd, and 4th spaces pass to the overlying breast tissue. Only about 18% of breasts are supplied by all three of these sources [46]. Branches from the internal thoracic artery are the only ones always present to some degree (Fig. 1.8). In most breasts, there are free anastomoses between the arteries supplying the breast; occasionally all three arterial sources remain separate [46].

1.4.4.2
Venous Drainage

The axillary, internal thoracic, and 3rd–5th intercostal veins drain the mammary gland (Fig. 1.11). Venous drainage corresponds to the arteries mentioned above, with the caveat that there are marked anatomic variations in human venous drainage. Breast surgeons are well aware of the variable distribution of the tributaries that drain into the axillary vein.

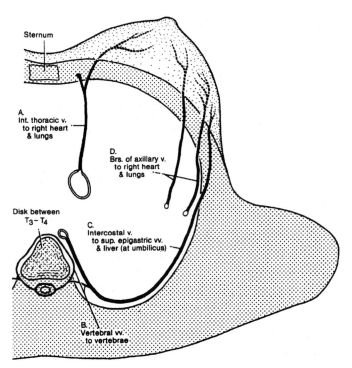

Fig. 1.11 Frontal section through the right breast showing pathways of venous drainage. Medial drainage through internal thoracic vein to the right heart (*A*). Posterior drainage to vertebral veins (*B*). Lateral drainage to intercostal vein, superior epigastric veins, and liver (*C*). Lateral superior drainage through axillary vein to the right heart (*D*). (From Skandalakis et al. [58], with permission)

The perforating tributaries from the medial half of the breast carry the greater part of the venous drainage. They enter the internal thoracic vein, which joins the brachiocephalic vein.

The axillary vein is formed by the junction of the basilic and brachial veins. It lies medial or superficial to the axillary artery and receives one or two pectoral branches from the breast. As it crosses the lateral border of the 1st rib, the axillary vein becomes the subclavian vein.

The intercostal veins communicate posteriorly with the vertebral venous system, which enters the azygos, hemiazygos, and accessory hemiazygos veins, which in turn drain to the superior vena cava. Anteriorly, they communicate with the brachiocephalic vein by way of the internal thoracic veins.

The principal vascular supply (arterial and venous) passes inferiorly and laterally from the upper intercostal spaces to reach the parenchyma and surrounding tissues superior to a horizontal plane through the nipple. The inferior parts of the breast below the level of the nipple are almost free of major vessels [45].

1.4.5
Lymphatics of the Breast

It is well known and accepted that the primary pathway of lymphatic drainage of the mammary gland is through lymph nodes in the axilla (Fig. 1.12). About three-quarters of all lymphatic drainage of the breast passes to the axillary nodes; the remainder drains principally to the internal thoracic group. Any part of the breast may drain to either group.

A plexus of lymphatic vessels lies in the interlobular connective tissue and communicates with a subareolar plexus around the nipple (subareolar plexus of Sappey). Efferent vessels pass from the breast tissue around the anterior axillary fold to the pectoral (anterior) group of axillary nodes, which lie along the lateral thoracic artery and vein at about the level of attachment of the pectoralis minor to the 5th rib. Some channels pass directly to the subscapular (posterior) group (Figs. 1.13, 1.14). Efferent vessels drain from the superior aspect of the breast directly to the apical axillary nodes deep to the clavipectoral fascia, just inferior to the clavicle, sometimes interrupted by small interpectoral and infraclavicular nodes (Fig. 1.15). From the medial part of the breast, lymphatics drain along the perforating vessels to the internal thoracic chain of nodes. Some drainage occurs along the lateral cutaneous branches of the posterior intercostal veins to the intercostal chain of nodes near the rib heads.

Lymphatic drainage of the breast typically accompanies the blood supply (Fig. 1.16). Drainage from any quadrant of the breast passes to axillary nodes (75%) or to the internal mammary chain (25%) [47]. Haagensen [48] traced the flow of lymph upward and laterally

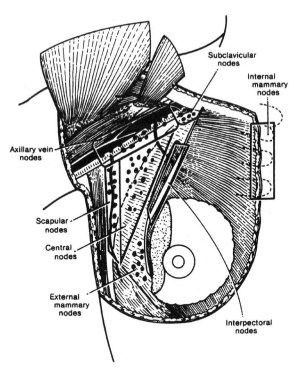

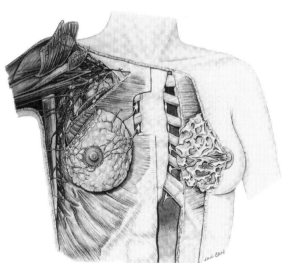

Fig. 1.12 Lymph nodes of the breast and axilla; classification of Haagensen and colleagues [48]. (From Skandalakis et al. [58], with permission)

Fig. 1.13 The anterior chest illustrating the structure of the chest wall, breast, and axilla. On the right side, the pectoralis major muscle has been cut lateral to the breast and reflected laterally to its insertion into the crest of the greater tubercle of the humerus. This exposes the underlying pectoralis minor muscle and the other muscles forming the wall of the axilla. The contents of the axilla, including the axillary artery and vein, components of the brachial plexus, and axillary lymph node groups and lymphatic channels are exposed. On the left side, the breast is cut to expose its structure in sagittal view. The lactiferous ducts and sinuses can be seen. Lymphatic channels passing to parasternal lymph nodes are also shown. (From Romrell and Bland [59], with permission)

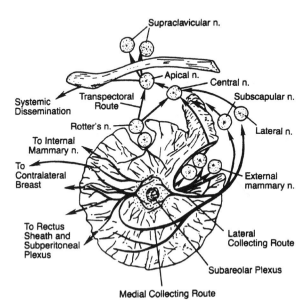

Fig. 1.14 Schematic drawing of the breast identifying the position of lymph nodes relative to the breast and illustrating routes of lymphatic drainage. The *clavicle* is indicated as a reference point. (From Romrell and Bland [59], with permission)

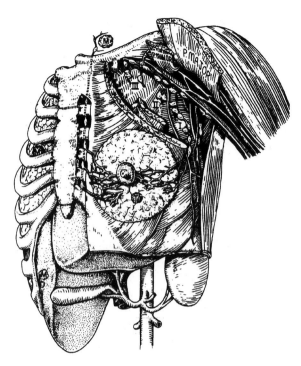

Fig. 1.15 Lymphatic drainage of the breast. The *Roman numerals* indicate lymph node groups as classified by Bland [43]. *M* metastasis, *T* tumor. (From Romrell and Bland [59], with permission)

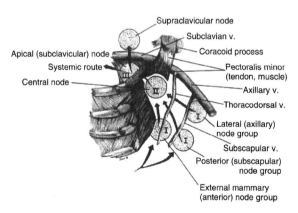

Fig. 1.16 Schematic drawing illustrating the major lymph node groups associated with the lymphatic drainage of the breast. The *Roman numerals* indicate three levels or groups of lymph nodes that are defined by their location relative to the pectoralis minor (classification of Bland [43]). Level I includes lymph nodes located lateral to the pectoralis minor; level II, lymph nodes located deep to the muscle; and level III, lymph nodes located medial to the muscle. The *arrows* indicate the general direction of lymph flow. (From Romrell and Bland [59], with permission)

through the tail of the breast to the central lymph nodes. Metastases are most frequently found at this location. Another drainage route follows lymphatics that pierce the pectoralis muscle and pass upward between the pectoralis major and minor to reach the axillary vein group or the subclavicular group of nodes. A few interpectoral nodes (of Rotter) may be encountered between the two muscles (Fig. 1.17).

Lymph nodes of the breast region occur in inconstant groups of varying numbers. The surgeon must keep in mind that many nodes are very small. Only the most careful search of the pathologic specimen will reveal all the lymph nodes present. This inconstancy is mirrored, if not magnified, by the terminology presented by different authors.

Anatomists describe four groups of axillary lymph nodes, whereas surgeons describe six groups [43]. Bland [43] presents the following grouping of the 24–38 nodes (Figs. 1.14–1.16):

1. Axillary vein group (lateral group): four to six lymph nodes
2. External mammary group (anterior or pectoral): four to five nodes
3. Scapular group (posterior or subscapular): six or seven nodes
4. Central group: three or four nodes
5. Subclavicular group (apical): six to twelve nodes
6. Interpectoral group (Rotter): one to four nodes

This author finds the terminology of Haagensen [48] most useful (Fig. 1.12). The major groups of Haagensen are 1) axillary, and 2) internal thoracic (mammary). The average number of nodes in each group follows.

1.4.5.1
Axillary Drainage (35.3 nodes)

Group 1: External mammary nodes, also called the anterior pectoral nodes (1.7 nodes). These lie along the lateral edge of the pectoralis minor, deep to the pectoralis major muscle, along the medial side of the axilla following the course of the lateral thoracic artery on the chest wall from the 2nd to the 6th rib. Deep to the areola is an extensive network of lymphatic vessels, the so-called subareolar plexus of Sappey. In the circumareolar region, large lateral and medial trunks receive much of the lymph from the breast parenchyma. The lateral trunk receives collaterals from the upper half of the breast, and the internal trunk drains the lower part of the breast. These vessels pass around the lateral border of the pectoralis major muscle to reach the external mammary nodes.

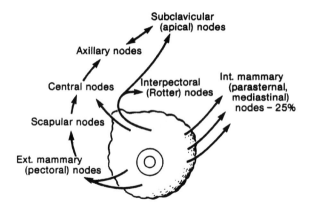

Fig. 1.17 Diagram of lymphatic drainage of the breast. (From Skandalakis et al. [58], with permission)

Group 2: Scapular nodes (5.8 nodes). These lie on the subscapular vessels and their thoracodorsal branches. Lymphatics from these intercommunicate with intercostal lymphatic vessels.

Group 3: Central nodes (12.1 nodes). This is the largest group of lymph nodes; they are the nodes most easily palpated in the axilla because they are generally larger in size. These nodes are embedded in fat in the center of the axilla. When they enlarge, they can compress the intercostobrachial nerve, the lateral cutaneous branch of the 2nd or 3rd thoracic nerve, causing accompanying pain.

Group 4: Interpectoral nodes, also called Rotter's nodes (1.4 nodes). These lie between the pectoralis major and minor muscles. Often there is a single node. They are

the smallest group of axillary nodes and will not be found unless the pectoralis major is removed.

Group 5: Axillary vein nodes (10.7 nodes). This is the second largest group of lymph nodes in the axilla. They lie on the caudal and ventral surfaces of the lateral part of the axillary vein.

Group 6: Subclavicular nodes (3.5 nodes). These lie on the caudal and ventral surfaces of the medial part of the axillary vein. Haagensen [48] considered them to be inaccessible unless the pectoralis minor muscle is sacrificed.

The axillary lymph nodes are defined in three levels according to their location in relation to the pectoralis minor muscle (Fig. 1.18):

- Level I: Lymph nodes located in the vicinity of the lower border of the pectoralis minor muscle. This level is formed by three groups: exterior mammary lymph nodes, axillary vein lymph nodes, and scapular lymph nodes.
- Level II: Lymph nodes located deep to (under) the pectoralis minor muscle. This level is formed by central lymph nodes and some subclavian nodes.
- Level III: Lymph nodes located at the medial border of the pectoralis minor. These are the subclavicular group.

1.4.5.2
Internal Thoracic (Mammary) Drainage (8.5 nodes)

Lymphatic vessels emerge from the medial edge of the breast on the pectoralis fascia. They accompany the perforating blood vessels, which, at the end of the inter-

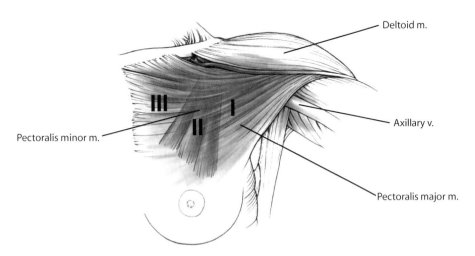

Fig. 1.18 Levels of axillary lymph nodes identified in relation to the pectoralis minor muscle: *I* lateral, *II* behind, *III* medial. (From Wood and Bostwick [62], with permission)

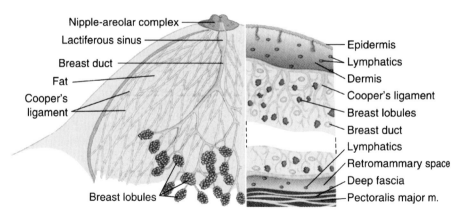

Fig. 1.19 The mature resting breast. The breast lies cushioned in fat between the overlying skin and the pectoralis major muscle. Both the skin and retromammary space under the breast are rich with lymphatic channels. (From Iglehart and Kaelin [63], with permission)

costal space, pierce the pectoralis major and intercostal muscles to reach the internal thoracic nodes. These nodes also receive lymphatic trunks from the skin of the opposite breast, the liver, the diaphragm, the rectus sheath, and the upper part of the rectus abdominis [48]. The nodes, about four or five on each side, are small and usually in the fat and connective tissue of the intercostal spaces. The internal thoracic trunks empty into the thoracic duct or the right lymphatic duct. This route to the venous system is shorter than the axillary route.

The student of breast anatomy should also remember that a few other lymph nodes are associated in an indirect way with the breast, such as intercostal lymph nodes, diaphragmatic nodes, and mediastinal nodes. Durkin and Haagensen [49] identified an average of 50 nodes in 100 specimens obtained from Halstead-type radical mastectomy.

The retromammary space is located between the pectoralis major muscle, the deep fascia, and the breast parenchyma (Fig. 1.19). The skin of the breast and the retromammary space under the breast are rich in lymphatic vessels.

Note: By definition, the sentinel lymph node of the breast is the first lymph node to accept drainage, either malignant or benign, from a breast tumor. This is the first site of metastasis.

1.4.6
Innervation

In 1840, the great English anatomist Sir Astley Cooper [50] described the nerves supplying the breast as arising

from the 2nd–6th intercostal nerves, with mammary branches passing on the surface of the gland and intercommunicating. He also described the two mammary branches from the 4th lateral cutaneous nerve and mentioned that the nipple receives its innervation through a "plexus under it." Sarhadi et al. [51], in a study of the innervation of the breast, stated that their findings "are uncannily like those of Cooper."

It is of some importance, especially to plastic surgeons, to remember that the nerve supply to the areola and nipple is attributable to the anterior ramus of the lateral cutaneous branch of the 4th thoracic (T4) or intercostal nerve (Figs. 1.20, 1.21). This branch, which

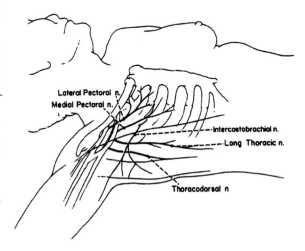

Fig. 1.20 Important peripheral nerves. (From Aitken and Minton [64], with permission)

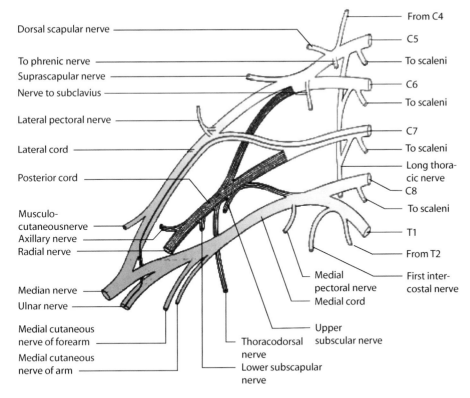

Dorsal scapular nerve

To phrenic nerve
Suprascapular nerve
Nerve to subclavius

Lateral pectoral nerve

Lateral cord

Posterior cord

Musculo-
cutaneousnerve
Axillary nerve
Radial nerve

Median nerve
Ulnar nerve

Medial cutaneous
nerve of forearm

Medial cutaneous
nerve of arm

From C4

C5

To scaleni

C6

To scaleni

C7

To scaleni

Long thora-
cic nerve
C8

To scaleni

T1

From T2

Medial
pectoral nerve
Medial cord

First inter-
costal nerve

Upper
subscular nerve

Thoracodorsal
nerve
Lower subscapular
nerve

Fig. 1.21 The brachial plexus. The posterior division of the trunks and their derivatives are shaded. The fibers from C7 that enter the ulnar nerve are shown as a *heavy black line. Letters* and *numbers C4–C8* and *T1–T2* indicate the ventral rami of these cervical and thoracic spinal nerves. (From Standring [57], with permission)

provides sensation for the nipple and areola and motor supply to the smooth muscle of the nipple, passes medially after turning about the lateral border of the pectoralis major muscle, within the superficial fascia. It can be spared in reconstructive procedures, thereby leaving the patient with a sensate and responsive nipple.

1.4.6.1
Thoracodorsal Nerve

The thoracodorsal nerve (middle subscapular) arises deeply from the posterior cord of the brachial plexus, ventral to the subscapularis muscle (Fig. 1.22). It passes downward and medially to reach and innervate the latissimus dorsi muscle. The nerve and its associated vessels can best be found near the medial border of the latissimus dorsi about 5 cm above a plane passing through the 3rd sternochondral junction [52]. Once located, the neurovascular bundle should be marked with umbilical tape for protection. If there is obvious involvement of lymph nodes around the nerve, it must be sacrificed.

Remember: Most injury to the brachial plexus is the result of stretching the nerves during surgery, although direct injury is possible.

1.4.6.2
Long Thoracic Nerve

The long thoracic nerve innervates the serratus anterior muscle and lies on it (Fig. 1.22). When the superficial fascia is reflected, the nerve or branches from it can be reflected also, making identification of the nerve difficult. Unless actually invaded by cancer, this nerve should be spared to avoid "winging" of the inferior angle of the scapula. The landmark for locating the nerve is the point at which the axillary vein passes over the 2nd rib. Careful dissection of this area will reveal the nerve descending on the 2nd rib posterior to the axillary vein [52].

1.4.6.3
Anterior Thoracic Nerves (Pectoral)

The importance of the medial and lateral pectoral (anterior thoracic) nerves has been emphasized by various authors (Fig. 1.23) [53–55]. The medial pectoral nerve is superficial to the axillary vein and lateral to the pectoralis minor muscle. The lateral pectoral nerve, which is larger than the medial nerve, is the nerve supply of the

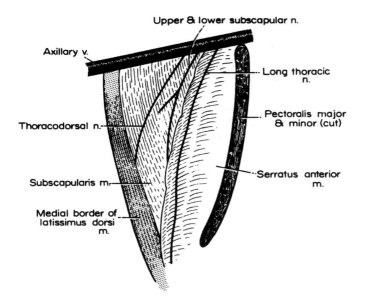

Fig. 1.22 Anatomic landmarks for location of thoracodorsal (medial subscapular) nerve during surgery (see text). (From Skandalakis et al. [65], with permission)

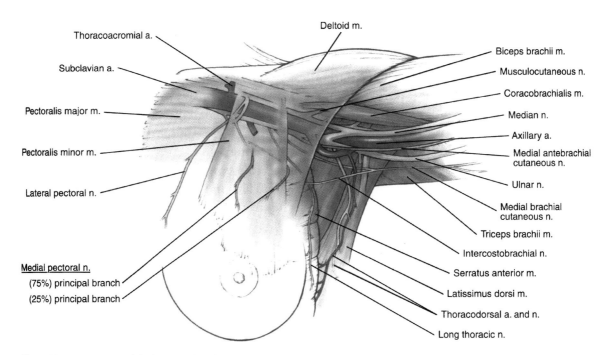

Fig. 1.23 Major nerves of the breast and axilla. (From Wood and Bostwick [62], with permission)

clavicular part of the muscle as well as the sternal portions of the pectoralis major muscle. It is also superficial to the axillary vein and lies at the medial edge of the pectoralis minor muscle. The branch of the lateral pectoral nerve to the clavicular head of the pectoralis major muscle arises proximal to, or beneath, the clavicle.

The medial pectoral nerve arises from the medial cord of the brachial plexus near the origin of the thoracoacromial artery from the axillary artery. The lower part of the lateral pectoral nerve crosses the axillary artery just distal to the origin of the thoracoacromial artery and joins the medial pectoral nerve, forming a neural loop of varying size. From this loop, several branches arise that pass into the pectoralis minor muscle, some penetrating that muscle to enter the overlying pectoralis major muscle. Such branches supply the sternal and costal parts of the pectoralis major muscle.

1.4.6.4
Intercostobrachial Nerve

The intercostobrachial nerve is the lateral cutaneous branch of the 2nd or 3rd intercostal nerve, or a combination of the two intercostal nerves. After crossing the fatty and lymphatic tissues of the axilla posteromedially, it reaches the medial area of the skin of the arm.

Dividing the intercostobrachial nerves causes an annoying dysesthesia of the inner aspect of the upper arm. It is usually possible to spare the intercostobrachial nerves during an axillary dissection unless the nerves pass through nodes matted with metastases. It is necessary to divide the axillary specimen to free the nerves, and care should be taken to look and palpate for lymph nodes in order to avoid dividing through a lymph node that might contain a metastasis.

1.5
Histology

Sakakura has noted, "Today, the mammary gland is one of the most studied organs because of its usefulness as a tool in such disciplines as developmental biology, biochemistry, endocrinology, cell biology, histology, oncology, virology, and molecular biology" [56].

The 15 or 20 mammary lobes are irregular and subdivided into several lobules. The breast parenchyma is supported by fibrous bands (suspensory ligaments of Cooper). The breast contains multiple ducts lined with columnar epithelium of one or more layers, according to their length (Fig. 1.24).

Gray's Anatomy [57] states that "Lactiferous ducts draining each lobe of the breast pass through the nipple and open onto its tip as 15–20 orifices. Near its orifice, each of these ducts is slightly expanded as a lactiferous sinus, which, in the lactating breast, is further dilated by the presence of milk. Each lactiferous duct is therefore connected to a system of ducts and lobules, surrounded by connective tissue stroma, collectively forming a lobe of the mammary gland. Lobules consist of the portions of the glands that have secretory potential."

The lobes of parenchyma and their ducts are arranged radially with respect to the position of the nipple, so that the ducts pass centrally toward the nipple like spokes of a wheel and terminate separately upon the summit of the nipple. The segment of the duct within the nipple is the narrowest portion of the duct. Therefore, secre-

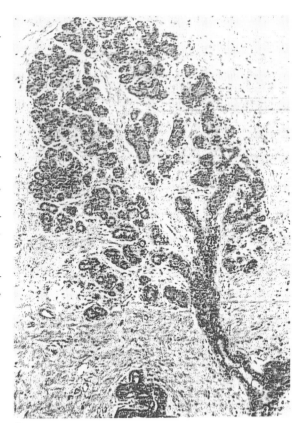

a

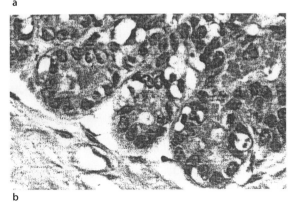

b

Fig. 1.24 **a** A glandular lobule surrounded by collagenous interlobular connective tissue in the mature resting breast. A terminal duct (*bottom right*) branches extensively to terminate in rudimentary acini, which are shown at higher magnification in the *lower panel* (**b**). (From Young and Heath [66], with permission)

tions or sloughed cells tend to collect within the part of the duct just deep to the nipple, resulting in apparent expansion of the ducts (Fig. 1.25).

In the fat-free area under the areola, the dilated portions of the lactiferous ducts (the lactiferous sinuses) are

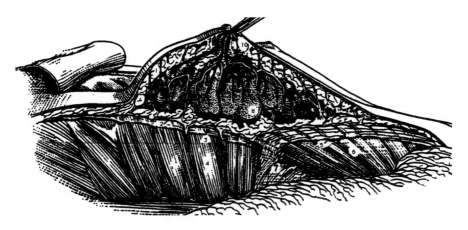

Fig. 1.25 Breast topography (from a dissection photograph). Retinacula cutis (*1*), membranous layer (*2*), serratus anterior fascia (*3*), serratus anterior muscle (*4*), pectoral fascia (*5*), pectoralis major muscle (*6*), suspensory ligament of axilla (*7*), lobe of breast parenchyma (*8*), lactiferous duct (*9*), ampulla (*10*). (From Colborn and Skandalakis [60], with permission)

the only sites of actual milk storage. Intraductal papillomas may develop here. The ducts are surrounded by a sheath of soft, cellular, intralobular connective tissue derived from the upper papillary layer of the dermis. Between the ducts is the denser, less cellular connective tissue from the reticular layer of the dermis. Because of the radial arrangement of the lobes with respect to the nipple, the site of production of serous or sanguineous fluid emerging upon the surface of the nipple can be determined by stroking the breast tissue with the tip of a finger, beginning peripherally and terminating at the nipple.

Remember: Each lobe of the gland ends at a lactiferous duct that empties at the terminus of the nipple.

The suspensory ligaments of Cooper form a network of strong, irregularly shaped connective tissue strands or bands connecting the dermis of the skin with the deep layer of superficial fascia, passing between the lobes of parenchyma and attaching to the parenchymal elements and ducts. Occasionally, the superficial fascia is fixed to the skin in such a way that ideal subcutaneous total mastectomy is impossible.

With malignant invasion, portions of the ligaments of Cooper may contract, producing a characteristic fixation and retraction or dimpling of the skin (Fig. 1.26). This must not be confused with the irregular, roughened appearance of the skin called peau d'orange, which is secondary to obstruction of the superficial subcuticular lymphatic vessels. In peau d'orange, the subdermal attachment of hair follicles and the edematous skin results in the pitted appearance of the skin. Skin dimpling due to Cooper's ligament retraction is also not to

be confused with direct invasion of the skin by tumor. Ligament retraction does not imply tumor extension to the skin and its association with poorer prognosis [3].

In the resting (nonlactating) breast, the main duct system is present, but there are few or no secretory acini. During pregnancy, the ducts proliferate, and secretory acini develop at the ends of each of the smaller branches. The intralobular connective tissue becomes thinned to form well-vascularized septa separating adjacent acini. Although there is a relative reduction in the quantity of adipose tissue present, there is an increase in the size of the breast because of duct and acinus formation.

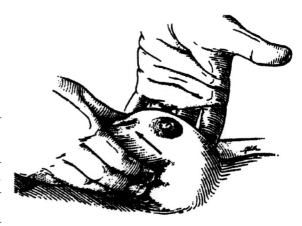

Fig. 1.26 Dimpling of the breast, resulting from involvement of Cooper's ligaments by invasive disease (from clinical photograph). Emphasized by pressure from examiner's hand. (From Colborn and Skandalakis [60], with permission)

1.6
Conclusions

With knowledge of the embryology and anatomy of the breast and its associated entities, and with the application of careful anatomic technique, the general and plastic surgeon will benefit the patient and avoid operative complications.

References

1. Andry de Bois-Regard N: Orthopaedia: Or, the Art of Correcting and Preventing Deformities in Children. London, A Millar 1758, pp 50–51

2. Kopans DB: Breast Imaging, 3rd edn. Philadelphia, Lippincott Williams & Wilkins 2007, pp 7–43

3. Skandalakis JE, Colborn GL, Skandalakis PN, Weidman TA, Skandalakis LJ: Breast. In: Skandalakis JE (ed). Skandalakis' Surgical Anatomy: The Embryologic and Anatomic Basis of Modern Surgery. Athens, Paschalidis Medical Publications 2004, pp 155–188

4. Howard BA, Gusterson BA: Human breast development. J Mammary Gland Biol Neoplasia 2000;5(2):119–137

5. Langebartel DA: The Anatomical Primer: An Embryological Explanation of Human Gross Morphology. Baltimore, University Park Press 1977, pp 78–79

6. Russo J, Russo IH: Development of the human breast. Maturitas 2004;49(1):2–15

7. Bland KI, Romrell LJ: Congenital and acquired disturbances of breast development and growth. In: Bland KI, Copeland EM III. The Breast: Comprehensive Management of Benign and Malignant Disorders. St. Louis, Saunders 2006, pp 199–220

8. Neville MC: Anatomy and physiology of lactation. Pediatr Clin North Am 2001;48(1):13–34

9. Neville MC, Medina D, Monks, Hovey RC: The mammary fat pad. J Mammary Gland Biol Neoplasia 1998;3(2):109–116

10. Sakakura T: Mammary embryogenesis. In: Neville MC, Daniel CW (eds). The Mammary Gland: Development, Regulation, and Function. New York, Plenum Press, 1987, pp 37–66

11. Robinson GW, Karpf AB, Kratochwil K: Regulation of mammary gland development by tissue interaction. J Mammary Gland Biol Neoplasia 1999;4(1):9–19

12. Froriep L: Beobachtung eines falle von mangel der brustdruse. Notizen aus dem Gebiete der Natur und Heilkunst 1839;1:9

13. Gilly E: Absence complete des mamelles chez une femme mere: atrophie de membre superior droit. Courrier Med 1882;32:27

14. Thompson J: On a form of congenital thoracic deformity. Teratology 1895;2:1

15. Deaver JB, McFarland J: The Breast: Anomalies, Diseases and Treatment. Philadelphia, P Blackiston's & Sons 1917

16. Skandalakis JE, Gray SW, Ricketts R, Skandalakis LJ: The anterior body wall. In: Skandalakis JE, Gray SW. Embryology for Surgeons (2nd edn). Baltimore, Williams & Wilkins, 1994, pp 540–594

17. Trier WC: Complete breast absence: case report and review of the literature. Plast Reconstr Surg 1965;36(4):431–439

18. Merlob P: Congenital malformations and developmental changes of the breast: a neonatological view. J Pediatr Endocrinol Metabol 2003;16(4):471–485

19. Jones KL: Smith's Recognizable Patterns of Human Malformation, 6th edn. Philadelphia, Elsevier Saunders 2006

20. OMIM—Online Mendelian Inheritance in Man. http://www.ncbi.nlm.nih.gov/sites/entrez?db=omim

21. Nelson MM, Cooper CKN: Congenital defects of the breast—an autosomal dominant trait. South Afr Med J 1982;61(12):434–436

22. Amesse L, Yen FF, Weisskoff B, Hertweck SP: Vaginal uterine agenesis associated with amastia in a phenotypic female with a de novo 46,XX,t(8;13)(q22.1;q32.1) translocation. Clin Genet 1999;55(6):493–495

23. Fraser FC: Dominant inheritance of absent nipples and breast. Novant'anne delle Leggi Mendeline. Rome, Instituto Gregorio Mendel 1956, pp 360–362

24. Goldenring H, Crelin ES: Mother and daughter with bilateral congenital amastia. Yale J Biol Med 1961;33:466–467

25. Kowlessar M, Orti F: Complete breast absence in siblings. Am J Dis Child 1968;115(1):91–92

26. Greydanus DE, Matytsina L, Gains M: Breast disorders in children and adolescents. Prim Care Clin Office Pract 2006;33(2):455–466

27. Huffman JW, Dewhurst CJ, Caprano VJ: The Gynecology of Childhood and Adolescence, 2nd edn. Philadelphia, WB Saunders 1981, pp 542–559

28. Lawrence RA, Lawrence RM: Breastfeeding: A Guide for the Medical Profession, 6th edn. Philadelphia, Elsevier Mosby 2005, pp 39–64

29. Ishida LH, Alves HRN, Munhoz AM, Kaimoto C, Ishida LC, Saito FL, Gemperlli R, Ferreira MC: Athelia: case report and review of the literature. Br J Plast Surg 2005;58(6):833–837

30. Latham K, Fernandez S, Iteld L, Panthaki Z, Armstrong MB, Thaller S: Pediatric breast deformity. J Craniofac Surg 2006;17(3):454–467

31. Schmidt H: Supernumerary nipples: prevalence, size, sex and side predilection—a prospective clinical study. Eur J Pediatr 1998;157(10): 821–823

32. Pellegrini JR, Wagner RF: Polythelia and associated conditions. Am Fam Physician 1983;28(3):129–132

33. Darwin C: The Descent of Man and Selection in Relation to Sex. New York, Appleton 1889

34. Chatterjee A, Kumar M: Supernumerary breast. J Indian Med Assoc 1980;75(10):202–203

35. Dixon J, Mansel R: ABC of breast diseases. Congenital problems and aberrations of normal breast development and involution. Br Med J 1994;309(6957):797–800

36. Mehes K, Pinter A: Minor morphological aberrations in children with isolated urinary tract malformations. Eur J Pediatr 1990;149(6);399–402

37. Meggyessy V, Mehes K: Association of supernumerary nipples with renal anomalies. J Pediatr 1987;111:412–413

38. Mehes K, Szule E, Torzsok F, Meggyesse V: Supernumerary nipples and urologic malignancies. Cancer Genet Cytogenet 1987;24(1):185–188

39. Goeminne L: Synopsis of mammo-renal syndromes. Humangenetik 1972;14;170–171

40. Araco A, Gravante G, Araco F, Gentile P, Castri F, Delogu D, Filingeri V, Servelli V: Breast asymmetries: a brief review and our experience. Aesth Plast Surg 2006;30(3):309–319

41. DeLuca-Pytell DM, Piazza RC, Holding JC, Snyder N, Hunsicker LM, Phillips LG: The incidence of tuberous breast deformity in asymmetric and symmetric mammaplasty patients. Plast Reconstr Surg 2005;116(7):1894–1899

42. Anastassiades OT, Choreftaki T, Ioannovich J, Gogas J, Papdimitriou CS: Megalomastia: histological, histochemical and immunohistochemical study. Virchows Arch A Pathol Anat Histopathol 1992;420(4):337–344

43. Bland K: Anatomy of the breast. In: Fischer JE (ed). Mastery of Surgery, 5th edn. Philadelphia, Lippincott Williams & Wilkins 2007, pp 482–491

44. Donegan WL: General considerations. In: Nora PF (ed). Operative Surgery: Principles and Techniques, 2nd edn. Philadelphia, Lea & Febiger 1980

45. Morehead JR: Anatomy and embryology of the breast. Clin Obstet Gynecol 1982;25(2):353–357

46. Maliniac JW: Arterial blood supply of the breast: revised anatomic data relating to reconstructive surgery. Arch Surg 1943;47:329–343

47. Hultborn AL, Hulten B, Roos M, Rosencrantz M, Rosengren B, Ahren C: Effectiveness of axillary lymph node dissection in modified radical mastectomy with preservation of pectoral muscles. Ann Surg 1974;179(3):269–272

48. Haagensen CD: Lymphatics of the breast. In: Haagensen CD, Feind CR, Herter FP, Slanetz CA Jr, Weinberg JA (eds). The Lymphatics in Cancer. Philadelphia, WB Saunders 1972, pp 300–398

49. Durkin K, Haagensen CD: An improved technique for the study of lymph nodes in surgical specimens. Ann Surg 1980;191(4):419–429

50. Cooper A: The Anatomy of the Breast. London, Longman 1840, pp 91–109

51. Sarhadi NS, Shaw-Dunn J, Soutar DS: Nerve supply of the breast with special reference to the nipple and areola: Sir Astley Cooper revisited. Clin Anat 1997;10(4):283–288

52. Feller I, Woodburne RT: The long thoracic and thoracodorsal nerves in radical mastectomy. Surg Gynecol Obstet 1958;107(6):789–791

53. Scanlon EF, Caprini JA: Modified radical mastectomy. Cancer 1975;35(3):710–713

54. Scanlon EF: The importance of the anterior thoracic nerves in modified radical mastectomy. Surg Gynecol Obstet 1981;152(6):789–791

55. Moosman DA: Anatomy of the pectoral nerves and their preservation in modified mastectomy. Am J Surg 1980;139(6):883–886

56. Sakakura T: New aspects of stroma–parenchyma relations in mammary gland differentiation. Int Rev Cytol 1991;125:165–202

57. Standring S (ed): Gray's Anatomy: The Anatomical Basis of Clinical Practice, 39th edn. Edinburgh, Elsevier Churchill Livingstone 2005, p 972

58. Skandalakis JE, Gray SW, Rowe JS Jr.: Anatomical Complications in General Surgery. New York, McGraw-Hill 1983

59. Romrell LJ, Bland KI: Anatomy of the breast, axilla, chest wall, and related metastatic sites. In: Bland KI, Copeland EM III. The Breast: Comprehensive Management of Benign and Malignant Disorders. St. Louis, Saunders 2006

60. Colborn GL, Skandalakis JE: Clinical Gross Anatomy: A Guide for Dissection Study and Review. New York, Parthenon 1993

61. Basmajian JV, Slonecker CE: Grant's Method of Anatomy, 11th edn. Baltimore, Williams & Wilkins 1989

62. Wood WC, Bostwick J III: Breast and axilla. In: Wood WC, Skandalakis JE (eds). Anatomic Basis of Tumor Surgery. St. Louis, Quality Medical Publishing 1999

63. Iglehart DJ, Kaelin CM: Diseases of the breast. In: Townsend CM (ed). Sabiston Textbook of Surgery: The Biological Basis of Modern Surgical Practice. Philadelphia, Saunders 2004

64. Aitken DR, Minton JP: Complications associated with mastectomy. Surg Clin North Am 1983; 63:1331–1352

65. Skandalakis LJ, Vohman MD, Skandalakis JE, et al.: The axillary lymph nodes in radical and modified radical mastectomy. Am Surg 1979; 45:522–525

66. Young B, Heath JW (eds): Wheater's Functional Histology: A Text and Colour Atlas, 4th edn. Edinburgh, Churchill Livingstone 2000

67. Skandalakis JE (ed): Skandalakis' Surgical Anatomy: The Embryologic and Anatomic Basis of Modern Surgery. Athens, Paschalidis Medical Publications 2004

CHAPTER 2

Nerves, Ligaments, and Vessels of the Chest and Breast

2

Elisabeth Würinger

2.1
Introduction

Understanding of the anatomical structures of the breast allows better understanding of breast augmentation.

2.2
Nerves, Ligaments, Vessels

The neurovascular supply of the nipple runs along a regularly located suspension apparatus, the ligamentous suspension (Figs. 2.1–2.3) [1–5]. This is a well-defined, coherent fibrous sling that shows a regular and predictable location. It models the breast and carries the weight of the breast by constant fibrous structures. It is composed of a horizontal septum, which originates at the inferior border of the pectoral fascia along the 5th rib and traverses the breast to the middle of the nipple.

At its medial and lateral borders, the horizontal septum curves upward into vertically directed ligaments. The strong medial vertical ligament is attached to the sternum. The lateral vertical ligament emerges from the lateral edge of the pectoral fascia. The horizontal septum and its vertical extensions thereby build a regular located sling of dense connective tissue, which connects the gland to the thoracic wall. The line of fixation of this ligamentous circle follows the borders of pectoralis major to a great extent.

This suspensory circle also has superficial extensions into the skin medially, caudally, and laterally, which define the extent and borders of the breast. The medial superficial ligament is rather weak. The firm lateral superficial ligament has a strong suspensory function by attaching to the axillary fascia along the midaxillary line. It produces the concavity of the armpit and thus corresponds to the suspensory ligament of the axilla. The vertical ligaments merge into the superficial mammary fascia in a cranial and anterior direction. Thus, the ligamentous suspension also connects with the ligamenta suspensoria, described by Cooper as stretching from the mammary fascia into the skin. The increased

density of Cooper's ligaments from the origin of the horizontal septum into the inframammary crease skin represents the superficial part of the horizontal septum; it builds the inframammary crease.

The ligamentous suspension allows location of the main vessels and nerves to the nipple. The horizontal septum guides two vascular layers. The smooth and even cranial neurovascular layer is composed of musculocutaneous branches of the thoracoacromial artery and branches of the lateral thoracic artery. The perforating branches of the 4th and 5th intercostal arteries run along the caudal vascular layer. The main nerve to the nipple, the deep branch of the 4th intercostal nerve, is guided by the horizontal septum.

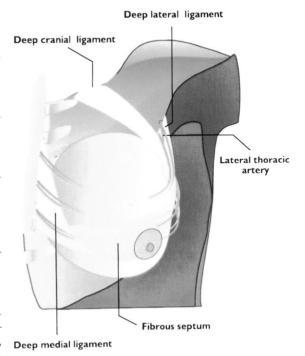

Fig. 2.1 Deep ligaments, lateral thoracic artery, and fibrous septum

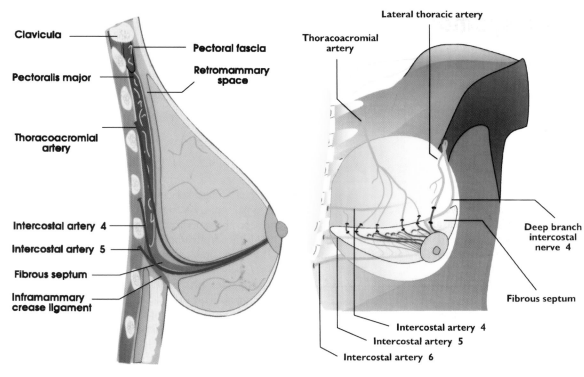

Fig. 2.2 Vessels, pectoralis major muscle, inframammary crease ligament, and retromammary space

Fig. 2.3 Vessels, deep branch of the 4th intercostal nerve, and fibrous septum

Also the vertical ligaments are guiding structures for main nerves and vessels. Perforating branches of the internal mammary artery run along the medial ligament together with the medial intercostal nerves. Branches of the lateral thoracic artery run along the lateral ligament together with the lateral intercostal nerves. The remaining parts of the breast receive no distinct vessels from the thoracic wall.

References

1.   Würinger E, Mader N, Posch E, Holle J: Nerve and vessel supplying ligamentous suspension of the mammary gland. Plast Reconstr Surg 1998;101(6):1486–1493

2.   Würinger E: Refinement of the central breast reduction by application of the ligamentous suspension. Plast Reconstr Surg 1999;103(5):1400–1410

3.   Würinger E, Tschabitscher M: New aspects of the topography of the mammary gland regarding its neurovascular supply along a regular ligamentous suspension. Eur J Morphol 2003;40(3):181

4.   Würinger E: Secondary reduction mammaplasty. Plast Reconstr Surg 2002;109(2):812–814

5.   Würinger E: Vertical scar mammaplasty with the inferocentral pedicle in vertical scar mammaplasty. In: Hamdi M, Hammond D, Nahai F (eds). Vertical Scar Mastopexy. Berlin, Springer Verlag 2005, pp 75–82

CHAPTER 3

Anthropomorphic Measurement of the Breast

Melvyn Westreich

3.1
Introduction

The female breast has a diverse physiognomy that makes accurate reproducible measurements of this organ very difficult. It is a three-dimensional soft tissue structure that is anchored to a bony and muscular framework but does not remain constant over time. Breast shape is affected by physiological changes associated with puberty, ovulation, gestation, lactation, and senescence. Although Maliniac [1, 2] described various "normal" values for measurements of the breast many years ago, there have been only five studies, using different protocols [3–7], that have actually attempted to develop a standardized method of measuring and recording the shape of the breast in a clinical setting . Several surgical techniques base their preoperative planning measurements on the "normal" values established by these studies. The author of this chapter will present some of the methods used for measuring and evaluating the difficult physiognomy of the female breast, suggest a simple protocol to measure the breast, and offer suggestions as to how these measurements may be beneficial in clinical practice.

Any protocol that attempts to record the shape of the breast must somehow note the following parameters: shape, volume, relative position to the trunk and the other breast, ptosis, projection, quality of the breast envelope, and any pathological morphology of the breast.

3.2
Shape

The breast is a structure made up of skin, breast tissue (lactiferous ducts along with breast stroma), and fat. It is positioned on the anterior chest along the embryonic milk line and begins to develop into a functional organ with puberty. Although conical during puberty, gravity seems to elongate and enhance the lower half of the breast until it becomes teardrop in shape. It is theorized that there are structures known as Cooper's ligaments that control the ptosis of the breast and. when lax, allow the breast parenchyma to drop below the inframammary line [8]. However, there is no real evidence that

Cooper's ligaments actually exist, and they may in fact just be the breast parenchyma between the lactiferous lobulations. There is evidence to suggest that the more fibrotic the breast parenchyma, the less it will become ptotic.

Although breast shape may vary quite a bit, certain universal concepts of breast aesthetics seem to be accepted by artists and the general public. A well-shaped breast will have little or no ptosis. The nipple will be at the anteriormost point of the breast mound. The inferior pole of the breast should be in the form of a half cone. A line from the clavicle to the nipple should be straight, without a marked "ski-jump" depression above the areola. The lateral breast should not extend more than a few centimeters posterior to the anterior axillary fold.

Undoubtedly the best way to record the shape of the breasts would be to make a cast or mold of these structures, either directly or by generating a computer model [4, 9]. However, these methods are either difficult to perform or extremely costly and are not readily adaptable to general clinical use. In recent years new technologies have emerged that allow excellent three-dimensional recording of the breast shape, but they do have drawbacks in that they do not demonstrate well the area beneath a ptotic breast, and they are still quite costly and certainly are not available in the average clinical setting. Therefore, anthropomorphic measurements, linear, curvilinear, and volumetric, will have to suffice for the practitioner studying the physiognomy of the breast.

3.3
Volume

The volume of the breast changes dramatically throughout a women's life. In some, the volume increases with gestation and lactation, and in others it decreases. Invariably, along with the normal aging process, the breast atrophies and becomes smaller. Three-dimensional (3D) computer-enhanced imaging methods (computed tomography, magnetic resonance imaging, 3D camera) can accurately determine the volume of the breast, but they have some difficulty in differentiating how much of the volume is determined by the breast tissue and how much by the underlying torso [10–24]. The biostereotactic method overcomes this problem by having the woman lie facedown over a study port. With this expensive apparatus, a stereotactic image is made of the breast hanging down in the study port [25–27]. Although this and the other 3D methods, are accurate, they all require expensive equipment, cameras, or lasers, and the author is not aware of any studies that have compared the values obtained by these methods with the conventional direct methods for determining breast volume in a clinical setting [15]. There have been reports that have compared "measured" volumes obtained by 3D imaging with the volumes measured of mastectomy specimens [15, 20]. The classic methods for determining breast volume that have been used in a clinical setting have been water displacement, breast casting [4, 9], and the Grossman–Roudner device [28–30]. Each method has been studied for accuracy and found to correlate one with the other. The Grossman–Roudner device was supplied free of charge by one of the implant companies over 20 years ago, but that company has since ceased to exist. At present the author is unaware of any company marketing the device. However, the three basic discs are shown here (Fig. 3.1).

The discs have a single radial slit which allows the circles to become cones of variable volumes and thus measure the breast. The smallest disc (measuring volumes of 125–200 cc) has a diameter of 15.85 cm. The mid-sized disc (measuring volumes of 200–300 cc) has a diameter of 18.00 cm. The largest disc (measuring volumes of 300–425–200 cc) has a diameter of 20.15 cm. Since the radii of the circles are fixed the volumes of the variable cones can be calculated and marked at the appropriate point on the periphery of the base of the cone.

3.4
Position

Anyone who has observed the transformation of a young girl into a young woman knows that the breast seems to move down on the chest wall until it reaches its attachment point on the anterior chest between the sternum and the anterior axillary fold in front of ribs 2–6. Its position is supposedly controlled by a unique structure called the inframammary fold/line, which is thought to be a fibrous attachment of the inferior breast skin to the subcutaneous fascia of the abdomen and chest and to the periosteum of the ribs [31]. Although histological studies have demonstrated the existence of this unique structure, it probably is more of a reactive fibrosis of the breast to the underlying tissues at that particular level rather than a separate anatomic entity; if it were a unique element of the anterior chest wall at a particular height, it would be hard to explain why we have recorded breast descent on the chest wall even into the 5th decade of life.

The best method to record the relative position of the breast on the anterior chest is by photographic documentation. If this is used, it is important to include other anatomic features in the photograph in order to orient the breast for size and spatial relationships (shoulders, umbilicus, etc.). It would also be beneficial to include a short piece of ruler in the photo so that, if necessary, actual measurements may be made from the

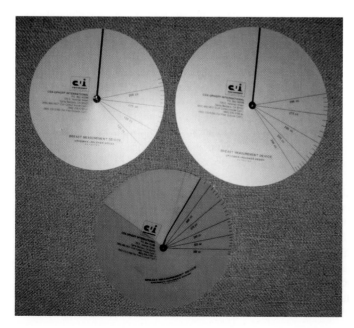

Fig. 3.1 Grossman–Roudner breast measurement discs

photo using this ruler as a guide. An alternative is to measure the positions of the various anatomic features of the breast in their relationship to the anatomic structures that surround them. The important features that must be recorded are the position of the nipple, the inframammary line, and the medial and lateral extent of the breast. These features need be measured in relationship to fixed anatomic structures such as the manubrial notch, acromion, clavicle, humerus, xyphoid, chest wall, and so on.

3.5
Ptosis and Projection

Projection is defined as the distance from the chest wall to the anterior most point on the breast mound (not the nipple). Ptosis is defined as the presence or absence of breast tissue below the inframammary line. Ptosis has been further graded by Regnault by the relative percentage of the total breast tissue that has fallen below the inframammary line. The interrelationship between the two can be seen in that it is almost impossible to determine the actual projection of a very ptotic breast because the tissue is often pushed forward by the abdominal wall. But even in such situations, when one is taking anthropomorphic measurements of the breast, the ptosis should be recorded and an estimate made of projection, making a note that it is an estimate. The interrelationship between these two parameters can also be seen in breast augmentation surgery to correct minimal ptosis. Whether one uses the newer anatomic implants or the round variety, this surgery corrects the ptosis by swinging the breast tissue like a pendulum into a more anterior position. By swinging up the tissue and filling the empty breast envelope, breast projection increases. When measuring the breast it is important to record the relative position of the nipple, projection at rest (passive), projection with traction (active—where the breast envelope is pulled forward by traction), and degree of ptosis if appropriate.

3.6
Breast Envelope Quality

The skin and soft tissue covering of the breast change with age. Many pubescence girls develop striae, and many postpartum women develop atrophy of the skin and subcutaneous structures. The presence or absence of striae or tonus of the skin should be recorded. The thickness of the covering skin and subcutaneous tissue should be measured with a caliper above and below the nipple. Any scars or previous surgery should be noted as well.

3.7
Pathological Morphology of the Breast

There are various common and not so common morphological variants of the breast. These include asymmetry, tuberous breasts, synmastia ("kissing breasts"), marked axillary extensions of the breast tissue, inverted nipples, abnormally large nipples, and outward- or inward-facing breasts. It is also important to record chest wall abnormalities that can affect the shape of the breast, such as Poland's syndrome, pigeon breast, pectus excavatum, and so on. In addition, if the breast has had previous surgery, such as augmentation or reduction, appropriate morphological changes should be recorded—capsular contracture, high-riding nipples, etc.

3.8
Protocol History

Maliniac [1, 2] was the first to attempt to collate the standards for measuring the breast while at the same time pointing out the enormous variety in breast shape among women. He was aware that various changes in the basic physiognomy of the breast will affect the success of aesthetic breast surgery. He cited numerous "standards" for breast morphology and even included the measurements of Venus de Milo. Surprisingly, since Maliniac's classic book was published there have been only five published studies that have measured a series of women's breasts using a standard protocol [3–7]. Although each study added information on the morphology of the breast, none of the protocols is complete enough to accurately record and study all breasts.

In Penn's classic article [3], 20 women with "aesthetically perfect breasts" were studied; however, he did not define the criteria he used to select the women studied. Many techniques for breast reduction base their preoperative measurement plans and nipple positioning on the distances published by Penn. The parameters studied by Penn were age, height, acromial span, "ideal nipple plane," midclavicle to "ideal nipple plane," midclavicle to nipple, nipple to nipple, nipple to submammary, and manubrium to nipple.

An article by Smith et al. [4] reports on 66 women who were studied using an interesting standard protocol. The article differed from Penn's in that the study by Smith and colleagues was not restricted to only those women with aesthetically perfect breasts. By analyzing their data, it can be seen that at least one-third of the women had marked hypertrophy, ptosis, or both. This flaws Smith et al.'s comprehensive study because they were interested in determining "normal" breast morphology, but that cannot be determined by including women with breast morphology that by definition would be considered "pathological." Although it is of some interest to determine and know what the proportions of the "average" breast are, it has little clinical importance. Because all cosmetic surgery is aimed at creating an aesthetically pleasing breast, it would have been more correct to determine what the proportions and components of the aesthetically pleasing breast were.

The parameters studied by Smith et al. were breast size, lateral breast crease, axilla to nipple, nipple to midline, nipple to inframammary crease, nipple to lowest point on breast, breast volume, and nipple to nipple. In addition, Smith et al. compared their results with the concept of the "ideal nipple plane."

Brown et al. [7] performed a study using a protocol similar to Smith et al.'s in a series of 60 subjects. They wanted to determine "normal" values for evaluating the breast. Although their protocol is thorough, they also included women with breast pathology and measured from soft tissue landmarks, which flaws the conclusions.

Qiao and colleagues [6, 32, 33] performed an interesting study in which they added recordings of the subjects' relative weight compared with the norm and measured the circumference of the chest at the height of the axilla, nipples, and abdomen as well as the circumference of the thigh. They found a correlation between breast volume and the difference in the circumference taken across the axilla and over the nipples and also with the amount that the patient was overweight. They also developed a method to determine breast volume based on measurements of the breast mound, but logically this formula would not be accurate in a markedly ptotic breast. The article also does not state whether they corroborated the actual volumes determined by their formulas with actual measured volumes of the subject's breasts. Finally, the article does not state if the subjects had perfect breasts, but from the material presented, it appears that most of the 125 young Asian subjects had small breasts [6].

When the author was designing and refining the present protocol to make it appropriate for all breasts, the parameters studied by the previous investigators were evaluated. Some seemed appropriate, whereas others did not. In the author's initial study, a protocol was used that reported on 50 women with aesthetically perfect breasts. "Aesthetically perfect" was defined as a nonptotic breast in which no common aesthetic procedure would be considered appropriate (excluding augmentation) to enhance the breast's form. All subjects were nulliparous Caucasians from a wide ethnic mix. The study was aimed at determining normal values for perfect breasts in the hope that the "normal values" obtained could be applied to aesthetic breast surgery. However, the author realized that that initial protocol was not appropriate for all breasts, and appropriate changes have been made.

Smith et al. [4] reported their results in centimeters taken to the second decimal place (i.e., to a 10th of a millimeter), whereas Penn reported to the nearest quarter-inch (equal to 0.68 cm). The author found that normal respirations or minor position changes caused fluctuations of a number of millimeters, making Smith et al.'s level of accuracy impractical in the clinical setting. Therefore, an accuracy level similar to that of Penn [3] seemed more appropriate. The author elected to use measurements to the nearest half-centimeter, performed with a simple measuring tape. An anthropometric caliper was reserved for obese patients and certain other measurements as noted in the protocol. The only additional paraphernalia needed for our measurements are the Grossman–Roudner device for volume [28, 29], a small tissue caliper, and a carpenter's level to assess the level of the nipple and inframammary crease in relationship to the humerus and midline. Although bra/cup size gives an indication of volume, it is not an exact measurement because cup size varies from one manufacturer to another and from one band size to another [34–36] (see below).

Smith et al. [4] performed volumetric analysis of the breasts by making a plaster cast of the subject's chest and then measuring the amount of sand needed to fill the mold. The author's volumetric measurements were made with the Grossman–Roudner device [28, 29]. This device, which utilizes a variable cone, does not measure all the breast tissue, since the tip of the cone is not always filled when a firm or very small breast is measured [30]. There are no standard cones for volumes above 450 ml, but they could be calculated and easily fashioned. In addition, some of the tissue lateral to the pectoral fold may not be within the cone. However, the sand fill and water displacement methods also do not adequately measure the tissue lateral to the pectoral folds. Probably the most accurate methods to determine breast volume are those described by Loughry and colleagues [25–27] using biostereometric analysis; Daly's Shape™ system [23]; and Malata's Body Map™ system [37]. Their major drawback is that they require special apparatus and are not portable. In contrast, the Grossman–Roudner cones come in a small flat envelope, are sterilizable, and may even be used intraoperatively. Although there may be a 5% variance using this device, the author feels that in the clinical setting in which a single individual takes the measurements, that should not be of any major significance. In addition, Smith has coauthored a paper [30] confirming the accuracy of the Grossman–Roudner method.

Another problem encountered in the other four protocols is that they do not exactly define their points of reference. Therefore, the author [4] arbitrarily specified that all measurements to the nipple are to the center.

Measurements to or from the clavicle, manubrium, umbilicus, and pubis are to the superior borders of each. The author also specifies that the body be in the normal anatomic position, with the elbows bent at 90° and the palms up. This position assists in standardizing the orientation of the arms, shoulders, and general posture of the upper trunk. The clavicular point is set at 5 cm lateral to the clavicular-manubrial joint, with the measurement to the nipple from this point running along the midbreast meridian.

All the parameters studied by Penn seem appropriate to us except for his measurement from the clavicle to the level of the "ideal nipple plane" on the midbreast meridian. The ideal nipple plane is a concept developed by Maliniac [1, 2] and adopted by Pitanguy, which assumes that the ideal level for the nipple in all women is a point on the midbreast meridian at the level of the midhumeral point (midpoint from olecranon to acromion). Penn's method for measuring this point is difficult to standardize or study because it will change with any movement of the shoulder and humerus in their relationship to the breast. Even temporarily bad posture will change this value. In our protocol we simply mark the level of the nipple along the length of the humerus using a carpenter's level and measure the distance from the acromion. Penn's measurement, if needed, can be calculated from this. In the author's initial study the protocol did not include height and weight, and it was felt that humeral length and trunk length, which have been shown to be directly proportional to height, would suffice. However, in the revised protocol they are included, and the body mass index can be calculated from these data.

The other protocols used in the past [3, 4, 6, 7] and Hauben et al.'s [38] study of the nipple–areola included certain measurements that the author felt were problematic. The most difficult are the measurements from the lateral breast crease to nipple and the axilla to nipple, and the measurements to or from the medial and lateral borders of the breast mound. In general, the soft tissue landmarks are too variable to be of any aid in studying the breast [39]. They will vary from woman to woman and change with the slightest motion, making them very imprecise. A distance taken from Smith's anterior axillary fold line to any of the points on the anterior chest could show differences of 15–20% because of minor position changes, irrespective of changes in the breast. In our protocol we elected not to use soft tissue landmarks at all. The only soft tissue structures that are studied are those that are directly related to the breast (nipple and inframammary crease), and we make no measurements from any soft tissue landmarks to the breast.

Another measurement that presents some difficulty is bra/cup size. This is extremely variable from manufacturer to manufacturer and was not needed in our original study. However, this should be recorded as part of the general information on the shape of the patient's breast. When reporting bra or cup size, the name of the manufacturer should be included as well, since there is no industry standard and this number can vary. The general rule to determine cup size is to measure the circumference in inches around the chest at the inframammary line and add 5 to determine the band size (taken to an even number, e.g., 34, 36, 38). Then the circumference is measured across the nipples, with the woman in a bra if necessary. A difference of 1 inch between the two equals an A cup, a difference of 2 inch is a B cup, etc. Thus, the volume of the breast in a 34A cup is not the same size as for a 36A cup [34–36].

The final problematic measurement encountered was the distance from the nipple to midline. Although this will give a relational assessment of the breast, in a rounded breast or ptotic breast or in obese women this is a curvilinear measurement and is difficult to record accurately. In addition, it seems redundant, since the nipple-to-nipple distance and breast projection are recorded. The author elected not to include this measurement in the protocol.

Qiao et al. [6] noted the difference between the circumference at the level of the axilla and across the nipples to determine breast volume. These measurements are part of the routine measurement recommended by bra manufacturers when determining the correct bra for women, and we have decided to include them in our new protocol. It is also important to record the other aspects of the subject's physiognomy that were, in addition to height and weight, included by the author:

1. Length from manubrium to xyphoid, umbilicus, and pubis
2. Chest width, depth, and circumference
3. Humeral length

The author [6] also included new parameters to more accurately describe the "pathological breast":

1. Lowest point on the breast
2. Width of the breast envelope
3. Thickness of the envelope above and below the nipple
4. Anterior extensibility of the envelope
5. Skin condition, including scars and previous surgeries
6. Recording of breast morphology and pathology
7. Regnault ptosis gradation
8. Age
9. Circumference at axilla and over nipples
10. Baker contracture classification if the breast has had implants

3.9
Protocol Method

The revised protocol gives an accurate reproducible assessment of the breast that can be very useful for patient evaluation in preoperative consultations and in assessing surgical goals and results (Table 3.1).

3.10
Definitions

All linear measurements are made with the subject standing in the normal anatomic position, with shoulders back and head straight ahead. Measurements on the arm are made with the elbow bent at 90° with palm facing upwards. Measurements to the nipple are made to the center of the nipple. Measurements to the umbilicus and pubis are to the superior border of each. The clavicular point is defined as a point on the upper border of the clavicle 5 cm lateral to the clavicular-manubrial joint. The suprasternal notch (manubrium), clavicular point, acromion, and xyphoid are all marked before measuring. Breast volume measurements are made using the Grossman–Roudner device [28–30]. Volume measurements are made in the manner specified by Grossman–Roudner with the subject standing with a posterior incline of the body to 45°. This is ac-

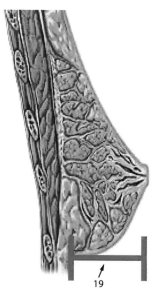

Fig. 3.3 Measurement of breast projection made just beneath the breasts

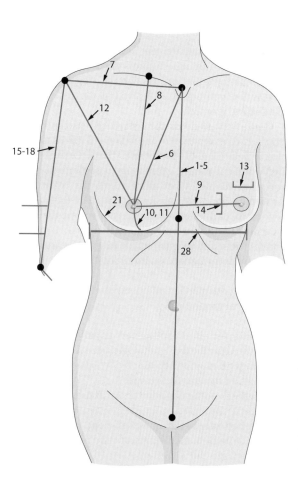

Fig. 3.2 Illustration showing the lines of measurement for the anterior chest, breast, and arm. To obtain "normal" breast volume using manubrium-to-nipple and nipple-to-nipple measurements, the distances are based on the results of anthropomorphic measurements of 50 women with aesthetically "perfect" breasts

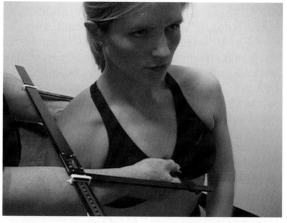

Fig. 3.4 Example of how to use anthropometric caliper. Note that the caliper position in this photo is not appropriate for our protocol. (Photo courtesy of Rosscraft Innovations, Vancouver, Canada)

complished by having the subject stand with her back to a heavy table 3 feet (approximate) distant. The subject carefully extends her arms posteriorly to lean and support her straight body at the desired angle. A carpenter's level is used to accurately assess point levels with the midline and humerus. An anthropomorphic caliper is used for chest width, chest depth, breast width, and sometimes nipple-to-nipple distance (Figs. 3.2–3.4).

3.11
Accuracy

All linear measurements are rounded to the nearest half-centimeter. Volumes are rounded to the nearest 5 ml.

Definitions of the parameters measured (Table 3.1; Figs. 3.2, 3.3) are as follows:

1. Manubrium (M; suprasternal notch, SSN) to infra-mammary crease (M–In): Vertical midline measurement from M to the point level with the most inferior point on the inframammary crease (use carpenter's level)
2. Manubrium to lowest point on breast (LPB; M–LPB): As in 1, to point equal to this height in midline
3. Manubrium to xyphoid (M–Xy): As in 1, to palpable tip of xyphoid
4. Manubrium to umbilicus (M–Um): As in 1, to upper border of umbilicus
5. Manubrium to pubis (M–Pub): As in 1, to superior edge of pubis
6. Manubrium to center of nipple (M–N)
7. Manubrium to point of maximum lateral prominence of acromion (M–Ac)
8. Nipple to clavicle (N–Cl): Vertical measurement from a point 5 cm lateral to the manubrial-clavicular joint to the center of the nipple
9. Nipple to nipple (N–N): Horizontal measurement from center of one nipple to the other
10. Areola to inframammary (Inf; Ar–In): Vertical measurement from inferior edge of areola to lowest point on inframammary crease
11. Areola to lowest point of breast (Ar–LPB): Vertical measurement from inferior edge of areola to most dependent point of breast
12. Nipple to acromion (Ac; N–Ac): Measurement from tip of acromion to center of nipple
13. Areolar width (A–Wi): Horizontal measurement of areolar width
14. Areolar height (A–He): Vertical measurement of areolar height
15. Acromion to olecranon (Ac–Ol): Vertical measurement from tip of acromion to tip of olecranon (elbow bent at 90°)
16. Acromion to inferior point (Ac–In): Vertical measurement on a line from tip of acromion to olecra-non to a point on the arm level with the inframam-mary line (use carpenter's level)
17. Acromion to nipple height (Ac–Ni): As in 15, to a point on the arm level with the nipple
18. Acromion to LPB height (Ac–LPB): As in 15, to a point on the arm level with the lowest point of breast
19. Breast projection (B–pr): Breast projection measured at 90° to chest wall just beneath breast (passive)
20. Breast distraction (B–D): Breast projection measured at 90° to chest wall just beneath breast (active) when grasping nipple and distracting anteriorly
21. Infra (Infra): Circumlinear measurement of the inferior 180° about the nipple on the inframammary crease
22. Width of breast envelope from lateral to median extent of inframammary fold (use caliper)
23. Thickness of breast envelope—upper: Caliper measurement 2 cm above areola
24. Thickness of breast envelope—lower: Caliper measurement 2 cm below areola
25. Volume: Volume of each breast using Grossman–Roudner device
26. Regnault ptosis gradation: 0-A-B-C [40]
27. Baker capsule classification if previous breast implants: 0-1-2-3-4 [41]
28. Chest circumference (Ch–ci): Chest circumference measured at the level of the most inferior point of the inframammary crease
    Chest circumference axilla (Ch–ci–ax): Chest circumference measured at the level of axilla
    Chest circumference nipples (Ch–ci–Ni): Chest circumference measured across and over the nipples; if the breast is ptotic, the woman should wear her bra for this measurement
29. Chest depth (Ch–de): Chest depth measured with anthropometric caliper at the level of the most inferior point of the inframammary crease (Fig. 3.4)
30. Chest width (Ch–wi): Chest width measured with anthropometric caliper at the level of the most inferior point of the inframammary crease
31. Breast envelope: Describe skin (striae and tonus), subcutaneous tissue, scars, and previous surgery
32. Morphological pathology of breast

In addition, the date and time of the exam and the procedure contemplated, if appropriate, are recorded. Pertinent personal identification information, height, and weight are recorded. The author does not recommend measuring or recording distances from or to the axillary fold or measurements of the various parameters of the breast mound itself, but these may be added by each investigator if deemed appropriate.

Table 3.1 Protocol sheet for anthropomorphic assessment of breast

Please Read Breast Morphology Protocol Instructions Prior to Measuring!!

Patient Information: _____ _____ _____
                           Family Name   First Name   Record Number

_____ _____ _____
Address   Phone   Procedure   Date of exam

_____ _____ _____ _____
Age   Height   Weight   Bra size and manufacturer

Right   **Left**   **Midline Measurements (*= use carpenter level)**

_____ _____   1. Manubrium to inframammary crease*

_____ _____   2. Manubrium to lowest point on breast*

_____ _____   3. Manubrium to xyphoid

_____ _____   4. Manubrium to umbilicus

_____ _____   5. Manubrium to pubis

                  Linear Measurements

_____ _____   6. Manubrium to nipple

_____ _____   7. Manubrium to acromion

_____ _____   8. Nipple to clavicle

_____ _____   9. Nipple to nipple

_____ _____   10. Areola to inframammary line

_____ _____   11. Areola to lowest (most dependent) point of breast

_____ _____   12. Nipple to acromion

_____ _____   13. Areolar width

_____ _____   14. Areolar height

Right   **Left**   **Arm Measurements**

_____ _____   15. Acromion to olecranon

_____ _____   16. Acromion to inframammary line height*

_____ _____ 17. Acromion to nipple height*

_____ _____ 18. Acromion to height of lowest point on breast*

_____ _____ 19. Breast projection (passive)

_____ _____ 20. Breast projection (active)

_____ _____ 21. Inframammary line length

_____ _____ 22. Width of breast envelope

_____ _____ 23. Thickness of breast envelope—upper

_____ _____ 24. Thickness of breast envelope—lower

_____ _____ 25. Volume

_____ _____ 26. Regnault ptosis gradation (0-A-B-C)

_____ _____ 27. Baker classification if previous implants (0-1-2-3-4)

_____ _____ 28. Chest circumference

_____ _____ 29. Chest depth—use anthropomorphic caliper

_____ _____ 30. Chest width—use anthropomorphic caliper

31. **Breast envelope** – Describe skin (striae and tonus), subcutaneous, scars, previous breast surgery:

_____

_____

32. **Morphological pathology** of breast: ☐ None ☐ Present – describe:

_____

_____

3.12
Clinical Application

The most important use of the breast measuring protocol is to assess the physiognomy of the breast and record any changes from previous measurements. These changes may be the result of surgeries performed or simply due to the vagaries of the passage of time. By including anthropomorphic measurements in the permanent record of every patient undergoing breast surgery, we have a tool to compare long-term and short-term results of surgical techniques. Even if the woman does not have surgery, we can assess how the breast changes as time progresses.

In addition, anthropomorphic measurements can help in the preoperative evaluation and can improve surgical outcomes [42]; if the surgeon fails to note that the anatomic features of a breast of a particular patient are not situated in a "normal" position, many types of "cookbook" surgery techniques can have disastrous results. If anatomic variants are discovered preoperatively, they can be discussed with the patient, and the surgical planning can be altered to accommodate the anomaly. For instance, if breast reduction surgery were planned for the young woman who modeled for the Venus de Milo, and the surgeon drew out a surgical plan for the procedure based on a suprasternal notch to nipple distance (M–N) of about 21 cm, as was suggested by Penn, the surgeon might find that the result was less than optimal, since Venus has a very short M–N distance of 16.51. This would have resulted in droopy ptotic breasts, which would not be considered aesthetically pleasing. This is often the consequence of using an inappropriate "cookbook" measurement to determine postoperative nipple position in such patients.

Because our goal in aesthetic surgery is to convert an "imperfect" breast into a "perfect" one, it is extremely enticing to think that we could simply determine nipple position by some arbitrary rule derived by one of the papers that studied perfect breasts. As mentioned previously, many methods use the results of Penn's classic study, but, unfortunately, subsequent studies have not corroborated these "normal" values. Other authors assume that in all women with perfect breasts, the M–Ni distances and the Ni–Ni distances will form an isosceles triangle. Equally problematic are those who assume, like Maliniac and Pitanguy, that in a perfect breast the nipple position will be above the horizontal line drawn at the midpoint between the acromion and olecranon on the humerus. Clinical experience has shown that none of these rules is true in all women. To avoid these discrepancies, the McKissock, LeJour, Hall-Findlay, and other breast reduction techniques (I. Pitanguy, personal communication, 1984; M. LeJour, personal communication, 1994) [43] determine the position of the nipple at the level of the inframammary fold irrespective of the distance from the suprasternal notch. This is not to say that it is not important to know the SSN–N distance; if surgeons take careful preoperative measurements, it will help alert them to possible problems with nipple positioning and in addition will allow them to follow the patient's postoperative progress.

The problem of determining nipple position in breast surgery is not restricted to the female breast. In two articles on the male breast physiognomy for female-to-male transsexual surgery, various methods for positioning the new breast on the chest wall were proposed. Beckenstein et al. [44] felt that positioning the nipple in relation to the inferior border of the pectoralis major was inaccurate. They found a direct correlation between subject height and the measurements M–Ni, Cl–Ni, and N–Ni, and suggested using a simple convergence formula to determine nipple position. In the author's study, a correlation was not found between body length and nipple position, but male breasts may be different. Hage and Van Kesteren [45], on the other hand, found that the rules used by artists [46–48] to determine nipple position cannot be used in transsexual surgery because the trunk of the male differs markedly from that of the female. That is, if a surgeon positions the nipple "as in a male" on a female torso, the position will be inaccurate. They felt it more reliable for the surgeon to consider the specific body habitus of each patient and to use the "ideal nipple plane" or the 4th or 5th rib and the inferior margin of the pectoralis major muscle to position the nipple.

Although the criteria for a perfectly shaped breast vary, certain concepts are accepted by all. The aesthetically pleasing breast will be of a size and fullness proportional to the body, have minimal ptosis, be conical to teardrop in shape, and have the nipple at the anterior-most position [47, 48]. Achieving this result through surgery is what aesthetic breast surgery is all about. Yet each surgical problem can be corrected by many techniques, with even more subtechniques. This multitude of methods indicates that with each procedure there is an element of difficulty in certain techniques in certain patients. Therefore, with just about every description of surgical technique, the surgeon is advised to make appropriate changes when needed. To make these decisions, the surgeon must rely on his or her inborn beauty sense and artistic skill [2].

Theoretically we should be able to turn to our artist friends for advice on what is normal for the shape and placement of the breast. Unfortunately, most sculptors and artists have almost always depicted a breast morphology that is more of an ideal than the real [47, 48]. The exaggerated high breasts of the Barbie doll, and those in classic and modern painting and sculpture, are examples of this. As a rule, the breasts depicted by artists will have minimal ptosis and will be high on the chest wall. Even Rubens, noted for the more robust women depicted in his works, adhered to this rule.

Usually the nipple will be the most prominent point on the breast, and there will be a straight (or minimally convex) line above it from clavicle to nipple. Also, each breast will rest in the approximate center of its half of the chest, and the inframammary crease will make an almost a perfect semicircle of 180°.

The surgeon must always be aware that a particular subject's anatomy may be inconsistent with these artistic rules and perhaps with a particular surgical method he or she is using. Only by knowing normal breast morphology, and realizing preoperatively that a particular subject is not "normal," can a surgeon avoid the pitfalls inherent to a particular technique [49–52].

When anyone with an artistic bend looks at a woman's breast, the computer that is the human brain analyzes the breast shape and determines whether the shape is appropriate. The human computer considers so many parameters that it is difficult to determine what it is that makes us decide that a certain shape and volume is appropriate and what is not. In search of some of these factors that correlate with appropriateness, we realized that one of the most important factors was volume. Therefore, in our initial study we analyzed our results, taking particular interest to see if there was any correlation between our various measurements and breast volume.

The author studied 15 of the variables measured in the 50 female subjects with perfect breasts and attempted to find a relationship between the linear variables and breast volume. Principle component analysis of the 15 variables failed to give a reduced set of factors. The scree plot of Eigen values suggested 11 factors, thus it did not give us a small number of predictors. Simple linear regression analysis of the 15 variables showed a significantly significant relationship between volume and nine of the variables listed below.

Measurements	r	p
M–In	0.459	<0.0008
M–NI	0.547	<0.00004
N–CL	0.484	<0.0004
N–Ni	0.507	<0.0002
AR–IN	0.582	<0.000009
AR–Wi	0.549	<0.00004
AR–He	0.588	<0.000008
B–pr	0.592	<0.000006
Infra	0.592	<0.00000001

However, the last five variables are measurements made of the breast shape and form directly. That is, if there were a bigger breast, these measurements would be automatically larger. Therefore, they would not be of any predictive value for determining appropriate breast size. This is similar to what Qiao et al. [6] found in their study, in that measurements of the breast mound can determine volume. However, our first four variables, M–In, M–Ni, N–CL, and N–Ni, are not a direct measurement of the breast itself but are a relationship of some anatomic point on the breast to a surrounding structure. In other words, there is a relationship between body physiognomy and breast volume. Because of the close interrelationship between these variables, we could not simply put them in a multiple regression analysis equation to determine volume. In addition, linear regression of volume on a set of linear measurements leads to skewed histograms of residuals, which is undesirable and unacceptable. The following formula, based on geometric logic, was proposed to determine volume:

$$\text{volume} = p_1^{a1} \times p_2^{a2} \ldots\ldots\ldots p_n^{an}$$

or

$$\log(\text{volume}) = [a_1 \times \log(p_1)] + [a_2 \times \log(p_2)] + \ldots + [a_n \times \log(p_n)]$$

where p = variables and a = regression coefficients

By evaluating the logs of the variables by a stepwise regression analysis for variable selection according to R-squared, we were able to determine that the same four variables were correlated to volume, with M–Ni and N–Ni the most significant. Because of the intimate interrelationships between the variables, we were able to propose several combinations of the variables to determine volume with insignificant differences. Therefore, for ease in the clinical setting, we propose the following multiple regression formula using only two variables to determine breast volume:

$$\text{volume} = (\text{M–Ni})^{1.103} \times (\text{N–Ni})^{0.811}$$

or
$$\log(\text{volume}) = [1.103 \times \log(\text{M–Ni})] + [0.811 \times \log(\text{N–Ni})]$$

Analysis of the variance of this equation shows an R-squared of 0.9988 and an error coefficient of variation of 0.0361. It has a probability of $p \leq 0.000001$. The results were acceptable under normality tests for skewness and kurtosis. All statistical work was done using the NCSS 6.0 computer program by Hintze (Kaysville, UT, USA).

Table 3.2 For calculating "appropriate" breast volume based on measurements of distance from manubrium to nipple (horizontal) and distance between the nipples (vertical)

	12	12.5	13	13.5	14	14.5	15	15.5	16
12	116.2928	121.6488	127.0268	132.4263	137.8463	143.2864	148.7458	154.224	159.7204
12.5	120.2073	125.7436	131.3027	136.8838	142.4863	148.1095	153.7527	159.4153	165.0967
13	124.0923	129.8075	135.5463	141.3078	147.0914	152.8963	158.7219	164.5674	170.4325
13.5	127.9492	133.842	139.7591	145.6998	151.6631	157.6484	163.655	169.6823	175.7296
14	131.7792	137.8484	143.9426	150.0611	156.2029	162.3674	168.5538	174.7615	180.9898
14.5	135.5834	141.8277	148.0979	154.393	160.7121	167.0546	173.4196	179.8065	186.2146
15	139.3628	145.7813	152.2262	158.6968	165.1921	171.7113	178.2537	184.8187	191.4055
15.5	143.1185	149.71	156.3286	162.9736	169.6439	176.3388	183.0576	189.7994	196.5637
16	146.8514	153.6148	160.4061	167.2243	174.0686	180.9382	187.8322	194.7499	201.6906
16.5	150.5624	157.4966	164.4595	171.4501	178.4673	185.5105	192.5786	199.6712	206.7873
17	154.2521	161.3563	168.4898	175.6516	182.8409	190.0566	197.298	204.5643	211.8549
17.5	157.9213	165.1945	172.4977	179.8299	187.1902	194.5776	201.9912	209.4304	216.8943
18	161.5708	169.0121	176.4841	183.9857	191.5161	199.0742	206.6592	214.2702	221.9067
18.5	165.2021	172.8097	180.4495	188.1198	195.8193	203.5472	211.3026	219.0847	226.8927
19	168.8131	176.5879	184.3948	192.2327	200.1006	207.9975	215.9225	223.8747	231.8534
19.5	172.407	180.3474	188.3205	196.3253	204.3607	212.4257	220.5194	228.6409	236.7895
20	175.9836	184.0887	192.2272	200.398	208.6001	216.8324	225.094	233.3841	241.7017
20.5	179.5433	187.8123	196.1155	204.4516	212.8196	221.2184	229.6471	238.1049	246.5907
21	183.0867	191.5189	199.9859	208.4865	217.0197	225.5842	234.1793	242.8039	251.4573
21.5	186.6141	195.2088	203.8389	212.5033	221.2009	229.9305	238.6911	247.4819	256.302
22	190.1261	198.8825	207.675	216.5025	225.3637	234.2576	243.1831	252.1394	261.1254
22.5	193.623	202.5404	211.4947	220.4846	229.5087	238.5662	247.6559	256.7769	265.9282
23	197.1052	206.1831	215.2984	224.4499	233.6364	242.8568	252.1099	261.3949	270.7108
23.5	200.5732	209.8108	219.0865	228.399	237.7471	247.1297	256.5457	265.994	275.4738
24	204.0273	213.4239	222.8593	232.3322	241.8413	251.3855	260.9636	270.5747	280.2178
24.5	207.4678	217.0228	226.6174	236.25	245.9195	255.6246	265.3642	275.1374	284.943
25	210.895	220.6079	230.361	240.1527	249.9819	259.8473	269.7479	279.6824	289.6501
25.5	214.3093	224.1795	234.0904	244.0407	254.029	264.0541	274.115	284.2104	294.3394
26	217.711	227.7378	237.8061	247.9143	258.0611	268.2554	278.4659	288.7216	299.0114
26.5	221.1003	231.2832	241.5082	251.7738	262.0786	272.4215	282.8011	293.2164	303.6664
27	224.4776	234.816	245.1972	255.6196	266.0818	276.5826	287.1208	297.6952	308.3048
27.5	227.843	238.3365	248.8733	259.452	270.0711	280.7293	291.4254	302.1584	312.9271
28	231.1969	241.8449	252.5368	263.2712	274.0466	284.8617	295.7153	306.6063	317.5335
28.5	234.5396	245.3414	256.188	267.0775	278.0087	288.9802	299.9907	311.0391	322.1243
29	237.8711	248.8264	259.827	270.8713	281.9577	293.0851	304.252	315.4573	326.7
29.5	241.1918	252.3001	263.4542	274.6527	285.8939	297.1766	308.4994	319.8612	331.2608
30	244.5019	255.7626	267.0698	278.422	289.8175	301.255	312.7332	324.2509	335.8069

16.5	17	17.5	18	18.5	19	19.5	20	20.5	21
165.2345	170.7659	176.3141	181.8786	187.459	193.0551	198.6663	204.2923	209.9329	215.5876
170.7964	176.514	182.2489	188.0008	193.7691	199.5535	205.3535	211.169	216.9994	222.8445
176.3165	182.2188	188.1391	194.0768	200.0315	206.0029	211.9904	217.9938	224.0127	230.0467
181.7965	187.8823	193.9866	200.1088	206.2486	212.4056	218.5792	224.7692	230.9751	237.1967
187.2383	193.5063	199.7932	206.0988	212.4224	218.7636	225.122	231.4973	237.889	244.2968
192.6434	199.0924	205.5609	212.0484	218.5546	225.0788	231.6208	238.1801	244.7563	251.3491
198.0135	204.6422	211.291	217.9594	224.6469	231.3531	238.0774	244.8196	251.5791	258.3556
203.3498	210.1571	216.9851	223.8332	230.701	237.5879	244.4934	251.4173	258.359	265.3181
208.6537	215.6386	222.6447	229.6714	236.7182	243.7847	250.8704	257.9749	265.0976	272.2383
213.9263	221.0877	228.2708	235.4751	242.7001	249.9451	257.2099	264.4938	271.7966	279.1177
219.1689	226.5058	233.8649	241.2457	248.6477	256.0704	263.5131	270.9756	278.4573	285.9578
224.3823	231.8937	239.4279	246.9843	254.5624	262.1616	269.7814	277.4214	285.0811	292.76
229.5677	237.2527	244.961	252.692	260.4452	268.22	276.0159	283.8325	291.6692	299.5256
234.7259	242.5836	250.4651	258.3699	266.2973	274.2468	282.2178	290.21	298.2228	306.2557
239.8579	247.8873	255.9412	264.0187	272.1195	280.2428	288.3881	296.555	304.743	312.9515
244.9643	253.1647	261.39	269.6396	277.9128	286.209	294.5278	302.8685	311.2308	319.6141
250.0461	258.4166	266.8126	275.2333	283.6781	292.1464	300.6377	309.1515	317.6873	326.2445
255.1039	263.6438	272.2095	280.8006	289.4162	298.0558	306.7189	315.4049	324.1133	332.8436
260.1385	268.8469	277.5817	286.3422	295.1279	303.938	312.7721	321.6295	330.5098	339.4124
265.1505	274.0266	282.9297	291.859	300.814	309.7939	318.7981	327.8262	336.8776	345.9517
270.1404	279.1836	288.2543	297.3517	306.4751	315.624	324.7977	333.9957	343.2174	352.4623
275.109	284.3185	293.556	302.8207	312.112	321.4291	330.7716	340.1387	349.5301	358.945
280.0568	289.4319	298.8355	308.2669	317.7252	327.2099	336.7204	346.256	355.8163	365.4005
284.9842	294.5243	304.0934	313.6907	323.3154	332.967	342.6449	352.3483	362.0767	371.8296
289.8919	299.5963	309.3302	319.0927	328.8832	338.701	348.5455	358.416	368.312	378.2328
294.7803	304.6484	314.5664	324.4735	334.4291	344.4125	354.423	364.4599	374.5227	384.6109
299.6499	309.681	319.7425	329.8336	339.9537	350.102	360.2778	370.4806	380.7096	390.9644
304.5011	314.6946	324.919	335.1735	345.4574	355.77	366.1106	376.4785	386.8732	397.294
309.3344	319.6896	330.0763	340.4936	350.9408	361.417	371.9217	382.4542	393.0139	403.6001
314.1501	324.6666	335.2149	345.7944	356.4042	367.0436	377.7118	388.4083	399.1323	409.8834
318.9487	329.6258	340.3353	351.0764	361.8482	372.6501	383.4813	394.3411	405.229	416.1442
323.7305	334.5677	345.4377	356.3398	367.2732	378.237	389.2306	400.2533	411.3044	422.3833
328.4959	339.4926	350.5227	361.5853	372.6796	383.8048	394.9602	406.1451	417.3589	428.6009
333.2453	344.401	355.5905	366.813	378.0677	389.3538	400.6705	412.0171	423.393	434.7975
337.9789	349.293	360.6415	372.0235	383.438	394.8844	406.3619	417.8697	429.4072	440.9737
342.6971	354.1692	365.6761	377.217	388.7909	400.3971	412.0347	423.7032	435.4017	447.1297
347.4003	359.0298	370.6946	382.3939	394.1266	405.8921	417.6895	429.5181	441.3772	453.2661

Table 3.2 (continued) For calculating "appropriate" breast volume based on measurements of distance from manubrium to nipple (horizontal) and distance between the nipples (vertical)

21.5	22	22.5	23	23.5	24	24.5	25	25.5	26
221.2563	226.9385	232.6341	238.3427	244.0641	249.789	255.5443	261.3027	267.0729	272.8548
228.7039	234.5774	240.4647	246.3655	252.2794	258.2064	264.1461	270.0983	276.0628	282.0393
236.0955	242.1588	248.2363	254.3278	260.4329	266.5515	272.6831	278.8277	284.9849	291.1546
243.4353	249.6835	255.9517	262.2325	268.5274	274.836	281.1583	287.4938	293.8424	300.2039
250.7203	257.1592	263.6132	270.082	276.5653	283.0628	289.5743	296.0995	302.6381	309.19
257.958	264.5828	271.2232	277.8787	284.5492	291.2343	297.9337	304.6473	311.3747	318.1157
265.1488	271.9582	278.7837	285.6247	292.4811	299.3526	306.2388	313.1395	320.0544	326.9833
272.2943	279.2873	286.2967	293.3221	300.3633	307.4199	314.4917	321.5784	328.6797	335.7953
279.3965	286.5718	293.764	300.9727	308.1975	315.4382	322.6945	329.966	337.2525	344.5537
286.4568	293.8135	301.187	308.5782	315.9856	323.4093	330.8489	338.3041	345.7748	353.2605
293.4767	301.0137	308.5684	316.1403	323.7292	331.3348	338.9567	346.5947	354.2484	361.9176
300.4578	308.1741	315.9084	323.6605	331.4299	339.2164	347.0196	354.8393	362.675	370.5267
307.4012	315.2958	323.2089	331.1401	339.0891	347.0556	355.0391	363.0395	371.0563	379.0894
314.3083	322.3803	330.4712	338.5806	346.7082	354.8536	363.0166	371.1967	379.3937	387.6072
321.1802	329.4287	337.6964	345.9832	354.2885	362.612	370.9534	379.3124	387.6886	396.0817
328.018	336.4421	344.8859	353.349	361.8311	370.3319	378.8508	387.3878	395.9423	404.5141
334.8227	343.4215	352.0405	360.6792	369.3373	378.0144	386.7101	395.4241	404.1561	412.9057
341.5954	350.3681	359.1614	367.9749	376.8081	385.6607	394.5323	403.4226	412.3312	421.2578
348.3369	357.2828	366.2496	375.237	384.2445	393.2718	402.3185	411.3843	420.4687	429.5715
355.0481	364.1663	373.3059	382.4665	391.6476	400.8488	410.0698	419.3102	428.5696	437.8478
361.7299	371.0197	380.3313	389.6643	399.0181	408.3925	417.7871	427.2014	436.6351	446.0879
368.3831	377.8437	387.3266	396.8312	406.3571	415.9039	425.4712	435.0587	444.6659	454.2926
375.0083	384.6392	394.2926	403.9681	413.6653	423.3838	433.1323	442.8831	452.6631	462.4629
381.6064	391.4067	401.23	411.0757	420.9436	430.8331	440.7438	450.6754	460.6275	470.5997
388.178	398.1471	408.1395	418.1548	428.1926	438.2524	448.3338	458.4365	468.5599	478.7038
394.7238	404.861	415.0219	425.2061	435.4132	445.6426	455.894	466.167	476.4612	486.7762
401.2444	411.549	421.8778	432.2302	442.6059	453.0043	463.4251	473.8678	484.332	494.8174
407.7404	418.2118	428.7078	439.2279	449.7715	460.3383	470.9277	481.5395	492.1731	502.8283
414.2123	424.85	435.5126	446.1996	456.9106	467.6451	478.4026	489.1828	499.9853	510.8095
420.6608	431.4641	442.2926	453.1461	464.0238	474.9254	485.8504	496.7985	507.769	518.7618
427.0863	438.0546	449.0486	460.0678	471.1117	482.1798	493.2717	504.387	515.5251	526.6856
433.4894	444.6221	455.7809	466.9653	478.1748	489.4088	500.667	511.9489	523.2541	534.5821
439.8704	451.1671	462.4901	473.8392	485.2137	496.6131	508.037	519.485	530.9565	542.4513
446.23	457.69	469.1768	480.6899	492.2288	503.7931	515.3821	526.9956	538.6331	550.294
452.5686	464.1913	475.8413	487.5179	499.2207	510.9493	522.703	534.4814	546.2841	558.1107
458.8865	470.6715	482.4841	494.3237	506.1899	518.0822	530	541.9428	553.9103	565.902
465.1842	477.1309	489.1056	501.1078	513.1368	525.1923	537.2736	549.3804	561.5121	573.6684

26.5	27	27.5	28	28.5	29	29.5	30	
278.6482	284.4528	290.2685	296.0952	301.9325	307.7804	313.6387	319.5073	**12**
28.0277	294.0277	300.0392	306.0619	312.0958	318.1405	324.196	330.2621	**12.5**
297.3365	303.5305	309.7362	315.9536	322.1825	328.4226	334.6738	340.936	**13**
306.5779	312.9644	319.363	325.7737	332.1961	338.6302	345.0757	351.5325	**13.5**
315.7549	322.3325	328.9227	335.5252	342.1399	348.7666	355.405	362.055	**14**
324.87	331.6375	338.418	345.2111	352.0168	358.8347	365.6648	372.5068	**14.5**
333.926	340.8821	347.8516	354.8341	361.8294	368.8347	375.8579	382.8906	**15**
342.925	350.0687	357.2259	364.3966	371.5805	378.7773	385.987	393.2093	**15.5**
351.8694	359.1993	366.5433	373.901	381.2722	388.6568	396.0545	403.4652	**16**
360.7611	368.2762	375.8058	383.3494	390.9069	398.4791	406.0628	413.6607	**16.5**
369.602	377.3013	385.0153	392.7438	400.4866	408.2433	416.0138	423.7979	**17**
378.3938	386.2763	394.1739	402.0862	410.0131	417.9543	425.9097	433.879	**17.5**
387.1384	395.203	403.283	411.3782	419.4883	427.6131	435.7523	443.9057	**18**
395.8371	404.0829	412.3445	420.6216	428.9139	437.2213	445.5433	453.88	**18.5**
404.4915	412.9176	421.3598	429.8179	438.2915	446.7805	455.2845	463.8034	**19**
413.1029	421.7084	430.3304	438.9685	447.6225	456.2922	464.9773	473.6776	**19.5**
421.6727	430.4568	439.2576	448.0749	456.9085	465.758	474.6233	483.504	**20**
430.2022	439.1639	448.1427	457.1384	466.1506	475.1791	484.2237	493.2841	**20.5**
438.6923	447.8309	456.987	466.1602	475.3503	484.557	493.78	503.0192	**21**
438.6923	456.4591	465.7915	475.1414	484.5086	493.8927	503.2934	512.7106	**21.5**
447.1444	465.0493	474.5574	484.0833	493.6267	503.1874	512.7651	522.3595	**22**
455.5594	473.6028	483.2857	492.9868	502.7058	512.4423	522.1962	531.9671	**22.5**
463.9383	482.1204	491.9775	501.8531	511.7468	521.6585	531.5877	541.5344	**23**
472.2821	490.6031	500.6336	510.6829	520.7508	530.8368	340.9408	551.0624	**23.5**
480.5917	499.0517	509.255	519.4774	529.7186	539.9783	550.2563	560.5522	**24**
488.8679	507.4671	517.8425	528.2372	538.6511	549.0839	559.5352	570.0047	**24.5**
497.1116	515.8502	526.3969	536.9634	547.5493	558.1544	568.7783	579.4208	**25**
505.3236	524.2016	534.919	545.6566	556.4139	567.1907	577.9866	588.8014	**25.5**
513.5045	532.5221	543.4097	554.3176	565.2457	576.1935	587.1608	598.1473	**26**
521.6553	540.8124	551.8695	562.9473	574.0455	585.1637	596.3018	607.4592	**26.5**
529.7764	549.0732	560.2992	571.5462	582.8139	594.102	605.4101	616.7381	**27**
537.8686	557.3051	568.6994	580.115	591.5517	603.009	614.4867	625.9845	**27.5**
545.9326	565.5088	577.0708	588.6545	600.2595	611.8855	623.5321	635.1991	**28**
553.9689	573.6849	585.4141	597.1652	608.938	620.7321	632.5471	644.3828	**28.5**
561.9781	581.8339	593.7297	605.6477	617.5877	629.5493	641.5322	653.536	**29**
577.9175	589.9564	602.0182	614.1026	626.2093	638.3379	650.4881	662.6595	**29.5**
585.8488	598.0529	610.2802	622.5305	634.8034	647.0984	659.4153	671.7537	**30**

In simple terms, in the clinical setting the appropriate volume for a particular woman can be determined using two measurements: the distance from the manubrium notch to the center of the nipple (M–Ni), and then the nipple-to-nipple distance (N–Ni). Then, using a simple scientific calculator, the log of M–Ni is multiplied by factor 1.103, and the log of N–Ni is multiplied by the factor 0.811. The results are added, and this represents the log of the volume. By performing the antilog function, the volume is determined.

Since publication of the original article, the author noted that most surgeons shy away from anything resembling higher mathematics, and the use of logarithms scares them even more. Therefore, we have compiled a table that allows the surgeon to simply plug in the appropriate M–Ni distance on the table and then go down the appropriate row until he or she finds where it crosses the appropriate Ni–Ni distance (see Table 3.2). The number in the square is the volume in cubic centimeters of the appropriate "ideal normal breast" for those measurements. To use this number, the preoperative breast volume (of the unoperated breast) is measured directly using the Grossman–Roudner device. By subtracting the subject's actual breast volume from the "appropriate" volume, we obtain the volume of the required prosthesis.

It is very important to take into account that the volume obtained by the formula or the chart will only give the "normal" breast volume for that particular subject. "Normal" is what Mother Nature would give that woman had she deemed to give her perfect breasts. But Mother Nature is limited by the laws of gravity and the inability of normal breast parenchyma to support tissue past a certain weight. With the use of breast implants, we can surpass this "normal" volume without impinging on the ideal shape. Therefore, in the clinical application of the formula, we have found that although the formula will give us the "normal," or the size that nature would select for a particular subject's physiognomy, our subjects almost invariably request a larger size, usually between one and two standard deviations above the volume predicted. This amounts to a volume between 25% and 50% greater than that which would be the "normal" for the subject's body build. The exact size for each patient is determined in the preoperative consultation between the patient and surgeon, in which they must reach an agreement as to the appropriate breast size. If it is determined that the patient wishes to be "average," we will use a prosthesis of a volume approximately 150% of the calculated "normal." If she wants to be "small," we will aim for a volume of about 125% of the calculated "normal." This clinical skewing of breast volume is a result of the restrictions we placed on our original study group, which was comprised only of women with aesthetically

perfect breasts. Because we excluded all "pathological" breasts from the study, all breasts with ptosis greater than grade I were not included. Thus, while the pathologically large breasts were excluded, the pathologically small breasts were not. Thus, these small breasts included in our study group skew the results and require that we factor in our clinical experience in the use of the formula.

In each woman, the breast is an organ with varied volume, width, height, projection, tissue density, composition, shape, and position on the chest wall. At the same time, the variability in the physiognomy of the trunk and limbs affects what we discern as the appropriateness of the shape and size of the breast. A large breast on a small woman, or a small breast on a large woman, would appear inappropriate, irrespective of the actual shape or size of the breast. A woman with a breast high on the chest wall would find a smaller breast more appropriate, while a woman with a low breast would need more volume. It is easy to see how this would affect our choice of goals in breast reduction or breast augmentation surgery. We must always strive to create the breast that is appropriate for the patient's body shape. Therefore, it is important to do anthropomorphic measurements on all women contemplating aesthetic breast surgery to see if we ultimately achieve our goals.

Even with the accuracy attainable with the tables and formulas presented, there is still no substitute for adequate preoperative evaluation and surgical talent, experience, and skill. Maliniac's statement (with a slight paraphrase) is as true today as it was in 1950 [2]: The surgeon's sense of sculptural form must dictate the ultimate decision as to the placement (and shape) of the breasts.

References

1. Maliniac JW: Sculpture in the Living. New York, Lancet Press 1934, p 112
2. Maliniac JW: Breast Deformities and Their Repair. New York, Grune & Stratton 1950:68–72
3. Penn J: Breast reduction. Br J Plast Surg 1955;7(4): 357–371
4. Smith DJ, Palin WE, Katch VL, Bennett JE: Breast volume and anthropomorphic measurements: normal values. Plast Reconstr Surg 1986;78(3):331–335
5. Westreich M: Anthropomorphic breast measurement: protocol and results in 50 women with aesthetically perfect breasts and clinical application. Plast Reconstr Surg 1997;100(2):468–479
6. Qiao Q, Zhou G, Ling Y: Breast volume measurement in young Chinese women and clinical applications. Aesthetic Plast Surg 1997;21(5):362–368

7. Brown TP, Ringrose C, Hyland RE, Cole AA, Brotherston TM: A method of assessing female breast morphometry and its clinical application. Br J Plast Surg 1999;52(5):355–359

8. Bostwick J: Plastic and Reconstructive Breast Surgery. St. Louis, Quality Medical Publishing 2000, p 93

9. Edsander-Nord A, Wickman M, Jurell G: Measurement of breast volume with thermoplastic casts. Scand J Plast Reconstr Surg Hand Surg 1996;30(2):129–132

10. Tepper OM, Small K, Rudolph L, Choi M, Karp N: Virtual 3-dimensional modeling as a valuable adjunct to aesthetic and reconstructive breast surgery. Am J Surg 2006;192(4):548–551

11. Garson S, Delay E, Sinna R, Carton S, Delaporte T, Chekaroua K: 3 D evaluation and breast plastic surgery: preliminary study. Ann Chir Plast Esthet 2005;50(4):296–308

12. Garson S, Delay E, Sinna R, Delaporte T, Robbe M, Carton S: 3D evaluation and mammary augmentation surgery. Ann Chir Plast Esthet 2005;50(5):643–651

13. Tanabe YN, Honda T, Nakajima Y, Sakurai H, Nozaki M: Intraoperative application of three-dimensional imaging for breast surgery. Scand J Plast Reconstr Surg Hand Surg 2005;39(6):349–352

14. Simon JR, Kalbhen CL, Cooper RA, Flisak ME: Accuracy and complication rates of US-guided vacuum-assisted core breast biopsy: initial results. Radiology 2000;215(3):694–697

15. Kovacs L, Eder M, Hollweck R, Zimmermann A, Settles M, Schneider A, Udosic K, Schwenzer-Zimmerer K, Papadopulos NA, Biemer E: New aspects of breast volume measurement using 3-dimensional surface imaging. Ann Plast Surg 2006;57(6):602–610

16. Kovacs L, Yassouridis A, Zimmermann A, Brockmann G, Wohnl A, Blaschke M, Eder M, Schwenzer-Zimmerer K, Rosenberg R, Papadopulos NA, Biemer E: Optimization of 3-dimensional imaging of the breast region with 3-dimensional laser scanners. Ann Plast Surg 2006;56(3):229–236

17. Isogai N, Sai K, Kamiishi H, Watatani M, Inui H, Shiozaki H: Quantitative analysis of the reconstructed breast using a 3-dimensional laser light scanner. Ann Plast Surg 2006;56(3):237–242

18. Losken A, Fishman I, Denson DD, Moyer HR, Carlson GW: An objective evaluation of breast symmetry and shape differences using 3-dimensional images. Ann Plast Surg 2005;55(6):571–575

19. Losken A, Seify H, Denson DD, Paredes AA Jr, Carlson GW: Validating three-dimensional imaging of the breast. Ann Plast Surg 2005;54(5):471–476; discussion 477–478

20. Hussain Z, Roberts N, Whitehouse GH, Garcia-Finana M, Percy D: Estimation of breast volume and its variation during the menstrual cycle using MRI and stereology. Br J Radiol 1999;72(855):236–245

21. Edstrom LE, Robson MC, Wright JK: A method for the evaluation of minor degrees of breast asymmetry. Plast Reconstr Surg 1977;60(5):812–814

22. Wilmore JH, Atwater AE, Maxwell BD, Wilmore DL, Constable SH, Buono MJ: Alterations in breast morphology consequent to a 21-day bust developer program. Med Sci Sports Exerc 1985;17(1):106–112

23. Daly SE, Kent JC, Huynh DQ, Owens RA, Alexander BF, Ng KC, Hartmann PE: The determination of short-term breast volume changes and the rate of synthesis of human milk using computerized breast measurement. Exper Physiol 1992;77(1):79–87

24. Lee HY, Hong K, Kim EA: Measurement protocol of women's nude breasts using a 3D scanning technique. Appl Ergon. 2004;35(4):353–359

25. Loughry CW, Sheffer DB, Price TE Jr, Lackney MJ, Bartfey RG, Morek WM: Breast volume measurement of 248 women using biostereometric analysis. Plast Reconstr Surg 1987;80(4):553–558

26. Loughry CW, Sheffer DB, Price TE, Einsporn RL, Bartfai RG, Morek WM, Meli NM: Breast volume measurement of 598 women using biostereometric analysis. Ann Plast Surg 1989;22(5):380–385

27. Sheffer DB, Price TE, Loughry CW, Bolyard BL, Morek WM, Varga RS: Validity and reliability of biostereometric measurement of the human female breast. Ann Biomed Eng 1986;14(1):1–14

28. Grossman AJ, Roudner LA: A simple means for accurate breast volume determination. Plast Reconstr Surg 1980;66(6):851–852

29. Grossman AJ, Roudner LA: Measurement of breast volume: comparison of techniques. Discussion. Plast Reconstr Surg 1986;77(2):255

30. Palin WE, von Fraunhofer JA, Smith DJ: Measurement of breast volume: comparison of techniques. Plast Reconstr Surg 1986;77(2):253–255

31. Bayati S, Seckel BR: Inframammary crease ligament. Plast Reconstr Surg 1995;95(3):501–508

32. Qiao Q: Breast volume measurement in 125 Chinese young women. Zhonghua Zheng Xing Shao Shang Wai Ke Za Zhi. 1991;7(1):1–3, 72

33. Qiao Q, Ling Y, Zhou G, Song R: Breast volume measurement in 125 young Chinese women. Chin Med Sci J. 1992;7(1):44–48

34. McGhee DE, Steele JR: How do respiratory state and measurement method affect bra size calculations? Br J Sports Med 2006;40(12):970–974

35. Turner AJ, Dujon DG: Predicting cup size after reduction mammaplasty. Br J Plast Surg 2005;58(3):290–298

36. Greenbaum AR, Heslop T, Morris J, Dunn KW: An investigation of the suitability of bra fit in women referred for reduction mammaplasty. Br J Plast Surg 2003;56(3):230–236

37. Malata CM, Boot JC, Bradbury ET, Ramli AR, Sharpe DT: Congenital breast asymmetry: subjective and objective assessment. Br J Plast Surg 1994;47(2):95–102

38. Hauben DJ, Adler N, Silfen R, Regev D: Breast-areola-nipple proportion. Ann Plast Surg 2003;50(5):510–513

39. Westreich M: Comment: a method of assessing female breast morphometry and its clinical application. Br J Plast Surg 2000;53(4):358

40. Regnault P: Breast ptosis: definition and treatment. Clin Plast Surg 1973;3:193

41. Little G, Baker JL: Results of closed compression capsulotomy for treatment of contracted breast implant capsules. Plast Reconstr Surg 1980;65(1):30–33

42. Tebbets JB: Augmentation mammoplasty; tissue assessment and planning. In: Spear S, Willey SC, Robb GL, Hammond DC (eds). Surgery of the Breast, Principle and Art, 2nd edn. Lippincott, Philadelphia, Williams & Wilkins 2005, p 1261

43. McKissock PK: McKissock mammaplasty caliper, Padgett Instruments, Instrument Bulletin, 1982

44. Beckenstein MS, Windle BH, Stroup RT: Anatomical parameters for nipple position and areolar diameter in males. Ann Plast Surg 1996;36(1):33–36

45. Hage JJ, Van Kesteren PJM: Chest-wall contouring in female-to-male transsexuals: basic considerations and review of the literature. Plast Reconstr Surg 1995;96(2):386–391

46. Broadbent TR, Mathews VL: Artistic relationships in surface anatomy of the face: application to reconstructive surgery. Plast Reconstr Surg 1957;20(1):1–17

47. Seghers MJ, Longacre JJ, De Stefano GA: The golden proportion of beauty. Plast Reconstr Surg 1964;34:382

48. Peck SR: Atlas of Human Anatomy for the Artist. Oxford, Oxford University Press 1951

49. Bostwick J: Aesthetic and Reconstructive Breast Surgery. St. Louis, Mosby 1983, pp 22–23

50. Goldwyn RM: Plastic and Reconstructive Surgery of the Breast. Boston, Lippincott, Williams & Wilkins 1976, p 196

51. Goldwyn RM: Plastic and Reconstructive Surgery of the Breast. Boston, Lippincott, Williams & Wilkins 1976, p 184

52. Ramselaar JM: Precision in breast reduction. Plast Reconstr Surg 1988;82(4):631–643

CHAPTER 4

Anatomy and Clinical Significance of the Pectoral Fascia

4

Lin Jinde

4.1
Introduction

Augmentation mammaplasties with implants are now widely performed all over the world. Using orthodox technique, the implant is usually placed in the submuscular or subglandular plane. Cronin and Gerow [1] began placing subglandular silicone gel implants in 1962. Subpectoral implantation was first reported by Dempsey and Latham in 1968 [2]. The subglandular plane usually has implant edge visibility, especially in thin women, and causes a high incidence of fibrous capsular contracture, while use of the submuscular plane can lead to implant distortion, a breast with two peaks and a relatively long recovery period. Since the initial use of implants for breast augmentation, surgeons have been looking for the proper plane for breast augmentation. Recently, Graf et al. [3] and Barbato et al. [4] have reported that the subfascial plane for breast augmentation has many advantages over the conventional plane, including rapid recovery, satisfactory breast shape, and lower fibrous capsular contracture.

4.2
Technique

Thirty side fasciae were dissected on 15 cadavers of adult females. A 3-cm transverse incision was made above the nipple, which reached the median anterior line medially, lateral to the midaxillary line and deep to the pectoralis major muscle. After the pectoral fascia was identified, it was then separated bluntly along the subglandular and subfascial planes. After successfully dissection, the thickness of the pectoral fascia at four different sites was measured with vernier calipers: The upper site was at the intersection of the midclavicular line and the 3rd rib; the lower site was at the intersection of the midclavicular line and the 5th rib; the medial site was at the intersection of the parasternal line and the 4th rib; and the lateral site was at the preaxillary line and the 4th rib. The pectoral fascia at each site was mea-

sured three times, and the average thickness of each site was considered to be the thickness of the pectoral fascia at this site.

Two other incisions were then made along the median anterior line and the midaxillary line. Nerves and vessels were dissected carefully. Another incision 2 cm below the inframammary crease and parallel to the crease was made to look for connections between the horizontal septum and the inframammary crease.

4.3
Results

The pectoral fascia was attached to the clavicle and sternum and covered the pectoralis major muscle. It was continuous inferiorly with the fascia of the abdominal wall and laterally with the fascia of the back. Numerous thin fibrous bundles from the upper pectoral fascia were found to attach to the deep layer of the superficial fascia of the breast (Fig. 4.1). At the level of the 4th intercostal space, a dense horizontal septum was found connecting the pectoral fascia and nipple. This septum extended medially and laterally to merge into the medial and lateral ligaments of the breast. Along the inframammary crease, a dense connective tissue connected the skin of the inframammary crease and the pectoral fascia (Fig. 4.2). A pocket could be made between the pectoralis major muscle and its pectoral fascia; the pectoralis major muscle remained intact, and integrity of the pectoral fascia could be preserved (Fig. 4.3).

The thicknesses of the pectoral fasciae studied varied from 0.2 mm to 1.14 mm. The average thickness was, respectively, 0.49 mm, 0.60 mm, 0.52 mm, and 0.68 mm at the upper, lower, medial, and lateral sites (Table 4.1). The direction of the pectoral fascia fibers was nearly vertical to the direction of the pectoralis major muscle fibers, from upper medial to lower lateral.

The lateral branches from the 2nd to 6th intercostal nerves passed through the serratus anterior muscle, the pectoralis major muscle, and the pectoral fascia or along the lateral edge of the pectoralis major muscle

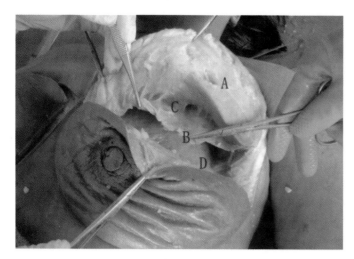

Fig. 4.1 Gland (*A*), pectoral fascia (*B*), thin fibrous bundles (*C*), pectoralis major muscle (*D*)

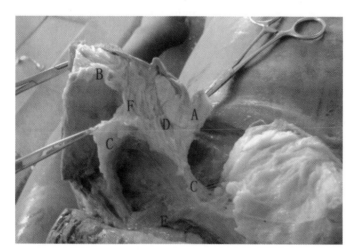

Fig. 4.2 Inframammary crease (*A*), gland (*B*), pectoral fascia (*C*), inframammary crease ligament connecting the skin of the inframammary crease and the pectoral fascia (*D*), pectoralis major muscle (*E*), horizontal fibrous septum connecting pectoral fascia and nipple (*F*)

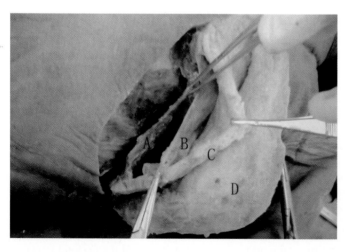

Fig. 4.3 Pectoralis major muscle (*A*), pectoral fascia (*B*), gland (*C*), skin (*D*)

into the breast. The anterior branches of the intercostal nerves emerged beside the sternum from the pectoralis major muscle and the pectoral fascia into the breast. The branches from the 3rd–5th intercostal nerves were relatively large. Perforating branches of the internal thoracic artery also emerged from the pectoralis major muscle and the pectoral fascia into the breast. Branches of the lateral thoracic artery at the 2nd–4th intercostal spaces passed through the pectoralis major and the pectoral fascia into the breast. No visible nerves or vessels were found at the upper or middle pectoral fascia. At the lower pectoral fascia, visible perforating branches of nerves and vessels emerging from the pectoral fascia into the breast were found (Fig. 4.4).

4.4
Discussion

Since the initial use of implants for breast augmentation, surgeons have been looking for the proper plane for breast augmentation. The orthodox plane of implant is the submuscular or subglandular plane. The subglandular plane usually has implant edge visibility, especially in thin women, and causes a high incidence of fibrous capsular contracture. The submuscular plane can lead to implant distortion, a breast with two peaks and a relatively long recovery period. Graf et al. [3] first reported that the subfascial plane for breast augmentation has some advantages over conventional technique, such as good breast shape and rapid recovery, and that it avoids some shortcomings such as implant edge visibility, implant distortion, a breast with two peaks and a relatively long recovery period. Furthermore, use of this plane can also provide the breast implant with

more soft tissue. The fascia originates from the clavicle and sternum. It covers the pectoralis major muscle and continues to cover the adjacent rectus abdominis, serratus anterior, and external oblique muscles. At the upper breast near the 2nd rib, the pectoral fascia tightly connects with superficial fascia of the breast and is difficult to dissect bluntly. Along the level of the 4th intercostal space, the horizontal septum originating from the pectoral fascia connects with the nipple. At the inframammary crease, a dense connective tissue is found connecting the crease skin and the pectoral fascia. Fascial thickness varies from 0.2 mm to 1.14 mm and differs at various sites. The average thickness of fascia is, respectively, 0.49 mm, 0.60 mm, 0.52 mm, and 0.68 mm in the upper, lower, medial, and lateral sites of the pectoral fascia. The lower fascia is thicker than the upper ($P1<0.05$), and the lateral fascia is thicker than the upper and medial ($P2<0.01$). The pectoral fascia is a dense connective tissue; its integrity can be preserved during dissection. Alhough the pectoral fascia is very thin, it is a dense tissue. It can provide implants with more soft tissue, just as the fascia of the dorsum nasi does for nasal implants. Before 1990 in China, nasal implants were usually placed in the subcutaneous plane for rhinoplasty. The implant could be easily pushed right and left, and it was more prone to being visible. Later, implants were inserted in the retrofascial space of the dorsum nasi. Although the fascia of the dorsum nasi is very thin, the chance of visibility of the implant edge is decreased, and the stability of the implant increases.

The direction of the pectoral fascia is vertical to the direction of the pectoralis major muscle fibers. Therefore, the pectoral fascia should be incised along its fibrous direction to preserve the integrity of the pectoral fascia during the operation. The thickness of the pec-

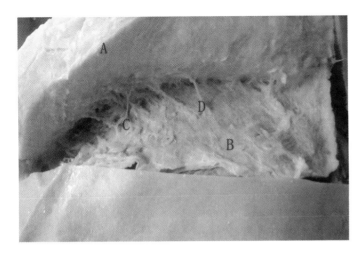

Fig. 4.4 Gland (*A*), pectoral fascia and underlying pectoralis major muscle (*B*), perforating branches of nerves and vessels passing through the pectoralis major muscle and its fascia (*C, D*)

Table 4.1 Thickness of pectoral fascia

	Upper (mm)	Lower (mm)	Medial (mm)	Lateral (mm)
1	0.38	0.29	0.45	0.72
2	0.42	0.58	0.43	0.49
3	0.21	0.30	0.34	0.48
4	0.88	0.99	0.87	0.62
5	0.53	0.72	0.49	0.82
6	0.65	0.49	0.74	0.98
7	0.46	0.67	0.41	0.53
8	0.78	0.59	0.65	0.64
9	0.40	0.50	0.39	0.62
10	0.38	0.70	0.45	0.69
11	0.78	0.82	0.56	0.93
12	0.72	0.82	1.02	1.01
13	0.48	0.41	0.29	0.60
14	0.31	0.45	0.4	0.59
15	0.42	0.59	0.80	0.65
16	0.40	0.69	0.40	0.80
17	0.35	0.57	0.64	0.87
18	0.35	0.45	0.59	0.62
19	0.51	0.66	0.42	0.91
20	0.60	0.70	0.39	0.58
21	0.25	0.38	0.22	0.40
22	0.27	0.41	0.30	0.37
23	0.30	0.56	0.30	0.52
24	0.61	0.85	0.58	0.72
25	0.20	0.24	0.45	0.35
26	0.24	0.30	0.20	0.39
27	0.91	0.84	0.64	0.80
28	0.74	0.76	0.82	1.00
29	0.62	0.85	0.70	1.14
30	0.59	0.79	0.70	0.62
Average	0.49	0.60	0.52	0.68

$P1 < 0.05$ (comparison between lower and upper)

$P2 < 0.01$ (comparison between upper and lateral and between medial and lateral)

toral fascia and the question of whether the integrity of the pectoral fascia can be preserved intraoperatively remain debated.

Tebbets [5] found that the thickness of the pectoral fascia was only 0.1–0.5 mm and that it was difficult to preserve its integrity during dissection. On the other hand, Graf et al. [3] investigated the anatomy of the pectoral fascia on a cadaver and found that the thickness of the pectoral fascia varied from 0.2 mm centrally to 1.0 mm laterally and medially and that it had more resistance than the gland or skin of the breast. The pectoral fascia could thus minimize the appearance of an implant's edges. The authors found that the integrity of the pectoral fascia could be preserved as long as the dissection was along the correct anatomic plane. At the upper and middle pectoral fascia, many thin fibers between the pectoral fascia and the deep layer of the superficial fascia of breast are found. At the level of the 5th rib is a horizontal fibrous septum that connects the nipple and pectoral fascia. The connection at this level between the pectoralis major muscle and pectoral fascia is very tight, the same as what Würinger and colleagues [6, 7] had reported. At the level of the inframammary crease, a dense connective tissue between skin and fascia is found. Controversy still exists regarding the ligament of the inframammary crease; many authors believe it was a part of Cooper's ligaments of the breast.

Yiping y et al. [8] investigated the breast with a histological technique and found that the connective tissue between the skin and pectoral fascia at the lower breast became denser than other areas and that Cooper's ligaments were represented as a membranous fibrous septum. Perhaps it was the horizontal fibrous septum, the ligament of inframammary crease, that was thought of as part of Cooper's ligaments. No visible perforating branches of nerve or vessel at the upper or middle pectoral fascia were found. But at the lower pectoral fascia, visible perforating branches of vessels and nerves emerged from the pectoralis major muscle and pectoral fascia into the breast.

Würinger and colleagues [6, 7] found that the perforating branches of vessels were from the thoracoacromial artery, branches of the lateral thoracic artery, the 4th–5th intercostal artery, and sometimes from the 6th intercostal artery. Branches of nerves were mainly from the 4th or 5th intercostal nerves [6]. These perforating branches are the main origins of bleeding or nerve injuries intraoperatively and postoperatively.

To minimize injuries of the vessels or nerves and to facilitate the surgical process, the optimal approach to the subfascial plane is a periareolar incision. An incision is made at the inferior side of the areola after the skin and subcutaneous tissue are incised, and then dissection through the subcutaneous plane around the inferior pole of the breast is performed to the inframammary crease. The inferior edge of the gland is retracted in a cranial direction to expose the pectoral fascia. After the pectoral fascia is identified, the fascia is then separated along its fibrous direction. The subfascial pocket is made by blunt dissection for breast augmentation.

4.5
Conclusions

The pectoral fascia can be dissected bluntly along the subfascial plane, keeping it intact. The potential pocket between the pectoralis major muscle and the pectoral fascia can be used as a plane for breast augmentation. The pectoral fascia may provide the breast implant with more soft tissue coverage.

References

1. Cronin T, Gerow F: Augmentation mammaplasty—a new "natural feel" prosthesis. In: Transactions of the Third International Congress of Plastic Surgeons. Amsterdam, Excerpta Medica 1964:41–49

2. Dempsey WC, Latham WD: Subpectoral implants in augmentation mammaplasty. Plast Reconstr Surg 1968;42(6):515–521

3. Graf RM, Bernardes A, Rippel R, Araujo LR, Demasio RC, Auersvald A: Subfascial breast implant: a new procedure. Plast Reconstr Surg 2003;111(2):904–908

4. Barbato C, Pena M, Triana C, Zambreno MA: Augmentation mammaplasty using the retrofascia approach. Aesth Plast Surg 2004;28(3):148–152

5. Tebbetts JB: Does fascia provide additional, meaningful coverage over a breast implant? Plast Reconstr Surg 2004;113(2):777–779; author reply 779–780

6. Würinger E, Mader N, Posch E, Holle J: Nerve and vessel supplying ligamentous suspension of the mammary gland. Plast Reconstr Surg 1998;101(6):1486–1493

7. Würinger E, Tschabitscher M: New aspects of the topographical anatomy of the mammary gland regarding its neurovascular supply along a regular ligamentous suspension. Eur J Morphol 2002;40(3):181–189

8. Yiping Y, Ji J, Senkai L, Dongming T: Re-assessment of the inframammary crease ligament. Zhong Hua Zheng Xing Shao Shang Wai Ke Za Zhi 1999;15(5):345–347

CHAPTER 5

The Inframammary Crease

5

Brooke R. Seckel, Shawkat A. Sati, W. Thomas McClellan

5.1
Introduction

The inframammary crease or fold is an essential landmark for an optimal result in aesthetic and reconstructive breast surgery. A well-defined inframammary crease and an appropriate areola to inframammary crease distance is arguably the most important component of a pleasing and aesthetically correct breast appearance following breast augmentation, reduction mammaplasty, and postmastectomy breast reconstruction.

Failure to preserve the inframammary crease during breast augmentation surgery creates an unacceptably abnormal breast profile often referred to as a "double-bubble" appearance or "Snoopy deformity," which patients find very disturbing (Fig. 5.1). Failure to create a well-defined inframammary crease symmetrical with the opposite breast is one of the most common problems following postmastectomy breast reconstruction, especially following the use of soft tissue expanders.

The anatomy of the inframammary crease has been the subject of significant debate in the plastic surgery literature. In 1845, Cooper [1] stated that "at the abdominal margin, the gland is turned upon itself at its edge, and forms a kind of hem." Since that time, many authors have attempted to define the structure and anatomy of this area in an effort to simplify its reconstruction. This chapter will present the findings of cadaver dissections [2] and relate the authors' clinical approach to reconstruction of the inframammary crease.

5.2
Anatomy

The inframammary fold is undetectable in the prepubescent breast; however, with the onset of puberty it comes to define the inferior aspect of the female breast. The crease is sited at the 5th rib medially, and its lowest potion reaches the 6th intercostal space (Fig. 5.2). The average distance from the inferior margin of the areola ranges from 5 cm to 9 cm. The presence of a true ligament at the fold is still the subject of many debates.

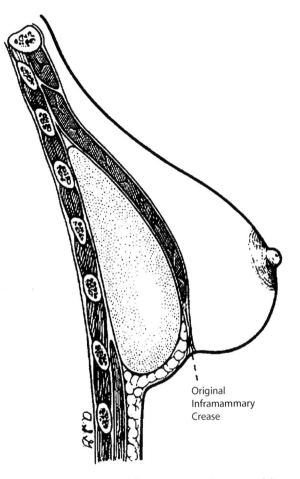

Original
Inframammary
Crease

Fig. 5.1 "Double-bubble" deformity. During the course of dissection of the subpectoral musculofascial pocket for prosthesis insertion, the ligament can be disrupted if the dissection is carried out too inferiorly. This will lead to inferior migration of the prosthesis and the double-bubble deformity. (Reproduced with permission from Bayati and Seckel [2])

According to Bayati and Seckel [2], there is a ligament that originates from the 5th rib's periosteum medially, from the fascia between the 5th and 6th ribs laterally, and inserts into the deep dermis of the submammary fold (Fig. 5.3). They believed it was a condensation of the rectus abdominis fascia medially and the fascia of the serratus anterior and external oblique laterally. Their study revealed a difference between

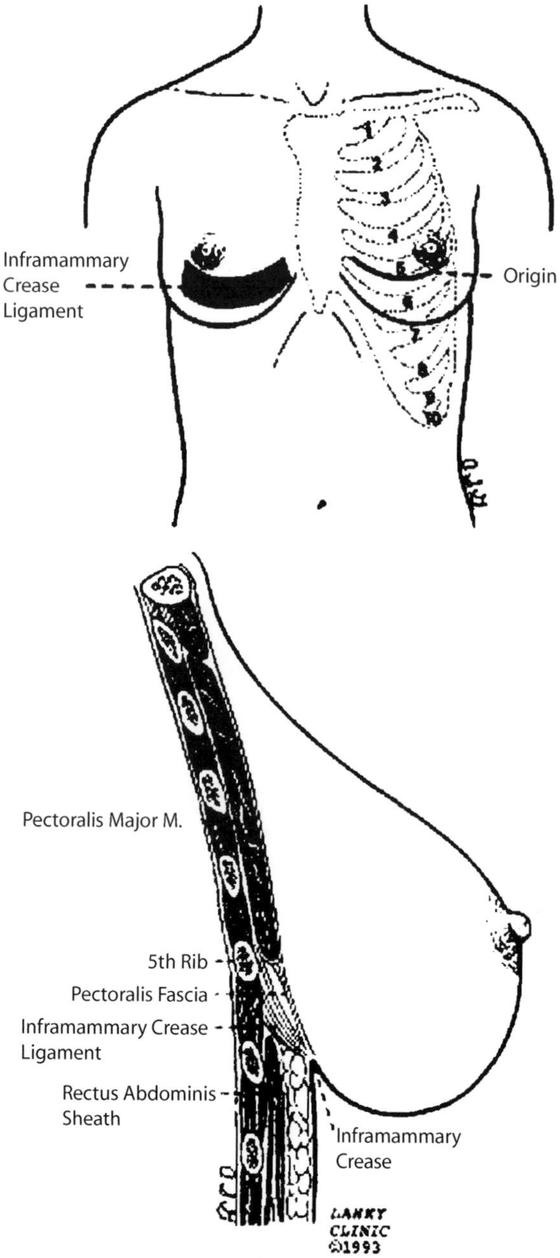

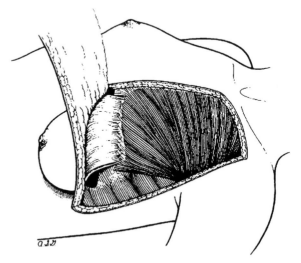

Fig. 5.2 The horizontal position of the inframammary ligament originating from the 5th rib periosteum medially and extending to the 5th–6th intercostal space laterally. The inframammary ligament originates from the 5th rib and inserts into the deep dermis of the skin. (Reproduced with permission from Bayati and Seckel [2])

Cooper's suspensory ligaments and the inframammary ligament. These authors emphasized that the presence of the double-bubble phenomenon is produced by the disruption of this ligament.

Maillard and Garey [3] had described a crescent-shaped ligament between the skin and the anterior surface of the pectoralis major, which is slightly lower than the anatomy described by Seckel. Van Straalen et al. [4] described a similar ligament found in the breasts of female-to-male transsexuals.

Nava et al. [5] disagreed, stating that the crease is devoid of a true ligament and instead has the usual two subcutaneous layers and one superficial fascia. This fascia deepens and the anterior breast envelope detaches, creating this fold. Garnier et al. [6] concluded that a subcutaneous inframammary ligament does not exist. Lockwood [7] described this superficial fascial system as a subdermal structure consisting of interwoven collagen fibers that support the skin by adhering to the underlying fascial layers. Boutros et al. [8] suggested that it is a dermal structure consisting of a collagen network arranged in arrays that run parallel to the skin surface along the long axis of the inframammary fold and that it is held in place by the condensation of the superficial fascial system.

Muntan et al. [9] did not demonstrate the presence of a ligament; they stated that the superficial fascia was connected to the dermis in the fold region in a variety of configurations. Lack of definition in this crease could

Fig. 5.3 The inframammary ligament extends to insert deep into the deep dermis of the inframammary skin fold. (Reproduced with permission from Bayati and Seckel [2])

be from breast hypoplasia or mastopathy or could be iatrogenic.

The male breast has neither a superficial layer of the fascia superficialis nor an inframammary ligamentous structure.

5.3
Reconstruction of the Inframammary Fold

5.3.1
History

In breast reconstruction, the inframammary fold is one of the most difficult anatomic structures to recreate. Nonetheless, it is a crucial element in achieving the optimal aesthetic outcome.

During mastectomy the inframammary crease should be preserved and, when possible, not be disturbed. Several studies have been done on the contents of the inframammary crease. Gui et al. [10] found that 28% of their inframammary fold specimens contained breast tissue and lymph nodes. However, Carlson et al. [11] confirmed that inframammary fold preservation is safe because it leaves less than 0.02% of the total breast tissue and hence does not appreciably affect the completeness of a mastectomy, as long as the patients are closely followed. However, the inframammary fold frequently needs to be violated during transverse rectus abdominis myocutaneous (TRAM) procedures to avoid compressing the pedicle.

In 1977, Pennisi [12] described a reliable external procedure that consisted of marking the lower thoracic skin, creating a dermal-fatty-superficial fascial flap, and turning up the flap and anchoring it to the muscular fascia. Ryan [13] added to that concept by fixing the flap to the periosteum. Bostwick [14] described an inframammary fold elevation technique through a short horizontal external approach, with the lower thoracic flap hypodermis sutured to the posterior capsule and deeper tissues. The procedure avoided an external scar and gave better definition than in previous repairs, but it had little projection and ptosis improvement.

Versaci [15] described a technique using an internal approach at the time of expander removal. An incision was made in the posterior capsule at the presumed position of the new fold. The lower third of the posterior capsule was detached. The undermined abdominal flap became the undersurface of the new breast, and the skin flap was secured to the periosteum. The disadvantages of this technique were a bulky inframammary region and an inframammary fold that appeared too deep. Pinella [16] described liposuctioning the lower thoracic bulkiness.

Nava et al. [5] described an internal approach in which the implant is removed through the previous mastectomy incision. The desired inframammary fold line is transposed by transfixing needles into the pocket. The superficial fascia is located and cut along the whole inframammary line, and a running stitch is used to secure the new fold. More recently, Chun and Pribaz [17] described a technique using a Steinmann pin to match the symmetry of the contralateral normal breast. The pin is introduced from lateral to medial underneath the skin so that it remains in the cavity. Permanent sutures are placed throughout the entire length of the pin. An external bolster is applied, and the pin is removed.

The authors have developed an "internal thoracic advancement flap" method that allows the surgeon to avoid the external scar of the original external procedure described by Pennisi [12] and Ryan [13].

5.3.2
Authors' Approach

5.3.2.1
The Internal Thoracic Advancement Flap

The most common and distressing disadvantages of previous techniques for reconstruction of the inframammary crease are the following:

1. Inferior migration of the reconstructed fold with flattening and loss of the fold and loss of the inferior pole of the reconstructed breast
2. A visible external scar, which is particularly unsatisfactory when deepithelialization has been performed as in the Ryan [13] and Pennisi [12] techniques and the deepithelialized skin migrates down beneath the fold into a visible location

The authors use a technique similar to that of Versaci [15] that utilizes an internal approach. However, we undermine and advance an inferior thoracoabdominal flap superiorly. The deep dermis of the undersurface of the flap is sutured to the periosteum of the ribs and intercostal fascia along the predetermined inframammary crease insertion point on the 5th rib and the 5th–6th intercostal space.

This technique may be applied during primary reconstruction, following the removal of a soft tissue expander, and in cases of breast augmentation in which "bottoming out" has occurred.

The anatomic location of the proposed inframammary crease is marked on the internal chest wall by using the Bovie cautery to coagulate a line along the appropriate landmarks outlined above (Fig. 5.2). The amount of skin that must be recruited to provide an adequate inferior pole of the breast is estimated. Dissection is carried out inferiorly below the 5th and 6th ribs, through the inferior capsule (in the case of a soft tissue expander or breast implant), or beneath the inferior mastectomy flap (in the case of a primary postmastectomy reconstruction). A crescent-shaped inferior thoracoabdominal flap is elevated down to a level 8–10 cm below the inferior skin edge of the mastectomy flap or the expander or implant pocket (Fig. 5.4).

With the operating room table flexed as for an abdominoplasty, the inferior thoracoabdominal skin flap is advanced superiorly. Size 0 Prolene buried sutures are placed into the undersurface of the deep dermis of the skin flap at a point 3–4 cm below the superior edge of the flap to allow for the advancement of sufficient skin superiorly to create an inferior pole of the new breast. The new inframammary crease is then sutured to the periosteum of the 5th and 6th ribs and the intervening intercostal fascia. Usually 8–10 sutures are required (Fig. 5.4).

This maneuver typically provides a significant amount of tissue to provide an adequate "inferior pole" to the reconstructed breast profile. In the case of a breast augmentation that has "bottomed out," the thoracoabdominal flap is not created or advanced. Instead, the inferior pocket capsule is opened, a 3-cm strip of capsule is resected, and the excess inferior pole breast skin is advanced internally with a running size 0 Prolene suture

to the periosteum and intercostal fascia along the landmarks of the inframammary crease.

5.3.2.2
Complications

Complications of this procedure are the same as those with any breast implant procedure. These include extrusion, capsular contraction, asymmetry, failure to achieve an adequate inferior pole of the breast, bleeding, infection, and scarring. The additional potential complication is a failure of the suspension sutures or long-term inferior migration of the flap and resultant loss of the fold. Inferior migration of the implant is another potential risk; however, in contrast to the procedures using an external approach with deepithelialization, the authors have not seen the latter event. When using this technique, there is less flattening and loss of fold compared with other methods of repair.

5.4
Discussion

The inframammary crease, an adequate inferior pole of the breast, an appropriate nipple position, and an appropriate areola-to-inframammary crease distance are

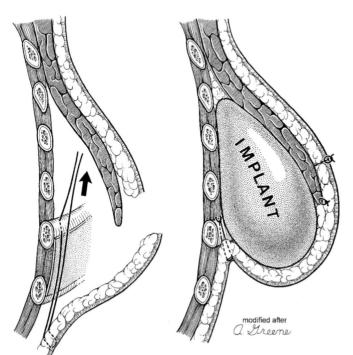

modified after
a. Greene

Fig. 5.4 Surgical technique: internal thoracic advancement flap

the essential components of an aesthetically appropriate breast appearance.

Failure to preserve or reconstruct the inframammary crease following breast reconstruction or in cosmetic breast augmentation causes one of the most unsatisfactory and distressing complications in aesthetic and reconstructive breast surgery.

The authors' opinion is that a crease ligament or other condensation of Scarpa's fascia and the posterior capsule of the breast constitutes a well-defined anatomic landmark that can be reconstructed. Reconstruction of this anatomic structure in the proper location can restore an appropriate and aesthetically acceptable inframammary crease both in postmastectomy breast reconstruction and in cosmetic breast augmentation when "bottoming out" or the "double bubble" has occurred.

References

1. Cooper AP: On the Anatomy of the Breast. London, Longmans 1845:10

2. Bayati S, Seckel BR: Inframammary crease ligament. Plast Reconstr Surg 1995;95(3):501–508

3. Maillard GF, Garey LJ: An improved technique for immediate retropectoral reconstruction after subcutaneous mastectomy. Plast Reconstr Surg 1987;80(3):396–408

4. van Straalen WR, Hage JJ, Bloemena E: The inframammary ligament: myth or reality? Ann Plast Surg 1995;35(2):237–241

5. Nava M, Quattrone P, Riggio E: Focus on the breast fascial system: a new approach for the inframammary fold reconstruction. Plast Reconstr Surg 1998;102(4):1034–1045

6. Garnier D, Angonin R, Foulon R, Chavoin JP, Ricbourg, B, Costagliola M: Le sillon sous-mammaire: mythe ou realite? Ann Chir Plast Esthet 1991;36(4):313–319

7. Lockwood TE: Superficial fascial system (SFS) of the trunk and extremities: a new concept. Plast Reconstr Surg 1991;87(6):1009–1018

8. Boutros S, Kattash M, Wienfeld A, Yuksel E, Baer S, Shenaq S: The intradermal anatomy of the inframammary fold. Plast Reconstr Surg 1998;102(4):1030–1033

9. Muntan CD, Sundine MJ, Rink RD, Acland RD: Inframammary fold: a histologic reappraisal. Plast Reconstr Surg 2000;105(2):549–556

10. Gui GP, Behranwala KA, Abdullah N, Seet J, Osin P, Nerurkar A, Lakhani SR: The inframammary fold: contents, clinical significance and implications for immediate breast reconstruction. Brit J Plast Surg 2004;57(2):146–149

11. Carlson GW, Grossl N, Lewis MM, Temple JR, Styblo TM: Preservation of the inframammary fold: what are we leaving behind? Plast Reconstr Surg 1996;98(3):447–450

12. Pennisi VR: Making a definite inframammary fold under a reconstructed breast. Plast Reconstr Surg 1977;60(4):523–525

13. Ryan JJ: A lower thoracic advancement flap in breast reconstruction after mastectomy. Plast Reconstr Surg 1982;70(2):153–160

14. Bostwick J III: Finishing Touches. Plastic and Reconstructive Breast Surgery. St. Louis, Quality Medical Publishing 1990, p 1126

15. Versaci AD: A method of reconstructing a pendulous breast utilizing the soft tissue expander. Plast Reconstr Surg 1987;80(3):387–395

16. Pinella JW: Creating an inframammary crease with a liposuction cannula (letter). Plast Reconstr Surg 1989;83(5):925

17. Chun YS, Pribaz JJ: A simple guide to inframammary-fold reconstruction. Ann Plast Surg 2005;55(1):8–11

CHAPTER 6

Breast Asymmetries: A Working Formulation

Gianpiero Gravante, Antonino Araco, Valerio Cervelli

6

6.1
Introduction

The first article regarding mammary asymmetry dates back to 1968 [1]. In the beginning of aesthetic surgery, this entity was named "Amazon's syndrome" and included only cases of unilateral amastia or hypoplasia of the breast [2, 3]. Edstrom et al. [4] were the first authors to recognize that different heterogeneous alterations were included under this definition and that "breast asymmetries," and not "breast asymmetry," would probably have been the correct way to describe them. These alterations of the breast consisted of asymmetries in the shape, volume, and position of the breasts and/or of the nipple–areola complex, and the term "Amazon's syndrome" soon appeared insufficient.

In the 1980s, surgeons felt the urgent need for classifications that could help in treatment planning and data sharing. The first introduced were based mainly on etiologic factors [5–8] and were not focused on breast appearance or on the type of operation needed. A "working formulation," useful because it is simple and practical for the aesthetic surgeon, was required and was introduced in 2006 [9].

6.2
Materials and Methods

The authors recorded all breast asymmetries operated in their practice. Inclusion criteria consisted of all women with primary breast asymmetry; exclusion criteria included incomplete breast growth due to prepubertal and pubertal age (less than 18–19 years old; preoperative physical examination), secondary asymmetries due to cancer or other benign pathologies that could change breast morphology (such as fibroadenomas), and previous breast surgery.

Based on our experience, we classified asymmetries of the breasts into six categories (Table 6.1). The first three groups represented hypertrophy-related breast asymmetry: Asymmetric hypertrophy of both breasts comprised group I (Fig. 6.1), hypertrophy with a normal contralateral breast comprised group II (Fig. 6.2), and hypertrophy with a hypoplastic contralateral breast comprised group III (Fig. 6.3). Two other groups represented hypoplastic-related breast asymmetry: Such asymmetry with a normal contralateral breast made up group IV (Fig. 6.4), and that with a hypoplastic contralateral breast made up group V (Fig. 6.5). The

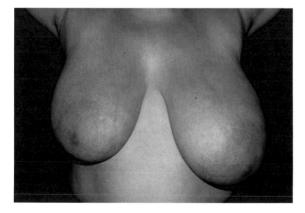

Fig 6.1 Group I

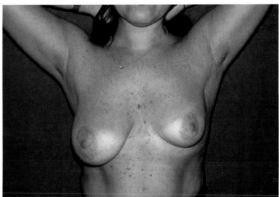

Fig 6.2 Group II

last group, group VI, included ptosis-related asymmetry (Fig. 6.6).

Bilateral asymmetric hypertrophy (group I) and unilateral hypertrophy with a normal contralateral breast (group II) were treated with reduction mammaplasty [10, 11] on the affected breasts (bilaterally for group I and only on the affected side for group II). Unilateral hypertrophy with amastia or hypoplasia of the contralateral side (group III) was treated with reductive mammaplasty on the hypertrophic breast and augmentation mammaplasty on the hypoplastic side. Unilat-

eral amastia or hypoplasia with a normal contralateral breast (group IV) included patients with Poland syndrome and was treated with muscular flap techniques (monopedicle TRAM flap). Asymmetric bilateral hypoplasia (group V) was treated with augmentation mammaplasty. Unilateral mammary ptosis (group VI) was treated with mastopexy and augmentation mammaplasty (Table 6.1).

Follow-up consisted of postoperative outpatient visits at 1 week, 6 months, and 1 year after the operation to control the aesthetic results.

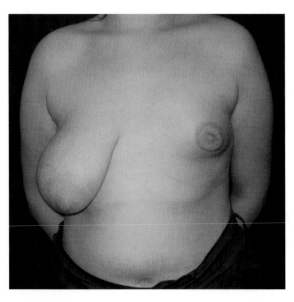

Fig 6.3 Group III

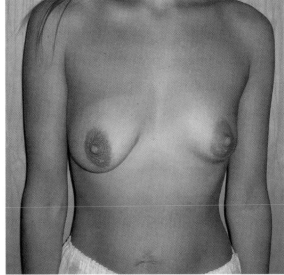

Fig 6.4 Group IV

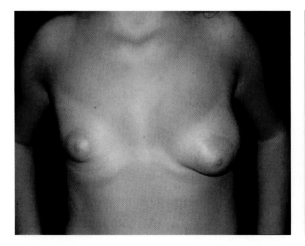

Fig 6.5 Group V

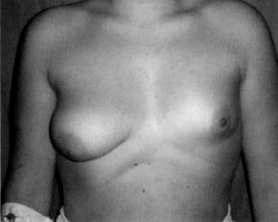

Fig 6.6 Group VI

Table 6.1 Morphological classification of mammary asymmetries and suggested treatments

Group	Description	Suggested treatment	Figures
I	Bilateral asymmetrical hypertrophy	Reduction mammaplasty	Fig. 6.1
II	Unilateral hypertrophy with normal contralateral breast	Reduction mammaplasty	Fig. 6.2
III	Unilateral hypertrophy with amastia or hypoplasia of the contralateral side	Reduction mammaplasty on the hypertrophic breast and augmentation mammaplasty on the hypoplastic breast	Fig. 6.3
IV	Unilateral amastia or hypoplasia with normal contralateral breast	Muscular flap techniques	Fig. 6.4
V	Asymmetric bilateral hypoplasia	Augmentation mammaplasty	Fig. 6.5
VI	Unilateral mammary ptosis	Mastopexy and augmentation mammaplasty	Fig. 6.6

6.3 Results

From January 1998 to January 2007, the authors observed 500 women referred for breast asymmetries. Fifty patients were excluded from this study because their breasts had not completed their growth (prepubertal). Thirty patients were excluded because an undiagnosed cancer was the cause of mammary asymmetry, and 243 patients were excluded because of previous breast surgery. We therefore recorded 177 patients for this study. No patient was lost to follow-up.

The patient age varied from 18 to 65 years (average 32 years). All patients were female. There were 30 patients in group I, 15 patients in group II, 10 patients in group III, five patients in group IV, 81 patients in group V, and 36 patients in group VI (Table 6.2). For patients in groups I and II, treated with reduction mammaplasty, reduction and perfect breast symmetry was achieved by removing more mammary parenchyma from the bulky breast. Patients in group III, treated with reduction mammaplasty on the hypertrophic breast and augmentation mammaplasty on the hypoplastic contralateral breast, achieved good results because of preparatory planning of the positioning and size of the prostheses to be inserted; a subglandular approach was preferred for mild hypoplasia and a retropectoral approach for severe hypoplasia. For group IV, the five patients with Poland syndrome, a monopedicle TRAM flap operation was used. Patients in group V were treated with the simple insertion of prostheses. Patients in group VI were treated with a mastopexy operation combined with the addition of prostheses to solve both the ptosis and the hypoplasia of the affected side. In this group, 14 patients also had a hypoplastic contralateral breast that was treated with a prosthetic insertion.

6.4 Discussion

Breast asymmetry refers to an asymmetric morphology of the shape, volume, and position of the breasts and/or of the nipple–areola complex. Since 1968 the real prevalence of this entity has not been precisely assessed, and it is has been stated that 5.2% of aesthetic breast operations are routinely performed to correct breast asymmetries [12]. Other authors believe that over half of the female population would be affected if screened for small deformities [13].

Causes are varied and can be roughly classified into congenital and acquired [5–8]. Among the congenital causes, Poland syndrome is one of the most important. This rare entity (1:30,000 cases per year) is probably due to an intrauterine vascular malformation that produces an ipsilateral breast and nipple hypoplasia and/or aplasia, a deficiency of subcutaneous fat and axillary hair, an absence of the sternal head of the pectoralis major, hypoplasia of the rib cage, and hypoplasia of the upper extremity to different degrees. The latissimus dorsi or the deltoid muscles are sometimes involved [14–22].

Apart from congenital causes, breast surgery is the first leading cause of acquired breast asymmetry. Every type of breast operation, whether performed for therapeutic or aesthetic reasons, can cause breast asymmetry to variable degrees. In some of these operations, asymmetry is a necessary consequence (such as lumpectomy for cancer) [23], whereas in others (such as reduction or

Table 6.2 Postoperative complications during follow-up (1 year)

Group	Number of patients	Prolonged pain	Hematomas	Seromas	Secondary cysts	Infections	Necrosis	Capsular contracture	Hypertrophic scars	Prosthesis substitution
I	30	1	2	—	—	—	—	—	—	—
II	15	—	—	—	—	—	—	—	2	—
III	10	1	—	—	—	1	—	—	—	—
IV	5	1	—	—	—	1	—	1	—	—
V	81	—	1	3	—	—	—	2	—	1
VI	36	—	1	—	—	—	—	1	—	1
Total	177	3	4	3	—	2	—	4	2	2

augmentation mammaplasty) it is an undesired complication leading to an additional surgical step to correct the defect [24]. Other reported causes include prepubertal trauma to the breast bud [25, 26].

Although etiology has been useful for introducing the heterogeneity of this condition and for providing initial classification criteria, the authors believe that it is not as helpful in treatment planning as morphology is. In fact, even if similar morphological defects have different causes, they require similar operations. For this reason, a morphological "working" classification was introduced in 2006. This described six different types of alterations based on breast appearance (Table 6.1). The first three groups define hypertrophic-related breast asymmetry: hypertrophy of one breast with asymmetry of the contralateral hypertrophic breast (group I), hypertrophy with a normal contralateral breast (group II), or hypertrophy with a hypoplastic contralateral breast (group III). Two other groups define hypoplastic-related breast asymmetry: with a normal contralateral breast (group IV) or with a hypoplastic contralateral breast (group V). The last group defines ptosis-related asymmetry (group VI).

Each group, once correctly classified, was treated with a specific operation. Bilateral asymmetrical hypertrophy (group I) was treated with a reduction mammaplasty [11]. Unilateral hypertrophy with a normal contralateral breast (group II) was treated with reductive mammaplasty only on the hypertrophic breast. Unilateral hypertrophy with amastia or hypoplasia of the contralateral side (group III) was treated with reductive mammaplasty on the hypertrophic breast and augmentation mammaplasty in the hypoplastic side. Unilateral amastia or hypoplasia with a normal contralateral breast (group IV) consisted of five patients with Poland syndrome; these patients were treated with muscular flap techniques (monopedicle TRAM flap). Asymmetric bilateral hypoplasia (group V) was treated with augmentation mammaplasty. Modest hypoplasia was treated with subglandular positioning of the prostheses; severe hypoplasia was treated with an expander device under major pectoral muscle [12, 22, 26]. Unilateral mammary ptosis (group VI) was treated with mastopexy combined with an augmentation mammaplasty.

This classification did not introduce new surgical techniques but helped the surgeons to correctly ascribe patients to each group and to find the consequent operation. Obviously, it did not substitute clinical judgment, but it helped the decision-making process and served as the beginning of a standardized and scientific approach to breast asymmetries. Good aesthetic results were achieved with the planned operations. Most of the time, one surgical step was enough to achieve the final planned breast volume and shape, and only patients affected by Poland syndrome required more procedures to correct this severe defect. Complication rates were, both for frequency and severity, similar to those in the literature for standard augmentation or reduction mammaplasty or mastopexy. Only a few cases of periprosthetic fibrosis and capsular contraction occurred after 1 year of follow-up, two of which required surgical substitutions (Table 6.2).

6.5 Conclusions

Aesthetic breast surgery has improved in the last 20 years with the introduction of new and different techniques, often used in combination. Many different procedures are now available to correct an asymmetric breast: reduction mammaplasty in cases of mammary hypertrophy; augmentation mammaplasty using prostheses for mammary hypoplasia; muscular and musculocutaneous flaps, free or with pedicles; and association of mastopexy and prosthesis in cases of asymmetry due to mammary hypoplasia and ptosis. Based on the authors' experience, the morphological working classification of breast asymmetries is useful to guide aesthetic surgeons in the choice of surgical approach. However, it could also be more useful to researchers to begin a worldwide standardized approach to this matter for data sharing and scientific debates.

References

1. Hueston JT: Surgical correction of breast asymmetry. Aust N Z J Surg 1968;38(2):112–116
2. Radlauer CB, Bowers DG Jr: Treatment of severe breast asymmetry. Plast Reconstr Surg 1971;47(4):347–350
3. Fischl RA, Rosenberg I, Simon BE: Planning unilateral breast reduction for asymmetry. Br J Plast Surg 1971;24(4):402–404
4. Edstrom LE, Robson MC, Wright JK: A method for the evaluation of minor degrees of breast asymmetry. Plast Reconstr Surg 1977;60(5):812–814
5. Beer GM, Kompatscher P, Hergan K: Poland's syndrome and vascular malformations. Br J Plast Surg 1996;49(7):482–484
6. Giacalone PL, Bricout N, Dantas MJ, Daures JP, Laffargue F: Achieving symmetry in unilateral breast reconstruction: 17 years experience with 683 patients. Aesthetic Plast Surg 2002;26(4):299–302
7. Elliot RA Jr, Hoehn JG, Greminger RF: Correction of asymmetrical breasts. Plast Reconstr Surg 1975;56(3):260–265
8. Vandenbussche F: Asymmetries of the breast: a classification system. Aesthet Plast Surg 1984;8(1):27–36
9. Araco A, Gravante G, Araco F, Gentile P, Castri F, Deogu D, Filingen V, Cervellio V: Breast asymmetries: a brief review and our experience. Aesthet Plast Surg. 2006;30(3):309–319
10. Planas J, Mosely LH: Improving breast shape and symmetry in reduction mammaplasty. Ann Plast Surg 1980;4(4):297–303
11. Gliosci A, Presutti F: Asymmetry of the breast: some uncommon cases. Aesthet Plast Surg 1994;18(4):399–403
12. Onesti MG, Mezzana P, Martano A, Scuden M: Breast asymmetry: a new vision of this malformation. Acta Chir Plast 2004;46(1):8–11
13. Rintala AE, Nordstrom RE: Treatment of severe developmental asymmetry of the female breast. Scand J Plast Reconstr Surg Hand Surg 1989;23(3):231–235
14. Marconi F, Gallucci A, Marra M, Pistorale T, Siden M: Idiopathic unilateral hypoplasia of the breast. Minerva Chir 1994;49(10):971–975
15. Trier WC: Complete breast absence. Plast Reconstr Surg 1965;36(4):431–439
16. Martin B, Emory RE: Symptomatic macromastia in a patient with Poland syndrome. Plast Reconstr Surg 2000;106(1):221–222
17. Tvdek M, Kletensky J, Svoboda S: Aplasia of the breast reconstruction using a free TRAM flap. Acta Chir Plast 2001;43(2):39–41
18. Beer GM, Kompatscher P, Hergan K: Poland's syndrome and vascular malformations. Br J Plast Surg 1996;49(7):482–484
19. Rohrich RJ, Hartley W, Brown S: Incidence of breast and chest wall asymmetry in breast augmentation: a retrospective analysis of 100 patients. Plast Reconstr Surg 2003;111(4):1513–1519
20. Hoffman S: Recurrent deformities following reduction mammaplasty and correction of breast asymmetry. Plast Reconstr Surg 1986;78(1):55–62
21. Smith DJ Jr, Palin WE Jr, Katch V, Bennett JE: Surgical treatment of congenital breast asymmetry. Ann Plast Surg 1986;17(2):92–101
22. Clough KB, O'Donoghue JM, Fitoussi AD, Nos C, Falcou MC: Prospective evaluation of late cosmetic results following breast reconstruction. I. Implant reconstruction. Plast Reconstr Surg 2001;107(7):1702–1709
23. Steele SR, Martin MJ, Place RJ: Gynecomastia: complications of the subcutaneous mastectomy. Am Surg. 2002;68(2):210–213
24. Goyal A, Mansel RE: Iatrogenic injury to the breast bud causing breast hypoplasia. Postgrad Med J 2003;79(930):235–236
25. Jansen DA, Spencer Stoetzel R, Leveque JE: Premenarchal athletic injury to the breast bud as the cause for asymmetry: prevention and treatment. Breast J 2002;8(2):108–111
26. Sadove AM, van Aalst JA: Congenital and acquired pediatric breast anomalies: a review of 20 years' experience. Plast Reconstr Surg 2005;115(4):1039–1050

CHAPTER 7

Benign Disorders of the Breast

7

Melvin A. Shiffman

7.1
Introduction

There are many benign disorders of the breast that may be encountered when performing breast augmentation. If mammography is performed prior to the surgery, some of these abnormalities may become apparent. Others may be diagnosed following a proper physical examination.

7.2
History

Prior to any cosmetic breast surgery it is essential that a thorough history of prior breast problems (lump, nipple discharge, nipple inversion, breast rash, breast surgery) and a family history of breast cancer and ovarian cancer be obtained. If there is a significant family history of breast and/or ovarian cancer in first-degree relatives, counseling should be considered because of the possible risk of hereditary breast cancer.

7.3
Physical Examination

There should be at least a complete examination of the breasts. This requires examining the breasts with the patient in a sitting position and in a supine position with arms overhead (which flattens the breasts against the chest wall). Observation includes evaluating the nipple and areola for abnormalities (inversion, rash, tumor), asymmetry, accessory nipples and areolas, erythema, and nevi. Each quadrant of both breasts should be examined carefully for any problem such as tumor, tenderness, or thickness (induration).

7.4
Mammography

Mammography should be performed at least on every patient 40 years and older if it was not already done within the prior 6 months. The author orders mammography for every patient, no matter the age, prior to elective breast surgery. Any abnormality found on mammography should be thoroughly investigated before surgery.

7.5
Benign Disorders

7.5.1
Rash

Dermatitis of the breast area can occur from allergic reactions to lotions, soaps, or perfume. Inflammation can occur from breastfeeding or from a partner who becomes too vigorous in attempts to stimulate the nipple. Treatment consists of steroid creams, and the rash should be resolved before surgery is performed.

A rash involving the nipple–areolar complex may be Paget's disease. If it is treated as dermatitis and does not respond quickly and completely to steroid treatment, then a biopsy needs to be performed. If the rash is associated with a breast lump, breast cancer must be considered. Paget's disease is almost always associated with an underlying breast cancer, whether palpable or not.

7.5.2
Nipple Discharge

A nipple discharge is not uncommon following pregnancy and may persist for 6 months after breastfeeding. Elective breast surgery should not be performed until at least 3 months after breastfeeding and after the milky discharge has subsided.

A clear discharge is most commonly benign and is usually noticed if the nipple is squeezed. A bloody discharge can be from ductal papilloma or papillomatosis and may have to be excised. This may require a ductogram to identify the problem duct system. Breast cancer can also result in a bloody discharge but is usually diagnosable on mammography. The author has encountered bloody discharge in a patient whose partners vigorously sucked on the nipples to stimulate the individual.

7.5.3
Mass

A breast mass may be from fibrocystic disorder, fibroadenoma, or cancer. Mammography, sonography, and/or magnification compression views can usually make the distinction, but biopsy may be necessary.

In a young patient under age 35, a well-defined, ballottable (squeezing the mass causes the mass to squirt out from the fingers and fall back to hit the fingers) mass is usually fibroadenoma. An apparent fibroadenoma on mammography in a patient over the age of 35 or one that is increasing in size in a patient under the age of 35 will need at least a large-core needle biopsy (preferably excision) to rule out cancer. Giant adenoma of the breast has been reported. Cystosarcoma phyllodes may appear on pathology to be a fibroadenoma, but it is a fast-growing tumor that frequently recurs if not adequately excised. There have been reports of malignant cystosarcoma phyllodes that have metastasized [2].

A nodular lesion of the nipple can be an adenoma or adenomatosis and may require biopsy or excision [3, 4].

7.5.4
Calcifications

Calcifications are usually observed on mammography. Magnification views may be necessary to define the type of calcification(s). Benign punctate round calcifications can occur in the breast at any age and are usually the result of a fibrocystic disorder. Stippled grouped calcifications may indicate cancer. If the calcifications are round on the craniocaudal view and teacup-shaped on the medial lateral oblique view, then they are considered benign. Other types of calcifications may require stereotactic needle biopsy to define the pathology. Diffuse calcifications of one or both breasts are usually from benign fibrocystic disorder.

Extensive ossification of the breast has been reported. This is a benign disorder associated with nonspecific chronic mastitis that appears as dense flakes of calcifications [5].

7.5.5
Cowden's Disease

Cowden's disease consists of facial trichilemmomas (benign tumors of the follicular epithelium), acral keratoses on the limbs, and oral mucosal papillomas and fibromas. This is a hereditary disorder with a high risk of breast cancer [6].

7.5.6
Weber–Christian Syndrome

Weber–Christian syndrome consists of relapsing non-suppurative nodular panniculitis. The disorder consists of crops of subcutaneous nodules of unknown etiology that are frequently tender and red and regress spontaneously with residual indentation of the overlying skin. This has been reported in the breast [7].

7.6
Discussion

It is up to the surgeon performing an elective procedure to make sure that a significant problem, such as cancer, is not present in the breast. Even benign disorders may need biopsy or excision prior to or during cosmetic breast surgery.

References

1. Block GE, Zlatnik PA: Giant fibroadenoma of the breast in a prepubertal girl: a case report with observations of hormonal influences. Arch Surg 1960;80:665–669
2. Rowell MD, Perry, RR, Jeng-Gwang H: Phyllodes tumors. Am J Surg 1993;165:376–379
3. Rawling Pratt-Thomas H: Erosive adenomatosis of the nipple. J South Carolina Med Assoc 1968;64:37049
4. Goldman RL, Cooperman H: Adenoma of the nipple: a benign lesion simulating carcinoma clinically and pathologically. Am J Surg 1970;119(3):322–325
5. France CJ, O'Connell JP: Osseous metaplasia in the human mammary gland. Arch Surg 1970;100:238–239
6. Brownstein MH, Wolf M, Bikowski JB: Cowden's disease: a cutaneous marker of breast cancer. Cancer 1978;44:2393–2398
7. Kaufman PA: Relapsing focal liponecrosis (Weber–Christian syndrome) of the breast. Arch Surg 1960;80: 219–223

CHAPTER 8

Malignant Breast Diseases

8

Melvin A. Shiffman

8.1
Introduction

Breast cancer has a major impact on women's health and is the second leading cause of cancer death. Risk factors include increasing age, hereditary genetic abnormalities, estrogens, dietary factors, benign breast disease, and environmental factors. The surgeon should be aware that breast cancer can occur at almost any age and is being detected at earlier ages and by smaller tumors because of the annual use of mammography.

8.2
Breast Augmentation

When a patient considers breast augmentation, the surgeon must obtain a family history concerning breast and ovarian cancer. He or she should ask whether the patient is taking estrogens, when her last mammogram was performed, and whether she has had any breast surgery. It would be wise to obtain any medical records of prior breast surgery, including the operative report, as well as mammogram reports.

The breast examination should be performed with the patient sitting and supine. The medical record should describe any breast asymmetry, nipple inversion, skin dimpling, or masses.

A preoperative mammogram should be considered in all patients but should always be obtained in a patient 40 years of age or older.

8.3
Cancer

Breast cancers are being diagnosed more frequently in earlier stages because of routine annual mammograms in patients over 40 years, but breast cancer can occur much earlier, especially in families with genetic abnormalities. Palpation alone may miss very early cancers that may be seen on mammogram.

Irregular, hard, nontender masses should be considered malignant. A mammogram followed by biopsy (needle) is necessary. When there are calcifications of a malignant character or architectural distortion, stereotactic needle biopsy will usually give the diagnosis. Open biopsy may be needed when the needle biopsy does not give a definitive diagnosis.

8.3.1
Types

Carcinoma in situ has several specific characteristics on biopsy. Although most do not metastasize, some types may spread to the lymph nodes (less than 4%). Lobular carcinoma in situ is a marker for possible future bilateral breast cancer.

Infiltrating ductal carcinoma is the most frequent type of breast cancer, and as the size increases, the probability of metastatic spread increases. Invasive lobular cancer does not usually become palpable at an early stage (<1 cm) because the tumor invades the tissues in strands ("Indian file").

8.3.2
Treatment

Treatment of breast cancer requires a definitive diagnosis. This means that needle, stereotactic needle, or open biopsy should be performed. Conservative therapy usually can be accomplished with small tumors, <3 cm, by the use of lumpectomy or quadrantectomy followed by radiotherapy. Mastectomy may be indicated in larger tumors or in patients who fear recurrence and wish the breast to be removed. Sentinel node excision may be used in breast cancer before more extensive axillary lymph node dissection. If the sentinel node is negative, a complete node dissection may be avoided.

Most cancers >1 cm in diameter will require chemotherapy as an adjunct to lumpectomy and radiotherapy or mastectomy. Many useful chemotherapeutic drugs are available that will prolong life in metastatic breast cancer. Spread to the bones alone has a better prognosis than when other organ systems are involved.

8.4
Genetic Testing

8.4.1
Breast Cancer Risk Assessment

There are features of familial breast cancer that can aid physicians in recognizing individuals who are at high risk because of inheriting a breast cancer susceptibility gene. The following individuals may have a high probability for mutations in BRCA1 or BRCA2:

1. Single affected relative with
   a. Breast cancer <30 years of age
   b. Ovarian cancer <30 years of age
2. Sister pairs:
   a. Breast cancer <50 years of age; breast cancer <50 years of age
   b. Breast cancer <50 years of age; ovarian cancer <60 years of age
   c. Ovarian cancer <60 years of age; ovarian cancer at any age
3. Families:
   a. Breast cancer only, more than three cases diagnosed <60 years of age
   b. More than two with breast cancer and more than one with ovarian cancer

BRCA1 is responsible for 28% of breast cancers under age 30 and 5% under age 50 and is associated with a 40–60% risk of breast cancer by age 60 and a 10–49% risk of ovarian cancer by age 60. BRCA2 is associated with female and male breast cancers, with less ovarian cancer than BRCA1, and with other cancers such as leukemia, lymphoma, gliomas, and upper gastrointestinal, prostate, colon, and brain cancers.

8.4.2
Molecular Genetic Testing

Genetic testing is not perfectly predictive. The absence of a mutation does not mean cancer will not occur. There is no substantial proof that screening for genetic defects leads to increased longevity.

Disclosure of results may be potentially psychologically distressing. Counseling about reproductive choices is needed if a gene with fatal consequences is potentially going to be passed on to a child. There is the problem of patient privacy versus the relatives' need to know, as well as the problem of patient autonomy versus the duty to warn third parties of potential harm. A potential for discrimination exists by employers and medical, life, and disability insurers.

8.5
Chromosome

The chromosome is divided into the short (petit) or p-arm and the long or q-arm. The regions and bands are numbered, proceeding from the proximal arm (near the centromere) to the distal arm (near the telomere; see Fig. 8.1). The region is the first number, and the band is the second number. Example: 1q23 = chromosome 1, q=long arm, 2=region, 3=band.

Genetic abnormalities can involve deletion (terminal or interstitial), duplication, mutation, transposition, or rearrangements (pericentric inversion, paracentric inversion).

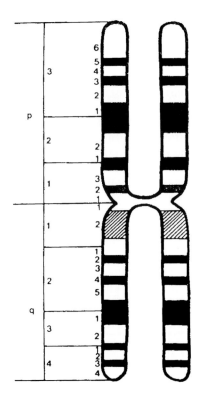

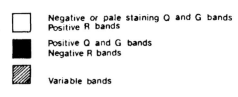

Negative or pale staining Q and G bands
Positive R bands

Positive Q and G bands
Negative R bands

Variable bands

Fig. 8.1 The chromosome with regions and bands

8.6
Breast Cancer Prevention Options

Breast cancer prevention options include the following:
1. Prophylactic mastectomy: 95–98% effective
2. Chemoprevention
    a. Tamoxifen
    b. Retinoids

8.7
Discussion

Any mass in the breast, no matter what the patient's age, should be considered as possible breast cancer. A ballottable mass in a patient under the age of 35 is usually a benign fibroadenoma. But even fibroadenomas can be cancerous, and if the mass is growing or the patient is over the age of 35, excision may be indicated.

A thorough breast examination in the sitting and supine positions should be performed before considering any cosmetic breast procedure.

After breast augmentation, it is incumbent on the surgeon to perform a thorough examination of the breast at each visit, and he or she should be cognizant of any unusual symptoms. Although breast cancer is usually not painful, there are cases of pain associated with breast cancer. Nipple inversion and skin indention should be suspicious for possible cancer. Any mass should be considered breast cancer until proven otherwise. The author has experienced one case in which the surgeon, who had performed a breast augmentation a few years before, was suspicious for cancer and performed a needle biopsy that was negative. It was suggested to the surgeon that the photos were typical of breast cancer and that recuts of the pathology specimen should be performed or an open biopsy done. The recuts showed the cancer.

Patients with a significant family history of breast cancer and/or ovarian cancer may be candidates for cancer counseling. Prophylactic mastectomy with reconstruction may be a better choice than augmentation.

8.8
Conclusions

Surgeons should always be suspicious of the possibility of cancer in a patient with a mass, skin dimpling, or nipple retraction. A patient under age 40 can still develop cancer; the youngest patient with breast cancer that the author has seen was 16 years old.

CHAPTER 9

Mammograms in Cosmetic Breast Surgery

9

Melvin A. Shiffman

9.1
Introduction

The use of preoperative and postoperative mammograms in cosmetic surgery has never been standardized. There appears to be some consensus that at least preoperative mammograms should be obtained according to the recommendations of the American Cancer Society for screening mammography. Women at average risk should begin monthly self-breast examination at age 20, receive a clinical breast examination every 3 years from age 20 to age 39, and receive an annual mammogram and clinical breast examination starting at age 40 [1]. There is no specific surveillance strategy for women at higher risk for breast cancer, but these patients may benefit by earlier initiation of screening, screening at shorter intervals, and screening with additional methods such as ultrasound or magnetic resonance imaging [1].

9.2
Preoperative Mammograms

The purpose of a preoperative mammogram is to detect any significant disorder of the breast(s) prior to cosmetic surgery so that the problem can be resolved before surgery or during surgery. Also, the mammogram is a baseline for detecting abnormalities after the cosmetic surgery.

The incidence of new breast cancer cases is increasing at a yearly rate and was estimated to be 203,500 in 2002 [2] and 211,300 in 2003 in the United States [3].

It is essential to detect an early cancer so that cosmetic procedures of the breast do not cut across, distort, diminish the opportunity for cure of, or limit the usefulness of lumpectomy in the treatment of the cancer. Breast cancer is now being detected—through the use of mammograms—earlier in the development of the tumor, at a smaller size, and with a better prognosis for cure.

The detection of a fibroadenoma is significant because carcinoma may occur within the fibroadenoma [4–10]. The average age for fibroadenoma is 23, whereas the average age for carcinoma in the fibroadenoma is 43 [4]. A new tumor after age 35 should be biopsied (most commonly with stereotactic needle biopsy). Under age 35, a fibroadenoma would need to be biopsied or excised if it continues to grow.

The 18–39-year-old patient is in the age group of most common debate concerning whether to perform preoperative mammograms. This age group has not had a high incidence of breast cancer, but because of earlier diagnosis, there is presently a higher incidence than previously reported. The average breast cancer tumor size in the author's practice was 3.0 cm from 1964 through 1984, but from 1985 to 2006 it was 2.0 cm, showing that earlier diagnosis was being made through mammographic screening methods and better patient awareness of the need for regular examinations. Breast cancer has been reported in patients under the age of 30 [11]. The youngest patient with cancer seen by this author was 16 years of age. An argument by radiologists has been that youthful breasts have marked dysplasia on mammography that prevents the detection of some abnormalities. But by increasing the radiation slightly to eliminate some of the dysplastic changes, a mammogram can be performed that will then focus on architectural distortion and calcifications.

Patients with a significant family history of breast cancer should begin to have annual mammograms 10 years before the youngest age of the individual(s) in the family with the cancer. If a patient with a significant family history desires breast augmentation, then the patient must be forewarned that the implant could possibly reduce the chance of early detection of cancer, and consideration must be given to placing the implants beneath the pectoralis major muscle.

9.3
Postoperative Mammograms Following Cosmetic Breast Surgery

Following cosmetic breast surgery, routine mammograms (6–12 months postoperatively) help formulate a baseline for future detection of breast cancer. Surgery involving the breasts can result in architectural distortion from scars and calcifications.

9.4
Cosmetic Surgeries

9.4.1
Breast Augmentation

The insertion of implants through the areola or periareolar incisions usually involves dissection through the breast tissues, which may result in architectural scars within the breast tissue. Axillary, inframammary, and umbilical approaches do not usually breach the breast tissue itself. Calcifications have been reported in the fibrous capsule (around the implant) but do not resemble the calcifications seen with breast cancer [12–17]. For implants in place for more than 12 years, 52.5% of those ruptured showed calcification, but only 10.0% of intact implants showed calcification [13].

Fat transfer into the breast parenchyma is no longer performed [18]. The fat for augmentation is now injected beneath, into, and above the pectoralis muscle, although the patient should be forewarned of the possibility of inadvertent injection into the breast itself. The calcifications around a fat cyst are easily diagnosed as benign [19]. Stippled calcifications of fat necrosis following fat injection appear circular and smooth and can usually be distinguished by an experienced mammographer from calcifications found with cancer. If there is any question, the calcified area can be sampled through stereotactic needle biopsy under local anesthesia.

Kinoshita et al. [20] stated that in some magnetic resonance (MR) findings of fat necrosis it was difficult to distinguish benign from malignant lesions. Kurtz et al. [21] studied MR findings in patients with fat necrosis and found that all of the 15 fat necroses displayed fat-isointense signal on T1-weighted and on proton-weighted, fat-suppressed sequences. They were delineated by a more or less wide rim of low signal intensity with a sharp border to the center. After intravenous injection of gadopenetate dimeglumine, they showed no increase in signal intensity in the center and no increase, or a minor increase, of the rim. Ultrasound could not distinguish fat necrosis from recurrent tumor in six cases, although seven looked like atypical cysts. MR mammography was felt to be a promising method for diagnosing fat necrosis.

Bilgen et al. [22] studied 126 fat necrosis lesions in 94 patients. On mammogram, they found radiolucent oil cysts (34 or 26.9%), round opacity (16% or 12.6%), asymmetric opacity or heretogenicity of the subcutaneous tissues (20% or 15.8%), dystrophic calcifications (5% or 3.9%), and suspicious spiculated mass (5% or 3.9%).

Follow-up mammograms showed curvilinear calcifications in five and decreased density in six rounded opacities, with another two disappearing. Eleven dystrophic calcifications became more course, six of the asymmetric opacities became vague, one developed an oil cyst and coarse calcifications, and one spiculated mass developed a small radiolucent oil cyst in the center. On sonogram, the lesions were solid in 18 (9.5%), anechoic with posterior acoustic enhancement in 21 (16.6%), anechoic with posterior acoustic shadowing in 20 (15.8%), cystic with internal echoes in 14 (11.1%), and cystic with mural nodule in five (3.9%). There was increased echogenicity of the subcutaneous tissues in 34 (26.9%), and 14 (11.1%) were normal. Follow-up ultrasound showed that 18 of the 29 that had increased subcutaneous tissue echogenicity turned back to normal, while small cysts formed in the remaining 11. In the 19 solid-appearing masses, 15 showed decreases in size, while four remained stable (biopsy disclosed fat necrosis). The four complex masses increased in size and appeared more cystic. It was concluded that knowledge of the mammographic and ultrasound appearance of fat necrosis and evolution of these patterns may enable imaging follow-up and reduce the number of biopsies.

9.4.2
Breast Reduction

Breast reduction involves cutting into and removing areas of breast tissue, which may result in significant scarring, architectural distortion, and calcifications, usually from fat necrosis [23]. Miller et al. [24] noted that after reduction mammoplasty, all patients are left with a linear scar between the nipple and inframammary fold that accounts for the frequent finding of skin thickening along the lower breast. Fat necrosis presents as an irregular calcified mass. Brown et al. [25] noted that asymmetric densities were present in approximately half of the patients. Parenchymal calcifications were apparent in 50% of patients after 2 years. Four out of 42 patients had biopsies for suspicious densities, which were benign on pathology.

Abboud et al. [26] reported that breast reduction using liposuction has been associated with calcifications from fat necrosis. Sixty patients with breast reduction—34 with and 26 without liposuction—were studied. There was a 6–30-month follow-up, and calcifications were noted in 11%. Deep intraparenchymal calcifications were more frequent after liposuction, and most (five of seven) were macrocalcifications. None could be confused with malignant calcifications because they were more scattered, more regular, and less numerous. (If there is any question as to the cause of calcifications, stereotactic needle biopsy should be performed.) Alterations in breast tissue resulting from the use of ultrasonic assisted liposuction were a thickened dermal undersurface and markedly thickened vertical collagenous fibers with intact lymphatic vessels and intact blood vessels [27].

The use of ultrasound-assisted liposuction for breast reduction has not been found to injure the breast tissue but still may be associated with calcifications [28, 29].

9.4.3
Mastopexy

Breast lift (mastopexy) does not usually disturb the breast parenchyma unless there is some breast tissue reduction. The lift is mainly a skin reduction with release of the breast from the underlying muscle to reorient the breast into a higher position.

9.5
Discussion

A preoperative mammogram is a screening technique to detect abnormalities before cosmetic surgery. There is some argument that cosmetic surgery is an elective procedure being performed on a healthy patient and that there should be a more detailed workup with mammography to protect the patient even in the young age group before breast surgery. This would mean that every patient, no matter what age, should have a preoperative mammogram prior to cosmetic breast surgery (R. Jackson, 24 April 2003, personal communication). Peras [30] reported that in 1,149 cases of cosmetic surgery, early diagnosis of breast cancer was possible in 34 cases by the use of mammography. He strongly recommended that a policy of mandatory preoperative mammography be implemented so that all patients can be protected from a potentially lethal disease by early detection.

It is the surgeon's choice whether to order a preoperative mammogram prior to cosmetic breast surgery on a patient under the age of 40. If requested to have a preoperative mammogram, patients who refuse may safely be operated upon, but the refusal should be noted in the medical record. This will help protect the physician if there is future litigation. It is also the physician's choice whether to do cosmetic breast surgery on a patient over the age of 40 who refuses a preoperative mammogram. The patient should be fully informed of the possible consequences of missing a significant abnormality.

Postoperative mammograms will protect the patient by providing a baseline for future reference. However, there are many patients who do not come back to the surgeon for follow-up mammography because they feel fine and do not wish to be bothered with the procedure or the cost. The surgeon probably should document in the medical record that the postoperative mammogram had been requested.

The patient who has a significant family history of breast cancer should be counseled on the possibility of future breast cancer and the possible need for genetic testing prior to any cosmetic procedure on the breast. If genetic testing is positive for BRCA1 or BRCA2, the individual has a 50–90% lifetime risk of developing breast cancer [31–34]. If the genetic abnormality is present, a variety of early detection and prevention programs are available [35]. Patients at any age with a significant family history should have a mammogram before any cosmetic breast surgery is contemplated. The problems of early diagnosis of breast cancer that may be present if augmentation mammoplasty or any other cosmetic procedure of the breast is performed should be thoroughly explained before making any decisions about surgery.

References

1. Smith RA, Saslow D, Sawyer KA, Burke W, Costanza ME, Evans WP III, Foster RS Jr, Eyre HJ, Sener S, et al.: American Cancer Society guidelines for breast cancer screening: update 2003. CA Cancer J Clin 2003;53(3):141–169
2. Jemal A, Thomas A, Murray T, Than M: Cancer statistics, 2002. CA Cancer J Clin 2002;52(1):23–47
3. Jemal A, Murray T, Samuels A, Ghafoor A, Ward E, Thun MJ: Cancer statistics. CA Cancer J Clin 2003;53(1):5–26
4. Durso EA: Carcinoma arising in fibroadenoma: a case report. Radiology 1972;102:565
5. Buzonowsaki-Konakry K, Harrison EG, Payne WS: Lobular carcinoma arising in fibroadenoma of the breast. Cancer 1975;35:450–456
6. Azzopardi JG: Problems in Breast Pathology. Philadelphia, WB Saunders 1979
7. Pick PW, Iossifides IA: Occurrence of breast carcinoma within a fibroadenoma. A review. Arch Pathol Lab Med 1984;108(7):590–594
8. Schnitt SJ, Connolly JL: Pathology of benign breast disorders. In: Harris JR (ed). Diseases of the Breast, 2nd edn. Philadelphia, Williams & Wilkins 2000, pp 75–93
9. Botta P-G, Cosimi MF: Breast lobular carcinoma in a fibroadenoma of the breast. Eur J Surg Pathol 1985;11:283–285
10. Diaz NM, Palmer JO, McDivitt RW: Carcinoma arising within fibroadenomas of the breast. A clinicopathologic study of 105 patients. Am J Clin Path 1991;95:614–622
11. Tabbane F, el May A, Hachiche M, Bahi J, Jaziri M, Cammoun M, Mourali N: Breast cancer in women under 30 years of age. Breast Cancer Res Treat 1985;6(2):137–144

12. Peters W, Smith D, Lugowski S, Pritzker K, Holmyard D: Calcification properties of saline-filled implants. Plast Reconstr Surg 2001;107(2):356–363

13. Peters W, Pritzker K, Smith D, Fornasier V, Holmyard D, Lugowski S, Kamel M, Visram F: Capsular calcification associated with silicone breast implants: incidence, determinants, and characterization. Ann Plast Surg 1998;41(4):348–360

14. Peter W, Smith D: Calcification of breast implant capsules: incidence, diagnosis, and contributing factors. Ann Plast Surg 1995;34(1):8–11

15. Schmidt GH: Calcification bonded to saline-filled implants. Plast Reconstr Surg 1993;92(7):1423–1425

16. Young VL, Bartell T, Destouet JM, Monsees B, Logan SE: Calcification of breast implant capsule. South Med J 1989;82(9):1171–1173

17. Nicoletis C, Wlodarczyk B: A rare complication of breast prosthesis: calcification of the periprosthetic retractile capsule. Ann Chir Plast Esthet 1983;28(4):388–389

18. Fulton JE: Breast contouring with "gelled" autologous fat: a 10-year update. Int J Cosm Surg Aesthet Derm 2003;5(2):155–163

19. Rocek V, Rehulka M, Vojacek K, Kral V: Fat necrosis of the breasts with ring calcification. Acta Univ Palacki Olomuc Fac Med 1982;102:143–147

20. Kinoshita T, Yashiro N, Yoshigi J, Ihara N, Narita M: Fat necrosis of breast: a potential pitfall in breast MRI. Clin Imaging 2002;26(4):250253

21. Kurtz B, Achten C, Audretsch W, Rezai M, Zocholl G: MR mammography of fatty tissue necrosis. Rofo Fortschr Geb Rontgenstr Neuen Bildgeb Verhfahr 1996;165(4):359–363

22. Bilgen IG, Ustum EE, Memis A: Fat necrosis of the breast: clinical, mammographic, and sonographic features. Eur J Radiol 2001;39(2):92–99

23. Baber CE, Libshitz HI: Bilateral fat necrosis of the breast following reduction mammoplasties. Am J Roent 1977;128:508–509

24. Miller CL, Feig SA, Fox JW: Mammographic changes in reduction mammoplasty. Am J Roent 1987;149:35–38

25. Brown FE, Sargent SK, Cohen SR, Morain WD: Mammographic changes following reduction mammaplasty. Plast Reconstr Surg 1987;80(5):691–698

26. Abboud M, Vadoud-Seyedi J, De May A, Cukierfajn M, Lejour M: Incidence of calcifications in the breast after surgical reduction and liposuction. Plast Reconstr Surg 1995;96(3):620–626

27. Di Giuseppe A: Ultrasound-assisted liposuction for breast reduction. In: Shiffman MA, Di Giuseppe A (eds). Textbook of Liposuction: Principles and Practice. Marcel Dekker 2004

28. Lejour M, Abboud M: Vertical mammoplasty without inframammary scar and with liposuction. Perspect Plast Surg 1990;4:67

29. Lejour M: Reduction of large breasts by a combination of liposuction and vertical mammoplasty. In: Cohen M (ed). Master of Surgery: Plastic and Reconstructive Surgery. Boston, Little, Brown 1994

30. Perras C: Fifteen years of mammography in cosmetic surgery of the breast. Aesthetic Plast Surg 1990;14(2):81–84

31. Taucher S, Gnant M, Jekesz R: Preventive mastectomy in patients at breast cancer risk due to genetic alterations in the BRCA1 and BRCA2 gene. Langenbecks Arch Surg 2003;388(1):3–8

32. Winer EP, Morrow M, Osborne CK, Harris JR: Malignant tumors of the breast. In: DeVita, VT, Hellman S, Rosenberg SA (eds). Cancer: Principles & Practice of Oncology, Philadelphia, Lippincott Williams & Wilkins 2001, pp 1651–1717

33. Ford D, Easton D, Bishop Narod SA, Goldgar DE: Risks of cancer in BRCA1 mutation carriers. Breast Cancer Linkage Consortium. Lancet 1994;343(8899):692–695

34. Struewing JP, Hartge P, Wacholder S, Baker SM, Berlin M, McAdams M, Timmerman MM, Brody LC, Tucker MA: The risk of cancer associated with specific mutations of BRCA1 and BRCA2: among Ashkenazi Jews. N Engl J Med 1997;336(20):1401–1408

35. Grann VR, Panegeas KS, Whang W, Antman KH, Neugut AI: Decision analysis of prophylactic mastectomy and oophorectomy in BRCA1-positive or BRCA2-positive patients. J Clin Oncol 1998;16(3):979–985

Part II
Preoperative Consultation

CHAPTER 10

Initial Consultation

Melvin A. Shiffman

10.1
Introduction

The initial consultation with a patient considering breast augmentation should be complete. The patient will be impressed if a proper history and examination are performed and will be more likely to schedule the surgery. Enough information from the patient should be requested to be able to evaluate whether or not to perform the surgery.

10.2
Subjective Reasons for Breast Augmentation

The patient is the only one to decide whether augmentation is necessary. Surgeons should avoid the patient who has a body dysmorphic disorder and is seeking a surgery that may minimally, if at all, improve the body. This becomes more important when revision may be necessary. Very minor corrections should be avoided.

A significant number of patients will need surgical correction of the augmentation for asymmetry, contracture, ptosis, infection, or necrosis. The more breast surgeries performed on a patient, the more likely the complications.

10.3
History

The patient's past history should be obtained, at least including past surgeries of the breast and chest, bleeding or bruising tendencies, pulmonary or heart disorders, and prior thromboembolism. The date of her last menstrual period should be requested.. Medications being taken should be listed, including aspirin, Coumadin, nonsteroidal anti-inflammatory drugs, estrogen, and herbals. If the patient presently smokes cigarettes, this may impact wound healing and may cause necrosis. A history of diabetes mellitus is important because uncontrolled diabetes increases the risk of slow healing and wound infection. The surgeon should have an internist check the blood sugar preoperatively and follow the blood sugar on a daily basis for at least 7 days postoperatively and then on a regular basis.

A history of breast cancer should be taken very seriously. The patient should have a checkup by the oncologist to make sure that metastases have not occurred, and any recent mammogram report should be obtained or a mammogram ordered to make sure there are no suspicious areas in either breast. If lumpectomy has been performed followed by radiation, there is a reasonable assumption that the breast tissues have a decreased blood supply from the radiation. Therefore, healing will be slower, and there is a greater risk of necrosis. Incisions near the area of the incision site for the lumpectomy, where increased radiation has been used, should be avoided because healing will be very prolonged, and the chance of wound breakdown increases.

The family history should include at least cancers of the breast, blood dyscrasias, and thromboembolism. Patients with a strong familial history of breast cancer should be counseled about the possibility of future breast cancer and the effects of the presence of an implant in the submammary position possibly decreasing the chance of early diagnosis.

10.4
Physical Examination

The physical examination should include at least the heart and lungs as well as the breast and axilla. The breasts should be examined both in the sitting and the supine position with the arms over the head (this flattens the breast against the chest wall). Observe the breast for skin or nipple indentations and asymmetry. Check for masses in the breast and axilla, tenderness, and induration.

Record the following measurements:
1. Sternal notch and/or midclavicle to nipples
2. Nipples to midline
3. Extent of ptosis: either the degree and/or measurement from nipple to inframammary fold and inframammary fold to lowest point of breast

10.5
Informed Consent

Informed consent requires that the patient receive enough information about the surgical procedure proposed and the alternatives as well as the possible risks and complications of each so that a knowledgeable decision can be made.

10.6
Implants

Evaluation for implant size may be performed in the office with the use of various sizes of implants, or baggies filled with water of different amounts, placed in the brassiere and using a mirror to determine what looks best. The patient can use baggies at home in order to consider the proper size, and she can bring in photos of topless women whose appearance she desires. The surgeon should make sure that the patient decides on the size and is not influenced by her spouse or boyfriend. The patient's own body image should be the determining factor. The surgeon and office staff should also not influence the patient as to size.

The type of implant—smooth or textured, silicone or saline—should be described along with its pros and cons. The position of the implants, above or below the muscle, should be discussed as well as the surgical incision site—axillary, periareolar, intraareolar, inframammary, and possibly the umbilical approach.

10.7
Discussion

The initial consultation should be taken seriously because the impression of the surgeon and the staff can influence the woman's decision about whether to have the surgery. The surgeon should take an active part in the discussion. A discussion should be held with the patient about the procedure's possible risks and complications as well as viable alternative procedures, and a statement of this being done should be included in the medical record.

Patients should not be influenced to have procedures that they did not initially request. The surgeon may suggest the types of surgery or other surgeries but should not try to convince the patient to have more than initially requested. If the patient has a surgery that was not initially requested and a complication occurs, there is a high likelihood that litigation will follow.

Rapport cannot usually be established easily on the first consultation. Another office visit and discussion are very helpful.

Preoperative and postoperative instructions should be given to the patient both orally and in writing. Preoperatively the patient should be taken off medications that may cause bleeding and estrogens that are a known cause of thromboembolism. She must stop smoking completely for at least 2 weeks before and 2 weeks after surgery. Herbals should be avoided before and after surgery.

Preoperative photos are a standard. Postoperative photos should be obtained after 6 months, but often the patient is happy with the result and does not wish to return just to have more photos.

Remember: The medical record is the physician's best defense. Records should be complete, detailed, and accurate. Make no changes; however, a single line can be made through an error. Write in the change, initial it, and date it.

CHAPTER 11

Method for Determining Bra Size and Predicting Postaugmentation Breast Size

11

Edward A. Pechter

11.1 Introduction

An article in the *London Daily Mail* in January 2006 headlined that "80 percent of women wear the wrong size bra," while at the same time an ad in the *Los Angeles Daily News* for a "bra fit event" by the JCPenney department store inquired, "Did you know 8 out of 10 of your friends are wearing the wrong bra size?" In the scientific literature, a British study found that all 102 of 102 women seeking reduction mammaplasty wore the wrong size bra [1]. If these numbers are accurate, why are so many women unable to select the correct bra size? The answer lies largely with shortcomings of the traditional method of bra sizing.

All traditional methods of bra measurement are variations of a scheme that determines cup size by the relationship of the circumference of the chest around the breasts to its circumference above or below the breasts. Experience has shown this method to be so inaccurate as to be useless, helping explain why so many women are said to wear the wrong size bra.

In response to this problem, a new system of bra measurement was developed. It is a modified version of a previously reported method of bra sizing that determines cup size by direct breast measurement [2] while now allowing for the fact that cup size varies with band size, e.g., the "C" cup of a size 36 bra is larger than the "C" cup of a size 34 bra yet smaller than the "C" cup of a size 38 bra.

With this system, brassiere band size is still determined by the industry standard of "underbust chest circumference plus 5," but cup size is determined by direct measurement of the breast in proportion to underbust circumference [3]. Although some women, for a variety of reasons, choose to wear a bra that does not fit properly by the usual criteria, virtually every woman measured with this system fits well into the bra determined to be her correct size. Most importantly to plastic surgeons, this method of measurement can be used during breast augmentation to help achieve the desired postaugmentation bra size.

11.2 Technique

Bra size is determined by two components, band size and cup size. Band size is expressed as a number, whereas cup size is represented by a letter, for example, "36C." In the traditional method of bra sizing, band size is determined by adding "5" to the underbust circumference (UBC), the circumference of the chest immediately below the breasts as measured snugly with a tape (Fig. 11.1). For example, if the UBC is 31 in, the band size is 36. If band size calculates to an odd number, the number is rounded up or down because bras are available only in even-numbered sizes.

Cup size is then determined by comparing band size to bust circumference, which is the circumference of the chest around the fullest part of the breasts, usually taken at the level of the nipples with the subject wearing a bra. A bust circumference 1 in greater than band size corresponds to an "A" cup, 2 in corresponds to a "B" cup, 3 in to a "C" cup, and so forth. For example, a woman who has a bust circumference of 39 in with a band size of 36 would fit a size 36C bra by this formula (39 – 36 = 3 = C cup).

That the traditional method of bra sizing is confusing is evidenced by uncertainty on the part of many lingerie fitters trying to use it, as well as by occasional erroneous instructions for its use in the lay press and on the Internet [4, 5]. More than one professional corsetiere has confided to me that they take measurements by this system but then disregard the numbers and "eyeball" the approximate bra size. Even when used properly, the traditional method is grossly inaccurate, usually indicating inappropriately small cup sizes or even "negative" cup sizes when the bust circumference is less than the band size. These limitations help explain why so many women are said to wear the wrong size of bra.

In the new method, bra size is determined by the relationship of breast size, or width, to the UBC. Breast width is determined independently for each breast and is measured with a tape from the point where the breast mound originates on the lateral chest wall to where it terminates in the parasternal area. The measurement

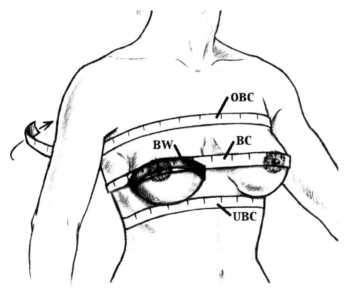

Fig. 11.1 Traditional method of bra sizing. *OBC* overbust circumference, the circumference of the chest above the breasts, under the arms, and high on the back. *BC* bust circumference, the circumference of the chest around the fullest part of the breasts, usually at the level of the nipples. *UBC* underbust circumference, the circumference of the chest immediately below the breasts. *BW* breast width, the distance across the breast from the point where the breast mound originates on the lateral chest wall to where it ends in the parasternal area

Table 11.1 Bra sizing chart (measurements are in inches)

Underbust Circumference	Breast Width									
	5	5.5	6	6.5	7	7.5	8	8.5	9	9.5
27	32AA	32AA/A	32A	32A/B	32B	32B/C	32C	32C/D	32D	32D/DD
28	32AA	34AA	32A	34A	32B	34B	32C	34C	32D	34D
29		34AA	34AA/A	34A	34A/AB	34B	34B/C	34C	34C/D	34D
30		34AA	36AA	34A	36A	34B	36B	34C	36C	34D
31			36AA	36AA/A	36A	36A/B	36B	36B/C	36C	36C/D
32			38AA	36A	38A	36B	38B	36C	38C
33			38AA	38AA/A	38A	38A/B	38B	38B/C	38C
34			38AA	40AA	38A	40A	38B	40B	38C
35				40AA	40AA/A	40A	40A/B	40B	40B/C
36				40AA	42AA	40A	42A	40B	42B
37					42AA	42AA/A	42A	42A/B	42B
38					42AA	44AA	42A	44A	42B
39						44AA	44AA/A	44A	44A/B
40						44AA	46AA	44A	46A

Table 11.1 *(continued)* Bra sizing chart (measurements are in inches)

Underbust Circumference	Breast Width									
	10	10.5	11	11.5	12	12.5	13	13.5	14	14.5
27	32DD	32DD/E	32E							
28	32DD	34DD	32E	34E						
29	34D/DD	34DD	34DD/E	34E						
30	36D	34DD	36DD	34E	36E					
31	36D	36D/DD	36DD	36DD/E	36E					
32	36D	38D	36DD	38DD	36E	38E				
33	38C/D	38D	38D/DD	38DD	38DD/E	38E				
34	40C	38D	40D	38DD	40DD	38E	40E			
35	40C	40C/D	40D	40D/DD	40DD	40DD/E	40E			
36	40C	42C	40D	42D	40DD	42DD	40E	42E		
37	42B/C	42C	42C/D	42D	42D/DD	42DD	42D/E	42E		
38	44B	42C	44C	42D	44D	42DD	44DD	42E	44E	
39	44B	44B/C	44C	44C/D	44D	44D/DD	44DD	44DD/E	44E	
40	44B	46B	44C	46C	44D	46D	44DD	46DD	44E	46E

passes over the fullest part of the breast, usually at the level of the nipple. Small or firm breasts can be accurately measured with a woman upright, whereas very large or ptotic breasts are better measured with the woman supine.

The relationship between breast width and UBC is shown in Table 11.1. Larger bra sizes can be extrapolated by noting that cup size advances by one letter for each 1-in increase in breast width. A notation such as "36B/C" indicates that the size falls between a "B" and a "C" cup in a size 36 bra, and a woman might wear one or the other size depending on the particular bra. Figs. 11.2 and 11.3 demonstrate the difference between the traditional and new methods of bra measurement in two representative patients.

11.3 Results

Rather than having breast augmentation patients choose an implant size, a task for which they generally have no experience, they were asked to name their desired postoperative bra size and to provide a representative

photograph. The information in Table 11.1 was used to achieve their goals, as illustrated in Figs. 11.4 and 11.5. Sizing implants filled with air were used intraoperatively to determine the implant volume that would give the desired breast dimension.

11.4 Discussion

The fact that bra cup size varies with band size is not a new observation [6–9], although disagreement exists over the degree of this variance, with some authors reporting that cup size changes by a full size with each incremental step in band size, e.g., the "C" cup of a size 36 bra is equal to the "D" cup of a size 34 bra and the "B" cup of a size 38 bra [6, 10]. From personally taking many hundreds of breast measurements and having women try on the corresponding bras, the author has discovered a more accurate finding to be that cup size changes by one increment only with every alternate band size change, e.g., the "C" cup of a 36 bra corresponds to the "D" cup of a size 32 bra and the "B" cup of a size 40 bra; this is reflected in Table 11.1.

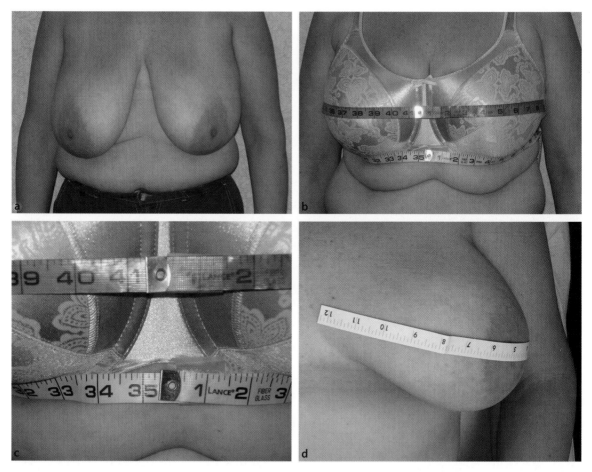

Fig. 11.2 a Woman with large, ptotic breasts. **b** Woman wearing a well-fitting 40DD brassiere. **c** Bust circumference is 41 in, underbust circumference is 35 in, and bra size by traditional measuring system is 40A. **d** Supine breast width is 12 in, and the bra size by the new measuring system is 40DD

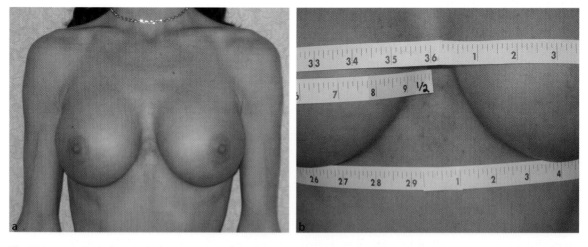

Fig. 11.3 a Woman with 500-ml silicone implants. **b** Bust circumference is 36 in, underbust circumference is 29 in, breast width is 9.5 in, bra size by traditional measuring system is 34B, and bra size by new measuring system is 34D

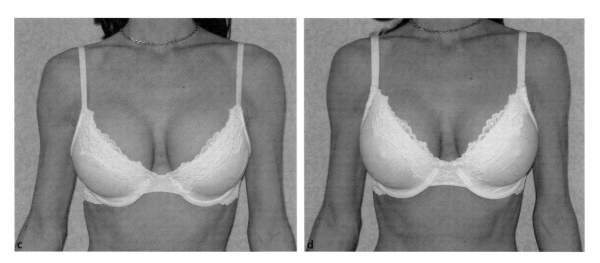

Fig. 11.3 *(continued)* **c** A 34B bra is too small, gapping across the lower chest and providing inadequate breast coverage. **d** A 34D bra fits perfectly

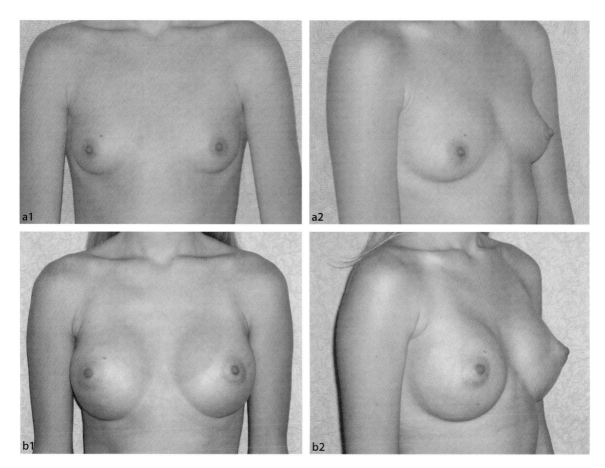

Fig. 11.4 a *1* Woman 5'6" tall weighing 115 lb seeking augmentation to "C" cup of size 34 bra. *2* Breast width is 6.5 in, underbust circumference is 29 in, and bra size is 34A. **b** *1* After augmentation. *2* The breast width has been increased to 8.5 in with 350-ml silicone implants, the underbust circumference remains 29 in, and the bra size is 34C

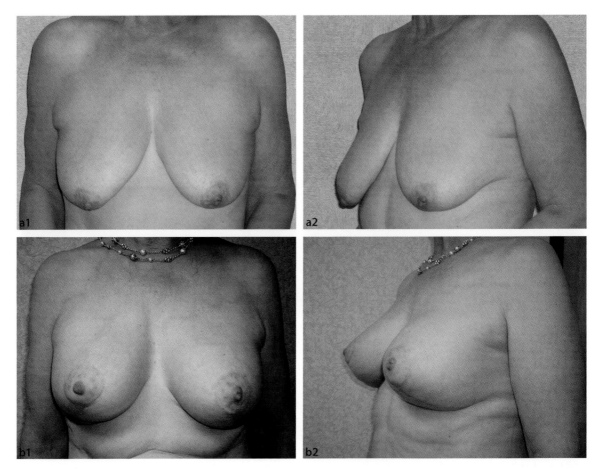

Fig. 11.5 a *1* Woman 5'7" in height weighing 142 lb with a size 36 bra seeking a breast lift and augmentation to a full C cup. *2* Breast width is 8.5 in, underbust circumference is 31 in, and bra size is 36 B/C ("full B"). **b** *1* After modified vertical mastopexy and simultaneous augmentation. *2* The breast width has been increased to 9.5 in with 280-ml saline implants, the underbust circumference remains 31 in, and the bra size is 36 C/D ("full C")

In one variation of the traditional measuring system, overbust circumference (OBC) is substituted for UBC+5. OBC is the circumference of the chest above the breasts, under the arms, and high on the back. If OBC is used, "5" is not added to the measurement to determine band size because OBC approximates UBC+5 in most women. This relationship may explain the custom of adding "5" to UBC to determine band size. Using OBC to calculate bra size is no more accurate than using band size because in either method the cup size is determined by an arbitrary comparison to bust circumference without direct breast measurement. Many individual modifications of the basic measuring system exist, as do other methods of breast measurement, both high-tech and low-tech [11–14].

Band size is not expected to change with breast surgery, although it might if the inframammary fold is surgically adjusted, changing the site of UBC measurement. Additionally, a woman between two band sizes may prefer one size before surgery and the other size afterward.

Experience has shown the bra sizing system described herein to be accurate and sensitive. A weight change of only a few pounds will often be reflected in the UBC or breast width, and the same measurements may change during the course of a woman's menstrual cycle and certainly during pregnancy. Breast measurements are helpful in breast augmentation and reduction [2, 10, 15] and in quantifying the difference in size in women with asymmetrical breasts, with each 1-in increment corresponding to a cup size.

Knowing how to determine bra size helps the plastic surgeon communicate with his or her patient about desired breast size. Despite use of this system, a postoperative bra size is not guaranteed because bras vary by style and manufacturer, and many women fit well into more than one size of bra. Preoperative photographs illustrating the patient's goals remain helpful in assuring that the patient's perception of a particular bra size matches the surgeon's.

11.5
Conclusions

It is important for plastic surgeons to be able to measure a woman's bra size since many women express their goals for breast surgery in such terms. Because the traditional system of bra measurement was found to be inaccurate, an improved technique was developed. Experience has shown that almost every woman will fit the size bra determined to be right for her by this new system, even if she chooses to wear a bra of a different size for personal reasons.

References

1. Greenbaum AR, Heslop T, Morris J, Dunn KW: An investigation of the suitability of bra fit in women referred for reduction mammaplasty. Br J Plast Surg 2003;56(3):230–236
2. Pechter E: A new method for determining bra size and predicting postaugmentation breast size. Plast Reconstr Surg 1998;102(4):1259–1265
3. Pechter E: An improved technique for determining bra size with applicability to breast surgery. Plast Reconstr Surg 2008;121(5):348e–350e
4. Wadyka S: Cosmo's boob bible. Cosmopolitan 2004, Jan:170–173
5. Bodas sizing guide. http://www.bodas.co.uk/sizing.php. Accessed 18 March 2007
6. Wise RJ: A preliminary report on a method of planning the mammaplasty. Plast Reconstr Surg 1956;17(5):367–375
7. Ramselaar JM: Precision in breast reduction. Plast Reconstr Surg 1988;82(4):631–643
8. Young VL, Nemecek JR, Nemecek DA: The efficacy of breast augmentation: breast size increase, patient satisfaction, and psychological effects. Plast Reconstr Surg 1994;94(7):958–969
9. Kanhai RC, Hage JJ: Bra cup size depends on band size. Plast Reconstr Surg 1999;104(1):300
10. Dal Cin A, Jeans ER: Can reduction mammoplasty patients be promised a particular size postoperatively? Canad J Plast Surg 2005;13:13–15
11. Bates RL: The efficacy of breast augmentation: breast size increase, patient satisfaction, and psychological effects. Plast Reconstr Surg 1995;96:1237–1238
12. Schnur PL, Schnur DP, Petty P, Hansen TJ, Weaver AL: Reduction mammaplasty: an outcome study. Plast Reconstr Surg 1997;100(4):875–883
13. Lee HY, Hong K, Kim EA: Measurement protocol of women's nude breasts using a 3D scanning technique. Applied Ergonomics 2004;35(4):353–359
14. Tezel E, Numanoglu A: Practical do-it-yourself device for accurate volume measurement of the breast. Plast Reconstr Surg 2000;105(3):1019–1023
15. Turner AJ, Dujon DG: Predicting cup size after reduction mammaplasty. Br J Plast Surg 2005;58(3):290–298

CHAPTER 12

Breast Assessment and Implant Selection Using the TTM Aesthetic Breast Chart

12

Toma T. Mugea

12.1
Introduction

In the introduction to an ambitious cultural history, which covers some 25,000 years of thought about the female breast, Yalom [1] declares, "I intend to make you think about women's breasts as you never have before." She explains the reverence with which the breast has been considered over the centuries. In the section on "The Sacred Breast," she points out, "For all but a fraction of human history, there was no substitute for a mother's milk… a maternal breast meant life or death for every newborn babe." In "The Erotic Breast," Yalom examines the breast as an object of sexual desire, beginning with the appearance of Agnes Sorel, mistress of the king of France, with one bare, voluptuous breast exposed in a late 15th-century painting. The section "The Domestic Breast" examines the perceived link between domestic harmony and maternal nursing. Further insights into the social undertones that contribute to modern opinion about the breast are provided in "The Political Breast," which explores the historical notion that what is natural in the human body is good for the body politic. Specific moments when dramatic changes in breast lore took place appear in "The Psychological Breast." Examples include the appearance of a nursing Madonna in 14th-century art and the breast's assumption of a critical role in Sigmund Freud's psychoanalytic theories at the turn of the 20th century. "The Medical Breast" examines the breast primarily in regard to lactation and disease, with emphasis on those moments when some new understanding of physiology or pathology occurred. Surgeons will be particularly interested in accounts of the earliest recording of breast cancer in an Egyptian papyrus and the evolution of breast cancer surgery, including a gripping account of a mastectomy endured by English writer Fanny Burney in 1811.

In our day, both plastic surgeons and patients involved in breast aesthetic surgery have very demanding expectations to create or have the best breast in terms of size, proportion, and position, with minimal scars, long-term shape maintenance, and few complications.

To achieve these expectations, the surgeon must know and document the exact situation of the breast before the surgery (breast and chest measurements, photos), the patient's desire, and, if this desire is realistic, how it can be achieved. Of course, the aimed-for result must also be documented and recorded in the patient file. The last step in aesthetic surgery is the method to obtain what is desired from the actual (physical) situation.

Breast surgery is one of the most difficult fields of aesthetic surgery because of the complexity of surgical procedures and the relative guidelines defining the aesthetically perfect breast. Authors have presented different dimensions as representative of the aesthetically perfect breast [2–8], referring to a breast that is ideal and could not be improved further.

The perfect breast is aesthetically best appreciated on a perfect trunk and on a perfect body. It is also important to correlate the aesthetically perfect breast with the idea of beauty in different cultures. Many of the famous nude statues' breasts that in ancient Greece that were perceived as aesthetic would nowadays be slightly criticized as too small and therefore proposed for augmentation surgery, whereas the breasts of the nude models painted by Rubens in the Renaissance period would undoubtedly require reduction, according to the contemporary view.

At the same time, it is impossible to impose a single standard of breast beauty to women who are so entirely different in height, weight, and constitutional type. Therefore, we need to discover the sizes that are aesthetically right for each particular woman, starting from her main parameters: height, weight, trunk height (the distance between the manubrium notch and the pubis), width across the shoulders, and pelvic width at the level of the anterior superior iliac spines.

12.2
Preoperative Assessment Using the TTM Chart

12.2.1
Subjects and Breast Categories

About 10 years ago, the author studied 380 consecutive 15–65-year-old female subjects with normal chests and

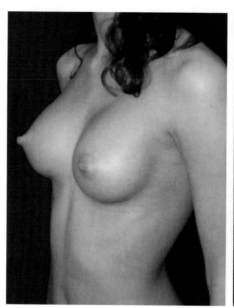 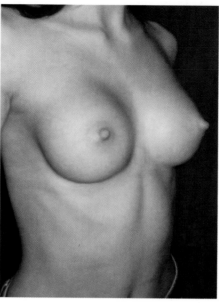

Fig. 12.1 a The aesthetically perfect breast (no common aesthetic procedures suggested). **b** Side view

no bone or spine deformities in order to collect different dimensions and find significant correlations between them in the cases of aesthetic breasts. Random cases were included, which consisted of women who came for consultations in aesthetic surgery, whether breast-related or not, and agreed to participate in the trial. All subjects were Caucasians representing a wide ethnic mixture.

Included were subjects in the following categories, in relation to female potential breast evolution in time:

1. Normal but unaesthetic breasts
2. Normal and aesthetic breasts
3. Aesthetically perfect breasts
4. Abnormal breasts

The author considered as normal a breast that was identified as such by the majority of women of the same age group and physiological status. A normal breast was estimated to have a volume somewhere between 300 ml and 500 ml, depending on the woman's physical build, and to be located sagitally between the 2nd and 7th ribs and transversely between the sternal edge and the anterior axillary line. The "tail" of the breast should extend toward the axilla, and the nipple should project at the height of the 4th intercostal gap [9].

The author considered as aesthetic the breast with a pleasant appearance, with a normal size and fullness, minimal ptosis, a conical to teardrop shape, and the nipple in the most anterior position, coming from a normal proportion, position, and projection.

The aesthetically perfect breast was one for which no common aesthetic procedures would be suggested. It is perfectly fit with a perfect body, in perfect harmony regarding proportion, position, and projection [10]. This is the "top model" situation (Fig. 12.1).

Because in normal life the female breast evolution is divided into five periods of time—teenager, young female, adult female, adult female age 40 and over, and elderly female—we admitted that a ptotic breast is normal in the last decades. Any modification in terms of hypertrophy, hypotrophy, or an early or advanced grade of ptosis according to the subject's biological status and age was considered abnormal.

Standards for the measurement technique were established as given below, and all measurements were made with the subject standing, with shoulders back and head straight ahead (Figs. 12.2, 12.3).

TTM® Chart

CODE:

Name: **XX**   Date: **YY**

Height: **1,64**   Weight: **50 kg**   Pregnancies: **0**   Weight Loss: **0**

Pinch Test: P= **2**   R= **4**

Chest problems: **NO**

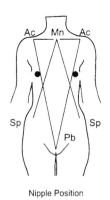

Nipple Position

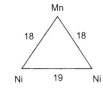

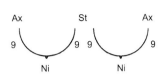

Areola Diameters

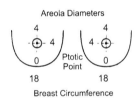

Breast Circumference

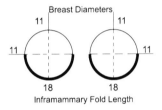

Inframammary Fold Length

Trunk measurements

Mn - Pb = 52

Ac - Ac = 30

Sp - Sp = 26

Chest Circumference

Ax Ch   = 80

Ni Ch   = 87

Infra Ch = 74

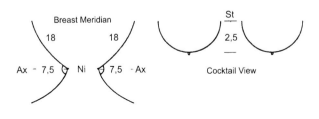

Notes:

Fig. 12.2 TTM chart

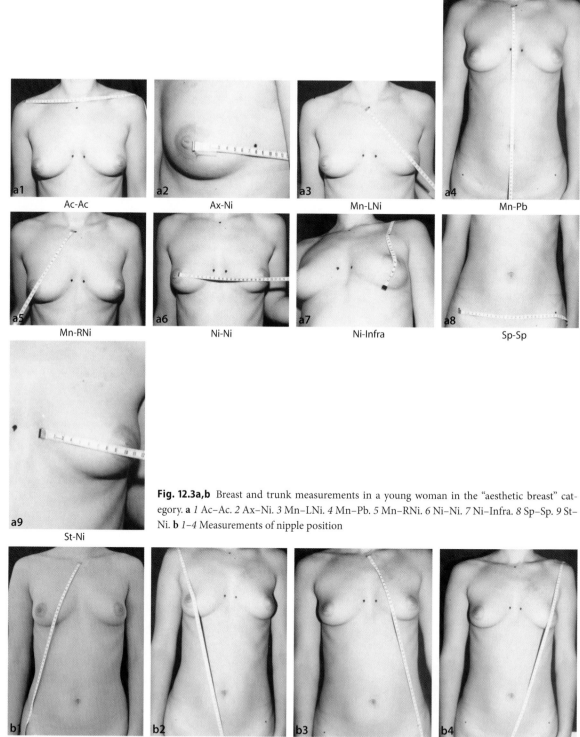

Ac-Ac

Ax-Ni

Mn-LNi

Mn-Pb

Mn-RNi

Ni-Ni

Ni-Infra

Sp-Sp

St-Ni

Fig. 12.3a,b Breast and trunk measurements in a young woman in the "aesthetic breast" category. **a** *1* Ac–Ac. *2* Ax–Ni. *3* Mn–LNi. *4* Mn–Pb. *5* Mn–RNi. *6* Ni–Ni. *7* Ni–Infra. *8* Sp–Sp. *9* St–Ni. **b** *1–4* Measurements of nipple position

Nipple position related to the inverted triangles (AcAcPb and SpSpMn)

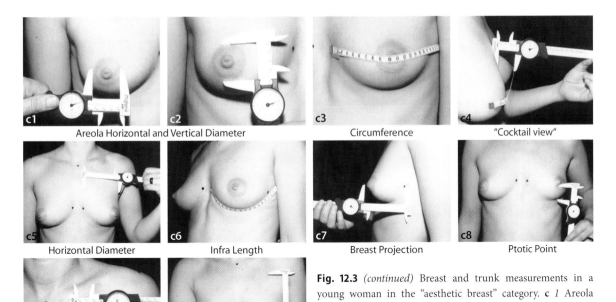

Fig. 12.3 *(continued)* Breast and trunk measurements in a young woman in the "aesthetic breast" category. **c** *1* Areola horizontal diameter. *2* Areola vertical diameter. *3* Circumference. *4* "Cocktail" view. *5* Horizontal diameter. *6* Inframammary crease length. *7* Projection. *8* Ptotic point. *9* Soft tissue thickness. *10* Vertical diameter

12.2.2
Use of the TTM Chart

Definitions of the points and measurements used in the TTM chart (Fig. 12.2) are as follows:

Mn (manubrium)	Suprasternal notch
Pb (pubis)	Superior edge of the pubis bone
Ac (acromion)	Lateral edge of the acromion bone
Sp (spinal)	Anterosuperior spine of the iliac bone
Ni (nipple)	Nipple
PP (ptotic point)	Lowest point of the ptotic breast in the standing position; on the chart we note the distance in centimeters between this point and the nipple
BUP (breast upper pole)	Anatomical landmark of the upper pole of the breast, corresponding to the 2nd rib space
Mn–Pb	Distance between the manubrium notch and the superior edge of the pubis, measured over the trunk and abdomen (in a thin female patient, this distance is a straight line, but in an obese one, it is a large curved line, and even the abdominal apron is measured)
Ac–Ac	Distance between the acromion points
Sp–Sp	Distance between the spine points (in a thin female patient, this distance is a straight line, and in an obese one, it is a large curved line)
Mn–RNi	Distance between the manubrium notch and the right nipple
Mn–LNi	Distance between the manubrium notch and the left nipple
Ni–Ni	Distance between the nipples
Ax–Ni	Distance between the axillary end of the inframammary fold and the nipple (in a normal breast, this is a straight line, but in a ptotic breast this line has an "S" shape)

St–Ni	Distance between the sternal end of the inframammary fold and the nipple
Ni–Infra	Distance between the nipple and the inframammary fold (the vertical measurement must follow the shape of the breast)
Ni–PP	Distance between the nipple to the ptotic point
AvD	Areolar vertical diameter (from margin to margin)
AhD	Areolar horizontal diameter (from margin to margin)
Infra length	Inframammary fold length, measured from the axillary end to the sternal end of the fold
BVM	Breast vertical meridian; the distance between the BUP and the inframammary fold level over the nipple
BHM	Breast horizontal meridian; the longer distance between the axillary end of the inframammary fold and the sternal end of the inframammary fold, following the shape of the breast, over the nipple
Breast mould meridians	Virtual lines between the nipple and the breast mould edges (Fig. 12.4)
BSM	Breast superior meridian; the virtual line between the upper edge of the breast mould and the nipple
BIM	Breast inferior meridian; the virtual line between the lower edge of the breast mould and the nipple (this corresponds to the Ni–Infra distance)
BMM	Breast medial meridian; the virtual line between the medial breast mould edge and the nipple (this corresponds to the St–Ni distance)
BLM	Breast lateral meridian; the virtual line between the lateral breast mould edge and the nipple (this corresponds to the Ax–Ni distance)
BC	Breast circumference; the longer distance between the axillary end

	of the inframammary fold and the sternal end of the inframammary fold, following the shape of the breast. In the aesthetic breast, breast circumference is identical to the BHM
BP	Breast projection; the distance between the nipple and the anterior axillary line, in standing position, measured as a straight line using a caliper
CW	Cocktail view; the distance between the sternum and the horizontal line connecting the most anterior points of the breasts in standing position, measured as a straight line using a caliper)
BVD	Breast vertical diameter; the distance between the breast anatomical landmarks in the sagittal plane, measured with a caliper
BHD	Breast horizontal diameter; the distance between the breast anatomical landmarks in the horizontal plane, corresponding to the medial and lateral edges of the inframammary fold
Ax–Ch	Axillary chest circumference; the chest circumference measured at the axillary level
Ni–Ch	Nipple chest circumference; the chest circumference measured over the most projected points of the breasts, which may correspond to the nipple in a normal aesthetic breast or may not correspond in a ptotic breast
Infra–Ch	Infrachest circumference; the chest circumference measured at the level of the inframammary fold
AcAcPb	Acromion pubic triangle, defined by the lines between the acromion points and the superior edge of the pubic bone
SpSpMn	Spinomanubrial triangle, defined by the lines between the manubrium notch and the anterior superior iliac spine points (Fig. 12.5)

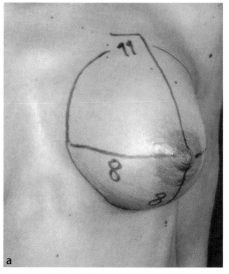
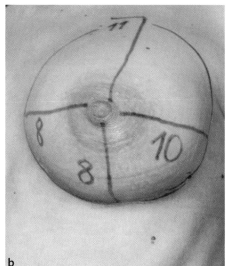
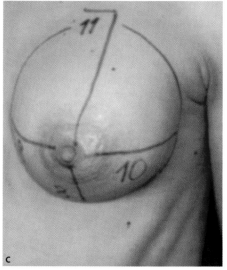
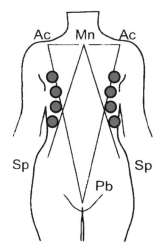

Fig. 12.4a–c Breast meridians from the nipple to the breast mould edges

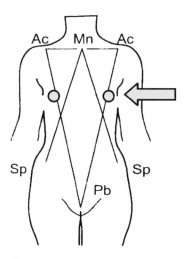

🔴 **Nipple Areola Complex gliding**   ⚪ **Aesthetic perfect position**

Fig. 12.5 Nipple–areola complex. **a** Natural gliding process. **b** The aesthetically perfect position related to the "inverted triangles"

Table 12.1 Age groups and breast types of subjects

Breast types	15–25 Years	26–35 Years	36–49 Years	50–65 Years	Total
Normal and unaesthetic breast	30	16	41	10	97
Normal and aesthetic breast	18	24	39	1	82
Aesthetically perfect breast	24	23	3	–	50
Abnormal breast	6	38	64	43	151
Total number of cases	**78**	**101**	**147**	**54**	**380**

Table 12.2 Measurement results (in centimeters) for the 50 cases of aesthetically perfect breasts found in a series of 380 consecutive female subjects age 15–65 years old

Nr.	age	H Cm	W Kg	Mn Pb	Ac Ac	Sp Sp	Mn RNi	Mn Lni	Ni Ni	Ax Ni
1	30	174	67	60	40	24	21	19	18	8
2	29	153	40	51	33	25	17	18	17	8
3	23	160	50	54	36	24	19	19	21	10
4	23	165	49	55	34	26	19	19	19	8
5	28	162	58	54	35	25	21	21	21	10
6	19	172	58	59	37	28	19	19	19	8
7	28	168	53	55	37	27	21	21	21	10
8	26	172	60	54	39	29	20	20	20	10
9	28	173	60	59	40	29	21	21	21	10
10	20	166	54	55	37	28	18	18	18	8
11	27	167	57	54	35	27	18	18	19	9
12	42	170	71	58	37	30	20	20	21	10
13	32	170	52	57	34	27	18	18	18	8
14	32	162	57	53	33	26	20	20	21	10
15	30	169	65	55	38	29	18	18	19	8
16	33	162	47	53	33	23	18	18	18	8
17	19	155	50	49	34	24	18	18	18	8
18	20	165	53	53	37	25	18	18	19	8
19	33	165	49	56	36	28	21	21	21	10
20	25	163	52	50	37	29	18	18	19	9
21	21	175	62	56	34	27	19	19	20	9
22	24	168	53	53	34	24	18	18	19	9
23	29	172	68	57	35	27	19	19	19	9
24	25	158	53	51	36	27	20	20	21	9

H height (cm), *W* weight (kg), *Mn* manubrium notch, *Pb* pubis, *Sp* spinal, *St* sternal, *Ni* nipple, *RNi* right nipple, *LNi* left nipple, *Ax–Ni* distance between axillary end of he inframammary fold and nipple, *Infra* inframammary fold length, *BHM* breast horizontal meridian, *BC* breast circumference, *BVM* breast vertical meridian, *AvD* areola vertical diameter, *AhD* areola horizontal diameter,

Considering the natural evolution with aging, normal nipple positions related to the "inverted triangles" are downward gliding on the external margins of the inverted triangles, corresponding to a high position in young teenagers and to a low position in elderly female patients.

The aesthetically perfect position was found to be in the upper part of the triangles, close to the junction point of the external margins (Fig. 12.5b).

The author classified the subjects into four age groups and four breast types (Table 12.1). Table 12.2 presents the results of the measurements (in centimeters) for the 50 cases of aesthetically perfect breasts that were found in the series of 380 consecutive female subjects age 15–65 years old.

The "K" number, representing the key to the aesthetic breast, or the "breast golden number," is the result of our calculations with a special program [10] designed to find and show the relationship between the breast and trunk dimensions.

The following connections between K and other distances were found in aesthetic breasts:

K = ideal aesthetic triangle
K= inframammary fold length
K = breast horizontal meridian (identical to breast circumference)
K= breast vertical meridian
K:2 = breast medial and lateral meridians (St–Ni, Ax–Ni)
K:3 = breast inferior meridian (Ni–Infra)

St Ni	Infra	Ni Infra	BHM BC	BVM	AvD	AhD	Ax Ch	Ni Ch	Infra Ch	BVD	BHD
8	19	7	20	19	6	6.3	81	82	77	12.5	12.5
8	18	5	18	18	5.5	5.5	75	78	70	10	10
10	21	7	21	20	5	5	85	90	82	12.5	12.5
8	19	7	19	19	5	5	84	89	78	12.5	12.5
10	21	7	21	21	5	5	87	91	82	12.5	12.5
8	19	6.5	19	19	5	5	83	87	78	11.5	11.5
10	20	7	21	21	5	5	83	86	77	12.5	12.5
10	20	6.5	20	20	4.5	4.5	91	93	85	11.5	11.5
10	21	7	21	21	4.7	4.7	84	91	80	12.5	12.5
8	18	6	18	17	4.4	4.4	81	83	76	11	11
9	19	6	19	19	4.5	4.5	83	86	80	11	11
10	20	6.7	21	21	5	5	86	89	81	11.5	11.5
8	18	6	18	18	4.5	4.5	81	85	78	11	11
10	21	7	21	21	5	5	84	89	76	12.5	12.5
8	19	6	18	18	4.3	4.3	82	86	78	11	11
8	19	6	18	18	4.5	4.5	79	84	74	11	11
8	19	6	19	19	4.7	4.7	78	83	75	11	11
8	19	6	19	19	4.5	4.5	80	85	79	11	11
11	21	7	22	21	5.2	5.2	78	85	71	12.5	12.5
9	18	6	19	19	4.7	4.7	79	82	75	11	11
9	19	6	19	19	5	5	83	84	77	11	11
9	19	6	19	19	4.7	4.7	79	83	76	11	11
9	19	6.5	19	19	5	5	82	86	77	11.5	11.5
9	20	6.5	20	20	4.7	4.7	86	94	86	11	11

Ax–Ch chest circumference at axillary level, *Ni–Ch* chest circumference at nipple level, *Infra–ch* chest circumference at inframammary fold level, *BVD* breast vertical diameter, *BHD* breast horizontal diameter

Table 12.2 *(continued)* Measurement results (in centimeters) for the 50 cases of aesthetically perfect breasts found in a series of 380 consecutive female subjects age 15–65 years old

Nr.	age	H Cm	W Kg	Mn Pb	Ac Ac	Sp Sp	Mn RNi	Mn Lni	Ni Ni	Ax Ni
25	32	180	68	51	35	29	19	19	20	9
26	20	173	57	54	34	27	19	19	19	8
27	26	168	50	55	29	23	18	18	18	9
28	22	164	65	51	34	29	20	20	20	10
29	27	170	50	53	33	26	18	18	18	9
30	19	175	57	59	35	25	19	19	20	8
31	26	170	60	57	38	28	21	21	21	10
32	17	173	54	57	29	25	18	18	18	9
33	24	170	52	53	34	23	18	18	19	9
34	20	170	58	53	34	28	19	19	19	9
35	22	162	49	52	34	24	18	18	18	9
36	25	176	61	57	38	24	21	21	21	10
37	20	165	50	54	37	24	19	19	19	9
38	22	168	68	56	37	32	21	21	21	10
39	27	164	53	55	33	27	19	19	19	8
40	23	170	57	54	34	25	18	18	19	9
41	25	162	56	51	37	26	19	19	19	9
42	19	170	48	50	32	26	18	18	18	8
43	19	156	60	54	37	27	20	20	20	10
44	36	169	60	55	35	28	19	19	19	9
45	32	173	65	59	39	26	20	20	20	9
46	36	162	48	55	33	26	19	19	20	9
47	31	164	52	53	32	25	18	18	18	9
48	27	164	59	49	39	30	21	21	21	10
49	30	166	54	51	36	23	18	18	18	9
50	30	168	54	57	32	27	19	19	19	9

H height (cm), *W* weight (kg), *Mn* manubrium notch, *Pb* pubis, *Sp* spinal, *St* sternal, *Ni* nipple, *RNi* right nipple, *LNi* left nipple, *Ax–Ni* distance between axillary end of he inframammary fold and nipple, *Infra* inframammary fold length, *BHM* breast horizontal meridian, *BC* breast circumference, *BVM* breast vertical meridian, *AvD* areola vertical diameter, *AhD* areola horizontal diameter,

St Ni	Infra	Ni Infra	BHM BC	BVM	AvD	AhD	Ax Ch	Ni Ch	Infra Ch	BVD	BHD
9	20	6.5	20	20	5	5	90	94	84	11.5	11.5
9	19	6	19	19	4.5	4.5	83	86	79	11	11
9	19	6	19	19	4.6	4.6	73	78	70	11	11
10	20	6.5	20	19	5	5	84	87	78	11.5	11.5
9	19	6	19	19	4.5	4.5	76	80	67	11	11
9	20	6.5	19	19	5	5	86	88	82	11.5	11.5
10	21	6.8	21	20	5	5	83	87	20	11.5	11.5
9	18	6	19	19	4.3	4.3	79	84	76	11	11
9	19	6	19	19	4.5	4.5	82	85	79	11	11
9	20	6.3	19	19	5	5	86	89	80	11	11
9	18	6.3	18	18	4.2	4.2	77	85	72	11	11
10	21	6.8	21	20	5.1	5.1	79	85	77	11.5	11.5
9	19	6.5	19	19	4.3	4.3	82	86	79	11.5	11.5
10	21	7	21	20	4.8	4.8	90	94	83	12	12
9	19	6.4	19	19	4.4	4.4	79	82	75	11.5	11.5
9	19	6	19	19	4.5	4.5	88	94	83	11	11
9	19	6	19	19	4.8	4.8	81	87	78	11	11
8	18	6	18	18	4.2	4.2	77	81	71	11	11
10	20	6.8	20	20	5	5	87	92	80	12	12
9	19	6.2	19	19	4.6	4.6	84	89	78	11	11
10	20	6.7	20	20	5	5	86	89	80	12	12
9	19	6	20	20	4.3	4.3	75	79	72	11	11
9	18	6	18	18	4.5	4.5	81	85	77	11	11
10	21	7	21	21	5	5	83	92	78	12.5	12.5
9	18	6	19	19	4.3	4.2	82	88	75	11	11
9	19	6.1	19	19	4.6	4.6	83	86	77	11	11

Ax–Ch chest circumference at axillary level, *Ni–Ch* chest circumference at nipple level, *Infra–ch* chest circumference at inframammary fold level, *BVD* breast vertical diameter, *BHD* breast horizontal diameter

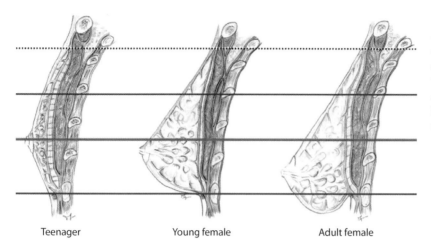

Fig. 12.6 Breast mould development and natural gliding on the chest wall. The *dotted line* represents the breast upper pole (anatomical landmark level), the *blue lines* represent the breast mould limits, and the *red line* represents the initial nipple level

The breast golden number shows, in the aesthetic breast, the identical length of the inframammary fold, breast circumference, breast vertical meridian, breast horizontal meridian, and ideal triangle. This is proof that the breast can be considered to have a hemispheric shape, with the nipple in the middle, in the most prominent point in the normal growing phase (Fig. 12.6). Because the breast will gain weight because of gravity and ligament tightening, the breast mould will translate in the lower two-thirds of the breast vertical meridian, together with the nipple–areola complex.

In the aesthetic breast, the nipple will be the center of this mould and will be located at two-thirds below the breast upper pole (anatomical landmark) and one-third superior to the inframammary fold level.

Because of the weight of the tissues, the upper two-thirds of the breast skin is stretched, and the tissues corresponding to the lower third of the breast meridian are compressed. If a significant part of the breast weight will be removed (as in breast reduction), it will retract. Any additional breast weight, natural or by implant, will stretch the soft tissue including the skin and ligaments and will led to a ptotic breast appearance.

In breast asymmetries, in some cases, an aesthetic situation and a ptotic breast can be found on the patient at the same time (Fig. 12.7). Pseudoptosis, glandular ptosis, and true ptosis [11, 12] are represented in Fig. 12.8.

The ideal breast measurements suggested by the computer program, based on trunk measurements, are suitable for thin or normal weight patients.

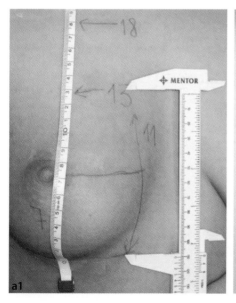

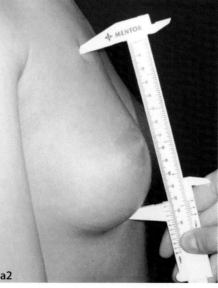

Fig. 12.7 a Right breast mould vertical diameters (13 cm in perimeter length = superior + inferior meridians, and 11 cm in straight length). *1* Note the breast vertical meridian length (18 cm), measured from the inframammary fold to the superior anatomical landmark, over the nipple. *2* Side view

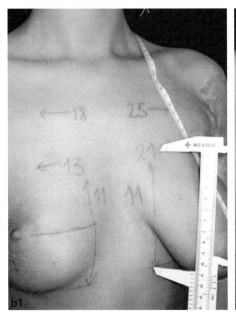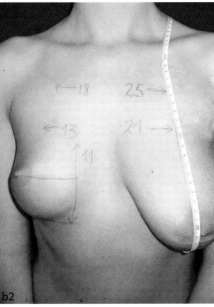

Fig. 12.7 (*continued*)
b *1* The left, ptotic breast shows the same breast mould vertical diameter value in straight length (11 cm), but 21 cm in perimeter length. *2* Note the breast vertical meridian length (25 cm), measured between the inframammary fold level and the superior anatomical landmark (breast upper pole), over the nipple

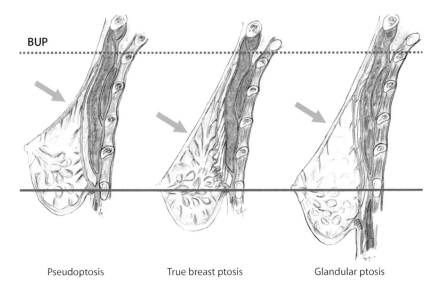

Fig. 12.8 Breast pseudoptosis (only the breast mould is hanging; the nipple and the inframammary fold are at the same level as in the normal situation). In glandular ptosis, the whole breast (including nipple, breast mould, and inframammary fold) glides over the chest, between the deep layer of the superficial fascia and the superficial layer of the deep fascia, because of the sustaining ligaments' laxity. In true breast ptosis, because of the breast weight, the breast organ hangs on the skin and the inframammary sustaining ligament [11, 12]. The *dotted line* shows the breast upper pole level (*BUP*; anatomical landmark), and the *lower line* shows the 6th rib level, where the inframammary fold level used to be. The *arrow* shows the upper pole of the breast mould

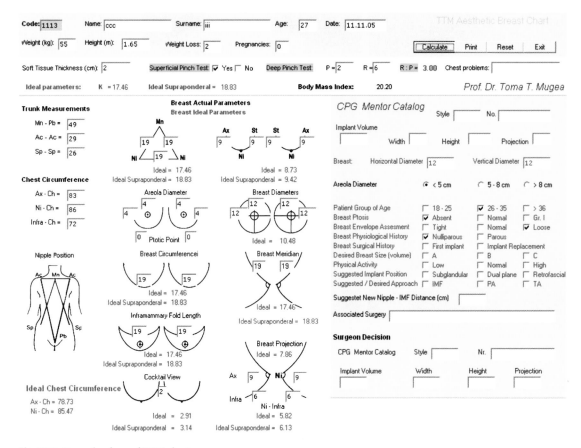

Fig. 12.9 Example of use of TTM chart

In the case of overweight patients, a correction factor is introduced that is related to the body mass index. Because in overweight patients we have to deal mainly with breast reduction or mastopexy, this new key is called key for breast reduction (KBR).

For the overweight patient, the ideal aesthetic triangle, inframammary fold length, breast vertical meridian, and breast circumference have the same value as the KBR. This is the breast golden number for overweight patients.

In Fig. 12.9, the trunk and breast dimensions of an overweight young female are shown. In her case, the dimensions correspond to her body weight, as can be seen on the TTM chart. In this case the breast golden number is 19 (ideal aesthetic triangle, inframammary fold length, breast circumference, and breast vertical meridian). Nipple location is at the junction of the upper two-thirds with the lower third on the breast vertical meridian.

To estimate skin tightening and elasticity, the superficial pinch test and the deep pinch test are used (Fig. 12.10). In the superficial pinch test, the smallest amount of skin and soft tissue that can be moved over the superficial fascia is grasped. If this test cannot be done, the skin is too tight and under tension, and breast augmentation cannot benefit from a full-projection implant.

In the deep pinch test, the largest amount of skin and soft tissues is grasped, without pectoralis musculofascial elements that can still be moved over the deeper structures (pectoralis fascia). If two dots are marked at the end of the stretched line and measurements are taken with the caliper arms, the two distances can be compared in the relaxed (R) and the pinched (P) situations.

If the deep pinch test shows an R:P ratio <2, this corresponds to a tight situation. The soft tissue is too tight, and the patient cannot benefit from a full-projection implant in breast augmentation. This situation can also be found in some candidates for breast reconstruction in whom tissue expansion is necessary.

If the deep pinch test shows the R:P ratio to be between 2 and 3, this corresponds to normal soft tissue elasticity. Breast augmentation can be done according to the chart suggestions, with midsize projection.

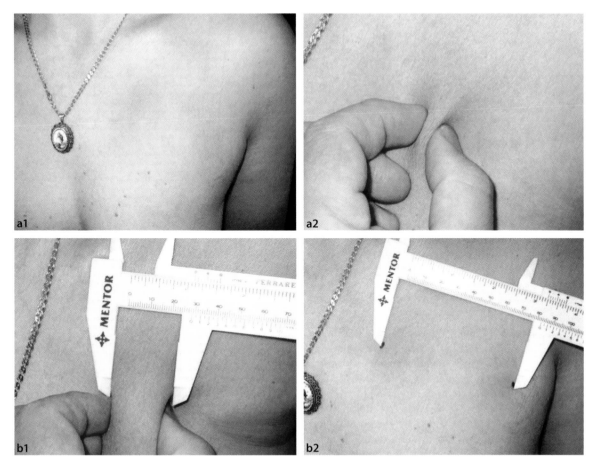

Fig. 12.10 a *1, 2* The superficial pinch test on the upper pole of the breast shows normal tension in the superficial subcutaneous layer. **b** The deep pinch test on the upper pole of the breast shows the soft tissue thickness and good skin elasticity. *1* The pinched distance is 2.5 cm. *2* The relaxed distance is 8 cm. The relaxed-to-pinched ratio (R:P) is >3, and a full-projection implant can be suggested

If the deep pinch test shows an R:P ratio >3, this corresponds to loose soft tissue or excess skin, as in the ptotic breast. The implant selected must have the largest projection for that specific breast diameter, or an associated mastopexy procedure may be necessary.

In some cases, the author observed different results of the superficial and deep pinch tests in different anatomical regions of the abdominal wall (Fig. 12.11). If in the epigastric area the soft tissues are tight, the hypogastric area that has been expanded by a pregnancy usually shows relaxed or even excessive soft tissues.

The challenge in plastic surgery is that there is no one implant, incision, or pocket plane that is appropriate to treat every patient. It is this notion that makes breast augmentation both an art and a science.

Although there is no one single technique for breast augmentation that is considered best, one must take the options that are available in conjunction with physical examination of the patient to create a sound surgical plan for achieving an aesthetic, natural-looking augmented breast.

Our approach to breast augmentation incorporates patient wishes with a detailed, individualized analysis of the chest wall and breast. Each patient receives a thorough physical examination and a photographic examination, even from the back, to detect asymmetries.

When critically examined using the TTM chart, nearly 80% of the women had asymmetries and more than one parameter of asymmetry. These data suggest that to obtain optimal results in breast augmentation, we should consider a highly individualized and comprehensive approach that takes into account breast and chest wall asymmetries. Also, appropriate preoperative counseling with each patient can eliminate the majority

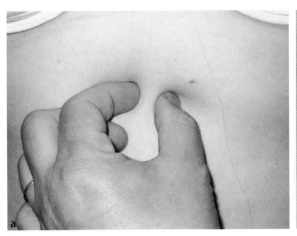
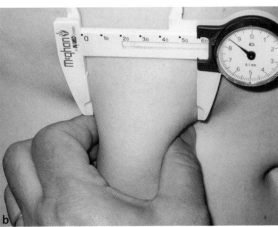

Fig. 12.11 a Superficial pinch test cannot be done in the epigastric area, in this case showing tension in the superficial subcutaneous layer. **b** Deep pinch test in the epigastric area shows the soft tissue thickness (6 cm) and low skin elasticity. The relaxed-to-pinched ratio (R:P) is <1.5

of postoperative complaints. By explaining that breast asymmetries are the rule rather than the exception and that subtle differences preoperatively may be more obvious after breast augmentation, patients will have a more realistic expectation for the final results.

The initial evaluation should focus on the chest wall itself for symmetry and shape. Any chest wall abnormalities, such as degrees of pectus excavatum or carinatum, should be noted on the chart and discussed with the patient using digital photographs to illustrate. If in pectus excavatum cases the nipples will be projected in a straight and parallel direction, in pectus carinatum cases the nipples will become more divergent as the breast volume will grow.

Any asymmetry or degree of rib flaring should be discussed. The presence and degree of breast ptosis should be documented, as any degree of ptosis greater than grade II may suggest a possible concomitant mastopexy and should be discussed. Also, breast asymmetries should be identified. These asymmetries include breast mound volume, inframammary fold position, the presence of base diameter constriction, and asymmetries of the nipple–areola complex size and position [13]. In our experience, unless a marked degree of asymmetry is observed, most patients benefit from using the same size implants on both sides. Minor tailoring may be achieved by adjusting fill volumes, whereas using implants with different diameters and volumes can often exacerbate an underlying asymmetry.

The procedure of breast augmentation confronts the surgeon with three distinct variables requiring decisions in the preoperative process: implant selection, incision location, and pocket plane.

12.3
Implant Selection

12.3.1
Surface Texture and Implant Fill

Historically, textured implants have been found to lower the capsular contracture rate [14, 15]. The differences between textured and nontextured implants seem to decrease when both are placed in the subpectoral position. The incidence of capsular contracture with saline-filled implants may decrease to nearly 1% when the implant is placed in the subpectoral position [16]. Therefore, surface texturing does not appear to offer a clear advantage in avoiding capsular contracture when the implants are placed submuscularly. Textured implants are recommended in patients with adequate soft tissue for whom subglandular positioning of the implant is desired.

The latest generation of silicone implants contains a soft cohesive gel that is slightly firmer than earlier silicone gel implants. This cohesive gel implant is a form-stable device that retains its anatomical shape (memory gel) even with some degree of capsular contracture or loss of integrity of the shell envelope. When cut or ruptured, the shape of the implant remains intact, and the silicone does not run out.

One aspect of these devices is that their use requires careful evaluation of the patient's chest dimensions to determine the appropriate style of implant [17]. The devices are available in a wide variety of dimensions that vary in height and projection.

12.3.2
Shape

Round implants can be considered to be more forgiving, enabling the creation of an aesthetically pleasing breast with a variety of patient shapes. In general, if there is an aesthetically shaped breast as well as relative volume to the existing breast, a round or shaped implant device is an appropriate choice. Round implants can appear somewhat anatomical, given a loose periprosthetic space in the setting of an underfilled device. This situation, however, carries an increased risk of shell folds, visible rippling, and possible early device failure [18].

Thin patients, patients with a high inframammary crease, patients with a vertically or horizontally deficient chest, and ptotic patients have a greater risk of excessive upper-pole fullness and distortion when augmented with round implants. In these cases, the anatomical implant provides valuable additional options to alter the breast shape.

Anatomically shaped implants refer to devices with a vertical axis that is different in dimension from the horizontal axis, and the biggest projection point is situated in the lower pole. Tall teardrop shapes are best suited for patients with a long chest or low breast position. A reduced-height-shaped device creates a relatively exaggerated width with abbreviated height to decrease upper-pole fullness [19]. With an anatomically shaped implant, there is a diminished tendency toward upper-pole bulges, roundness, or distortion, and there is greater volume support for the lower breast.

In our experience, anatomic implants retain their basic shape, whether recumbent or upright, because of the shape built into the device. A caveat unique to using these shaped devices is implant rotation [16]. Meticulous attention must be paid to not over-dissect the implant pocket, which would make rotation more likely. In difficult cases, we recommend postoperative use of a support brassiere with a binder strip placed across the superior pole of the breasts for 10–14 days to minimize the risk of rotation.

12.3.3
Dimensions

Usually, a wrong decision made in planning breast augmentation is related to wrong selection of implant size. Whether this is attributable to poorly managed patient expectations or to surgeon ignorance, it produces implant malposition conditions that are difficult to correct. The most important landmark for the breast is the inframammary fold and the associated breast width. This determines the natural limits of the breast. Size is ultimately determined by the base diameter of the breast, whereas shape is determined by projection in relation to base diameter. In general, we have found that a breast with a narrow base diameter does better with a round or anatomical implant with a smaller base diameter that yields slightly greater projection per unit volume than with a wider base diameter implant.

In breast augmentation aesthetic surgery, the author likes to respect several principles:

– Do not touch an aesthetically perfect breast. A breast augmentation operation means at least one surgery.
– Do not fall into the trap of a patient who wants to have large breasts outside the dimension (diameters) of the breast, if they are normal.
– Do not make the cocktail view too deep and narrow by moving the medial pocket location onto the sternum even slightly.
– Do not change the inframammary fold position by surgery unless significant inframammary fold abnormalities exist (as in the case of a tuberous breast deformity).
– Select the inframammary approach as the first option.
– Select the retrofascial position as the first option for the implant pocket if the quality of the soft tissues allows good coverage for the upper pole of the implant.
– Select an anatomical implant with memory gel as the first option, using the TTM chart and computer program.

12.3.4
TTM Chart and Computer Program for Anatomical Implant Selection

All the patient-collected data and desired cup sizes (A, B, C) were introduced into the chart and computer program (Fig. 12.12, with patient in Fig. 12.13 as the example) specially designed to calculate the ideal aesthetic parameters for the patient in her specific condition, even if she is thin or overweight. Note the correspondence between the aesthetic dimensions defined by the TTM chart and the end result of surgery (Fig. 12.14).

On the right side of the screen, the program will automatically suggest the implant selected from the CPG Mentor catalog, according to the breast diameters, soft tissue coverage and elasticity, and patient cup desire. The augmented breast must also look natural and fit the patient's body. Patients with demands for with extra size are not included in this program, being outside the aesthetic rules. Also, we can simulate for the patient what the aesthetic breast situation will be according to the different conditions of her body weight.

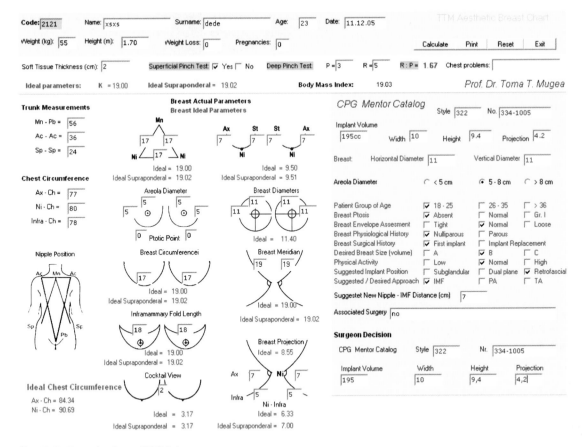

Fig. 12.12 Example of use of TTM chart

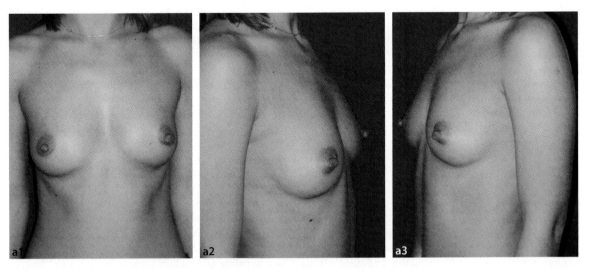

Fig. 12.13 Patient with breast augmentation. **a** *1–3* Preoperative views

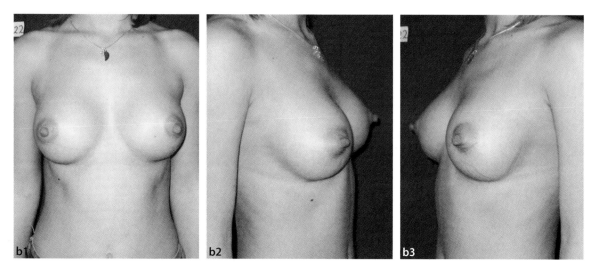

Fig. 12.13 *(continued)* Patient with breast augmentation. **b** *1–3* Postoperative views

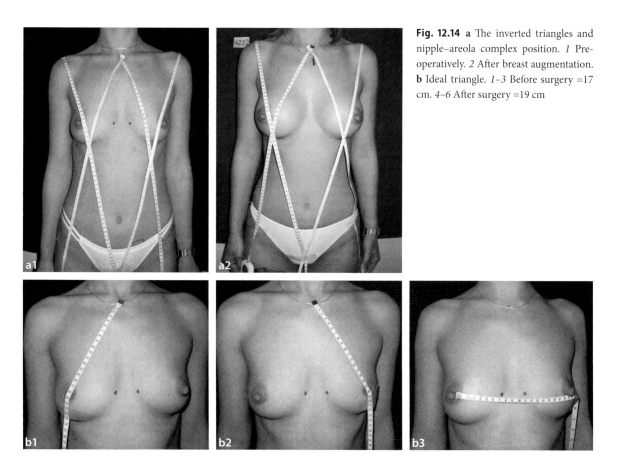

Fig. 12.14 a The inverted triangles and nipple–areola complex position. *1* Preoperatively. *2* After breast augmentation. **b** Ideal triangle. *1–3* Before surgery =17 cm. *4–6* After surgery =19 cm

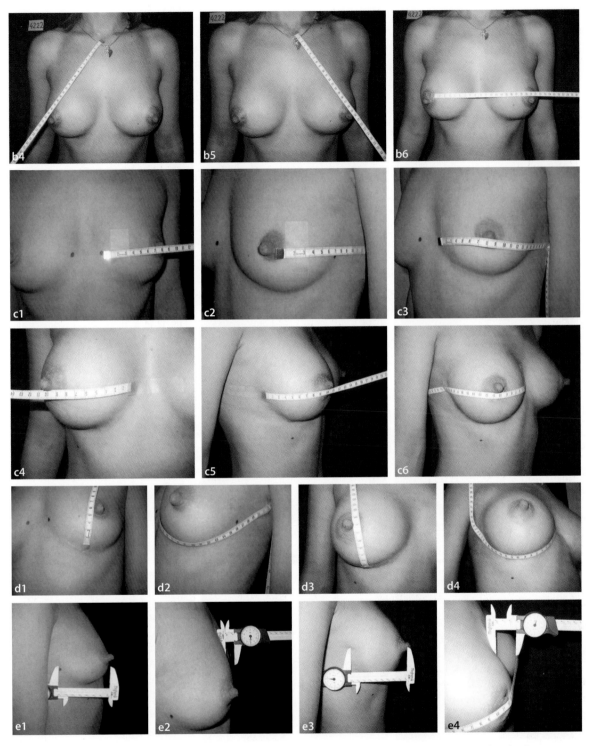

Fig. 12.14 *(continued)* **b** Ideal triangle. *1–3* Before surgery =17 cm. *4–6* After surgery =19 cm. **c** St–Ni and Ax–Ni distances and breast circumference. *1–3* St–Ni and Ax–Ni distances (7 cm) and breast circumference (17 cm) before surgery. *4–6* St–Ni (9 cm) and Ax – Ni (10 cm) distances and breast circumference (19 cm) after surgery. **d** Ni–Infra distance and inframammary fold length. *1, 2* Ni–Infra distance (5 cm) and inframammary fold length (17 cm) before surgery. *3, 4* Ni–Infra distance (7 cm) and inframammary fold length (19 cm) after surgery. **e** Breast projection and "cocktail view." *1, 2* Breast projection (7 cm) and "cocktail view" (2 cm) before surgery. *3, 4* Breast projection (9 cm) and "cocktail view" (3 cm) after surgery

If the surgeon selects another implant, he or she will fill in the section "surgeon decision" and can later compare the differences. This is also a comparative prospective study, allowing surgeons to correct even the algorithm of implant selection.

12.3.5
Additional Measurements for Anatomical Implants

Implant companies provide surgeons with detailed tables of implant dimensions, including the length, width, and height of any given implant volume. For anatomically shaped implants, they also describe high, moderate, and low projections for different implant heights at the same diameter.

To find more data about anatomical implant dimensions useful in operative planning and implant selection, the author did additional measurements, using a regular caliper and measuring in centimeters.

Because the sagittal length of the inner soft tissue covering of the implant is a very important dimension for implant accommodation, we consider this a fourth dimension of the anatomical implants, called the perimeter height. (See Fig. 12.15.) This fourth dimension of the implant is found by measuring the longer distance between the lower and the upper poles of the implant, corresponding to the vertical diameter, over the most projected point.

For implants with similar diameters, the perimeter height is greater in high-projection implants and smaller in low-projection devices.

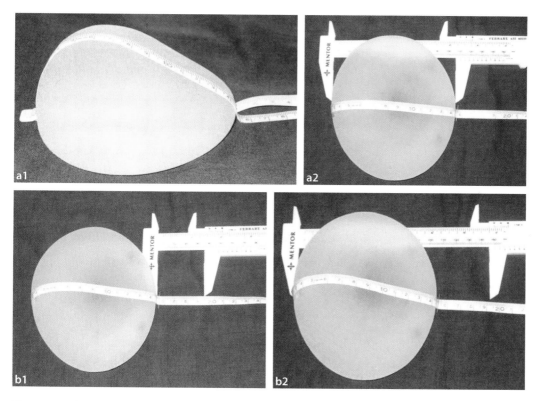

Fig. 12.15 a The implant measurement is 16 cm in perimeter height (*1*) and 11 cm in straight height (*2*). Mentor implant, CPG 323 style, high projection, volume 300 ml. (Catalog device dimensions are width 11.0 cm, height 10.3 cm, projection 5.6 cm.) **b** The difference between the perimeter (*1*: 15 cm) and the straight height (*2*: 11 cm) dimensions is 4 cm

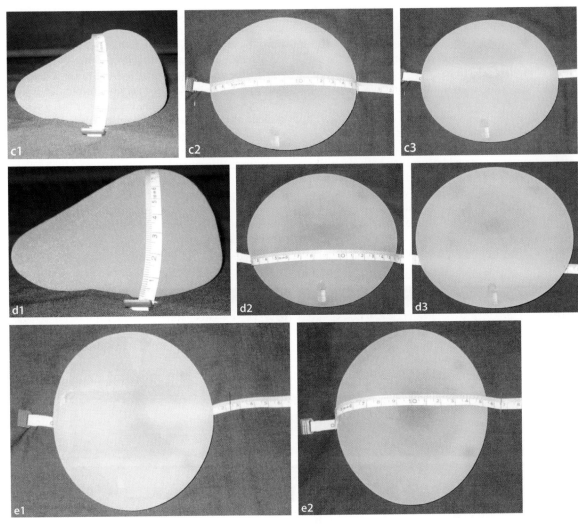

Fig. 12.15 *(continued)* **c** Perimeter diameter (17 cm) of the implant at maximum straight horizontal diameter level (*1*); implant labeled as width 13 cm (*2*). **d** *1, 2* Perimeter diameter (17 cm). *3* The straight horizontal diameter length (12 cm) at the maximum projection level. **e** *1* Simulation of a normal soft tissue cover length draping the implant. *2* In this example, 15 cm

The perimeter diameter is the fifth dimension of the anatomical implant and is found by measuring the distance between the left and right edges of the implant, over the convex face. This dimension can be measured corresponding to the horizontal diameter, or labeled implant width, or at the maximum projection level. Note the similar perimeter diameters of the implant at the maximum straight diameter and maximum projection level (17 cm). These dimensions came from "clinical" rough measurements, with a "soft" centimeter.

12.4
Soft Tissue Cover Tension and Capsule Formation

To obtain a well-accommodated implant as well as good tension over the implant, the pocket needs to have 1 cm of extra length in the straight height (in our example, 11 + 1 = 12 cm), and the soft tissue cover must provide at least 4 cm of extra length to the straight height, provided by soft tissue excess and elasticity, to match the implant perimeter height (Fig. 12.15).

In practice, to find the soft tissue cover length before surgery, we have to determine the difference between R and P (relaxed and pinched deep pinch test values) and add this to the breast mould vertical diameter (BMVD), which is usually smaller than the anatomical breast diameter defined by anatomical landmarks. This value [BMVD + v] represents the soft tissue cover length and must fit the implant perimeter height. The author has suggested to the implant device companies to put these implants' additional dimensions on the box label to help surgeons in implant selection.

Implant cover length that is too tight leads to a smaller implant projection and implant deformity, with lateral fullness and rippling. An implant with similar diameters but lower projection (smaller perimeter height) is required.

Choosing an implant with a greater base diameter will lead to unnatural fullness, both superiorly and inferiorly, and can lead to restrictions in arm motion laterally with synmastia medially.

The ideal aesthetic result in breast augmentation is obtained when there is a perfect match between implant selection and breast pocket dimensions, leading to good tension of the covering soft tissue over the implant [18]. In this situation the implant will be kept in position, maintaining the shape. Without dead space in the pocket, the fibrotic capsule [19] surrounding the implant will be thinner and capsule contraction unlikely [20].

The implant device is a foreign body. For every foreign body, the host will develop an inflammatory reaction [19], which is normal for a healthy organism. If the foreign body cannot be eliminated, the inflammatory reaction will become chronic, and fibroblasts will form a fibrotic capsule, placing the new volume in the surrounding soft tissue.

The textured implant will have one thin fibrotic capsule growing in strong connections with the textured surface, being adherent to its shell, and another capsule that is thicker and denser in fibrotic tissue, with a high density of fibroblasts and closely connected with the covering soft tissues. Between these two capsules, a synovial-like fluid can be found in different amounts. This means that between the textured implant device and the soft tissues, the host organism will develop a three-layer capsule. Sometimes fibrotic bands can be found connecting the first and third capsular layers, suggesting the abdominal postoperative adherent strap. For smooth implants, the first layer of the capsule is absent. No tissue will adhere to the device.

If the implant pocket is too large, the implant will slide inside, and the surrounding soft tissues will not be able to adhere to close the space. If the tension of the covering soft tissues is not appropriate to maintain the device's shape, the myofibroblasts from the surrounding capsule will start to contract, and the capsule will become thicker and firmer and include calcifications.

The aim of capsule contraction (foreign body reaction) is to obtain a smaller contact surface between the host and the foreign body (implant device), maintaining the volume. The original shape of the implant will become more spherical. This is the geometric form with the smallest surface for the same volume.

12.5
Conclusions

Perhaps one of the most important aspects of providing excellent outcomes to patients is our ability to customize a procedure to the individual. Just as there is no one procedure that is ideal for every patient, there is no one implant that is ideal for every woman.

Presently, there are around 100 different implant options. This large number of options is a tremendous advantage when trying to treat breast asymmetries or asymmetry within the chest wall. The surgeon can use our specific measurements of breast width, height, and projection along with the computer program to select an implant specific to each breast.

The anatomical cohesive gel implant adds a very important option to the list of available implants and will make it easier for surgeons to provide excellent results in a more predictable and customized manner.

The TTM chart allows aesthetic breast surgery to be more scientific, with predictable results. This chart, attached to the patient's file, provides a very good testimony about the preoperative situation and can also document the breast evolution at every follow-up visit. Difficult cases of breast asymmetry, before or after the surgery, can also be documented.

The TTM chart could be a useful tool for both younger and experienced plastic surgeons.

References

1. Yalom M: A History of the Breast. Knopf, New York 1997
2. Penn J: Breast reduction. Br J Plast Surg 1955;7(4): 357–371
3. Smith DJ Jr, Palin WE Jr, Katch VL, Bennet JE: Breast volume and anthropomorphic measurements: normal values. Plast Reconstr Surg 1986;78(3):331–335
4. Stark N, Olivari N: Breast asymmetry: an objective analysis of post-operative results. Eur J Plast Surg 1991;14:173
5. Brown RW, Cheng YC, Kurtay M: A formula for surgical modifications of the breast. Plast Reconstr Surg 2000;106(6):1342–1345

6.   Sommer NZ, Zook LG, Verhulst SJ: The prediction of breast reduction weight. Plast Reconstr Surg 2002; 109(2):506–511

7.   Westreich M: Anthropomorphic breast measurements protocol and results in 50 women with aesthetically perfect breasts and clinical application. Plast Reconstr Surg 1997;100(2):468–479

8.   Mugea TT: A new system for breast assessment using TTM chart. The 17th International Congress of the French Society of Aesthetic Surgery, Paris, 19–21 May 2001

9.   Georgiade NG, Georgiade GS: Reduction mammoplasty utilizing the inferior pyramidal dermal pedicle. In: Georgiade NG (ed). Aesthetic Breast Surgery. Baltimore, Williams & Wilkins 1983

10. Mugea TT: Aesthetic breast assessment—TTM chart. The 3rd International Congress of Cosmetic Medicine and Surgery, South American Academy of Cosmetic Surgery, 19–21 Oct 2001

11. Nava M, Quattrone P, Riggio E: Focus on the breast fascial system: a new approach for inframammary fold reconstruction. Plast Reconstr Surg 1998;102(4):1034–1035

12. Muntan CD, Sundine MJ, Rink RD, Acland RD: Inframammary fold: a histologic reappraisal. Plast Reconstr Surg 2000;105(2):549–556

13. Spear S: *Surgery of the Breast: Principles and Art.* Philadelphia, Lippincott-Raven 1998, pp 845–849

14. Hakelius L, Ohlsen LA: Clinical comparison of the tendency to capsular contracture between smooth and textured gel-filled silicone mammary implants. Plast Reconstr Surg 1992;90(2):247–254

15. Pollack H: Breast capsular contracture: a retrospective study of textured versus smooth silicone implants. Plast Reconstr Surg 1993;91(3):404–407

16. Mladick RA: No-touch submuscular saline breast augmentation technique. Aesthetic Plast Surg 1993;17(3):183–192

17. Heden P, Jernbeck J, Hober M: Breast augmentation with anatomical cohesive gel implants. Clin Plast Surg 2001;28(3):531–552

18. Spear SL, Mardini S: Alternative filler materials and new implant designs: what's available and what's on the horizon? Clin Plast Surg 2001;28(3):435–443

19. Spear SL: Breast augmentation with reduced-height anatomic implants: the pros and cons. Clin Plast Surg 2001;28(3)561–565

20. Camirand A, Doucet J, Harris J: Breast augmentation: compression—a very important factor in preventing capsular contracture. Plast Reconstr Surg 1999;104(2):529–538

21. Carpaneda CA: Inflammatory reaction and capsular contracture around smooth silicone implants. Aesthetic Plast Surg 1997;21(2):110–114

22. Becker H, Springer R: Prevention of capsular contracture. Plast Reconstr Surg 1999;103(6):1766–1768

CHAPTER 13

The Golden Ratios of the Breast

13

Richard Moufarrège

13.1
Introduction

Many artists have established the ratios of the human body. Among them, Leonardo Da Vinci presented his very famous man whose umbilicus is the center of a circle passing at the limit of his four outstretched limbs (Fig. 13.1). In the 20th century, the French architect Le Corbusier gave us the relative dimensions of the whole human body (Fig. 13.2.)

The author has never found, in the past artistic or anatomic literature [1–18], any rule or study establishing the proportions of the breast measurements that would allow a mathematical mean to delineate which proportions lead to a harmonious or, conversely, a deformed breast.

13.2
Method

The three dimensions of the breast were studied:
1. Height (H)
2. Projection (P)
3. Width (W)

Two ratios were developed from studying thousands of breast shapes in the author's plastic surgery practice:
1. Height over projection, or H/P
2. Height over width, or H/W

The best way to figure all kinds of proportions is to maintain one of the measurements constantly the same and have the other change. Two graphics were created

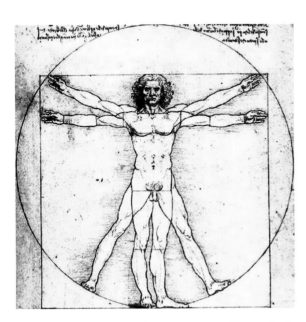

Fig. 13.1 Leonardo DaVinci's representation of human body lengths

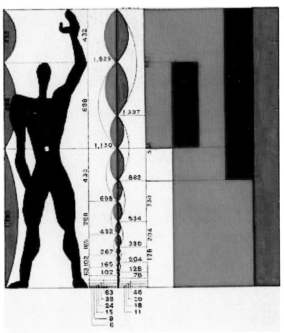

Fig. 13.2 Le Courbusier's study on body proportions

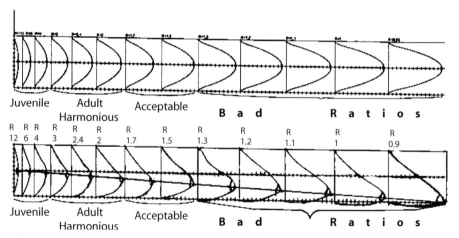

Juvenile   Adult   Acceptable   **B a d**   **R a t i o s**
                Harmonious

R	R	R	R	R	R	R	R	R	R	R	R	R
12	6	4	3	2.4	2	1.7	1.5	1.3	1.2	1.1	1	0.9

Juvenile   Adult   Acceptable   **B a d**   **R a t i o s**
                Harmonious

Fig. 13.3 The *upper row* represents a series of breast heights with progressively increasing projection. The *lower row* represents the same breast profiles with variation according to the factor of gravity

in which the height of the breast is always the same. The first graphic (Fig.13.3) is dedicated to the profile dimensions, i.e. the height and the projection. The second graphic (Fig. 13.4) is dedicated to the front dimensions, i.e. the height and the width.

In the first graphic, a series of breast profiles were represented, all with the same height and with a progressive projection from very small to very large. The H/P ratio was calculated for each profile, from 0.9 to 12 (Fig. 13.3). The second line of the first graphic represents the effect of gravity on the position of the nipple and breast. It is obvious that the first two profiles (H/P = 12 and H/P = 6) are those of juvenile breasts; the next four profiles (H/P = 4 to H/P = 2) correspond to adult harmonious breasts. The next two profiles (H/P = 1.7 and H/P = 1.5) are not the most harmonious, but they are acceptable. The next three profiles (H/P = 1.3, H/P = 1.1, and H/P = 0.9) are disharmonious and should not be acceptable as results of mammoplasties, augmentations, mastopexies, or reductions.

In the second graphic (Fig. 13.4), the frontal aspect of the breast was represented by a series of breasts with the same height and with a progression of width from very narrow to very wide. It is obvious that the first two breasts (H/W = 4 and H/W = 2) are not acceptable.

These are the ratios obtained in some capsular deformities or in some prosthesis augmentations that are placed too high (Fig. 13.5). The next three breasts (H/W = 1.3, H/W = 1, and H/W = 0.7) are harmonious

breasts, and mammaplasty results should always be within these ratios between H/W = 0.7 and H/W = 1.3. The next four breasts are not harmonious and are encountered in some prosthesis displacements but mainly in the very long vertical incisions of reduction mammoplasties and in other techniques that drastically amputate the upper quadrant of the breast.

13.3
Results

It becomes obvious through these graphics that breast dimensions and the ratios of these dimensions are important factors to consider to obtain harmonious results in mammoplasties. The author calls the ratios corresponding to harmonious breasts the Golden Ratios of the breast. These ratios are as follows:

1. In the lateral view, H/P ≥ 2. A lower ratio is acceptable until H/P ≥ 1.5.
2. In the frontal view, H/W should be between 0.7 and 1.3; i.e., 0.7 ≤ H/W ≤ 1.3.

13.4
Discussion

Currently the trend is toward big breasts, and there is a dangerous tendency to favor the volume, neglecting the

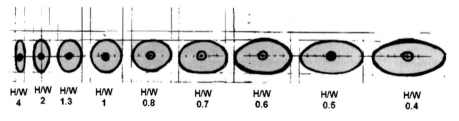

H/W	H/W	H/W	H/W	H/W	H/W	H/W	H/W	H/W
4	2	1.3	1	0.8	0.7	0.6	0.5	0.4

Fig. 13.4 Frontal dimension ratio progression height over width. Ratios from 0.7 to 1.3 are harmonious

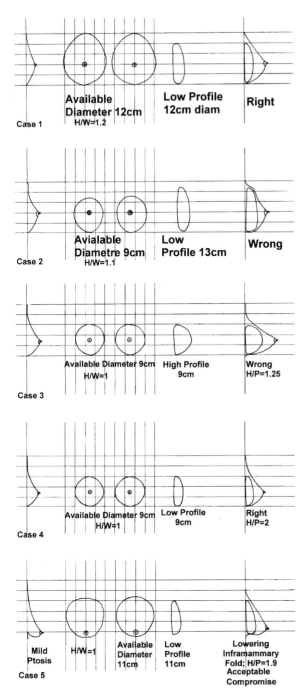

Fig. 13.5 Evaluation of the patient for breast augmentation

and extension are defined by a specific space from the 3rd to the 7th ribs and between the sternum medially and the anterior axillary line laterally. Consequently, the implementation base of the breast is limited.

With society's infatuation with big breasts, expansion of the breast can develop in the following three ways:

1. Medially and laterally, by exceeding the regular limit of the breast, with a mushroom deformity as a consequence (Fig. 13.6). This will also induce a poor ratio, H/W <0.7. The exceeding of the limit could eventually occur on one side more than other. This will lead to an asymmetrical breast (Fig. 13.6).
2. Superiorly and inferiorly, by exceeding the upper and lower limits of the breast, resulting in either a level of the upper quadrant that is too high (Fig. 13.5) or a downward migration of the prosthesis under the inframammary fold. Both situations will correspond to a frontal ratio of H/W>1.3.
3. Frontal expansion with an exaggeration of the breast projection (Figs. 13.7, 13.8)

Prosthesis manufacturers have, in order to remedy the problem of tight breasts, created a high-profile prosthesis with a small base diameter. This, in fact, would prevent the mushroom deformity, or the upward or downward exceeding of the augmented breast, by forward expansion of the breast volume. When too exaggerated, this frontal expansion will lead to an abnormal breast shape with a very low profile ratio, H/P <1.5 (Figs. 13.3, 13.5, 13.7, 13.8).

13.5
Choosing the Right Prosthesis

All types of prostheses can find an application in correct chests. The availability of a large variety of styles and dimensions of prostheses is an advantage we should use properly. A wide-based prosthesis is indicated in wide prethoracic spaces. One should not use them in very tight breasts or in a small prethoracic space with a very projected breast, and high-profile prostheses should be avoided. In such cases, the patient's insisting on having larger breasts than acceptable will lead to an inevitable deformity (Figs. 13.5–13.8).

In a tall woman with a wide chest, one should not use small prostheses with large projection, especially on very tight and tuberous breasts. In this case, the use of a wide prosthesis could partially correct the deformity, especially by mildly lowering the inframammary fold (Figs. 13.5, 13.8).

The first actions of a plastic surgeon when confronted with a patient asking for a breast augmentation (Figs. 13.5, 13.8) should be to:

shape. We as surgeons are solicited more and more for large breasts. Today's collective female unconscious is heavily bombarded by images of bulging breasts overflowing from low-cut dresses, images that are generously supported by "ultraspecialized" magazines.

The breast is a glandular appendix whose position

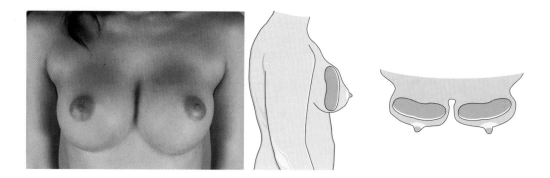

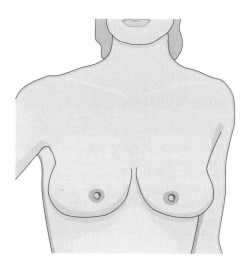

1. Evaluate the client's height and the weight. The author personally refuses to do breast augmentation on a very overweight patient.
2. Measure the available width of the frontal hemithorax. The prosthesis chosen must not be wider than that space.
3. Evaluate the projection. It is imperative to avoid prostheses that will change the breast into a "banana" or a "squash." That is, one should avoid getting a result with too much projection compared with the height (the H/P ratio should be >1.5, if not 2).

13.6
Conclusions

There is no single prosthesis that fits all breasts. One should take into consideration the patient's height and weight. The dimensions of the prosthesis should not be greater than the available diameter of the chest, and the final result should not be determined as a function of the volume but as a function of shape. This latter should correspond to the Golden Ratios of the breast (Figs. 13.9, 13.10).

Fig. 13.6 a Mushroom deformity due to a prosthesis too large in diameter. **b** Excessive lateral position of prostheses, leading to asymmetrical breasts

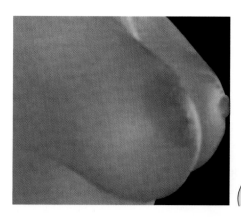

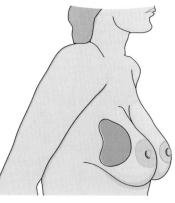

Fig. 13.7 The squash deformity due to a prosthesis with a too-high profile in a tight breast without lifting

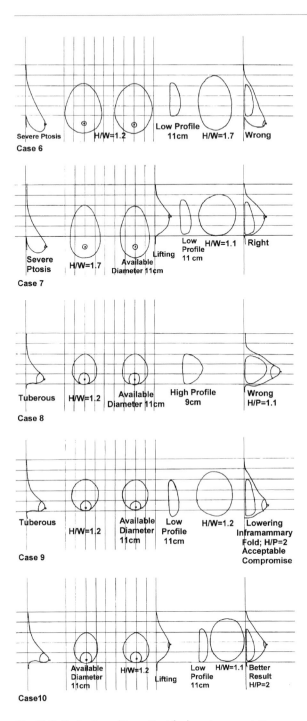

Fig. 13.8 Evaluation of the patient for breast augmentation

Fig. 13.9 Breast augmentation respecting the Golden Ratios of the breast. H/P =2, H/W =1. **a** *1, 2* Preoperative views. **b** *1, 2* Postoperative views

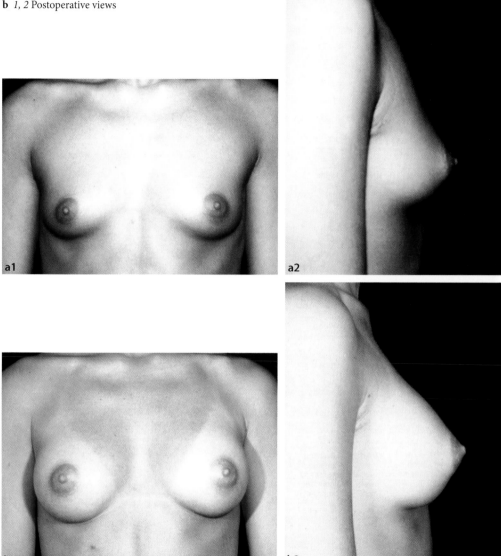

Fig. 13.10 Breast augmentation respecting the Golden Ratios of the breast. H/P =2.1, H/W =1. **a** *1, 2* Preoperative views. **b** *1, 2* Postoperative views

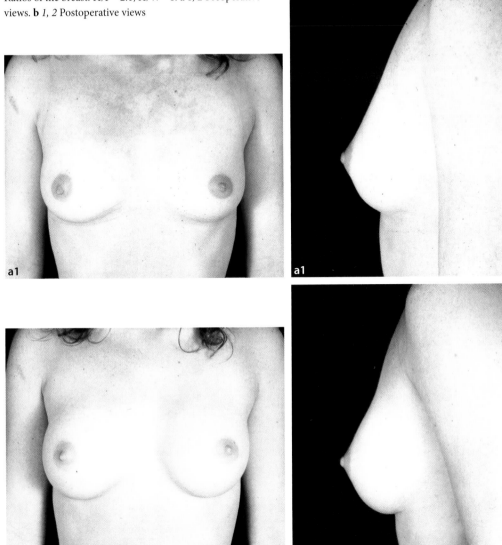

References

1. Aufricht G: Mammoplasty for pendulous breasts: empiric and geometric planning. Plast Reconstr Surg 1949;4:13

2. Drzewiecki A: Breast reduction by central pedicle technique. Plast Reconstr Surg 1986;78(6):830 (letter)

3. McKissock PK: Reduction mammaplasty with a vertical dermal flap. Plast Reconstr Surg 1972;49(3):245–252

4. Moufarrège R, Muller GH, Beauregard G, Bosse JP, Papillon J: Mammaplasty with a lower dermo-glandular pedicle. Ann Chir Plast 1982;27(3):249–254

5. Moufarrège R, Beauregard G, Bosse JP, Muller G, Papillon J, Pedras C: Reduction mammaplasty by the total dermoglandular pedicle. Aesthetic Plast Surg 1985;9(3):227–232

6. Moufarrège R: A new reduction mammaplasty with a vertical posterior pedicle. Quebec Society of Plastic Surgery Convention 1979

7. Ducommun N: La beauté du sein des femmes… d'aprés l'Éloge des tétons. Bibliothéque des Curieux 1914

8. De Compiègne M: Éloge du sein des femmes, coffret du bibliophile. Bibliothèque des Curieux 1920

9.   Reynaud J-P, Tassin X: Passé, présent et... avenir des prothèses mammaires. Ann Chir Plast Esthét 2003;48(5): 389–398

10. Glicenstein J: Histoire de l'augmentation mammaire. Ann Chir Plast Esthét 1994;38(6):647–655

11. Flageul G, Elbaz J-S: Les prothèses mammaires texturées. Ann Chir Plast Esthét 1994;38(6):711–720

12. Chavoin J-P, Costagliola M: Les implants mammaires inadaptés. Ann Chir Plast Esthét 1994;38(6):735–741

13. Hidalgo DA: Breast augmentation: choosing the optimal incision, implant and pocket plane. Plast Reconstr Surg 2000;105(6):2202–1226

14. Muller GH: Les indications et les voies d'abord de l'augmentation mammaire. Ann Chir Plast Esthét 1994;38(6):726–734

15. Flageul G, de Corado E, Olivier F: Analyse Morphologique du sein: le rêve et la réalité. In: Rapport du XXXIVᵉ Congrès de la SOF. CPRE, pp 29–38. Paris, October 1989

16. Moufarrège R: Anatomical and artistic breast considerations. Ann Chir Plast Esthét 2005;50((5):365–370

17. Muller G-H: Breast implants and silicone: silicone crisis' history. Ann Chir Plast Esthét 2005;50(5):350–356

18. Flageul G: Mammary augmentation surgery: reconstructive surgery of femininity. Ann Chir Plast Esthét 2005;50(5):333–336

CHAPTER 14

Body Image and Other Psychological Issues in Breast Augmentation

14

David B. Sarwer, Alison L. Infield

14.1
Introduction

As the popularity of cosmetic breast augmentation has surged in the past decade, so has interest in the psychological aspects of the procedures. A growing literature has investigated the preoperative characteristics of women who seek cosmetic breast augmentation. These studies have investigated both the preoperative personality characteristics of these women as well as their motivations for surgery. Body image dissatisfaction, and dissatisfaction with breast size and/or shape, is thought to serve as a primary motivation for surgery. Although some body image dissatisfaction is common among these women, a sizable minority suffer from excessive dissatisfaction consistent with the psychiatric diagnosis of body dysmorphic disorder, which is believed to contraindicate cosmetic surgical treatment.

Following breast augmentation, women typically report high levels of satisfaction with the procedure and improvements in body image. The impact of the procedure on other areas of functioning, such as self-esteem and quality of life, is less clear. These positive outcomes have been tempered by epidemiological studies that have identified a previously unanticipated relationship between cosmetic breast implants and subsequent suicide. In this chapter, we review the existing literature in all of these areas and use it to provide recommendations for the psychological assessment of the breast augmentation candidate.

14.2
Preoperative Psychosocial Status of Breast Augmentation Candidates

14.2.1
Demographic and Descriptive Characteristics

No "typical" breast augmentation candidate patient exists. The mass media often stereotypes the breast augmentation patient, frequently depicting her as a European-American woman in her early to mid-20s who is interested in the procedure to help facilitate the development of a romantic relationship [1, 2]. This stereotype, however, has been challenged by several studies that suggest that although the typical patient is European-American, she is frequently in her late 20s or early 30s, married, and has children [3–13]. The specific characteristics of women interested in cosmetic breast augmentation likely vary based on the region of the country, characteristics of a surgeon's practice, and a variety of other variables. Nonetheless, women from their late teens to mid-40s with various ethnic backgrounds and relationship status present for breast augmentation surgery [14].

Despite this variability, women who receive breast implants have been found to differ from other women on a variety of unique personality characteristics. Women with breast implants are more likely to have had more sexual partners over their lifetimes, report a greater use of oral contraceptives, be younger at their first pregnancy, and have a history of terminated pregnancies [15–18]. They are more frequent users of alcohol and tobacco [16–18] and have a higher rate of dissolved marriages [4, 10]. A number of women with breast implants have a below average body weight [15–20], leading to concern that some may be suffering from eating disorders. The rate of eating disorders among women interested in breast implants is, somewhat surprisingly, unknown.

14.2.2
Motivations for Breast Augmentation

The motivations for undergoing cosmetic surgery have been categorized as internal (undergoing the surgery to improve one's self-esteem) or external (undergoing the surgery for some secondary gain) [21, 22]. Although a distinction between internal and external motivations is difficult to ascertain in clinical practice, patients internally motivated are thought to be more likely to meet their postoperative goals [23].

Women interested in breast implants for cosmetic purposes are likely motivated by several factors [2]. Intrapsychic factors describe the anticipated effects of surgery on psychological status as well as on romantic and other social relationships. Women who seek breast augmentation report anticipating an improved quality of life, body image, and self-esteem, as well as increased marital and sexual satisfaction following surgery [2, 3, 5–7, 9]. Informational and medical factors also are thought to play a role in the decision to seek breast augmentation [2, 8, 11, 13, 19]. Women who undergo breast augmentation typically report obtaining a great deal of information about the risks and benefits of breast implants from the mass media [19, 24–27].

Body image dissatisfaction is thought to be the central motivation for cosmetic surgery [28–32]. Several empirical studies of breast augmentation and other cosmetic surgery patients have found that patients report heightened body image dissatisfaction preoperatively [33–37]. More specifically, breast augmentation candidates report greater dissatisfaction with their breasts compared with other small-breasted women not seeking breast augmentation [19, 20].

14.2.3
Preoperative Psychopathology

The presence of formal psychopathology among breast augmentation patients has been the focus of a number of studies [1, 2, 29, 31, 32]. The first studies of this issue, from decades ago, relied heavily on clinical interviews of prospective patients and described them as having high rates of formal psychiatric disorders, predominately mood, anxiety, and personality disorders [4, 6, 7, 9, 10, 12]. Other studies described patients as experiencing increased symptoms of depression, anxiety, and low self-esteem [4, 10, 12, 38]. More recent studies, many of which have used standardized psychometric measures rather than clinical interviews, described far less psychopathology among women pursuing breast augmentation [3, 13, 18–20].

The literature in this area unfortunately suffers from a range of methodological issues that make drawing anything more than tentative conclusions difficult [1, 31, 32]. The clinical interviews were generally not standardized, and the degree of psychopathology observed may have been influenced by the theoretical biases of the psychiatrist(s) conducting the interviews. Many of the studies that used paper-and-pencil measures of psychiatric symptoms relied on small sample sizes and often failed to use appropriate comparison groups.

Several recent studies have investigated the use of psychiatric treatment among breast augmentation candidates, with treatment serving as a potential marker of

psychopathology. Women with breast implants, compared with other cosmetic surgery patients or women from the general population, have been found to report a higher rate of outpatient psychotherapy [20], psychopharmacologic treatments [39], and psychiatric hospitalizations [40]. At least one study, however, found no differences between breast augmentation patients and controls in self-reported treatment for depression [18]. Again, these conflicting results make it difficult to make firm statements about the rate of psychopathology among breast augmentation candidates.

A number of studies have suggested that at least one form of psychopathology occurs with increased frequency among persons who present for cosmetic surgery [41]. Body dysmorphic disorder (BDD) is characterized as a preoccupation with a slight or imagined defect in appearance that leads to substantial distress or impairment in social, occupational, or other areas of functioning [42]. A number of studies conducted throughout the world have found that between 7% and 15% of cosmetic surgery and dermatology patients have some form of the disorder [35, 43–47]. Although the most common areas of concern are centered around the head and face, any body part, including the breasts, can be a source of concern [41]. While many patients with BDD believe that cosmetic surgery or other cosmetic medical treatments may improve their condition, retrospective studies have found that greater than 90% of persons with BDD report either no change or a worsening in their BDD symptoms following these treatments [48, 49]. As a result, BDD is believed to be a contraindication to cosmetic surgery [29, 32, 41, 50].

14.3
Changes in Psychosocial Status Following Breast Augmentation

The vast majority of women who undergo cosmetic breast augmentation report that they are satisfied with the postoperative result [13, 51, 52]. The impact of breast augmentation on psychosocial functioning is less clear. Postoperative expectations have been categorized as surgical, psychological, and social. Recent studies have suggested that women's expectations about the aesthetic result following breast augmentation often differ from those of the plastic surgeon; patients desire more upper pole fullness, whereas surgeons try to achieve a more natural, teardrop shape to the breast [53, 54]. Psychological expectations include anticipated improvements in psychological functioning postoperatively. The majority of women who receive breast implants report improvements in body image in the first 2 postoperative years [12, 13, 24, 55, 56]. The impact of breast augmentation on other areas of functioning, or over longer periods of time, are less clear. Some studies have found improvements in self-esteem and depressive symptoms, for example, whereas other investigations have not replicated these findings. Many women interested in breast augmentation believe that the procedures will change their social and romantic relationships by making them more attractive to current or potential romantic partners. Individuals who have undergone facial procedures have been judged as being more physically attractive [57, 58]. It is unclear whether such positive judgments occur after cosmetic breast augmentation.

The experience of a postoperative complication may compromise both postoperative satisfaction as well as the psychological benefits associated with breast augmentation [24, 59, 60]. This latter issue has received surprisingly little attention. At least one study has found that women who experienced postoperative complications, particularly complications that were detectable, reported less favorable changes in body image within the first 2 postoperative years [31].

14.4
Cosmetic Breast Augmentation and Suicide

Within the past decade, seven epidemiological studies conducted throughout the world and designed to investigate the relationship between silicone-gel-filled breast implants and all-cause mortality have found an association between cosmetic breast implants and suicide. This unanticipated relationship has received a great deal of media attention, was part of the U.S. Food and Drug Administration's 2006 decision to lift the restrictions on the use of silicone-gel-filled breast implants for cosmetic purposes, and left investigators scrambling for potential explanations of the relationship.

The first study to identify a relationship between breast implants and suicide was published in 2001 [61]. Investigators from the National Cancer Institute reviewed the medical records of 13,488 women who received breast implants from 18 surgical practices throughout the United States in a study designed to examine all-cause mortality associated with breast implants. There were 225 deaths among women with breast implants [standardized mortality ratio (SMR) 0.69; 95% confidence interval (CI) 0.6–0.8] compared with 125 deaths among 3,936 women who underwent other cosmetic procedures in the same practices (SMR 0.58; 95% CI 0.5–0.7). Women who received breast implants were found to have a higher rate of suicide (SMR 1.54), although this finding was not statistically significant between the two groups. Death by suicide was associated with an older age at implantation, with a greater than two-fold elevation in suicides in women more than 10 years from the date of surgery.

Three Scandinavian investigations subsequently found a similar association between breast implants and suicide. Koot and colleagues [62] reviewed the death records of 3,521 Swedish women who received cosmetic breast implants starting in 1965. Fifteen of the 85 deaths in these women were attributed to suicide when, based on age and calendar-year specific death rates, 5.2 would have been expected (SMR 2.9; 95% CI 1.6–4.8). In a study of 2,166 Finnish women who received cosmetic breast implants, Pukkala and colleagues [63] found 10 suicides where 3.13 were expected (SMR 3.19; 95% CI 1.53–5.86). Jacobsen and colleagues [40] similarly found an increased rate of death by suicide among 2,761 Danish women (SMR 3.1; 95% CI 1.7–5.2).

The study by Jacobsen and colleagues [40] was the first to provide any information on the psychiatric history of these women. Eight percent of women with cosmetic breast implants were found to have a history of psychiatric hospitalization prior to surgery (95% CI 7.0–9.0%). This was almost double the rate of psychiatric hospitalizations for women who underwent breast reduction (4.7%; 95% CI 4.2–5.2%) or other cosmetic procedures (5.5%; 95% CI 4.5–6.7%).

In 2006, Brinton and colleagues reported on an additional 5 years of follow-up of their American cohort of patients [64]. Twenty-nine deaths were categorized as suicides [SMR 1.63; 95% CI 1.1–2.3; relative risk (RR) 2.58, 0.9–7.8]. As in their initial study, the highest SMR for suicide was found for women who received their implants at age 40 or older, with the risk of suicide increasing after the first postoperative decade.

The largest study of this issue to date was published in 2006. In a cohort of 24,558 Canadian women with breast implants, there were 58 deaths attributed to suicide (SMR 1.73; 95% CI 1.31–2.24), where 33.5 were expected [65]. Among 15,893 women who underwent other forms of surgery, there were 33 suicides, which also represents a higher rate of suicide (SMR 1.55; 95% CI 1.07–2.18). The rate of suicide between women with breast implants and those who underwent other forms of cosmetic surgery did not differ, which is in contrast to other studies [61, 64], However, replicating previous investigations, the SMRs for suicide were higher for those women who received breast implants at age 40 or later and for those women who had their implants for longer periods of time.

Recently, Lipworth and colleagues [66] reported on an additional 8 years of follow-up of their earlier study of Swedish women [62]. Among women with cosmetic beast implants, they observed an increased rate of death by suicide (SMR 3.0; 95% CI 1.9–4.5). They also observed an increased number of deaths attributed to alcohol or drug dependence as well as from accidents or injuries that could have resulted from substance abuse. The authors suggest that several of these deaths may not have been accidental but rather deaths from suicide, a hypothesis also suggested by Brinton and colleagues in their more recent report [64].

Across the seven studies, the rate of suicide is two to three times greater than what would be expected from estimates from the general population. While the initial study in this area suggested that the rate of suicide among women with breast implants was greater than that of women who underwent other forms of cosmetic surgery, the larger investigation by Villeneuve et al. [65] found no difference in the rate of suicide between the two groups of cosmetic surgery patients. Several studies, however, suggest that the suicide rate is higher for women who received their implants at age 40 or later and that it increases with the life of the implant.

Several potential explanations of the relationship between beast implants and suicide have been offered. Most of the attention in this area has focused on the psychosocial status and functioning of the women who receive breast implants [67–69]. As detailed previously, women with breast implants have been shown to have a number of distinctive personality characteristics and life experiences. Many of these characteristics, such as alcohol and tobacco use, have been found to be risk factors for suicide in both the general population and psychiatric samples [70–75]. In reviewing the relationship between these characteristics and suicide among women with breast implants, Joiner has proposed that the suicide rate could be even higher than that found in the epidemiological studies [76]. In making this claim, he suggests that postoperative improvements in body image following breast augmentation may produce a "protective effect" for women who otherwise may be at risk for suicide.

Another possible explanation of the relationship between cosmetic breast augmentation and suicide may be unmet postoperative expectations. Some women may present for breast augmentation surgery with unrealistic expectations about the effect that surgery will have on their daily lives. When these expectations are not met, they may become despondent, depressed, and potentially suicidal. The occurrence of a postoperative complication should also be considered. The physical discomfort associated with capsular contracture or other complications could, in theory, contribute to a depressed mood, increased anxiety, and a decline in quality of life. The absence of a proactive response to a complication from the patient's surgeon could further contribute to the psychological reaction. Whether the stress of a postoperative complication could lead to a cascade of events that ultimately could contribute to suicide is unknown.

Perhaps the most intuitively pleasing of the potential explanations of the relationship is the occurrence of preexisting psychopathology. One of the epidemiologi-

cal studies in this area found a higher rate of previous psychiatric hospitalizations among women with breast implants compared both with women who underwent other cosmetic procedures and with those who underwent breast reduction [40]. A history of psychiatric hospitalizations is a strong predictor of suicide among women in the general population [77–79]. Unfortunately, the investigation by Jacobsen et al. [40] provided no information on diagnosis, history of illness, or other psychiatric treatments. However, as noted above, other studies have shown that women with breast implants report a higher rate of outpatient psychotherapy or psychopharmacological treatment compared with other women [20, 39].

Further research on the relationship between breast implants and suicide is imperative. The epidemiological investigations have provided only limited information on the psychosocial status of women with breast implants. In the absence of more definitive data, the assessment of preexisting psychopathology and potential suicidality takes an even more central role in the preoperative psychological assessment of women interested in cosmetic breast implants.

14.5
Preoperative Psychological Assessment of Breast Augmentation Patients

The preoperative psychological assessment of breast augmentation patients should focus on three areas: motivations for and expectations about surgery, physical appearance and body image, and psychiatric history and status [28, 50, 69, 80]. In addition, the surgeon should monitor patients' behavior with other employees in the office and be prepared to make referrals to qualified mental health professionals when appropriate.

14.5.1
Preoperative Motivations and Postoperative Expectations

The initial consultation with the surgeon should be used to evaluate the patient's motivations for surgery. Asking a new patient why she is interested in breast implants at this point in her life may help determine if she is interested in surgery for herself and her own sense of self-esteem, or if the interest in surgery is motivated by a current or hoped-for romantic partner. Being motivated for cosmetic surgery in order to please a romantic partner may put a patient at risk for a poor psychological outcome.

As detailed earlier, women present for breast augmentation with a range of postoperative expectations. The surgeon should inquire about these specific expectations and ensure that they are realistic. Additionally, patients should be reminded that, although breast augmentation may lead to improvements in body image and other areas of psychosocial functioning, it is impossible to predict the social responses of others. While some women may be pleased with increased attention related to their larger breasts, others may find the attention uncomfortable and unsettling. Thus, it may be useful to begin the conversation about postoperative expectations by asking breast augmentation candidates how they anticipate their lives to be different following surgery.

14.5.2
Physical Appearance and Body Image

The assessment of prospective patients' body image concerns is a central part of the initial consultation [50]. Patients should be asked what, specifically, they dislike about their breasts. They should be able to articulate concerns that are readily visible to the surgeon. The degree of dissatisfaction with the breasts should also be assessed. Studies throughout the body image and cosmetic surgery bodies of literature have shown that there is little relationship between one's physical appearance and her subjective body image. Women who report significant distress with comparatively "normal" breasts may be suffering from BDD. Similarly, women who report thinking about their breasts obsessively throughout the day may be suffering from BDD. Some women may reveal the extent of their preoccupation with their breasts by presenting the surgeon with numerous photographs of models or celebrities with breasts they desire. Although these pictures may be instructive to the surgeon in specific circumstances, such behavior likely only hints at the hours that patients have spent thinking about their breasts. Breast augmentation candidates should also be asked how their feelings about their breasts impact their daily behavior. Although it is common for many women to use padded bras, those who report excessive camouflaging of their breasts, avoidance of activity (particularly being seen undressed or in a swimsuit), or an inability to maintain relationships or employment because of their breasts may be suffering from BDD.

14.5.3
Psychiatric Status and History

It is not clear to what extent plastic surgeons routinely assess the psychiatric status and history of their patients, but this assessment should be a routine part of the initial consultation. In addition to assessing for BDD, mood and eating disorders may be overrepresented among women who seek breast augmentation. A patient's mood, affect, and overall presentation will provide important clues to the presence of a mood disorder. If one is suspected, neurovegetative symptoms, including sleep, appetite, and concentration, should be assessed. Patients who endorse these symptoms should be asked about the frequency of crying, irritability, social isolation, feelings of hopelessness, and the presence of suicidal thoughts. The presence of depressive symptoms likely warrants a mental health consultation prior to surgery, particularly given the association between breast implants and suicide as detailed above.

Eating disorders such as anorexia and bulimia nervosa also may occur with greater frequency among women who seek body-contouring procedures such as breast augmentation and liposuction [1, 29]. To screen for the presence of an eating disorder, the height and weight of all patients should be obtained and used to calculate body mass index (the patient's weight in kilograms divided by her height in square meters). Patients with a BMI $<20\,kg/m^2$ should be asked about recent weight fluctuations, amenorrhea, ongoing dieting efforts, binge eating, purging, and other compensatory behaviors.

The treating surgeon should also obtain a psychiatric treatment history. This should include directed questions about both outpatient psychopharmacological and psychotherapeutic treatments as well as psychiatric hospitalizations. Approximately 20% of cosmetic surgery patients report ongoing psychiatric treatment, most commonly pharmacologic treatment with antidepressant medications [81]. Many of these patients probably received these medications from their primary care physicians, who often prescribe subtherapeutic dosages of these medications [39]. Therefore, plastic surgeons should not assume that a low dosage of an antidepressant medication is appropriately controlling depressive symptoms. Referral for additional psychiatric assessment is warranted when the surgeon does not believe that the depressive symptoms are well controlled.

Women with a history of psychopathology who are not currently engaged in mental health treatment also warrant a preoperative psychiatric consultation to further assess their psychological status and appropriateness for breast augmentation. Patients currently in treatment should be asked if their mental health professional is aware of their interest in surgery. Surgeons should contact these professionals to confirm that surgery is appropriate. Some patients who have been dissatisfied with their postoperative results have used their psychiatric history as part of their legal action against the surgeon, claiming that their psychiatric condition prevented them from fully understanding the procedure and potential outcomes [50, 82].

14.5.4
Observation of Office Behavior

Patients' interactions with the surgeon's staff should be closely monitored during all office visits and other contacts. In their efforts to make themselves appear as appropriate for surgery as possible, patients typically are on their best behavior with the surgeon and may neglect to share important information, such as their psychiatric history, out of concern that they will be judged to be inappropriate for surgery. Nursing staff and office assistants may witness different aspects of patients' behavior that may alert the surgeon to a potential psychological problem. Patients who have difficulty following the standard office routine, in terms of scheduling and other preoperative assessments, warrant further attention. Patients who raise concerns among the staff should, at a minimum, be seen for a second consultation. If concerns persist, a mental health evaluation is merited.

14.5.5
Mental Health Referrals

A trusted psychologist or psychiatrist can be a valuable consultant to the successful cosmetic surgery practice. Such a mental health professional should have a working knowledge of the psychological aspects of cosmetic surgery as well as disorders with a body image component, including BDD and eating disorders. Most of the consultations to the mental health professional likely will occur preoperatively, to help assess a patient's appropriateness for surgery. A patient may also be referred postoperatively if 1) the patient is dissatisfied with what the surgeon considers to be a successful procedure, or 2) the patient experiences an exacerbation of psychopathology that was not detected preoperatively. In either scenario, cosmetic surgery patients may react to a referral to a mental health professional with anger, and many will likely refuse to go to the consultation. To increase the likelihood that the patient will accept the referral, it should be treated like a referral to any other mental health professional. The surgeon should communicate to the patient the specific areas of concern and the reason for the referral. This information should also be communicated to the mental health professional.

14.6
Conclusions

A relatively large body of literature has investigated the psychological aspects of cosmetic breast augmentation. Many of these studies have focused on the presence of psychiatric symptoms or formal psychopathology among prospective patients as well as improvements in psychosocial status following surgery. With the exception of BDD, the rate of psychopathology among breast augmentation candidates is not yet firmly established. Nevertheless, concern remains that other diagnoses, such as eating disorders and mood disorders, may be relatively common among women who receive breast implants.

These issues have taken on greater relevance because of the previously unknown association between cosmetic breast implants and subsequent suicides. This relationship should be considered in the clinical care of women interested in cosmetic breast augmentation. However, this relationship should be balanced with studies that show high levels of postoperative satisfaction and improvements in body image in the majority of women. Furthermore, with the exception of BDD, there is a dearth of information on the relationship between preoperative psychopathology and postoperative outcomes. Thus, there is currently little evidence to support a recommendation that all women who present for cosmetic breast augmentation be required to undergo a psychiatric evaluation prior to surgery. Nonetheless, breast augmentation candidates who present with a history of psychopathology, or those whom the plastic surgeon suspects as having some form of psychopathology, should undergo mental health consultation before surgery.

Conflicts of interest: Dr. Sarwer is a consultant for Allergan. Dr. Sarwer receives grant support from the National Institute of Diabetes and Digestive and Kidney Diseases (grant numbers R03-DK067885 and R01-DK072452), as well as the American Society of Plastic Surgeons/ Plastic Surgery Educational Foundation (grant number DR06-04).

References

1. Sarwer DB, Didie ER, Gibbons LM: Cosmetic surgery of the body. In: Sarwer DB, Pruzinsky T, Cash TF, Goldwyn RM, Persing JA, Whitaker LA (eds). Psychological Aspects of Reconstructive and Cosmetic Plastic Surgery: Empirical, Clinical, and Ethical Issues. Philadelphia, Lippincott Williams & Wilkins 2006, pp 251–266
2. Sarwer DB, Nordmann JE, Herbert JD: Cosmetic breast augmentation surgery: a critical overview. J Womens Health Gend Based Med 2000;9(8):843–856
3. Baker JL, Kolin IS, Bartlett ES: Psychosexual dynamics of patients undergoing mammary augmentation. Plast Reconstr Surg 1974;53(6):652–659

4. Beale S, Lisper H, Palm B: A psychological study of patients seeking augmentation mammaplasty. Br J Psychiatry 1980;136:133–138

5. Druss RG: Changes in body image following augmentation breast surgery. Int J Psychoanal Psychother1973;2: 248–256

6. Edgerton MT, McClary AR: Augmentation mammaplasty: psychiatric implications and surgical indications. Plast Reconstruct Surg 1958;21(4):279–305

7. Edgerton MT, Meyer E, Jacobson WE: Augmentation mammaplasty II: Further surgical and psychiatric evaluation. Plast Reconstruct Surg 1961;27:279–302

8. Goin JM, Goin MK: Changing the Body: Psychological Effects of Plastic Surgery. Baltimore, Williams & Wilkins 1981

9. Schlebusch L: Negative bodily experience and prevalence of depression in patients who request augmentation mammaplasty. S Afr Med J 1989;75(7):323–326

10. Schlebusch L, Levin A: A psychological profile of women selected for augmentation mammaplasty. S Afr Med J 1983;64(13):481–483

11. Shipley RH, O'Donnell JM, Bader KF: Personality characteristics of women seeking breast augmentation. Plast Reconstr Surg 1977;60(3):369–376

12. Sihm F, Jagd M, Pers M: Psychological assessment before and after augmentation mammaplasty. Scan J Plast Surg 1978;12(3):295–298

13. Young VL, Nemecek JR, Nemecek DA: The efficacy of breast augmentation: breast size increase, patient satisfaction, and psychological effects. Plast Reconstr Surg 1994;94(7):958–969

14. 2001 National Plastic Surgery Procedural Statistics. Arlington Heights, IL, American Society of Plastic Surgeons 2008

15. Brinton LA, Brown SL, Colton T, Burich MC, Lubin J: Characteristics of a population of women with breast implants compared with women seeking other types of plastic surgery. Plast Reconstr Surg 2000;105(3):919–927

16. Cook LS, Daling JR, Voigt LF, deHart MP, Malone KE, Stanford JL, Weiss NS, Brinton LA, Gammon MD, Brogan D: Characteristics of women with and without breast augmentation. J Amer Med Assoc 1997;277(20):1612–1617

17. Fryzek JP, Weiderpass E, Signorello LB, Hakelius L, Lipworth L, Blot WJ, McLaughlin JK, Nyren, O: Characteristics of women with cosmetic breast augmentation surgery compared with breast reduction surgery patients and women in the general population of Sweden. Ann Plast Surg 2000;45(4):349–356

18. Kjoller K, Holmich LR, Fryzek JP, Jacobsen PH, Friis S, McLaughlin JK, Lipworth L, Henriksen TF, Jorgensen S, Bittmann S, Olsen JH: Characteristics of women with cosmetic breast implants compared with women with other types of cosmetic surgery and population-based controls in Denmark. Ann Plast Surg 2003;50(1):6–12

19. Didie ER, Sarwer DB: Factors that influence the decision to undergo cosmetic breast augmentation surgery. J Womens Health 2003;12(3):241–253

20. Sarwer DB, LaRossa D, Bartlett SP, Low DW, Bucky LP, Whitaker LA: Body image concerns of breast augmentation patients. Plast Reconstr Surg 2003;112(1):83–90

21. Edgerton MT Jr, Knorr NJ: Motivational patterns of patients seeking cosmetic (esthetic) surgery. Plast Reconstr Surg 1971;48(6):551–557

22. Pruzinsky T. Cosmetic plastic surgery and body image: critical factors in patient assessment. In: Thompson JK (ed). Body Image, Eating Disorders, and Obesity: An Integrative Guide for Assessment and Treatment. Washington, DC, American Psychological Association 1996, pp 109–127

23. Honigman R, Phillips KA, Castle DJ: A review of psychosocial outcomes for patients seeking cosmetic surgery. Plast Reconstr Surg 2004;113(4):1229–1237

24. Cash TF, Duel LA, Perkins LL: Women's psychosocial outcomes of breast augmentation with silicone gel-filled implants: a 2-year prospective study. Plast Reconstr Surg 2002;109(6):2112–2121

25. Handel N, Wellisch D, Silverstein MJ, Jensen JA, Waisman E: Knowledge, concern and satisfaction among augmentation mammaplasty patients. Ann Plast Surg 1993;30(1):13–22, discussion 21–22

26. Larson DL, Anderson RC, Maksud D, Grunert BK: What influences public perceptions of silicone breast implants? Plast Reconstr Surg, 1994;94(2):318–325

27. Palcheff-Wiemer M, Concannon MJ, Cohn VS, Puckett CL: The impact of the media on women with breast implants. Plast Reconstr Surg, 1993;92(5):779–785

28. Sarwer DB: The psychological aspects of cosmetic breast augmentation. Plast Reconstr Surg 2007;120(7 suppl 1):110S–117S

29. Sarwer DB, Crerand CE: Body image and cosmetic medical treatments. Body Image 2004;1:99–111

30. Sarwer DB, Crerand CE, Gibbons LM: Body dysmorphic disorder and aesthetic surgery. In: Nahai F (ed). The Art of Aesthetic Surgery: Principles and Techniques. St. Louis, Quality Medical Publishing 2005, pp 33–57

31. Sarwer DB, Pertschuk MJ, Wadden TA, Whitaker LA: Psychological investigations in cosmetic surgery: a look back and a look ahead. Plast Reconstr Surg 1998;101(4):1136–1142

32. Sarwer DB, Wadden TA, Pertschuk MJ, Whitaker LA: The psychology of cosmetic surgery: a review and reconceptualization. Clin Psychol Rev 1998;18(1):1–22

33. Pertschuk MJ, Sarwer DB, Wadden TA, Whitaker LA: Body image dissatisfaction in male cosmetic surgery patients. Aesth Plast Surg 1998;22(1):20–24

34. Sarwer DB, Bartlett SP, Bucky LP, LaRossa D, Low DW, Pertschuk MJ, Wadden TA, Whitaker LA: Bigger is not always better: body image dissatisfaction in breast reduction and breast augmentation patients. Plast Reconstr Surg. 1998;101(7):1956–1961

35. Sarwer DB, Wadden, TA, Pertschuk MJ, Whitaker LA: Body image dissatisfaction and body dysmorphic disorder in 100 cosmetic surgery patients. Plast Reconstr Surg 1998;101(6):1644–1649

36. Sarwer DB, Whitaker LA, Wadden TA, Pertschuk MJ: Body image dissatisfaction in women seeking rhytidectomy or blepharoplasty. Aesthet Surg J 1997;17:230–234

37. Simis KJ, Verhulst FC, Koot HM: Body image, psychosocial functioning, and personality: how different are adolescents and young adults applying for plastic surgery? J Child Psychol Psychiatry 2001;42(5):669–678

38. Ohlsen L, Ponten B, Hambert G: Augmentation mammaplasty: a surgical and psychiatric evaluation of the results. Ann Plast Surg 1978;2(1):42–52

39. Sarwer DB, Zanville HA, LaRossa D, Bartlett SP, Chang B, Low DW, Whitaker LA: Mental health histories and psychiatric medication usage among persons who sought cosmetic surgery. Plast Reconstr Surg 2004;114(7):1927–1933

40. Jacobsen PH, Holmich LR, McLaughlin JK, Johansen C, Olsen JH, Kjoller K, Friis S: Mortality and suicide among Danish women with cosmetic breast implants. Arch Intern Med 2004;164(22):2450–2455

41. Crerand CE, Franklin ME, Sarwer DB: Body dysmorphic disorder and cosmetic surgery. Plast Reconstr Surg. 2006;118(7):167e–180e

42. Diagnostic and Statistical Manual of Mental Disorders, 4th edn, text revision. Washington, DC, American Psychiatric Association 2000

43. Aouizerate B, Pujol H, Grabot D, Faytout M, Suire K, Braud C, Auriacombe M, Martin D, Baudet J, Tignol J: Body dysmorphic disorder in a sample of cosmetic surgery applicants. Eur Psychiatry 2003;18(7):365–368

44. Castle DJ, Molton M, Hoffman K, Preston NJ, Phillips KA: Correlates of dysmorphic concern in people seeking cosmetic enhancement. Aust N Z J Psychiatry 2004;38(6):439–444

45. Crerand CE, Sarwer DB, Magee L, Gibbons LM, Lowe MR., Bartlett SP, Becker, DG, Glat PM, LaRossa D, Low DW, Whitaker LA: Rate of body dysmorphic disorder among patients seeking facial plastic surgery. Psychiatric Ann 2004;34:958–965

46. Ishigooka J, Iwao M, Suzuki M, Fukuyama Y, Murasaki M, Miura S: Demographic features of patients seeking cosmetic surgery. Psychiatry Clin Neurosci 1998; 52(3):283–287

47. Veale D, De Haro L, Lambrou C: Cosmetic rhinoplasty in body dysmorphic disorder. Br J Plast Surg 2003;56(6):546–551

48. Crerand CE, Phillips KA, Menard W, Fay C: Nonpsychiatric medical treatment of body dysmorphic disorder. Psychosomatics 2005;46(6):549–555

49. Phillips KA, Grant JE, Siniscalchi J, Albertini RS: Surgical and nonpsychiatric medical treatment of patients with body dysmorphic disorder. Psychosomatics 2001;42(6):504–510

50. Sarwer DB: Psychological assessment of cosmetic surgery patients. In: Sarwer DB, Pruzinsky T, Cash TF, Goldwyn RM, Persing JA, Whitaker LA (eds). Psychological Aspects of Reconstructive and Cosmetic Plastic Surgery: Empirical, Clinical, and Ethical Issues. Philadelphia, Lippincott Williams & Wilkins 2006, pp 267–283

51. Park AJ, Chetty U, Watson ACH: Patient satisfaction following insertion of silicone breast implants. Brit J Plast Surg 1996;49(8):515–518

52. Schlebusch L, Marht I: Long-term psychological sequelae of augmentation mammaplasty. S Afr Med J 1993;83(4):267–271

53. Adams WP, Bengston BP, Glicksman CA, Gryskiewicz JM, Jewell ML, McGrath MH, Reisman NR, Teitelbaum SA, Tebbetts JB, Tebbetts T: Decision and management algorithms to address patient and Food and Drug Administration concerns regarding breast augmentation and implants. Plast Reconstr Surg. 2004;114(5):1252–1257

54. Hsia HC, Thomson JG: Differences in breast shape preferences between plastic surgeons and patients seeking breast augmentation. Plast Reconstr Surg. 2003;112(1):312–320

55. Banbury J, Yetman R, Lucas A, Papay F, Graves K, Zins JE: Prospective analysis of the outcome of subpectoral breast augmentation: sensory changes, muscle function, and body image. Plast Reconstr Surg 2004;113(2):701–707

56. Sarwer DB, Gibbons LM, Magee L, Baker JL, Casas LA, Glat PM, Gold, AH, Jewell ML, LaRossa D, Nahai F, Young VL: A prospective, multi-site investigation of patient satisfaction and psychosocial status following cosmetic surgery. Aesthetic Surg J 2005;25:236

57. Cash TF, Horton CE: Aesthetic surgery: effects of rhinoplasty on the social perception of patients by others. Plast Reconstr Surg 1983;72(4):543–550

58. Kalick SM: Aesthetic surgery: how it affects the way patients are perceived by others. Ann Plast Surg 1979;2(2):128–134

59. Fiala TG, Lee WP, May JW: Augmentation mammoplasty: results of a patient survey. Ann Plast Surg 1993;30(6):503–509

60. Honigman R, Phillips KA, Castle DJ: A review of psychosocial outcomes for patients seeking cosmetic surgery. Plast Reconstr Surg 2004;113(4):1229–1237

61. Brinton LA, Lubin JH, Burich MC, Colton T, Hoover RN: Mortality among augmentation mammoplasty patients. Epidemiology 2001;12(3):321–326

62. Koot VC, Peeters PH, Granath F, Grobbee DE, Nyren O: Total and cause specific mortality among Swedish women with cosmetic breast implants: prospective study. Br Med J 2003;326(7388):527–528

63. Pukkala E, Kulmala I, Hovi SL, Hemminki E, Keski-maki I, Pakkanen M, Lipworth L, Boice JD Jr, McLaughlin JK: Causes of death among Finnish women with cosmetic breast implants, 1971–2001. Ann Plast Surg 2003;51(4):339–342

64. Brinton LA, Lubin JH, Murray MC, Colton T, Hoover RN: Mortality rates among augmentation mammoplasty patients: an update. Epidemiology 2006;17(2):162–169

65. Villeneuve PJ, Holowaty EJ, Brisson J, Xie L, Ugnat AM, Latulippe L, Mao Y: Mortality among Canadian women with cosmetic breast implants. Am J Epidemiol 2006;164(4):334–341

66. Lipworth L, Nyren O, Ye W, Fryzek JP, Tarone RE, McLaughlin JK: Excess mortality from suicide and other external causes of death among women with cosmetic breast implants. Ann Plast Surg 2007;59(2):119–123

67. McLaughlin JK, Wise TN, Lipworth L: Increased risk of suicide among patients with breast implants: do the epidemiologic data support psychiatric consultation? Psychosomatics 2004;45(4):277–280

68. Sarwer DB: Discussion of causes of death among Finnish women with cosmetic breast implants, 1971–2001. Ann Plast Surg 2003;51:343–344

69. Sarwer DB, Brown GK, Evans DL: Cosmetic breast augmentation and suicide: a review of the literature. Am J Psychiatry 2007;164(7):1006–1013

70. Angst J, Clayton PJ: Personality, smoking and suicide: a prospective study. J Affect Disord 1998;51(1):55–62

71. Berglund M: Suicide in alcoholism. A prospective study of 88 suicides: I. The multidimensional diagnosis at first admission. Arch Gen Psychiatry 1984;41(9):888–891

72. Malone KM, Waternaux C, Haas GL, Cooper TB, Li S, Mann JJ: Cigarette smoking, suicidal behavior, and serotonin function in major psychiatric disorders. Am J Psychiatry 2003;160(4):773–779

73. Miller M, Hemenway D, Bell NS, Yore MM, Amoroso PJ: Cigarette smoking and suicide: a prospective study of 300,000 male active-duty Army soldiers. Am J Epidemiol 2000;151(11):1060–1063

74. Miller M, Hemenway D, Rimm E: Cigarettes and suicide: a prospective study of 50,000 men. Am J Public Health 2000;90(5):768–773

75. Nielsen AS, Bille-Brahe U, Hjelmeland H, Jensen B, Ostamo A, Salander-Renberg E, Wasserman D: Alcohol problems among suicide attempters in the Nordic countries. Crisis 1996;17(4):157–166

76. Joiner TE: Does breast augmentation confer risk of or protection from suicide? Aesthetic Surg J 2003;23:370–375

77. Appleby L, Shaw J, Amos T, McDonnell R, Harris C, McCann K, Kiernan K, Davies S, Bickley H, Parsons R: Suicide within 12 months of contact with mental health services: national clinical survey. Br Med J 1999;318(7193):1235–1239

78. Goldacre M, Seagroatt V, Hawton K: Suicide after discharge from psychiatric inpatient care. Lancet 1993;342(8866):283–286

79. Qin P, Agerbo E, Mortensen PB: Suicide risk in relation to socioeconomic, demographic, psychiatric, and familial factors: a national register-based study of all suicides in Denmark, 1981–1997. Am J Psychiatry 2003;160(4):765–772

80. Sarwer DB: Psychological considerations in cosmetic surgery. In: Goldwyn RM, Cohen M (eds). The Unfavorable Result in Plastic Surgery: Avoidance and Treatment. Philadelphia, Lippincott Williams & Wilkins 2001, pp 14–23

81. Sarwer DB, Grossbart, TA, Baker A: Psychosocial evaluation of the cosmetic surgery patient. In: Kaminer MS, Dover JS, Arndt KA (eds). Atlas of Cutaneous Aesthetic Surgery. Philadelphia, WB Saunders, in press

82. Gorney M: Professional and legal considerations in cosmetic surgery. In: Sarwer DB, Pruzinsky T, Cash TF, Goldwyn RM, Persing JA, Whitaker LA (eds). Psychological Aspects of Reconstructive and Cosmetic Plastic Surgery: Empirical, Clinical, and Ethical Issues. Philadelphia, Lippincott Williams & Wilkins 2006, pp 315–327

CHAPTER 15

Body Dysmorphic Disorder

15

Melvin A. Shiffman

15.1
Introduction

The patient with body dysmorphic disorder (BDD) should be avoided in performing breast augmentation. Understanding the disorder is essential for every cosmetic surgeon.

15.2
Definition

BDD is defined as a preoccupation with an imagined or a very slight defect in physical appearance that causes significant distress to the individual. It was first described in 1886 by Morselli, who called it "dysmorphophobia." The disorder is manifested in people who dislike some aspect of how they look to such an extent that they cannot stop thinking and worrying about it. To other people, these reactions may seem excessive because the supposed problem may not even be noticeable or may be related to a very minor blemish such as a mole or mild acne scarring that anyone else may not notice. But to sufferers of the syndrome, the "defects" are very real, very obvious, and very severe.

15.3
Symptoms

Symptoms of BDD include the following:
1. The individual is preoccupied with the supposed appearance problem.
2. The patient takes actions to "hide" the defect or avoid situations because he or she feels ugly and does not want to be seen by others.

Some patients with BDD do realize they look worse to themselves than to others and that their view of their appearance is exaggerated and distorted. Others are convinced that their view of their physical defect is accurate. Some have the feeling that other people are taking special notice of the "defect" and that people are staring at it and making fun of it or laughing about it behind the person's back, when in reality, no one may even notice it. Many sufferers feel ashamed and fear being rejected by others.

Most patients with BDD perform one or more repetitive and often time-consuming behaviors, also known as rituals, that are usually aimed at examining, "improving," or hiding the perceived flaw in appearance. They usually spend a lot of time checking themselves in the mirror to see whether their "defect" is noticeable or has changed in some way. Others will frequently compare themselves with other people or images in magazines or on billboards. Some will spend hours grooming themselves by applying make-up, changing clothes, or rearranging their hair to "correct" or cover up the perceived problem. Others attempt to camouflage or hide their "defect" by wearing a hat, a wig, or sunglasses. In extreme cases, the individual will wear a mask or hood over the head. Some try, by acting or standing in a certain way in public, to make the "defect" seem less noticeable. Others weigh or measure themselves continually or wear big and baggy clothing to hide what they think are "huge" hips or large breasts. Some may wear many layers of clothing to make them appear larger or more muscular, and some men (especially those who suffer from "muscle dysmorphia") lift weights or exercise excessively to try to increase muscle bulk. They may eat special diets or use drugs such as anabolic steroids to try to build up their muscles.

Patients with body dysmorphia may approach cosmetic surgeons or dermatologists, seeking surgery or medical treatments.

15.4
Consequences of BDD

Some patients with BDD function well despite their distress. Others are severely impaired by their symptoms, often becoming socially isolated by not going to school or work, and extreme cases refuse to leave home for fear of being embarrassed about their appearance. It can be especially difficult for sufferers to go to places such as beaches, hair salons, shopping malls, or places where the person may feel anxious about how he or she looks. It is not uncommon for patients with BDD to feel depressed about their problem and the negative impact this has on their life. Some become so desperate that they attempt suicide.

Relationship problems are common, and many BDD sufferers have few friends, avoiding dates and other social activities or even getting divorced because of their symptoms.

15.5
Associated Disorders

Many patients with BDD also suffer from depression at some point in their life, and there is a high rate of depression in families of patients who develop BDD. The patient develops low self-esteem, heightened sensitivity, and feelings of rejection and unworthiness.

Other disorders include obsessive compulsive disorders such as eating disorders, anxiety disorders, trichotillomania (hair pulling), and abuse of drugs or alcohol.

There is a high rate of suicidal ideation (mean of 57.8% of 185 subjects over 4 years) and a mean of 2.6% attempted suicides per year [1, 2].

15.6
Treatment

Serotonin-reuptake inhibitors (SRIs) are a group of medications that appear to be useful and effective in patients with BDD. The SRIs are a type of antidepressant used successfully for treating both depression and obsessive compulsive disorder. These include Prozac, Zoloft, Cipramil, and Aropax.

Cognitive behavioral therapy appears to be an effective treatment for BDD [3]. The behavioral component consists of "exposure and response prevention," in which patients expose their "defects" in situations that they would usually avoid, while response prevention involves helping patients stop carrying out the compulsive behavior related to their perceived defects. The aim over time is to decrease anxiety involved with that particular avoided situation. The cognitive component addresses the range of intrusive thoughts that accompany the behaviors or rituals, such as mirror checking, in BDD. This focuses on exploring beliefs and values that support and strengthen a person's perceptions about his or her body. Cognitive restructuring is aimed at developing an understanding of how these strongly held values impact the person's sense of self and at progressively building up alternative ways of thinking about the intrusive thought rather than going through the usual range of behaviors such as mirror checking and reassurance seeking. Restructuring consists of a range of techniques involving making changes to a person's values while not directly questioning the repetitive and intrusive thoughts the person has about his or her body.

15.7
Discussion

Understanding BDD and recognizing the patient with this disorder will prevent many misunderstandings between patient and physician, especially the dermatologist or cosmetic surgeon. The BDD patient presenting for treatment of minimally abnormal skin findings, if recognized, will prevent unnecessary and potentially unsuccessful treatments [4–6]. Many patients with BDD seek cosmetic surgery, and the unwary surgeon will invariably have to deal with a dissatisfied patient. Many eventually fall into the cosmetic surgery victim category of "overoperation." Recognition and deferral of surgery for BDD patients is advised because findings have shown the propensity of these patients to litigate, threaten, and even harm or kill their surgeons [7].

15.8
Conclusions

Failure to diagnose BDD in a preoperative cosmetic surgery patient will almost always lead to a dissatisfied patient. The surgeon will have a patient who is continuously dissatisfied with results no matter what is done to correct the perceived deformity. The treatment for patients with BDD is medication, usually SRIs, or psychiatric care with cognitive behavioral therapy. The surgeon has to identify BDD patients before surgery, tell them that surgery is not the solution for their problems, and refer them to a psychiatrist for treatment.

References

1. Phillips KA, Menard W: Suicidality in body dysmorphic disorder: a prospective study. Am J Psychiatry 2006;163(7):1280–1282
2. Phillips KA, Coles ME, Menard W, Yen S, Fay C, Weisberg RB: Suicidal ideation and suicide attempts in body dysmorphic disorder. J Clin Psychiatry 2005;66(6):717–725
3. Honigman R, Castle DJ: Body dysmorphic disorder—a guide for people with BDD. Collaborative Therapy Unit, Mental Health Research Institute 2003

4. Buescher LS, Buescher KL: Body dysmorphic disorder. Dermatol Clin 2006;24(2):251–257

5. Glaser DA, Kaminer MS: Body dysmorphic disorder and the liposuction patient. Dermatol Surg 2005;31(5):559–560

6. Mackley CL: Body dysmorphic disorder. Dermatol Surg 2005;31(5):553–558

7. Hodgkinson DJ: Identifying the body-dysmorphic patient in aesthetic surgery. Aesthetic Plast Surg 2005;29(6):503–509

CHAPTER 16

Use of Decision and Management Algorithms in a Breast Augmentation Practice

16

Caroline A. Glicksman

16.1
Introduction

This is an initiative to advance patient education, informed consent, and outcomes and to reduce operation rates.

Over the last 16 years, the U.S. Food and Drug Administration (FDA), patient advocate groups, patients, and the public have all expressed concerns regarding the safety and efficacy of silicone breast implants. Although the FDA approved the release of the 4th-generation silicone implants in November 2006, they did so with "conditions for approval." Large postapproval studies are required of both Mentor and Allergan, and data concerning rupture rates, reoperation rates, and local complications will be reviewed by the FDA at 1, 4, and 10 years [1].

Despite advances in implant technology over the last 40 years, reoperation in the breast augmentation core studies remains the most common complication reported, with rates as high as 21% within 3 years. These rates have remained unacceptably high and are independent of any specific breast implant [2]. The decision and management algorithms presented in this chapter are the result of the combined work of nine plastic surgeons from diverse backgrounds. Utilizing the combined individual clinical experience and the best clinical evidence, the Breast Augmentation Surgeons for Patients Initiative (BASPI) focused on a single objective: reducing reoperation rates in breast augmentation [3]. The decision and management algorithms are the result of this initiative and are designed as templates. They are optional, additional resources for surgeons to consider and are not intended to define standards of practice. In addition, they cannot address all the individual variables of each clinical problem or those within the doctor patient relationship. The algorithms also do not include unanticipated findings during surgery.

16.2
Incorporating the Algorithms in Patient Education and Informed Consent

When patients present with unfavorable results from breast augmentation, they are more likely to understand their alternatives if their surgeon had prepared them preoperatively for the risks of an adverse event. Preoperative informed consent materials are available online [4] and are now included in the preoperative planners provided by the breast implant manufactures [5]. Patients who did not receive preoperative education that included the potential risks and trade-offs of their decisions often become even more stressed in learning that they may encounter new risks associated with a revision surgery, in addition to new costs.

Before any reoperation is undertaken, detailed information and informed consent documentation are even more critical and challenging than for the primary operation. The detailed decision and management algorithms presented in this chapter contain essential summary information about the potential benefits and risks of each decision and help clarify the realistic choices or alternatives. They contain spaces where a patient may sign or initial understanding and acceptance of choices at each decision-making stage.

More importantly, the documents can be useful in their ability to prevent unnecessary reoperation, such as size change, when the patient receives detailed information with regard to risks and long-term trade-offs. By demanding that patients accept responsibility for their decisions, informed consent documents may encourage patients to reconcile their decisions with the limitations of their individual tissues.

16.3
Practical Clinical Use of Algorithms in the Office

When a problem occurs in the augmented patient, she may return to her primary surgeon or seek revision elsewhere. Decision and management algorithms are invaluable in the training of office personnel—not necessarily to deliver definitive answers, but to develop a basic knowledge of how problems will be approached. The scheduling of a new patient with an implant problem will require the office staff or patient to collect old records if available. Records may include all operative reports; implant manufacture information; size, style, and fill of current implants; and up-to-date mammography or magnetic resonance imaging (MRI) results when applicable. This information, in addition to the physical exam, is then applied to the appropriate algorithm for all patients presenting with an implant complication. Unfortunately, some valuable information may not be obtained until the patient is in the operating room. All explanted implants should be weighed. Discrepancies between the actual fill of a saline implant at explantation and the weight documented in previous operative reports are common. These findings are relevant in revision procedures and should be documented.

Each flowchart has six specific objectives:

1) To minimize reoperation
2) To prioritize alternatives that are most likely to reduce reoperation
3) To define realistic choices for the surgeon and patient
4) To involve the patient in the decision-making process
5) To define "out" points for implant removal without replacement in specific clinical situations
6) To provide thorough documentation of choices and assumption of responsibility for those choices

Each of the six flowcharts addresses a specific clinical problem or issue. Patients may present with the following clinical issues or problems: grade 3 or 4 capsular contracture (see Table 16.1), stretch deformities (implant bottoming or displacement; see Table 16.2), possible implant failure or rupture (see Table 16.3), implant size exchange (see Table 16.4), infection (see Table 16.5), or an undefined symptom complex (see Table 16.6). Each algorithm is designed to provide both the surgeon and the patient with a basic set of alternatives from which to evolve better solutions. In addition, the flowcharts incorporate two additional components: 1) a summary of potential benefits and trade-offs associated with each decision and 2) a space for the patient to specifically accept or decline alternatives at each stage of the decision-making process, documented in writing by the patient's initials.

The decision and management algorithms are clinically useful for all patients with implant issues, regardless of who the initial surgeon was or over how many years the problem has progressed. They are not intended to be definitive; however, difficult problems demand difficult choices.

Table 16.1 Alternatives for management of capsular contracture grades 3 and 4

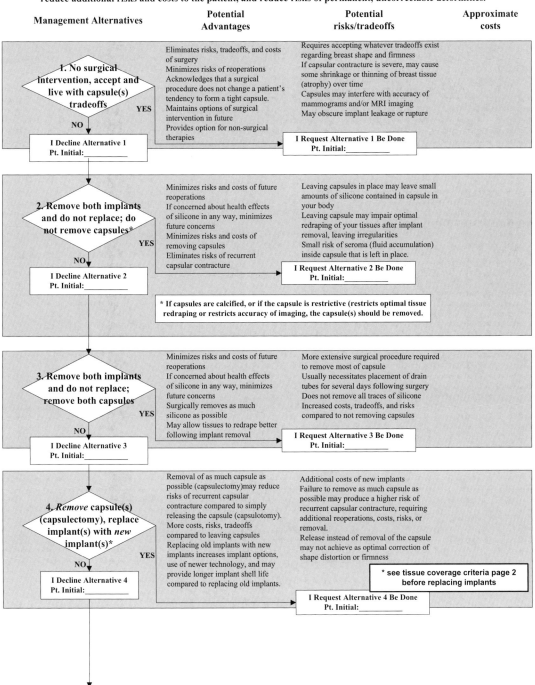

Alternatives for Management of Capsular Contracture Grades 3 and 4
The BASPI Workgroup, John B. Tebbetts, M.D., Moderator
Copyright 2004

**Management alternatives are listed prioritizing alternatives most likely to reduce risks of additional operations, reduce additional risks and costs to the patient, and reduce risks of permanent, uncorrectable deformities.

Management Alternatives	Potential Advantages	Potential risks/tradeoffs	Approximate costs

1. No surgical intervention, accept and live with capsule(s) tradeoffs — YES / NO

I Decline Alternative 1
Pt. Initial:_____

Eliminates risks, tradeoffs, and costs of surgery
Minimizes risks of reoperations
Acknowledges that a surgical procedure does not change a patient's tendency to form a tight capsule.
Maintains options of surgical intervention in future
Provides option for non-surgical therapies

Requires accepting whatever tradeoffs exist regarding breast shape and firmness
If capsular contracture is severe, may cause some shrinkage or thinning of breast tissue (atrophy) over time
Capsules may interfere with accuracy of mammograms and/or MRI imaging
May obscure implant leakage or rupture

I Request Alternative 1 Be Done
Pt. Initial:_____

2. Remove both implants and do not replace; do not remove capsules* — YES / NO

I Decline Alternative 2
Pt. Initial:_____

Minimizes risks and costs of future reoperations
If concerned about health effects of silicone in any way, minimizes future concerns
Minimizes risks and costs of removing capsules
Eliminates risks of recurrent capsular contracture

Leaving capsules in place may leave small amounts of silicone contained in capsule in your body
Leaving capsule may impair optimal redraping of your tissues after implant removal, leaving irregularities
Small risk of seroma (fluid accumulation) inside capsule that is left in place.

I Request Alternative 2 Be Done
Pt. Initial:_____

* If capsules are calcified, or if the capsule is restrictive (restricts optimal tissue redraping or restricts accuracy of imaging, the capsule(s) should be removed.

3. Remove both implants and do not replace; remove both capsules — YES / NO

I Decline Alternative 3
Pt. Initial:_____

Minimizes risks and costs of future reoperations
If concerned about health effects of silicone in any way, minimizes future concerns
Surgically removes as much silicone as possible
May allow tissues to redrape better following implant removal

More extensive surgical procedure required to remove most of capsule
Usually necessitates placement of drain tubes for several days following surgery
Does not remove all traces of silicone
Increased costs, tradeoffs, and risks compared to not removing capsules

I Request Alternative 3 Be Done
Pt. Initial:_____

4. Remove capsule(s) (capsulectomy), replace implant(s) with new implant(s)* — YES / NO

I Decline Alternative 4
Pt. Initial:_____

Removal of as much capsule as possible (capsulectomy) may reduce risks of recurrent capsular contracture compared to simply releasing the capsule (capsulotomy).
More costs, risks, tradeoffs compared to leaving capsules
Replacing old implants with new implants increases implant options, use of newer technology, and may provide longer implant shell life compared to replacing old implants.

Additional costs of new implants
Failure to remove as much capsule as possible may produce a higher risk of recurrent capsular contracture, requiring additional reoperations, costs, risks, or removal.
Release instead of removal of the capsule may not achieve as optimal correction of shape distortion or firmness

* see tissue coverage criteria page 2 before replacing implants

I Request Alternative 4 Be Done
Pt. Initial:_____

Table 16.1 *(continued)* Alternatives for management of capsular contracture grades 3 and 4

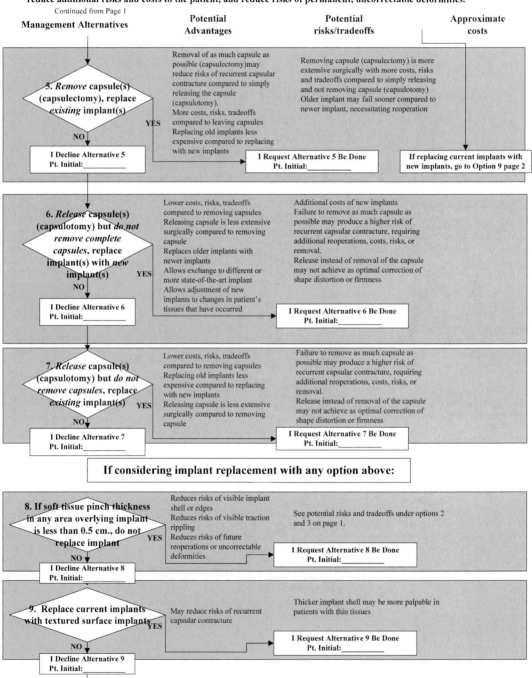

Alternatives for Management of Capsular Contracture Grades 3 and 4
The BASPI Workgroup, John B. Tebbetts, M.D., Moderator, Page 2
Copyright 2004

**Management alternatives are listed prioritizing alternatives most likely to reduce risks of additional operations, reduce additional risks and costs to the patient, and reduce risks of permanent, uncorrectable deformities.

Continued from Page 1

Management Alternatives	Potential Advantages	Potential risks/tradeoffs	Approximate costs

5. *Remove* capsule(s) (capsulectomy), replace *existing* implant(s)

YES / NO

I Decline Alternative 5 Pt. Initial:_____

Removal of as much capsule as possible (capsulectomy) may reduce risks of recurrent capsular contracture compared to simply releasing the capsule (capsulotomy).
More costs, risks, tradeoffs compared to leaving capsules
Replacing old implants less expensive compared to replacing with new implants

Removing capsule (capsulectomy) is more extensive surgically with more costs, risks and tradeoffs compared to simply releasing and not removing capsule (capsulotomy)
Older implant may fail sooner compared to newer implant, necessitating reoperation

I Request Alternative 5 Be Done Pt. Initial:_____

If replacing current implants with new implants, go to Option 9 page 2

6. *Release* capsule(s) (capsulotomy) but *do not* remove complete capsules, replace implant(s) with *new* implant(s)

YES / NO

I Decline Alternative 6 Pt. Initial:_____

Lower costs, risks, tradeoffs compared to removing capsules
Releasing capsule is less extensive surgically compared to removing capsule
Replaces older implants with newer implants
Allows exchange to different or more state-of-the-art implant
Allows adjustment of new implants to changes in patient's tissues that have occurred

Additional costs of new implants
Failure to remove as much capsule as possible may produce a less risk of recurrent capsular contracture, requiring additional reoperations, costs, risks, or removal.
Release instead of removal of the capsule may not achieve as optimal correction of shape distortion or firmness

I Request Alternative 6 Be Done Pt. Initial:_____

7. *Release* capsule(s) (capsulotomy) but *do not* remove capsules, replace *existing* implant(s)

YES / NO

I Decline Alternative 7 Pt. Initial:_____

Lower costs, risks, tradeoffs compared to removing capsules
Replacing old implants less expensive compared to replacing with new implants
Releasing capsule is less extensive surgically compared to removing capsule

Failure to remove as much capsule as possible may produce a higher risk of recurrent capsular contracture, requiring additional reoperations, costs, risks, or removal.
Release instead of removal of the capsule may not achieve as optimal correction of shape distortion or firmness

I Request Alternative 7 Be Done Pt. Initial:_____

If considering implant replacement with any option above:

8. If soft tissue pinch thickness in any area overlying implant is less than 0.5 cm., do not replace implant

YES / NO

I Decline Alternative 8 Pt. Initial:_____

Reduces risks of visible implant shell or edges
Reduces risks of visible traction rippling
Reduces risks of future reoperations or uncorrectable deformities

See potential risks and tradeoffs under options 2 and 3 on page 1.

I Request Alternative 8 Be Done Pt. Initial:_____

9. Replace current implants with textured surface implants

YES / NO

I Decline Alternative 9 Pt. Initial:_____

May reduce risks of recurrent capsular contracture

Thicker implant shell may be more palpable in patients with thin tissues

I Request Alternative 9 Be Done Pt. Initial:_____

Continued on Page 3

Table 16.1 *(continued)* Alternatives for management of capsular contracture grades 3 and 4

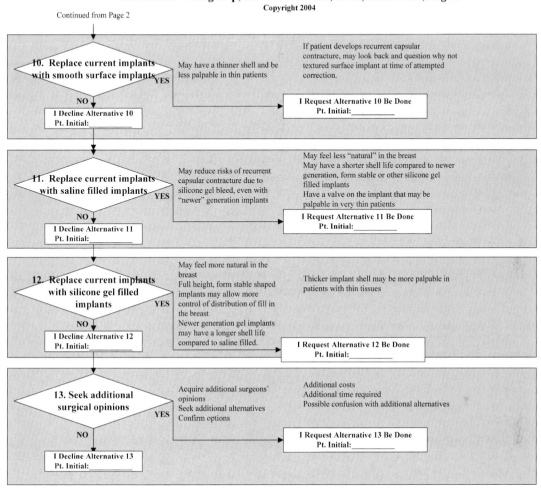

Alternatives for Management of Capsular Contracture Grades 3 and 4
The BASPI Workgroup, John B. Tebbetts, M.D., Moderator, Page 3
Copyright 2004

OUT POINTS

1) Recurrent capsular contracture after one complete capsulectomy and replacement with textured surface implants, or one conversion from submammary to dual plane or subpectoral
2) Soft tissue coverage over any area of the implant is less than 0.5cm. pinch thickness
3) Patient requests implant removal without replacement at any time

**If patient, surgeon, or patient's family are concerned about any aspect of silicone causing symptoms or possible associated conditions, see additional information and flowchart alternatives entitled "If Patient Has Symptoms or Concerns Related to Silicone"

Patient Name (please print):_____   Witness Name (please print): _____

Patient Signature: _____   Witness Signature: _____
Date: _____   Date: _____

Table 16.2 Alternatives for management of implant size exchange

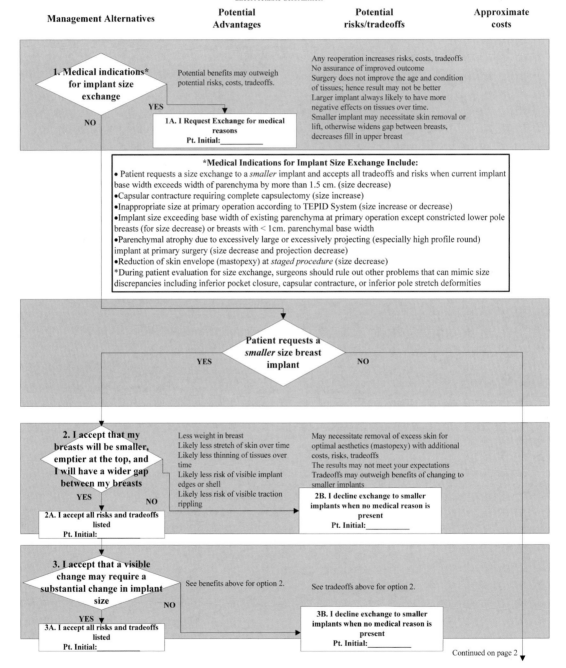

Alternatives for Management of Implant Size Exchange
The BASPI Workgroup, John B. Tebbetts, M.D., Moderator
Copyright 2004

The larger a patients' breasts, augmented or not, the worse the breasts are likely to look over time. Also, the larger the breasts following a breast augmentation, the greater the risks of additional operations, additional risks costs to the patient, and additional risks of permanent, uncorrectable deformities.

Management Alternatives	Potential Advantages	Potential risks/tradeoffs	Approximate costs

1. Medical indications* for implant size exchange

YES / NO

Potential benefits may outweigh potential risks, costs, tradeoffs.

1A. I Request Exchange for medical reasons
Pt. Initial:_____

Any reoperation increases risks, costs, tradeoffs
No assurance of improved outcome
Surgery does not improve the age and condition of tissues; hence result may not be better
Larger implant always likely to have more negative effects on tissues over time.
Smaller implant may necessitate skin removal or lift, otherwise widens gap between breasts, decreases fill in upper breast

*Medical Indications for Implant Size Exchange Include:
• Patient requests a size exchange to a *smaller* implant and accepts all tradeoffs and risks when current implant base width exceeds width of parenchyma by more than 1.5 cm. (size decrease)
•Capsular contracture requiring complete capsulectomy (size increase)
•Inappropriate size at primary operation according to TEPID System (size increase or decrease)
•Implant size exceeding base width of existing parenchyma at primary operation except constricted lower pole breasts (for size decrease) or breasts with < 1cm. parenchymal base width
•Parenchymal atrophy due to excessively large or excessively projecting (especially high profile round) implant at primary surgery (size decrease and projection decrease)
•Reduction of skin envelope (mastopexy) at *staged procedure* (size decrease)
*During patient evaluation for size exchange, surgeons should rule out other problems that can mimic size discrepancies including inferior pocket closure, capsular contracture, or inferior pole stretch deformities

Patient requests a *smaller* size breast implant

YES / NO

2. I accept that my breasts will be smaller, emptier at the top, and I will have a wider gap between my breasts

YES / NO

2A. I accept all risks and tradeoffs listed
Pt. Initial:_____

Less weight in breast
Likely less stretch of skin over time
Likely less thinning of tissues over time
Likely less risk of visible implant edges or shell
Likely less risk of visible traction rippling

May necessitate removal of excess skin for optimal aesthetics (mastopexy) with additional costs, risks, tradeoffs
The results may not meet your expectations
Tradeoffs may outweigh benefits of changing to smaller implants

2B. I decline exchange to smaller implants when no medical reason is present
Pt. Initial:_____

3. I accept that a visible change may require a substantial change in implant size

NO / YES

3A. I accept all risks and tradeoffs listed
Pt. Initial:_____

See benefits above for option 2.

See tradeoffs above for option 2.

3B. I decline exchange to smaller implants when no medical reason is present
Pt. Initial:_____

Continued on page 2 ▼

Table 16.2 *(continued)* Alternatives for management of implant size exchange

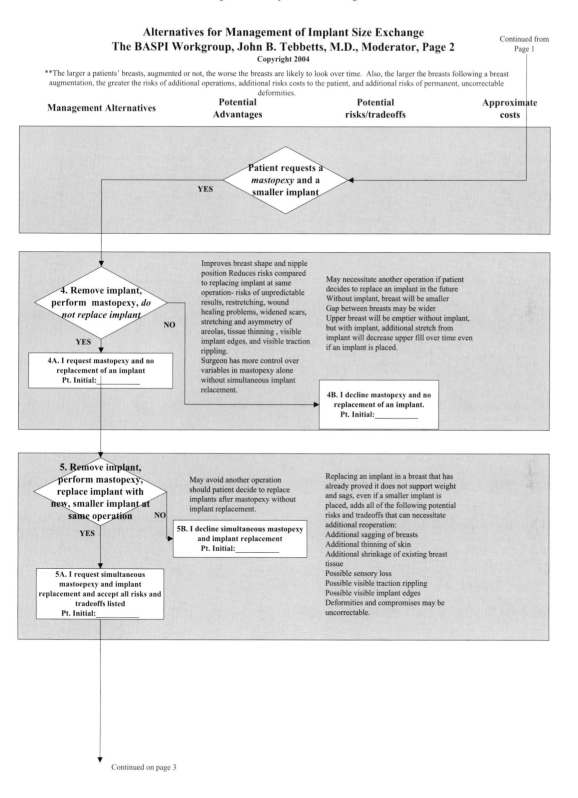

Alternatives for Management of Implant Size Exchange
The BASPI Workgroup, John B. Tebbetts, M.D., Moderator, Page 2
Copyright 2004

Continued from Page 1

**The larger a patients' breasts, augmented or not, the worse the breasts are likely to look over time. Also, the larger the breasts following a breast augmentation, the greater the risks of additional operations, additional risks costs to the patient, and additional risks of permanent, uncorrectable deformities.

Management Alternatives	Potential Advantages	Potential risks/tradeoffs	Approximate costs

Patient requests a *mastopexy* and a smaller implant

YES

4. Remove implant, perform mastopexy, *do not replace implant*

NO

YES

Improves breast shape and nipple position Reduces risks compared to replacing implant at same operation- risks of unpredictable results, restretching, wound healing problems, widened scars, stretching and asymmetry of areolas, tissue thinning , visible implant edges, and visible traction rippling.
Surgeon has more control over variables in mastopexy alone without simultaneous implant relacement.

May necessitate another operation if patient decides to replace an implant in the future
Without implant, breast will be smaller
Gap between breasts may be wider
Upper breast will be emptier without implant, but with implant, additional stretch from implant will decrease upper fill over time even if an implant is placed.

4A. I request mastopexy and no replacement of an implant Pt. Initial:_____

4B. I decline mastopexy and no replacement of an implant. Pt. Initial:_____

5. Remove implant, perform mastopexy, replace implant with new, smaller implant at same operation

NO

YES

May avoid another operation should patient decide to replace implants after mastopexy without implant replacement.

5B. I decline simultaneous mastopexy and implant replacement Pt. Initial:_____

Replacing an implant in a breast that has already proved it does not support weight and sags, even if a smaller implant is placed, adds all of the following potential risks and tradeoffs that can necessitate additional reoperation:
Additional sagging of breasts
Additional thinning of skin
Additional shrinkage of existing breast tissue
Possible sensory loss
Possible visible traction rippling
Possible visible implant edges
Deformities and compromises may be uncorrectable.

5A. I request simultaneous mastoepexy and implant replacement and accept all risks and tradeoffs listed Pt. Initial:_____

Continued on page 3

Table 16.2 *(continued)* Alternatives for management of implant size exchange

Alternatives for Management of Implant Size Exchange
The BASPI Workgroup, John B. Tebbetts, M.D., Moderator, Page 3

Continued from Page 2

Copyright 2004

**The larger a patients' breasts, augmented or not, the worse the breasts are likely to look over time. Also, the larger the breasts following a breast augmentation, the greater the risks of additional operations, additional costs to the patient, and additional risks of permanent, uncorrectable deformities.

Management Alternatives	Potential Advantages	Potential risks/tradeoffs	Approximate costs

Patient requests a *larger* size breast implant

YES ——— NO ———→ I decline exchange of my implant(s) to either a smaller or larger size
Pt. Initial:_____

6. No medical reason for exchange to larger implants

May make patient happier with breast size

NO

YES

6A. I request exchange to larger implants when no medical reason is present
Pt. Initial:_____

6B. I decline exchange to larger implants when no medical reason is present
Pt. Initial:_____

Larger implant causes many more long-term negative effects on tissues
Risks: Tissue thinning, tissue stretch, shrinkage of breast tissue, additional and more rapid sagging, palpable implant edges and shell, visible implant edges, visible traction rippling, possible additional sensory loss
All additional risks associated with a first time augmentation
May decrease accuracy of mammograms
Additional costs, time off normal activities

7. I accept additional tissue stretch that is not reversible

No potential benefits from additional tissue stretch

NO

YES

7A. I accept all risks and tradeoffs listed
Pt. Initial:

7B. I decline exchange to larger implants when no medical reason is present
Pt. Initial:

Additional sagging of breasts
Additional thinning of skin
Additional shrinkage of existing breast tissue
Possible sensory loss
Possible visible traction rippling
Possible visible implant edges
Deformities and compromises may be uncorrectable.

8. I accept additional thinning of my skin that is not reversible

No potential benefits from additional thinning of skin

NO

YES

8A. I accept all risks and tradeoffs listed
Pt. Initial:

8B. I decline exchange to larger implants when no medical reason is present
Pt. Initial:

Implant edges and shell will be easier to feel
May see implant edges and shell
Effects on tissues may not be apparent for several years
May see rippling caused by implant pulling on thin overlying tissues (traction rippling)
All above listed problems are uncorrectable

9. I accept that I may develop visible implant edges that can't be corrected

No potential benefits from visible implant edges

YES ——— NO

9A. I accept all risks and tradeoffs listed
Pt. Initial:

9B. I decline exchange to larger implants when no medical reason is present
Pt. Initial:_____

As the skin thins due to stretch caused by larger implants, implant edges may become visible.
This deformity is often not correctable.

Continued on page 4

Table 16.2 *(continued)* Alternatives for management of implant size exchange

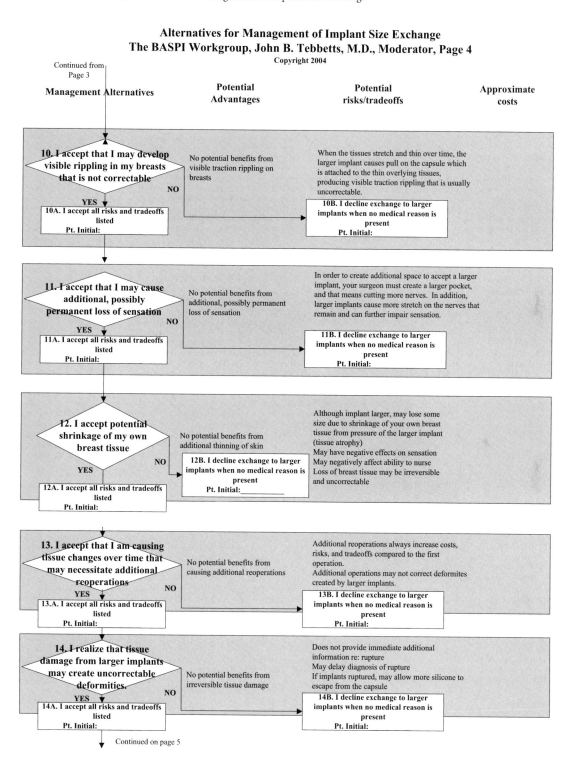

Alternatives for Management of Implant Size Exchange
The BASPI Workgroup, John B. Tebbetts, M.D., Moderator, Page 4
Copyright 2004

Continued from Page 3

Management Alternatives	Potential Advantages	Potential risks/tradeoffs	Approximate costs

10. I accept that I may develop visible rippling in my breasts that is not correctable   NO

YES
10A. I accept all risks and tradeoffs listed
Pt. Initial:

No potential benefits from visible traction rippling on breasts

When the tissues stretch and thin over time, the larger implant causes pull on the capsule which is attached to the thin overlying tissues, producing visible traction rippling that is usually uncorrectable.

10B. I decline exchange to larger implants when no medical reason is present
Pt. Initial:

11. I accept that I may cause additional, possibly permanent loss of sensation   NO

YES
11A. I accept all risks and tradeoffs listed
Pt. Initial:

No potential benefits from additional, possibly permanent loss of sensation

In order to create additional space to accept a larger implant, your surgeon must create a larger pocket, and that means cutting more nerves. In addition, larger implants cause more stretch on the nerves that remain and can further impair sensation.

11B. I decline exchange to larger implants when no medical reason is present
Pt. Initial:

12. I accept potential shrinkage of my own breast tissue   NO

YES
12A. I accept all risks and tradeoffs listed
Pt. Initial:

No potential benefits from additional thinning of skin

12B. I decline exchange to larger implants when no medical reason is present
Pt. Initial:_____

Although implant larger, may lose some size due to shrinkage of your own breast tissue from pressure of the larger implant (tissue atrophy)
May have negative effects on sensation
May negatively affect ability to nurse
Loss of breast tissue may be irreversible and uncorrectable

13. I accept that I am causing tissue changes over time that may necessitate additional reoperations   NO

YES
13.A. I accept all risks and tradeoffs listed
Pt. Initial:

No potential benefits from causing additional reoperations

Additional reoperations always increase costs, risks, and tradeoffs compared to the first operation.
Additional operations may not correct deformites created by larger implants.

13B. I decline exchange to larger implants when no medical reason is present
Pt. Initial:

14. I realize that tissue damage from larger implants may create uncorrectable deformities.   NO

YES
14A. I accept all risks and tradeoffs listed
Pt. Initial:

No potential benefits from irreversible tissue damage

Does not provide immediate additional information re: rupture
May delay diagnosis of rupture
If implants ruptured, may allow more silicone to escape from the capsule

14B. I decline exchange to larger implants when no medical reason is present
Pt. Initial:

Continued on page 5

Table 16.2 *(continued)* Alternatives for management of implant size exchange

Continued from Page 4

Alternatives for Management of Implant Size Exchange
The BASPI Workgroup, John B. Tebbetts, M.D., Moderator, Page 5
Copyright 2004

**The larger a patients' breasts, augmented or not, the worse the breasts are likely to look over time. Also, the larger the breasts following a breast augmentation, the greater the risks of additional operations, additional risks costs to the patient, and additional risks of permanent, uncorrectable deformities.

Management Alternatives	Potential Advantages	Potential risks/tradeoffs	Approximate costs
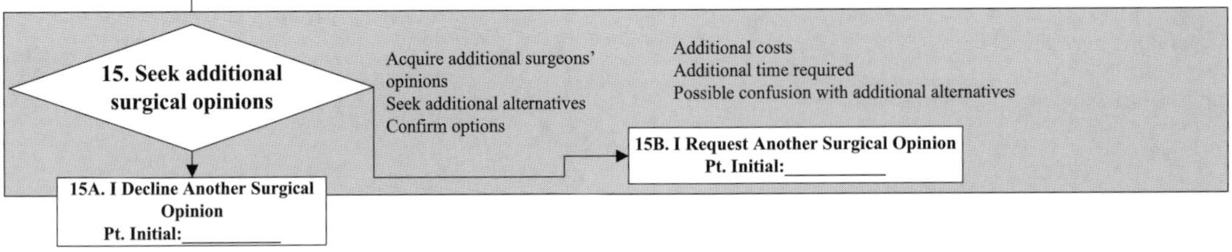 **15. Seek additional surgical opinions**	Acquire additional surgeons' opinions Seek additional alternatives Confirm options	Additional costs Additional time required Possible confusion with additional alternatives	

15A. I Decline Another Surgical Opinion
Pt. Initial:_____

15B. I Request Another Surgical Opinion
Pt. Initial:_____

OUT POINTS
1) If soft tissue coverage in any area of the breast is less than 0.5cm. pinch thickness, decline to replace with larger implants
2) If N:IMF is increased more than 20% compared to N:IMF set at primary surgery, decline to replace with larger implants
3) If any portion of the implant is visible or if visible rippling is present in any portion of the breast, decline to replace with larger size implants.

Patient Name (please print):_____   Witness Name (please print): _____

Patient Signature: _____   Witness Signature: _____
Date: _____   Date: _____

Table 16.3 Alternatives for management of concerns of shell disruption or leaking silicone implant

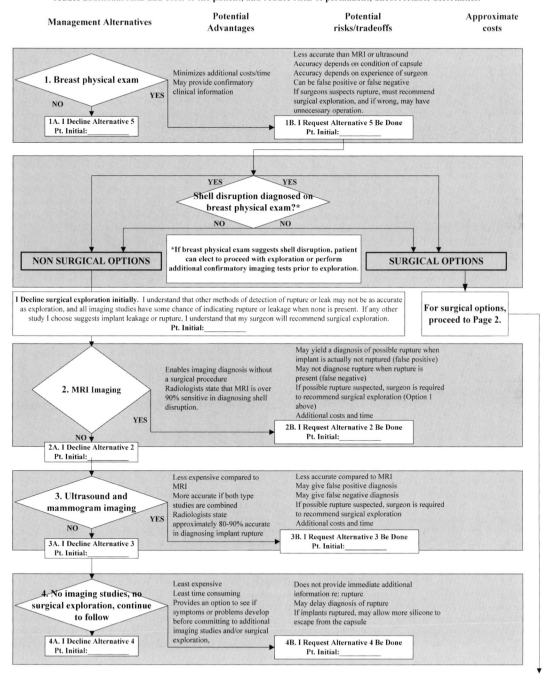

Alternatives for Management of Concern of Shell Disruption or Leaking Silicone Gel Implant
The BASPI Workgroup, John B. Tebbetts, M.D., Moderator
Copyright 2004
**Management alternatives are listed prioritizing alternatives most likely to reduce risks of additional operations,
reduce additional risks and costs to the patient, and reduce risks of permanent, uncorrectable deformities.

Management Alternatives	Potential Advantages	Potential risks/tradeoffs	Approximate costs

1. Breast physical exam
NO
YES

1A. I Decline Alternative 5
Pt. Initial:_____

Minimizes additional costs/time
May provide confirmatory clinical information

Less accurate than MRI or ultrasound
Accuracy depends on condition of capsule
Accuracy depends on experience of surgeon
Can be false positive or false negative
If surgeons suspects rupture, must recommend surgical exploration, and if wrong, may have unnecessary operation.

1B. I Request Alternative 5 Be Done
Pt. Initial:_____

YES   YES
Shell disruption diagnosed on breast physical exam?*
NO   NO

*If breast physical exam suggests shell disruption, patient can elect to proceed with exploration or perform additional confirmatory imaging tests prior to exploration.

NON SURGICAL OPTIONS   **SURGICAL OPTIONS**

I Decline surgical exploration initially. I understand that other methods of detection of rupture or leak may not be as accurate as exploration, and all imaging studies have some chance of indicating rupture or leakage when none is present. If any other study I choose suggests implant leakage or rupture, I understand that my surgeon will recommend surgical exploration.
Pt. Initial:_____

For surgical options, proceed to Page 2.

2. MRI Imaging
YES
NO
2A. I Decline Alternative 2
Pt. Initial:_____

Enables imaging diagnosis without a surgical procedure
Radiologists state that MRI is over 90% sensitive in diagnosing shell disruption.

May yield a diagnosis of possible rupture when implant is actually not ruptured (false positive)
May not diagnose rupture when rupture is present (false negative)
If possible rupture suspected, surgeon is required to recommend surgical exploration (Option 1 above)
Additional costs and time

2B. I Request Alternative 2 Be Done
Pt. Initial:_____

3. Ultrasound and mammogram imaging
NO
YES
3A. I Decline Alternative 3
Pt. Initial:_____

Less expensive compared to MRI
More accurate if both type studies are combined
Radiologists state approximately 80-90% accurate in diagnosing implant rupture

Less accurate compared to MRI
May give false positive diagnosis
May give false negative diagnosis
If possible rupture suspected, surgeon is required to recommend surgical exploration
Additional costs and time

3B. I Request Alternative 3 Be Done
Pt. Initial:_____

4. No imaging studies, no surgical exploration, continue to follow
4A. I Decline Alternative 4
Pt. Initial:_____

Least expensive
Least time consuming
Provides an option to see if symptoms or problems develop before committing to additional imaging studies and/or surgical exploration,

Does not provide immediate additional information re: rupture
May delay diagnosis of rupture
If implants ruptured, may allow more silicone to escape from the capsule

4B. I Request Alternative 4 Be Done
Pt. Initial:_____

Table 16.3 *(continued)* Alternatives for management of concerns of shell disruption or leaking silicone implant

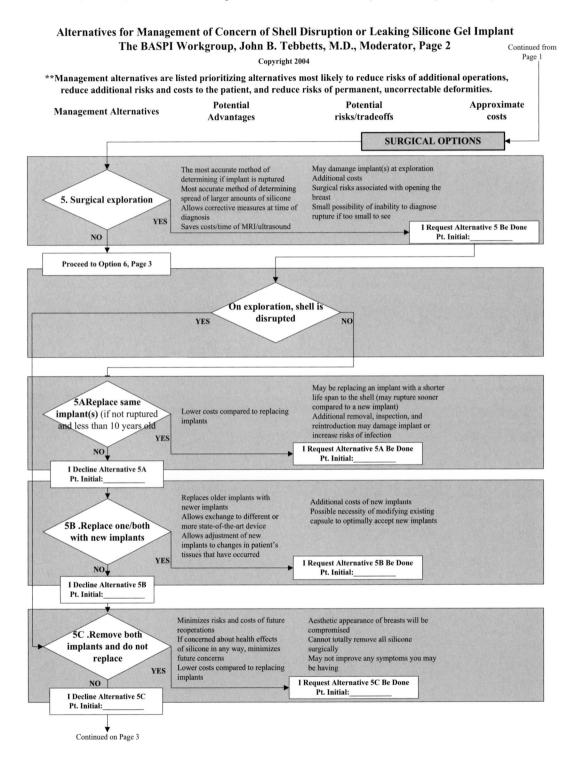

Alternatives for Management of Concern of Shell Disruption or Leaking Silicone Gel Implant
The BASPI Workgroup, John B. Tebbetts, M.D., Moderator, Page 2

Continued from Page 1

Copyright 2004

**Management alternatives are listed prioritizing alternatives most likely to reduce risks of additional operations, reduce additional risks and costs to the patient, and reduce risks of permanent, uncorrectable deformities.

Management Alternatives	Potential Advantages	Potential risks/tradeoffs	Approximate costs

SURGICAL OPTIONS

5. Surgical exploration   YES / NO

The most accurate method of determining if implant is ruptured
Most accurate method of determining spread of larger amounts of silicone
Allows corrective measures at time of diagnosis
Saves costs/time of MRI/ultrasound

May damage implant(s) at exploration
Additional costs
Surgical risks associated with opening the breast
Small possibility of inability to diagnose rupture if too small to see

I Request Alternative 5 Be Done
Pt. Initial:_____

Proceed to Option 6, Page 3

On exploration, shell is disrupted   YES / NO

5A Replace same implant(s) (if not ruptured and less than 10 years old   YES

Lower costs compared to replacing implants

May be replacing an implant with a shorter life span to the shell (may rupture sooner compared to a new implant)
Additional removal, inspection, and reintroduction may damage implant or increase risks of infection

I Request Alternative 5A Be Done
Pt. Initial:_____

I Decline Alternative 5A
Pt. Initial:_____

5B. Replace one/both with new implants   YES / NO

Replaces older implants with newer implants
Allows exchange to different or more state-of-the-art device
Allows adjustment of new implants to changes in patient's tissues that have occurred

Additional costs of new implants
Possible necessity of modifying existing capsule to optimally accept new implants

I Request Alternative 5B Be Done
Pt. Initial:_____

I Decline Alternative 5B
Pt. Initial:_____

5C. Remove both implants and do not replace   YES / NO

Minimizes risks and costs of future reoperations
If concerned about health effects of silicone in any way, minimizes future concerns
Lower costs compared to replacing implants

Aesthetic appearance of breasts will be compromised
Cannot totally remove all silicone surgically
May not improve any symptoms you may be having

I Request Alternative 5C Be Done
Pt. Initial:_____

I Decline Alternative 5C
Pt. Initial:_____

Continued on Page 3

Table 16.3 *(continued)* Alternatives for management of concerns of shell disruption or leaking silicone implant

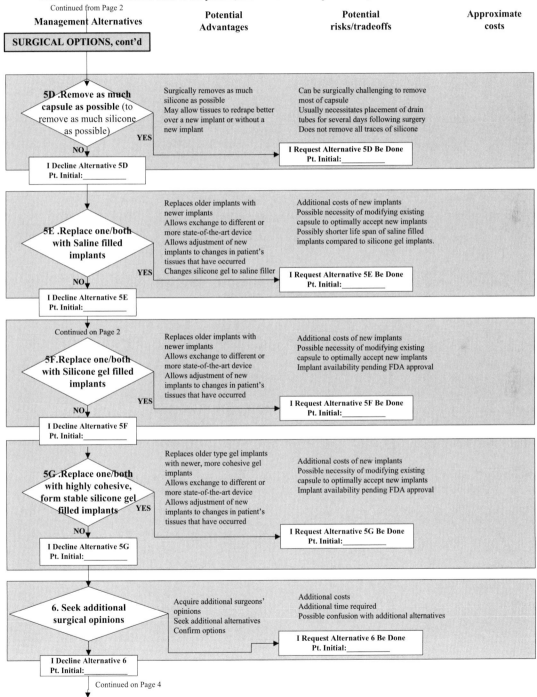

Alternatives for Management of Concern of Shell Disruption or Leaking Silicone Gel Implant
The BASPI Workgroup, John B. Tebbetts, M.D., Moderator, Page 3
Copyright 2004
**Management alternatives are listed prioritizing alternatives most likely to reduce risks of additional operations,
reduce additional risks and costs to the patient, and reduce risks of permanent, uncorrectable deformities.

Continued from Page 2

Management Alternatives	Potential Advantages	Potential risks/tradeoffs	Approximate costs

SURGICAL OPTIONS, cont'd

5D .Remove as much capsule as possible (to remove as much silicone as possible) — **YES**

Surgically removes as much silicone as possible
May allow tissues to redrape better over a new implant or without a new implant

Can be surgically challenging to remove most of capsule
Usually necessitates placement of drain tubes for several days following surgery
Does not remove all traces of silicone

I Request Alternative 5D Be Done
Pt. Initial:_____

NO → I Decline Alternative 5D Pt. Initial:_____

5E .Replace one/both with Saline filled implants — **YES**

Replaces older implants with newer implants
Allows exchange to different or more state-of-the-art device
Allows adjustment of new implants to changes in patient's tissues that have occurred
Changes silicone gel to saline filler

Additional costs of new implants
Possible necessity of modifying existing capsule to optimally accept new implants
Possibly shorter life span of saline filled implants compared to silicone gel implants.

I Request Alternative 5E Be Done
Pt. Initial:_____

NO → I Decline Alternative 5E Pt. Initial:_____

Continued on Page 2

5F.Replace one/both with Silicone gel filled implants — **YES**

Replaces older implants with newer implants
Allows exchange to different or more state-of-the-art device
Allows adjustment of new implants to changes in patient's tissues that have occurred

Additional costs of new implants
Possible necessity of modifying existing capsule to optimally accept new implants
Implant availability pending FDA approval

I Request Alternative 5F Be Done
Pt. Initial:_____

NO → I Decline Alternative 5F Pt. Initial:_____

5G .Replace one/both with highly cohesive, form stable silicone gel filled implants — **YES**

Replaces older type gel implants with newer, more cohesive gel implants
Allows exchange to different or more state-of-the-art device
Allows adjustment of new implants to changes in patient's tissues that have occurred

Additional costs of new implants
Possible necessity of modifying existing capsule to optimally accept new implants
Implant availability pending FDA approval

I Request Alternative 5G Be Done
Pt. Initial:_____

NO → I Decline Alternative 5G Pt. Initial:_____

6. Seek additional surgical opinions

Acquire additional surgeons' opinions
Seek additional alternatives
Confirm options

Additional costs
Additional time required
Possible confusion with additional alternatives

I Request Alternative 6 Be Done
Pt. Initial:_____

I Decline Alternative 6 Pt. Initial:_____

Continued on Page 4

Table 16.3 *(continued)* Alternatives for management of concerns of shell disruption or leaking silicone implant

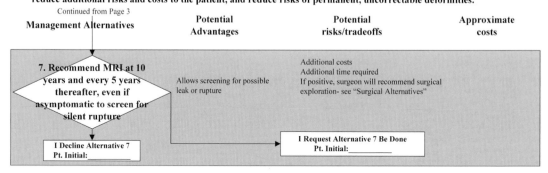

Alternatives for Management of Concern of Ruptured or Leaking Silicone Gel Implant

Continued from Page 3

The BASPI Workgroup, John B. Tebbetts, M.D., Moderator, Page 4

Copyright 2004

**Management alternatives are listed prioritizing alternatives most likely to reduce risks of additional operations, reduce additional risks and costs to the patient, and reduce risks of permanent, uncorrectable deformities.

Continued from Page 3 **Management Alternatives**	**Potential Advantages**	**Potential risks/tradeoffs**	**Approximate costs**
7. Recommend MRI at 10 years and every 5 years thereafter, even if asymptomatic to screen for silent rupture	Allows screening for possible leak or rupture	Additional costs Additional time required If positive, surgeon will recommend surgical exploration- see "Surgical Alternatives"	
I Decline Alternative 7 **Pt. Initial:_____**		**I Request Alternative 7 Be Done** **Pt. Initial:_____**	

Surgeon actions:
1) Return all implants with shell disruption to manufacturer for analysis
2) Request a written report with results of analysis within 3 months from manufacturer

**If patient, surgeon, or patient's family are concerned about any aspect of silicone causing symptoms or possible associated conditions, see additional information and flowchart alternatives entitled "If Patient Has Symptoms or Concerns Related to Silicone"

Patient Name (please print):_____   Witness Name (please print): _____

Patient Signature: _____   Witness Signature: _____
Date: _____   Date: _____

OUT POINTS   1) Patient requests removal without replacement at any time
2) When available soft tissue coverage in any area of the breast is less than 0.5cm pinch thickness (0.25cm overlying implant)

Table 16.4 Alternatives for management of possible periprosthetic space infection or seroma

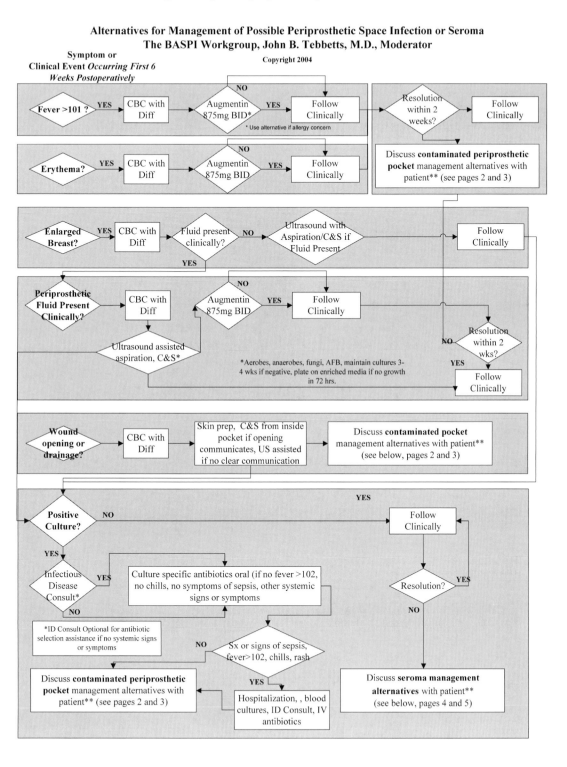

Table 16.4 *(continued)* Alternatives for management of possible periprosthetic space infection or seroma

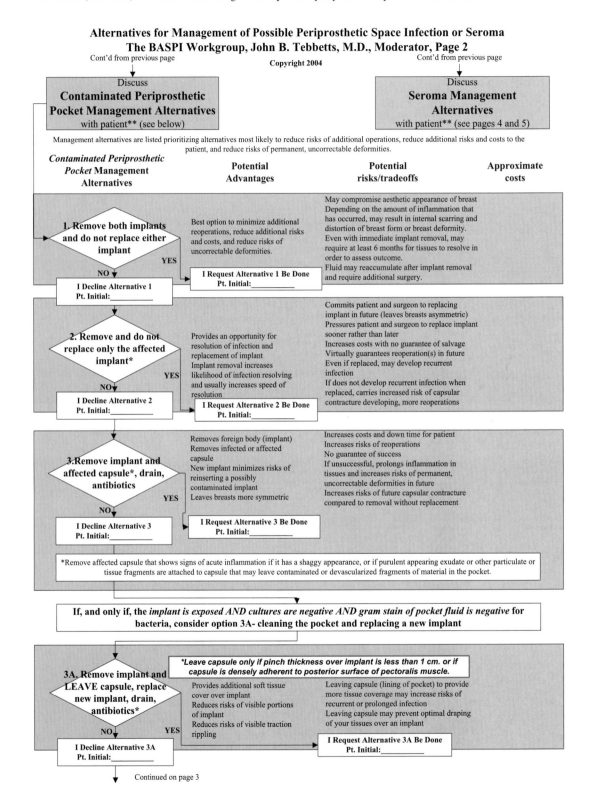

Continued on page 3

Table 16.4 *(continued)* Alternatives for management of possible periprosthetic space infection or seroma

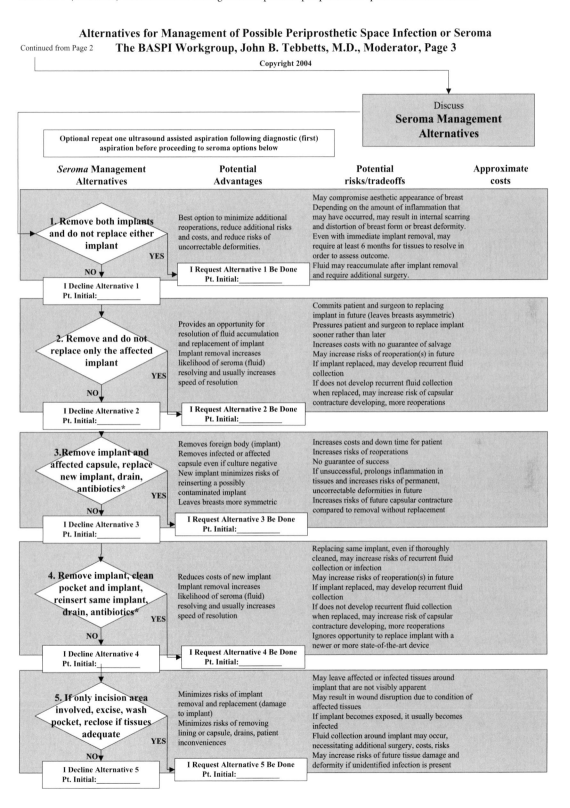

Alternatives for Management of Possible Periprosthetic Space Infection or Seroma
Continued from Page 2   **The BASPI Workgroup, John B. Tebbetts, M.D., Moderator, Page 3**
Copyright 2004

Discuss
**Seroma Management
Alternatives**

Optional repeat one ultrasound assisted aspiration following diagnostic (first) aspiration before proceeding to seroma options below

Seroma Management Alternatives	Potential Advantages	Potential risks/tradeoffs	Approximate costs
1. Remove both implants and do not replace either implant YES	Best option to minimize additional reoperations, reduce additional risks and costs, and reduce risks of uncorrectable deformities.	May compromise aesthetic appearance of breast Depending on the amount of inflammation that may have occurred, may result in internal scarring and distortion of breast form or breast deformity. Even with immediate implant removal, may require at least 6 months for tissues to resolve in order to assess outcome. Fluid may reaccumulate after implant removal and require additional surgery.	
NO → I Decline Alternative 1 Pt. Initial:_____	I Request Alternative 1 Be Done Pt. Initial:_____		
2. Remove and do not replace only the affected implant YES	Provides an opportunity for resolution of fluid accumulation and replacement of implant Implant removal increases likelihood of seroma (fluid) resolving and usually increases speed of resolution	Commits patient and surgeon to replacing implant in future (leaves breasts asymmetric) Pressures patient and surgeon to replace implant sooner rather than later Increases costs with no guarantee of salvage May increase risks of reoperation(s) in future If implant replaced, may develop recurrent fluid collection If does not develop recurrent fluid collection when replaced, may increase risk of capsular contracture developing, more reoperations	
NO → I Decline Alternative 2 Pt. Initial:_____	I Request Alternative 2 Be Done Pt. Initial:_____		
3. Remove implant and affected capsule, replace new implant, drain, antibiotics* YES	Removes foreign body (implant) Removes infected or affected capsule even if culture negative New implant minimizes risks of reinserting a possibly contaminated implant Leaves breasts more symmetric	Increases costs and down time for patient Increases risks of reoperations No guarantee of success If unsuccessful, prolongs inflammation in tissues and increases risks of permanent, uncorrectable deformities in future Increases risks of future capsular contracture compared to removal without replacement	
NO → I Decline Alternative 3 Pt. Initial:_____	I Request Alternative 3 Be Done Pt. Initial:_____		
4. Remove implant, clean pocket and implant, reinsert same implant, drain, antibiotics* YES	Reduces costs of new implant Implant removal increases likelihood of seroma (fluid) resolving and usually increases speed of resolution	Replacing same implant, even if thoroughly cleaned, may increase risks of recurrent fluid collection or infection May increase risks of reoperation(s) in future If implant replaced, may develop recurrent fluid collection If does not develop recurrent fluid collection when replaced, may increase risk of capsular contracture developing, more reoperations Ignores opportunity to replace implant with a newer or more state-of-the-art device	
NO → I Decline Alternative 4 Pt. Initial:_____	I Request Alternative 4 Be Done Pt. Initial:_____		
5. If only incision area involved, excise, wash pocket, reclose if tissues adequate YES	Minimizes risks of implant removal and replacement (damage to implant) Minimizes risks of removing lining or capsule, drains, patient inconveniences	May leave affected or infected tissues around implant that are not visibly apparent May result in wound disruption due to condition of affected tissues If implant becomes exposed, it usually becomes infected Fluid collection around implant may occur, necessitating additional surgery, costs, risks May increase risks of future tissue damage and deformity if unidentified infection is present	
NO → I Decline Alternative 5 Pt. Initial:_____	I Request Alternative 5 Be Done Pt. Initial:_____		

Table 16.4 *(continued)* Alternatives for management of possible periprosthetic space infection or seroma

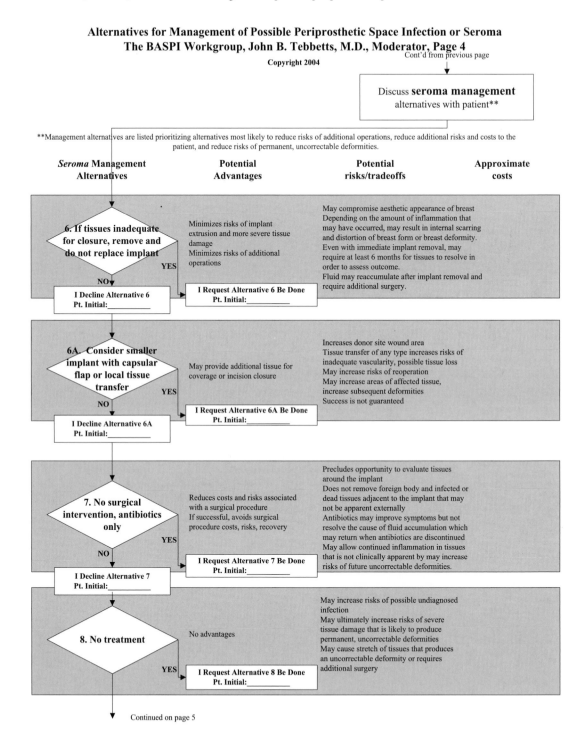

Continued on page 5

Table 16.4 *(continued)* Alternatives for management of possible periprosthetic space infection or seroma

**Alternatives for Management of Possible Periprosthetic Space Infection or Seroma
The BASPI Workgroup, John B. Tebbetts, M.D., Moderator, Page 5**

Copyright 2004

Cont'd from page 4

9. Seek additional surgical opinions

Acquire additional surgeons' opinions
Seek additional alternatives
Confirm options

Additional costs
Additional time required
Possible confusion with additional alternatives

I Request Alternative 9 Be Done
Pt. Initial:_____

I Decline Alternative 9
Pt. Initial:_____

Patient Name (please print):_____

Patient Signature: _____
Date: _____

Witness Name (please print): _____

Witness Signature: _____
Date: _____

OUT POINTS 1) Culture proved infection of the periprosthetic pocket
2) Inadequate (<0.5cm thick or severely indurated or inflammed) soft tissue coverage at the incision site for safe reclosure
3) Any time patient requests removal without replacement

Implant Replacement Criteria 1) No replacement for 3-6 months with no evidence of infection AND complete tissue resolution- normal soft tissues in all areas of the breast
2) No replacement if the patient has had more than 1 episode of infection in the affected breast
3) No replacement if soft tissue pinch thickness in any area overlying the implant is less than 0.5cm pinch thickness

Table 16.5 Alternatives for management of stretch deformities and implant malposition

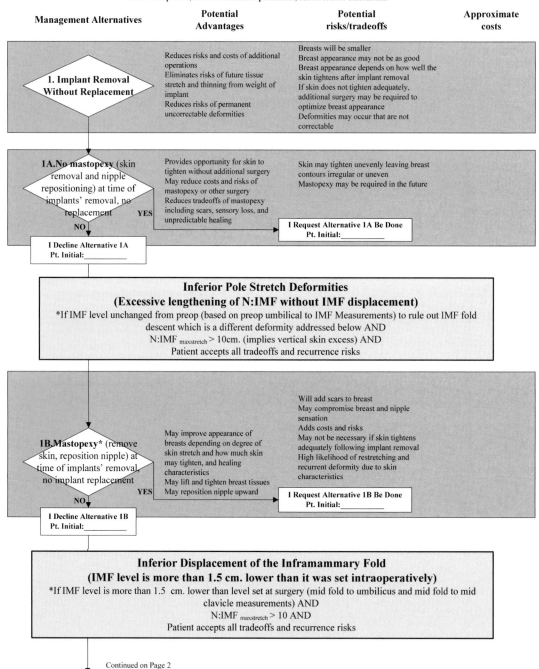

Alternatives for Management of Stretch Deformities and Implant Malposition
The BASPI Workgroup, John B. Tebbetts, M.D., Moderator

Copyright 2004
**Management alternatives are listed prioritizing alternatives most likely to reduce risks of additional operations, reduce additional risks and costs to the patient, and reduce risks of permanent, uncorrectable deformities.

Management Alternatives	Potential Advantages	Potential risks/tradeoffs	Approximate costs

1. Implant Removal Without Replacement

Reduces risks and costs of additional operations
Eliminates risks of future tissue stretch and thinning from weight of implant
Reduces risks of permanent uncorrectable deformities

Breasts will be smaller
Breast appearance may not be as good
Breast appearance depends on how well the skin tightens after implant removal
If skin does not tighten adequately, additional surgery may be required to optimize breast appearance
Deformities may occur that are not correctable

1A. No mastopexy (skin removal and nipple repositioning) at time of implants' removal, no replacement   **YES**   **NO**

Provides opportunity for skin to tighten without additional surgery
May reduce costs and risks of mastopexy or other surgery
Reduces tradeoffs of mastopexy including scars, sensory loss, and unpredictable healing

Skin may tighten unevenly leaving breast contours irregular or uneven
Mastopexy may be required in the future

I Request Alternative 1A Be Done
Pt. Initial:_____

I Decline Alternative 1A
Pt. Initial:_____

Inferior Pole Stretch Deformities
(Excessive lengthening of N:IMF without IMF displacement)
*If IMF level unchanged from preop (based on preop umbilical to IMF Measurements) to rule out IMF fold descent which is a different deformity addressed below AND
N:IMF $_{maxstretch}$ > 10cm. (implies vertical skin excess) AND
Patient accepts all tradeoffs and recurrence risks

1B. Mastopexy* (remove skin, reposition nipple) at time of implants' removal, no implant replacement   **YES**   **NO**

May improve appearance of breasts depending on degree of skin stretch and how much skin may tighten, and healing characteristics
May lift and tighten breast tissues
May reposition nipple upward

Will add scars to breast
May compromise breast and nipple sensation
Adds costs and risks
May not be necessary if skin tightens adequately following implant removal
High likelihood of restretching and recurrent deformity due to skin characteristics

I Request Alternative 1B Be Done
Pt. Initial:_____

I Decline Alternative 1B
Pt. Initial:_____

Inferior Displacement of the Inframammary Fold
(IMF level is more than 1.5 cm. lower than it was set intraoperatively)
*If IMF level is more than 1.5 cm. lower than level set at surgery (mid fold to umbilicus and mid fold to mid clavicle measurements) AND
N:IMF $_{maxstretch}$ > 10 AND
Patient accepts all tradeoffs and recurrence risks

Continued on Page 2

Table 16.5 *(continued)* Alternatives for management of stretch deformities and implant malposition

Alternatives for Management of Stretch Deformities and Implant Malposition
The BASPI Workgroup, John B. Tebbetts, M.D., Moderator, Page 2

Copyright 2004
**Management alternatives are listed prioritizing alternatives most likely to reduce risks of additional operations, reduce additional risks and costs to the patient, and reduce risks of permanent, uncorrectable deformities.

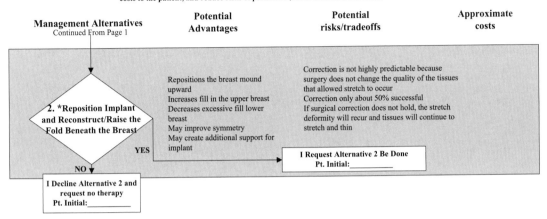

Management Alternatives Continued From Page 1	Potential Advantages	Potential risks/tradeoffs	Approximate costs
2. *Reposition Implant and Reconstruct/Raise the Fold Beneath the Breast	Repositions the breast mound upward Increases fill in the upper breast Decreases excessive fill lower breast May improve symmetry May create additional support for implant	Correction is not highly predictable because surgery does not change the quality of the tissues that allowed stretch to occur Correction only about 50% successful If surgical correction does not hold, the stretch deformity will recur and tissues will continue to stretch and thin	

YES → **I Request Alternative 2 Be Done** Pt. Initial:_____

NO → **I Decline Alternative 2 and request no therapy** Pt. Initial:_____

Synmastia
(Periprosthetic pockets connect medially or are within 1 cm. of connecting)

Attempted surgical correction with replacements of implants at the same procedure is NOT recommended if the implant is partially retropectoral AND the medial origins of the pectoralis along the sternum have been divided. If the synmastia is retromammary, and all medial origins of the pectoralis along the sternum are intact, may consider reconstructing the synmastia and replacing implants to a subpectoral position at the same procedure, accepting that replacing implants at the same procedure may add risks and tradeoffs.

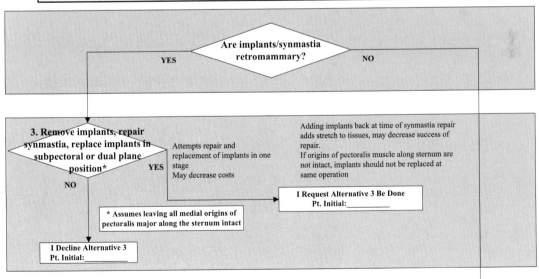

Are implants/synmastia retromammary?

YES ← → NO

3. Remove implants, repair synmastia, replace implants in subpectoral or dual plane position*	Attempts repair and replacement of implants in one stage May decrease costs	Adding implants back at time of synmastia repair adds stretch to tissues, may decrease success of repair. If origins of pectoralis muscle along sternum are not intact, implants should not be replaced at same operation	

YES → **I Request Alternative 3 Be Done** Pt. Initial:_____

NO

* Assumes leaving all medial origins of pectoralis major along the sternum intact

I Decline Alternative 3 Pt. Initial:_____

Continued on Page 3

Table 16.5 *(continued)* Alternatives for management of stretch deformities and implant malposition

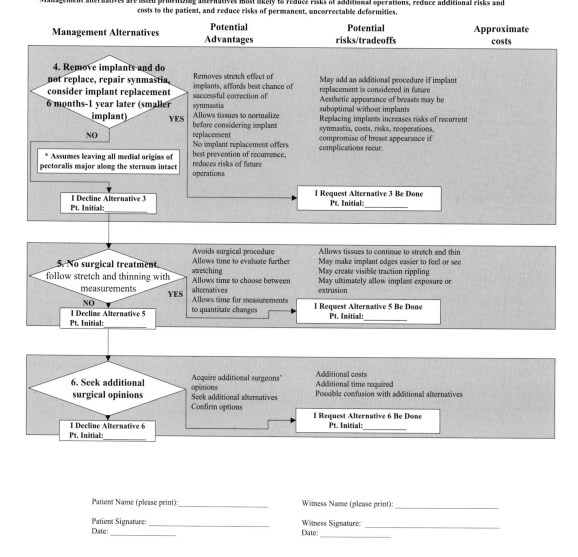

Alternatives for Management of Stretch Deformities and Implant Malposition
The BASPI Workgroup, John B. Tebbetts, M.D., Moderator, Page 3

Copyright 2004
**Management alternatives are listed prioritizing alternatives most likely to reduce risks of additional operations, reduce additional risks and costs to the patient, and reduce risks of permanent, uncorrectable deformities.

Management Alternatives	Potential Advantages	Potential risks/tradeoffs	Approximate costs
4. Remove implants and do not replace, repair synmastia, consider implant replacement 6 months-1 year later (smaller implant) YES NO * Assumes leaving all medial origins of pectoralis major along the sternum intact I Decline Alternative 3 Pt. Initial:_____	Removes stretch effect of implants, affords best chance of successful correction of synmastia Allows tissues to normalize before considering implant replacement No implant replacement offers best prevention of recurrence, reduces risks of future operations	May add an additional procedure if implant replacement is considered in future Aesthetic appearance of breasts may be suboptimal without implants Replacing implants increases risks of recurrent synmastia, costs, risks, reoperations, compromise of breast appearance if complications recur. I Request Alternative 3 Be Done Pt. Initial:_____	
5. No surgical treatment, follow stretch and thinning with measurements YES NO I Decline Alternative 5 Pt. Initial:_____	Avoids surgical procedure Allows time to evaluate further stretching Allows time to choose between alternatives Allows time for measurements to quantitate changes	Allows tissues to continue to stretch and thin May make implant edges easier to feel or see May create visible traction rippling May ultimately allow implant exposure or extrusion I Request Alternative 5 Be Done Pt. Initial:_____	
6. Seek additional surgical opinions I Decline Alternative 6 Pt. Initial:_____	Acquire additional surgeons' opinions Seek additional alternatives Confirm options	Additional costs Additional time required Possible confusion with additional alternatives I Request Alternative 6 Be Done Pt. Initial:_____	

Patient Name (please print):_____   Witness Name (please print): _____

Patient Signature: _____   Witness Signature: _____
Date: _____   Date: _____

OUT POINTS
1) If pinch thickness of soft tissues overlying implant in any area is <0.5cm
2) Implant shell visibility in any area where more soft tissue coverage is not available without tissue transfer
2) Recurrence of any stretch deformity after a one or two-stage attempt at correction
3) Patient request at any time

Table 16.6 Alternatives for management of undefined symptoms

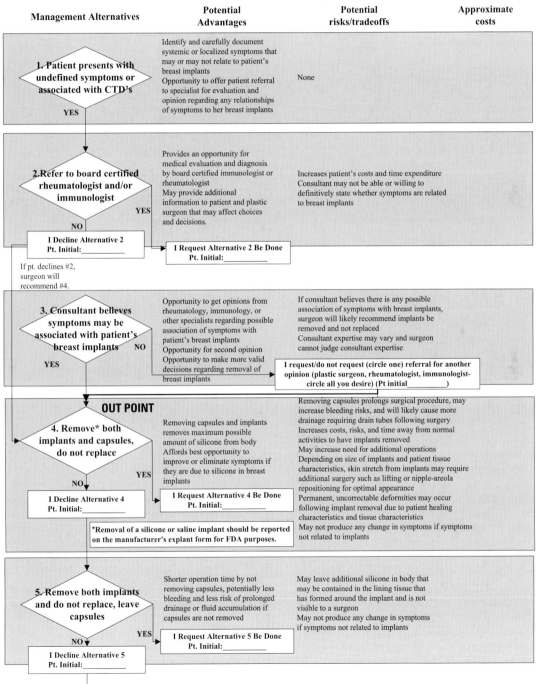

Alternatives for Management of Undefined Symptom
Complexes
The BASPI Workgroup, John B. Tebbetts, M.D., Moderator
Copyright 2004

Management alternatives are listed prioritizing alternatives most likely to reduce risks of additional operations, reduce additional risks and costs to the patient, and reduce risks of permanent, uncorrectable deformities.

Table 16.6 *(continued)* Alternatives for management of undefined symptoms

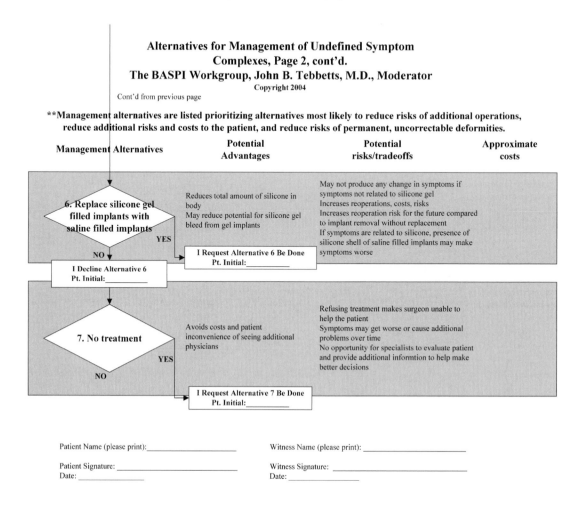

**Alternatives for Management of Undefined Symptom
Complexes, Page 2, cont'd.
The BASPI Workgroup, John B. Tebbetts, M.D., Moderator**
Copyright 2004

Cont'd from previous page

**Management alternatives are listed prioritizing alternatives most likely to reduce risks of additional operations, reduce additional risks and costs to the patient, and reduce risks of permanent, uncorrectable deformities.

Management Alternatives	Potential Advantages	Potential risks/tradeoffs	Approximate costs
6. Replace silicone gel filled implants with saline filled implants YES	Reduces total amount of silicone in body / May reduce potential for silicone gel bleed from gel implants	May not produce any change in symptoms if symptoms not related to silicone gel / Increases reoperations, costs, risks / Increases reoperation risk for the future compared to implant removal without replacement / If symptoms are related to silicone, presence of silicone shell of saline filled implants may make symptoms worse	
NO / I Decline Alternative 6 Pt. Initial:____	I Request Alternative 6 Be Done Pt. Initial:____		
7. No treatment YES	Avoids costs and patient inconvenience of seeing additional physicians	Refusing treatment makes surgeon unable to help the patient / Symptoms may get worse or cause additional problems over time / No opportunity for specialists to evaluate patient and provide additional informtion to help make better decisions	
NO	I Request Alternative 7 Be Done Pt. Initial:____		

Patient Name (please print):_____   Witness Name (please print): _____

Patient Signature: _____   Witness Signature: _____
Date: _____   Date: _____

OUT POINTS 1) Board certified rheumatologist relates symptoms, findings or diagnosis to breast implants, or diagnoses CTD.
2) Patient desires implant removal, regardless of findings of rheumatologist.

16.4
Implant Size Change

When comprehensive preoperative patient education and informed consent are combined with sound preoperative planning, reoperation for a change in implant size can be dramatically reduced [6]. There are, however, a great number of plastic surgeons who ignore these tissue characteristics and measurements. Although the vast majority of patients request a larger device when electing an implant exchange, it is not uncommon to see patients requesting a size change to remove excessively large implants placed by another surgeon.

Replacing an implant to a larger size may require capsulectomy or capsulotomy, and possible adjustment to the inframmary fold. In addition, the patient must be aware that the larger device will inevitably produce further negative effects on the tissues over time. These include continued stretching and thinning of the overlying skin and parenchyma and increased visibility or palpability, which may not be apparent for several years.

Replacing the implant with a smaller device may be even more complicated. The pocket must be reduced by either capsulorrhaphy or creation of a new pocket (position change or Neo-pocket; S. Spear S and B. Bengston, personal correspondence). In addition, issues of skin excess may need to be addressed by some form of mastopexy. Physicians may choose to correct these problems in one or multiple stages. Trade-offs may include additional sagging of breasts, palpable implant edges, or visible rippling. Patients need to be aware of the risks and trade-offs associated with each procedure as well as the additional costs.

In addition to size change alone, the issue of a saline-to-silicone switch has now become a relevant part of the decision-making algorithm. When a medical problem exists in one breast or capsular contracture or deflation of a saline device, the choice to replace both devices with a newer-generation silicone implant is logical. However, more and more patients are requesting a switch to silicone from saline, for no other reason than an "upgrade," where no medical problem exists and the change is solely for feel and comfort. Although this procedure inarguably increases costs to the patient and may be considered medically unnecessary, it is an inevitable result of our quest to prove silicone devices safe and effective. We can expect to see an increase in the number of patients requesting an implant exchange to the newer round and cohesive devices as a result of the release of silicone devices to the U.S. market and of manufacturers increasing their direct-to-consumer marketing. In addition, many women may not have been given the preoperative choice between silicone and saline devices but may have preferred a silicone device if given that choice. The patient, however, needs to understand the clear risks and trade-offs associated with even a "simple" implant exchange. Patients must be made aware of the hard data and accept the risk of a significantly higher capsular contracture rate in any revision augmentation [7].

16.5
Alternatives for Managing Capsular Contracture Grades 3 and 4

Advanced preoperative planning and improved surgical techniques that provide an atraumatic dissection, combined with practices that reduce bacterial contamination intraoperatively and selection of the latest generation of silicone gel devices, have been shown to dramatically reduce capsular contracture rates [3]. Unfortunately, capsular contracture rates have been reported to be as high as 17.2% at 3 years in recent premarket approval data [8]. In addition, patients with older-generation devices may have lost contact with their primary plastic surgeon and may present up to 30 years following primary breast augmentation, often with grades 3 and 4 capsular contractures that have been neglected for years. The management algorithm for capsular contracture grades 3 and 4 prioritizes alternatives that are most likely to reduce the risks of additional operations and costs to the patient, as well as reduce the risks of permanent, uncorrectable deformities.

Of all of the management alternatives outlined in the algorithms, only explantation without replacement offers the patient a guarantee of no future implant revision procedures. These "out points" have been shown to reduce reoperation rates. Removal without replacement must be a joint decision of the patient and the surgeon when both agree that removing the implants is preferable to possible recurrent deformities, additional surgeries, and costs [9]. The algorithm provides for alternative management of capsular contractures, should the patient and physician decide to replace the devices, and allows patients to participate in the decision-making process. Traditional procedures designed to treat capsular contracture should, like primary augmentation, be performed in conjunction with a system of quantifiable implant selection for replacement and a surgical technique that reduces bleeding and tissue trauma. (See Fig. 16.1.)

16.6
Alternatives for Managing Possible Periprosthetic Space Infection

Signs and symptoms of a periprosthetic infection may develop acutely, within the first 6 weeks postoperatively, or years after breast augmentation as either an infection or periprosthetic fluid collection or seroma. Indications for removal of the implant may include culture-proven infection of the periprosthetic pocket, inadequate tissue for implant coverage, or patient choice.

The use of ultrasound needle-guided drainage of the periprosthetic space provides necessary cultures and is well tolerated and accepted by patients. If successful, antibiotic management can reduce the costs and risks associated with a surgical procedure, although the results may be temporary. Recurrent seroma formation and continued tissue inflammation are likely to produce permanent uncorrectable deformities and capsular contracture. If explantation is required, the implant should not be replaced for 3–6 months after complete resolution of symptoms. The implant should not be replaced if the patient has experienced more than one episode of documented infection in the same breast (Fig. 16.2).

16.7
Alternatives for Managing Stretch Deformities and Implant Malposition

A method of breast implant selection that preoperatively includes quantified measurements of the patient's existing tissue characteristics has been shown to reduce stretch deformities and implant malposition and to lower reoperation rates [6]. The larger the device, the

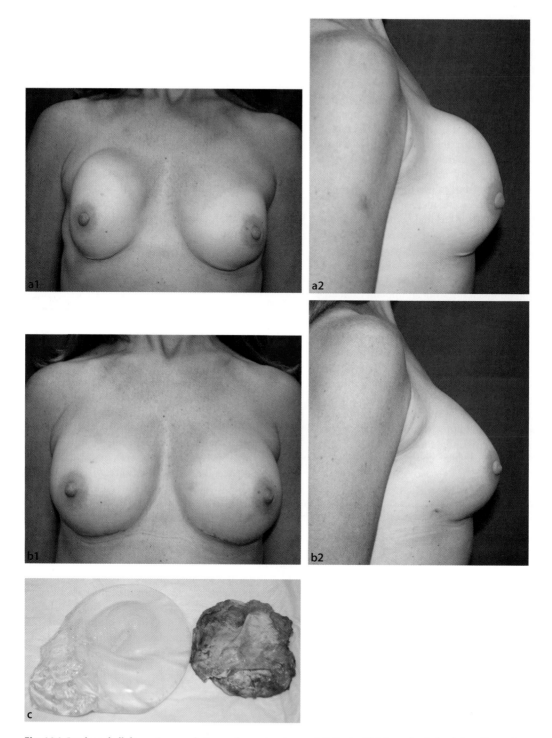

Fig. 16.1 Implant shell disruption, grade 4 capsular contracture. **a** *1* Patient with bilateral subglandular silicone implants (1988) with rupture on the right, with a grade 4 capsular contracture. *2* Side view. **b** *1* Explantation, bilateral complete capsulectomies, and replacement with partial submuscular 410 cohesive gel implants. *2* Side view. **c** Removed implant and excised capsule

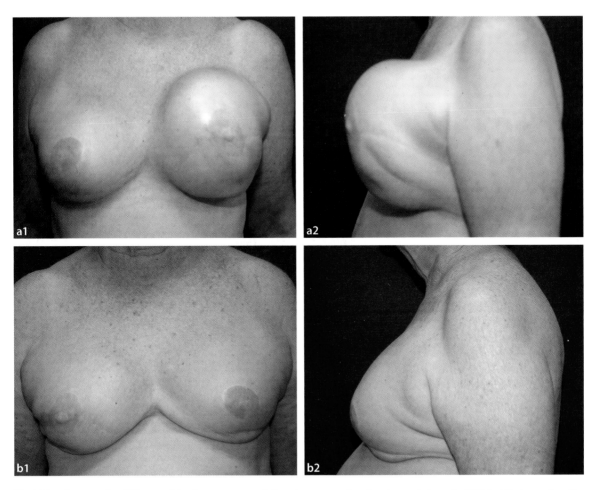

Fig 16.2 **a** Preoperative. Silicone gel implant rupture and chronic seroma after closed capsulotomy in 1998. **b** *1* Postoperative. Patient 10 years after open capsulectomy and replacement with highly cohesive gel implants. *2* Lateral view

more likely the patient will develop stretch deformities and malposition over time. Preoperative planning, surgical technique, and factors related to wound healing, as well as the patient's genetic tissue characteristics, all play a role in the long-term persistence maintenance of implant position. Using the decision-making algorithm, patients and physicians can prioritize the alternatives most likely to reduce additional operations. Capsulorrhaphy or alternative pocket procedures may be used in conjunction with implant size change, and procedures that correct the associated acquired skin deformities may be necessary. Patients may elect to delay a skin-tightening procedure but may be left with uneven breast contours requiring future mastopexy. Patients and physicians should consider no further surgery if there is recurrence of the deformity after a one- or two-staged attempt at surgical correction or if tissues overlay the implant by <0.5 cm. (See Figs. 16.3, 16.4.)

16.8
Management of Shell Disruption or Leaking Silicone Gel Implant

Perhaps no other area in the long debate on the safety of silicone gel implants has produced as much concern by plastic surgeons, patients, and the FDA as the identification and management of silicone gel implant ruptures. The FDA now recommends that all women undergo their first MRI at 3 years after implant surgery and every 2 years thereafter [10]. Patients with older-generation implants are at higher risk for implant shell disruption. Rupture rates as reported in the Inamed Core Study were estimated to be 14% at 10 years. Physical examination has been found to be less accurate than MRI for detecting silent ruptures, with rupture rates of 3.4% at 4 years by MRI and 1.1% without MRI [11]. The sensitivity of clinical exams for diagnosing implant rup-

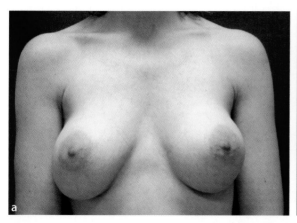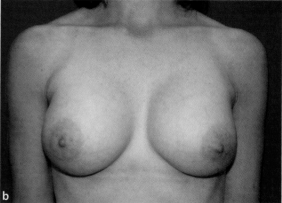

Fig. 16.3 Malposition: stretch deformity. **a** Patient has subglandular saline implants with malposition and inferior stretch deformity. **b** Bilateral position change to partial submuscular, capsulorrhaphies, and replacement with 410 cohesive gel implants

ture is only 30% [12]. MRI enables diagnosis without a surgical procedure, but it may lead to false positives or negatives. If the breast MRI is positive for rupture or the physician has a high level of suspicion that implant shell disruption has occurred, surgical exploration is the most reliable method to detect device failure.

If the patient and physician have decided to replace a ruptured device, the patient should be aware that a complete capsulectomy will surgically remove as much silicone as possible, but it may not remove all if the silicone. This may be very important for future mammography. It may also allow the tissues to drape with fewer contour irregularities over the new device. The trade-offs associated with complete capsulectomy are the need for postoperative drains and no guarantee of complete removal of all old silicone gel. A ruptured device should be sent back to the manufacturer for analysis when applicable. (See Fig. 16.5.)

16.9
Alternatives for Managing Undefined Symptom Complexes

In 1999, the Institute of Medicine's Safety of Silicone Breast Implants Committee found no convincing evidence for atypical connective tissue or rheumatic disease or a novel constellation of signs and symptoms in women with silicone breast implants [13]. Despite these conclusions, the FDA, patients, and patient advocate groups continue to demonstrate concern. It is therefore important to document any development of connective tissue disease or other undefined symptom complex in patients who have undergone breast augmentation. The 10-year

prospective postmarket studies required of the manufacturers will also continue to collect relevant data.

Localized or systemic symptoms that may be related to a connective tissue disease or undefined symptom complex should be carefully documented. In addition, patients should be referred to a board-certified rheumatologist or immunologist for further specialized evaluation and testing. The patient must understand that consultant expertise may vary, and conclusions may or may not aid in the decision to remove breast implants. The decision-making algorithm can be used to determine "out points" when implant removal is suggested by the consultant or requested by the patient.

16.10
Conclusions

The concerns of the FDA and patient advocate groups resulted in a 15-year moratorium on the sale of silicone breast implants in the United States. Despite the evolution of the devices, reoperation rates for primary breast augmentations have remained as high as 21% at 3 years. The FDA's decision to release silicone gel breast implants to the market in November 2006 came with very clear rulings and requirements for postmarket surveillance. Both Allergan and Mentor are required to each enroll over 40,000 patients in a 10-year prospective study to evaluate the safety and efficacy of silicone gel implants. These studies will focus on complication and reoperation rates, as well as on rare adverse events, MRI and rupture rates, mammography, and childbearing issues.

The contributors to the BASPI workgroup collaborated to refine the decision and management algorithms

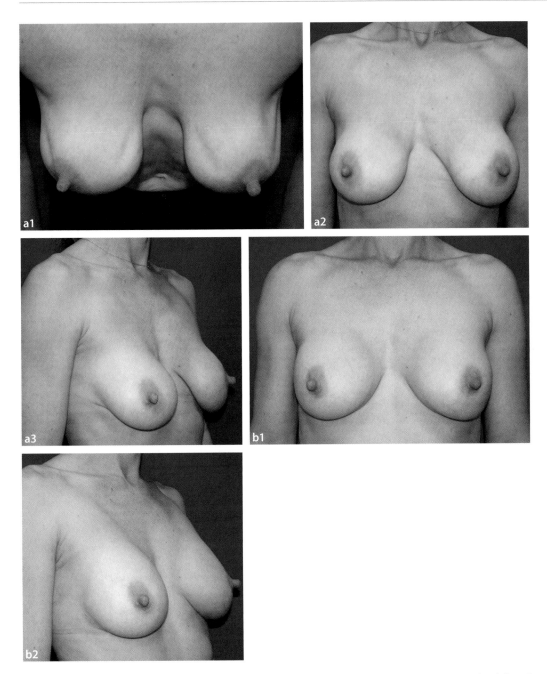

Fig. 16.4 Malposition: stretch deformity and excessive thinning of the overlying tissue. **a** *1–3* Patient has bilateral subglandular saline round implants with stretch deformities and bottoming out. **b** *1, 2* Bilateral capsulectomies, position change to partial submuscular 410 cohesive gel and inferior crescent mastopexy

already in use by the senior author. The flowcharts have proved successful in each of the contributor's practices for over 10 years. When combined with preoperative patient education and a system of implant selection based on quantifiable, individual patient tissue characteristics, the decision and management algorithms contribute to a dramatically lower reoperation rate in the management of breast implant patients.

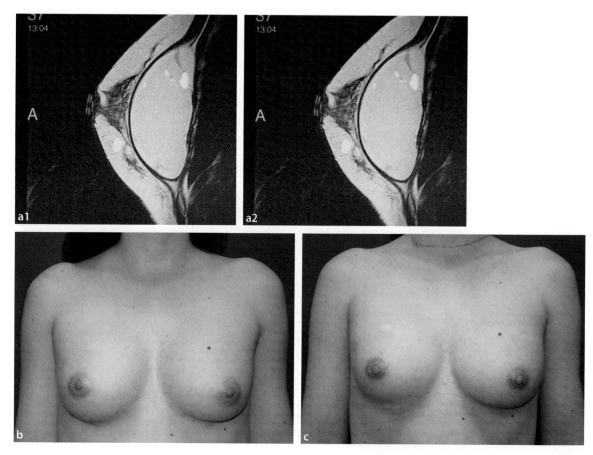

Fig. 16.5 Implant shell disruption, capsular contracture. **a** *1* Magnetic resonance imaging (MRI) of right breast before repair. *2* MRI after repair. **b** Patient with bilateral submuscular round silicone gel implants (1983) with rupture after biopsy of right breast. Grade 3 capsular contracture on right. **c** Bilateral capsulectomies and replacement with 410 cohesive gel implants

References

1. U.S. Food and Drug Administration: FDA approves silicone gel-filled breast implants after in-depth evaluation. Press release, 7 November 2006. http://www.fda.gov/bbs/topics/NEWS/2006/NEW01512.html

2. Adams WP, Potter: Breast implants: materials and manufacturing past, present, and future. In: Spear S (ed). Surgery of the Breast Principals and Art, Lippincott, Williams and Wilkins 2006

3. Adams WP, Bengston BP, Glicksman CA, Gryskiewicz JM, Jewell ML, McGrath MH, Reisman NR, Teitelbaum SA, Tebbetts J.B., Tebbetts T: Decision and management algorithms to address patient and Food and Drug Administration concerns regarding breast augmentation and implants. Plast Reconstr Surg 2004;114(5):1252–1257

4. Tebbetts JB: An approach that integrates patient education and informed consent in breast augmentation. Plast Reconstr Surg. 2002;110(3):971–978

5. Allergan. Augmentation surgery with silicone-filled breast implant patient planner, 2006. http://www.allergan.com

6. Tebbetts JB, Adams WB: Five critical decisions in breast augmentation using five measurements in 5 minutes: the high five decision support process. Plast Reconstr Surg 2005;116(7):2005–2016

7. Inamed premarketing approval data. Updated 20 April 2005. http://www.fda.gov/cdrh/panel

8. Mentor premarketing approval data. Updated 20 April 2005. http://www.fda.gov/cdrh/panel

9. Tebbetts JB: "Out points" criteria for breast implant removal without replacement and criteria to minimize reoperations following breast augmentation. Plast Reconstr Surg 2004;114(5):1258–1262

10. Augmentation patient labeling for Allergan. http://www.fda.gov/cdrh/breastimplants, p 31

11. U.S. Food and Drug Administration Center for Devices and Radiological Health. Breast implants home page. http://www.fda.gov/cdrh/breastimplants. Accessed 15 March 2007

12. Holmich LR: The diagnosis of silicone breast implant rupture: clinical findings compared with findings at magnetic resonance imaging. Ann Plast Surg 2005;54(6):583–589

13. Bondurant S, Ernster V, Herdman R (eds), Committee on the Safety of Silicone Breast Implants, Institute of Medicine: Safety of Silicone Breast Implants. Washington, DC, National Academy Press 1999v

Part III
Implants

Chapter 17

Silicone Versus Saline Implants

17

Robert S. Reiffel

17.1
Introduction

Multiple factors can influence the decision of whether to use either saline-filled or silicone-gel-filled implants for cosmetic breast augmentation. There are differences in three basic areas: implant performance and appearance; the patient's anatomy, desires, and concerns; and the surgeon's preference. All three categories must be considered in order to make the proper choice of which implant is best for which patient.

Silicone (polydimethylsiloxane) is a polymeric compound that can be manufactured with different properties, depending on the number of molecules in the polymer chain and the amount of cross-linking between the chains. By increasing the amount of cross-linking, the material can be changed from a liquid to a more viscous gel or a more rubber-like elastomer.

All gels are, by definition, more cohesive than liquids. However, within the broad category of gels, the degree of cohesiveness can be engineered to be thinner or more rubbery by modifying the amount of cross-linking between the polymer chains. Cohesive-I type implants are softer, more like liquids. However, because they are cohesive, the gel does not flow out of the implant if the shell fails. Cohesive-II implants are firmer and more resistant to pressure and gravity (Fig. 17.1).

Cohesive-III implants are more rubbery still, like the "gummy bear" candy they have been nicknamed after. To lessen the confusion between different degrees of cohesiveness, these latter implants are described as "shape stable," which means they are the most resistant to deformation under the influence of gravity or the overlying soft tissue envelope (Fig. 17.2).

The first silicone implants, made by Dow Corning from approximately 1964 to 1968, were made of Silastic 0, containing a thick elastomer shell, a viscous gel, and a Dacron patch for fixation. These were an improvement over the types of sponges and other devices that had been in use, but they were unnaturally firm and had a high incidence of capsular contracture [1, 2].

The second generation of silicone implants, Silas-

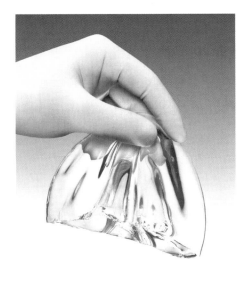

Fig. 17.1 Gel-filled Mentor implant cut open to show the gel stays inside because it is "cohesive"

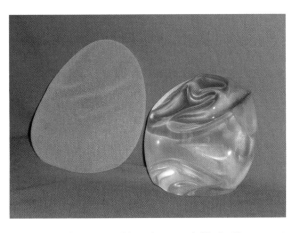

Fig. 17.2 *Left:* Shape-stable cohesive gel-filled Allergan 410 implant maintains its shape when upright. *Right:* Standard gel-filled implant sags toward the bottom

tic II, was introduced in 1972. These had a thinner shell and a less viscous gel. However, they reportedly did not decrease the incidence of capsular contracture, and they had a higher rate of rupture than the previous model. Because gel "bleed" of non-cross-linked silicone was noted across the intact shell, manufacturers changed the shells again in the 1970s to try to combat this problem, creating the third generation of silicone-gel-filled implants [2].

In 1992, because of increasing allegations of medical injuries and diseases from implants that had never been subject to testing before they were originally released, the U.S. Food and Drug Administration (FDA) removed them from public use and made them investigational in the United States. Around that time, manufacturers began to improve the nature of the gel, making it more cohesive, and they also improved the shells further, thus creating the fourth generation of gel-filled devices. The fifth generation of devices is the form-stable, highly cohesive ones, containing the cohesive-III type of gel.

In 1964, the first saline-filled implant was made in France. Unfortunately, it had a high rate of failure. The U.S. product was first made in 1968, using high-temperature platinum-catalyzed shells, which also failed too often. With a change to thicker, room-temperature vulcanized (RTV) shells, the performance has improved. The shell, however, is still made out of the same basic substance as in the gel-filled model. Some implants have been sold prefilled with saline, but the only ones available in the United States now are delivered empty, meaning there is a valve that must remain competent for the life of the implant and not be vulnerable to leakage.

17.2
Implant Characteristics

There are several important characteristics to consider with regard to each implant. Of great importance is its "feel" or softness and how closely it mimics normal breast tissue. Of equal importance is how accurately and reliably the implant can produce the shape it is designed to simulate. As with every procedure, the risk of negative effects must be considered, from capsular contracture to more systemic diseases such as connective tissue disorders. Finally, the different implants dictate different procedures for their insertion, based on their inherent nature.

Gel-filled implants are manufactured in different degrees of cohesiveness in order to impart different characteristics to them. A softer gel feels more like normal breast tissue than a more cohesive gel. As one progresses to the more cohesive types of gel-filled im-

plants, the advantage of shape stability must be weighed against the disadvantage of a firmer and less natural feel. By contrast, a saline-filled implant will, in general, feel more firm than a soft gel, and this firmness becomes even more pronounced as a saline-filled implant has more solution added to it.

The softness of the implant is of greatest importance when the amount of native breast tissue under which it is placed is less voluminous. If there is ample breast (and sometimes muscle) tissue to cushion the feel of the implant, even a firmer implant will not be palpated as such. However, when an implant is placed under thinner soft tissues, the final product will be, relatively, more implant and less soft tissue, so the implant's characteristics will be more readily evident. Obviously, the larger the implant for a given patient, the more this becomes a problem. It tends to be especially evident at the edges and bottom of the implant, where there is usually less breast tissue for coverage [3].

Another issue occurs when a secondary procedure becomes necessary. The natural tendency of soft tissues, even underlying ribs, is to yield to pressure from the implants and to stretch and thin out over time. Therefore, the amount of coverage is usually diminished in secondary procedures, making saline-filled implants even more palpable. Hence, gel-filled implants are usually better under such circumstances [3].

In addition, some patients need to have their inframammary fold lowered in order to centralize the implant on the nipple–areola complex. Therefore, whether the implant is placed above or below the muscle or fascia, the inferior hemisphere of the finished product is, basically, the implant. Under such circumstances, the characteristics of the implanted device will be more palpable, so a softer one will generally feel more natural.

The shape of an implant is determined by the native shape of its shell, the degree of distension of that shell by the fill material, the nature of the material inside, the effect of compression by the overlying soft tissues, and the effect of gravity. Gel-filled implants come prefilled by the manufacturer, so their volume is fixed. However, saline-filled implants, for the most part, are filled in the operating room, leaving room for variability. Both the gel-filled and saline-filled types are manufactured in different base diameters and sometimes heights with respect to projection.

When a saline-filled implant is designed, a certain range of fill volumes is specified by the manufacturer, from "minimal fill" to "maximum fill." However, surgeons are free to use volumes outside the recommended range. At a lower fill volume, because the pressure in the implant is less, it will have a wider stance and a softer feel. But because it is incompletely filled, it will

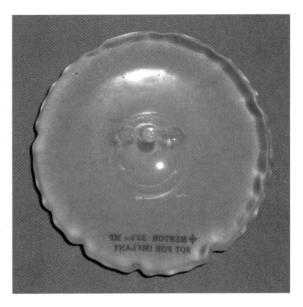

also have rippling on its anterior surface when it is lying flat on a surface or the patient is lying down (Fig. 17.3).

As more saline is instilled into the implant, it becomes narrower at the base and acquires more projection, and the anterior ripples fill out. As filling increases and pressure within the implant increases, new folds begin to develop on the edges, causing scalloping, and the implant becomes more firm to palpation (Fig. 17.4) [4].

The other issue that occurs with variability in implant filling is the overall change in the base diameter and projection. With less fill, the base diameter will be wider and the projection less, whereas with increased fill, the diameter decreases and the projection increases (Fig. 17.5).

The tendency for this change of shape to occur depends on the characteristics of the elastomeric shell, which can vary from manufacturer to manufacturer (Fig. 17.6).

The volume of saline that will produce the best shape is obviously somewhere in the middle between anterior rippling and side scalloping. This is termed the "optimum fill" volume [4].

The "minimum fill" and "maximum fill" volumes of saline implants were initially estimated by the manufacturers based on how much gel they had been placing in similar implant shells. However, it was subsequently learned that, for some implants, the optimum fill volume may be 5–10% above the stated maximum fill" volume. That additional amount that can be instilled is known as overfill. While, technically, it is above the recommended volume as stated by the manufacturer, it may be a necessary addition in order to optimize the aesthetic result. This varies from implant to implant (Figs. 17.5, 17.6) and should be discussed with the manufacturer and the patient [4].

The reason the manufacturers do not simply change their recommended fill ranges is that the specifications for each implant are filed with the FDA at the time each

Fig. 17.4 An overfilled implant will lose the anterior rippling but develop scalloping on the edges

implant is initially manufactured. Any changes would require an entire new filing and approval process. For some implants, changes in design, such as the valve, have been made, so the changes in fill range are incorporated in the new filing and approval. This varies from implant to implant.

As can be seen from the above examples, for the implants pictured, the Mentor implant has a stated fill range of 50 ml (325–375 ml), but at the higher range it is already beginning to show some scalloping, so the optimal fill volume of that implant would be less than the stated maximum. However, for the Allergan implant, which has a stated range of only 30 ml (330–360 ml) even at the maximum stated amount the implant is not overfilled because it still has some mild anterior rippling and no side scalloping.

Gel-filled implants are, obviously, filled by the manufacturer and are not subject to these issues. For a given volume, the gel-filled implants have less rippling on the surface and no scalloping on their edges. The new form-stable implants address this problem even more effectively because they are designed to not change shape at all under the influence of gravity or thin or tight overlying soft tissues (Fig. 17.7).

The softer the implant, the less its inherent shape will influence the configuration of the final product. Both saline-filled implants and less cohesive gel-filled implants will be influenced by gravity, with the filler material spread more evenly when the patient is supine and

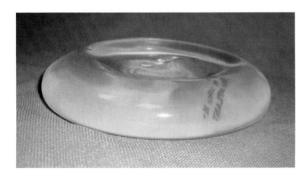

Fig. 17.3 An underfilled saline implant will have increased rippling on the anterior surface

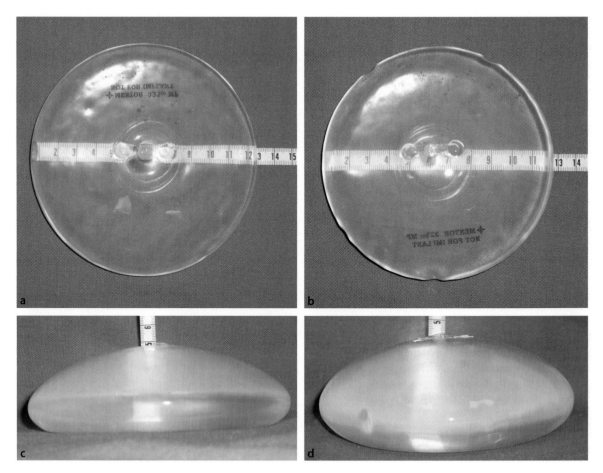

Fig. 17.5 a A moderate-profile Mentor 325-ml implant filled with stated minimum of 325 ml. Edges are smooth, and diameter is 13 cm. **b** Same implant filled with stated maximum of 375 ml. Edges are starting to scallop, and diameter has de-creased to 12.8 cm. **c** Moderate-profile Mentor 325-ml implant filled to stated minimum of 325 ml. Projection is 2.6 cm. **d** Same implant filled to stated maximum of 375 ml. Note increased projection to 4.3 cm

tending to migrate to the bottom of the implant when the patient is erect (Fig. 17.2). An implant filled with a more cohesive type of gel will be less subject to this type of deformation. Therefore, if a patient has a deficiency in the superior portion of the breast, even with submuscular or subfascial placement of the implant, a highly cohesive gel-filled implant will give a better and more reproducible shape than a soft gel or a saline-filled one. Of course, this comes with the disadvantage of a firmer feel [5].

The advantage of the shape-stable implant becomes even more obvious in secondary procedures in which rippling, thin skin, and shape deformities must be corrected. The highly cohesive implants can be thought of more as a shape-altering device than just a volume-altering device, allowing for correction of such various problems.

When an implant shell folds repeatedly in the same location, that movement can cause it to split and fail in what is termed a fold-flaw or crease-fold failure. While the true failure rate of silicone-gel-filled prostheses may not be known because a number of such failures remain asymptomatic, when a saline-filled prosthesis deflates, it is almost always evident to the patient and the physician. Numerous studies have demonstrated that the failure rate of saline-filled implants increases if the implant is underfilled [6–10]. This increased rate may be secondary to the increased rippling, in general, of saline-filled implants when compared with gel-filled ones, causing more folding of the implant shell, or it may be due to the abrasive effect of the saline on the shell as compared with the lubricant effect of gel [11]. Whatever the reason, if a saline implant is filled to a lower volume, it will have a softer feel but a higher incidence of shell failure. Although choosing to fill the saline implant to a higher volume will diminish the likelihood of failure, it

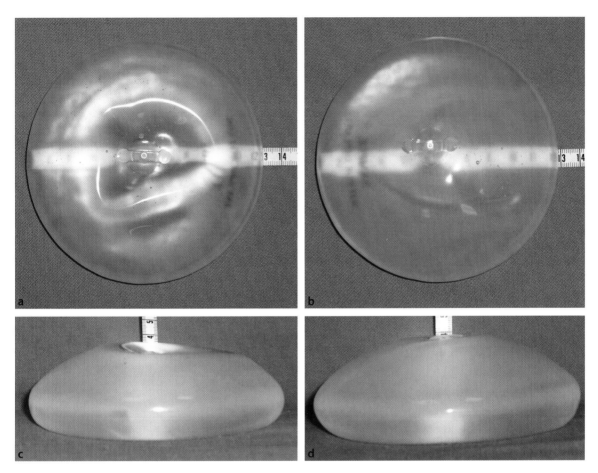

Fig. 17.6 a Allergan 330-ml implant filled to stated minimum of 330 ml. Diameter is 13 cm. **b** Same implant filled to stated maximum of 360 ml. Diameter has decreased to 12.9 cm. **c** Allergan 330-ml implant filled to stated minimum of 330 ml. Projection is 3.5 cm. **d** Same implant filled to 360 ml. Projection has increased to 3.8 cm

Fig. 17.7 a Gel-filled implant has no ripples on surface or scallops on edges. **b** Gel-filled implant maintains smooth contour when patient is lying down

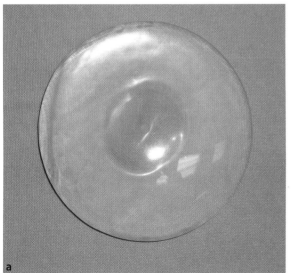

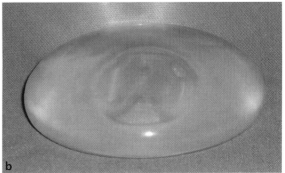

will also increase the implant's firmness and the palpability of its edges.

For gel-filled implants, shell failure may be symptomatic to the patient or it may be detected only on imaging studies. For the shape-stable devices, the incidence is lower still, because even if the implant ruptures, the material stays inside. In addition, there is a lower incidence of symptomatic capsular contracture [5].

Naturally, except for the very few models that come prefilled and are not available in the United States, the saline-filled models have a valve through which saline is instilled in the operating room. This valve is also subject to failure. Capsular tissue can grow around the strap and sealing plug, covering the fill valve (Fig. 17.4). With movement of the implant in the pocket, traction and deformation of the valve can occur, causing failure and leakage [12, 13]. This is less of a problem with textured implants, which move around in the pocket less. In addition, a large study comparing deflation rates between standard and prefilled implants showed significantly more deflations in the prefilled group, so valve failure cannot be considered a significant long-term problem [7].

In addition, although surgical trauma can just as easily be inflicted upon a gel-filled implant as a saline-filled one, the results of such injury may not be evident in the case of a gel-filled implant, especially the more cohesive types. As noted, however, when a saline-filled implant deflates, it is almost always the cause of great consternation on the part of the patient and the surgeon (Fig. 17.8). In one study, nearly 7% of the implants returned to a major manufacturer in a 30-month period because of early deflation were found to have needle damage (Fig. 17.9) [14].

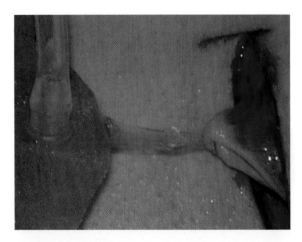

Fig. 17.8 Tissue has grown around protective strap of a saline-filled implant that was removed and replaced for aesthetic reasons

Other factors that can lead to excessive implant failure are the instillation of either antibiotics or steroids into the lumen, although those medications have also been shown to decrease the rate of capsular contracture [8]. In addition, in 2000 the FDA banned the use of povidone-iodine during breast augmentation. Although some subsequent studies have shown that it does not have a deleterious effect on shell integrity and does diminish the rate of capsular contracture, other studies have concluded that povidone-iodine can weaken silicone, depending on the method of vulcanization used in manufacturing the shell. Until conclusive data are available, the use of povidone-iodine during either filling of the implant or irrigation of the pocket should be avoided [15–17].

Another obvious difference between the saline and gel-filled implants is the ease of insertion. Because the saline ones are inserted empty, they can easily be inserted through a much smaller incision and also through a remote incision, such as the umbilicus [18–21]. Gel-filled implants will always require a larger incision for their safe insertion, and the shape-stable ones require still larger incisions than the standard gel-filled ones [22].

Once the implant is inserted into the patient, the different types of devices behave differently over the long term. The elastomeric shell is not totally impervious, so it is susceptible to migration of material both into and out of the implant. Some surgeons take advantage of this characteristic and place antibiotics or steroids into the implant, where they can exert their influence over an extended time course.

Not all migration across the shell is advantageous. There have been reports of spontaneous autoinflation of saline-filled implants. The exact cause of this condition, or its true incidence, is not known, but it may be more common than initially suspected [23, 24].

Migration or "bleed" of the contents outward has been recognized for a long time, and manufacturers have changed not only the characteristics of the gel but also the characteristics of the envelope in an effort to combat it [1, 25]. The effects of gel bleed outside the implant have been studied extensively. Although previous studies showed an increased incidence of capsular contracture in gel-filled implants as compared with saline-filled implants, this may not be as prevalent with the newer devices. In addition, there has been much publicity and concern about the possibility of serious connective tissue disorders resulting from long-term implantation of silicone-gel-filled implants. However, there is now a significant body of data that demonstrates no increased incidence of major local or systemic disease compared with the general population [26–33].

Whenever an implant of any type is inserted in a patient, the body naturally forms a capsule around it.

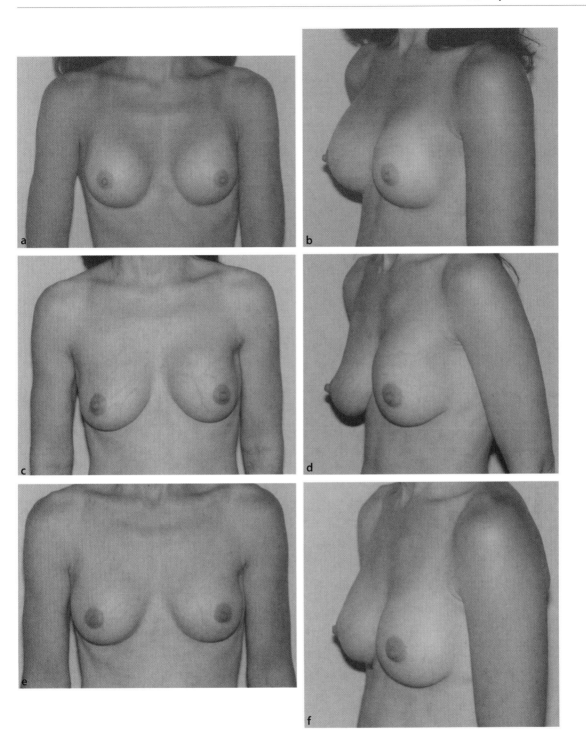

Fig. 17.9 **a** A 31-year-old patient with 255-ml submuscular saline-filled implants with Baker III capsular contracture. **b** The implants feel firm, and the superior hemispheres are visibly protruding. **c** The right-side implant has deflated. **d** Deflated right implant and Baker III contracture on left side. The same contracture on the right probably caused the fold-flaw failure and deflation. **e** After insertion of new size 240-ml submuscular saline-filled implants. **f** Baker I result. Implant feels soft, and superior hemisphere is no longer convex

For devices such as pacemakers, this is of no aesthetic consequence. However, for breast implants, a firm or hard capsule will make the result cosmetically deforming. The earlier gel-filled implants, with their Dacron fixation patches, had a high incidence of calcification in their surrounding capsules. The newer devices are not subject to this same high incidence. However, even saline-filled devices can still develop calcification on their surface and in the surrounding capsules (Figs. 17.9, 17.10) [32, 34].

From 1992 until 2006, breast implants were classified as investigational by the FDA in the United States. Although they have since been released for general use in cosmetic augmentation (with the exception of the most cohesive shape-stable devices that are part of a separate study and not yet released), some patients will still not qualify for them because of age (under 22) or preexisting connective tissue disorders [35]. Moreover, some patients still may feel concerned about the safety of those devices. For them, only saline-filled implants should be used.

17.3
Patient Characteristics

Each patient presents her own anatomical challenge to the surgeon, who must assess not only the absolute volume deficiency that must be corrected but also the shape and distribution of the desired correction and how that will change under the effects of clothing and gravity. In addition, the quantity and quality of the soft tissue coverage available will affect the final outcome. Therefore, one must first assess the patient's physical characteristics, and then use the knowledge of implant performance to choose the most appropriate device.

One must remember that the appearance of the implant after placement in the patient will be different than in its native state. The tightness of the overlying soft tissue envelope will compress and distort the implant. This obviously worsens with increasing volume. The thinner and less robust the native soft tissue coverage, the more the implant will be visible and palpable as a component of the final result. The larger the implant diameter for a given patient's chest size, the more the edges will be palpable, especially if the soft tissue coverage is poor. If the nipple is not centered on the breast mound and the inframammary fold must be lowered, the bottom hemisphere of the final mound will be, essentially, implant covered by skin, even in a partially submuscular or subfascial procedure.

For a patient with good quality and distribution of soft tissue who does not desire a significant change in volume relative to her own native breast tissue, almost any implant will suffice. However, for patients with a narrow chest diameter, a narrower-based implant must be used, or the edge of the implant will be more palpable. To achieve a larger size, the patient must accept more projection for the edge of the implant to be kept hidden. With larger volume implants and thinner soft tissue coverage, the edge of a saline-filled implant, with its inherent tendency to ripple, will be more visible and palpable (Fig. 17.11). Under such circumstances, a gel-filled implant would be a better choice [3].

Similarly, for patients with poor upper pole fullness that is only made worse upon standing, a more form-stable device would not lose its shape when going from supine to erect. However, such devices come with a firmer feel, which might be less desirable at the edge or inferior pole of the breast in a thin patient with poor coverage [22].

Placing the implant beneath the pectoralis muscle and/or fascia tends to blunt the inherent shape of the implant, thereby diminishing, but not eliminating, the tendency to ripple or feel firm. However, such placement carries the expectation of deformation of the breast during activity of that muscle, which can be a significant visual problem under various circumstances, such as in models, bodybuilders, and athletic individuals. Therefore, if the decision is made to place the implant in a prepectoral location, a saline-filled device is more likely to display any negative characteristics than a gel-filled one. A shape-stable highly cohesive device, with its minimal tendency to show surface folds, is particularly suited to such a situation [20, 22, 36, 37].

The location of the incision exerts a significant influence on the choice of implant. Any implant can be placed through an inframammary or transaxillary incision, although the shape-stable ones are usually placed only through the larger inframammary incision. For a patient with a large areola, even a moderately large gel-filled implant can be placed without undue difficulty (Fig. 17.10). However, placing a sizeable gel-filled implant through a small areola risks sufficient trauma, and the implant could easily be damaged. There are incision modifications that attempt to circumvent this difficulty, but they may cause scars that do not coincide with the natural margin of the areola and can be more visible [7, 38–40]. For the transumbilical approach, only saline-filled implants are used because the amount of trauma imparted upon a gel-filled implant during insertion would be excessive [18, 19, 21]. Therefore, if a patient has a small nipple–areola complex, she must usually accept either a saline-filled implant through an areolar incision or an inframammary incision for a gel-filled device. If there is a degree of ptosis or pseudop-

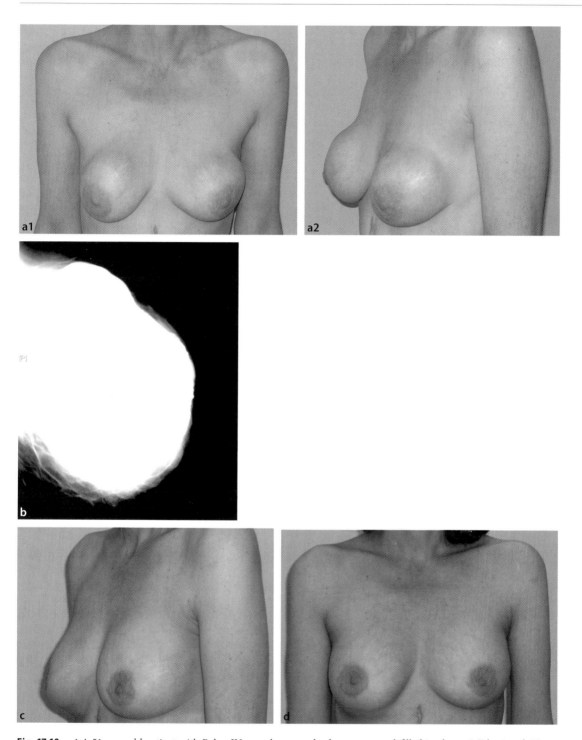

Fig. 17.10 a *1* A 51-year-old patient with Baker IV capsules around submammary gel-filled implants. *2* Side view. **b** Mammogram showing calcified capsule around implant. **c** After complete capsulectomy and insertion of smooth gel-filled 240-ml implants beneath pectoralis muscle. **d** Baker I result

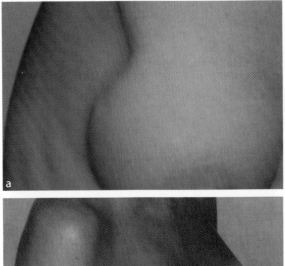

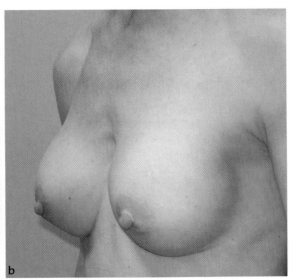

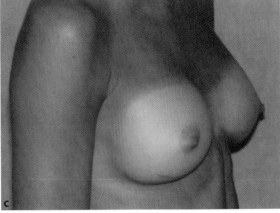

Fig. 17.11 a Thin patient with saline-filled implants who has minimal soft tissue coverage. Scalloping of implants can be seen. **b** Patient with edges of implants highly visible and palpable. **c** Patient with gel-filled implants in whom the edges are not prominent

tosis, the latter incision will not show, but for patients with no ptosis, the incision will be visible for a number of months, until the pink color fades (Fig. 17.10).

Although the voluminous body of scientific data has not demonstrated a link between gel-filled implants and systemic disease, the issue is not yet settled, especially in the minds of a number of patients. The manufacturers are still required to collect and submit data on patients previously enrolled in the adjunct investigational studies for the full terms of those studies. Physicians using gel-filled devices on new patients are required to submit data for a postapproval study, and new patients must also agree to follow-up examinations. In addition, patients with known connective tissue disease, such as lupus, scleroderma, rheumatoid arthritis, or fibromyalgia, and patients under 22 years of age are still not eligible to have gel-filled devices.

17.4
Conclusions

The final result is a product of the surgeon's skill in taking the patient's anatomical condition and using the available implants to shape a final result that is, hopefully, pleasing to all parties. The surgeon's experience and results with previous procedures will naturally influence the recommendation as to which implant or approach might be best under which circumstances.

In general, the gel-filled implants have the advantage of a more natural feel in the case of the softer gels, which is important for patients with less robust soft tissue coverage. This is especially true for thin patients or for those who wish a larger volume augmentation relative to their own inherent size and shape, especially if the edge of the implant will be palpable. For prepectoral placement and avoidance of the potential problem of implant distortion from muscle activity, the shape-stable highly cohesive gel implant will give a more natural appearance, although with a slightly firmer feel.

For those patients who start out with a shape that is more abnormal and will, therefore, be more reliant upon the implant to create a more normal breast mound, the more shape-stable highly cohesive gel implants will be advantageous. They are more effective for altering the shape of patients with issues such as thin soft tissue coverage, rippling, contractures, or upper pole or lower hemisphere deficiencies.

The saline-filled implants have the advantage of some variability in fill volume and shape on the operating table, as well as the ability to be placed through a smaller incision and inserted from a more remote location. This comes with a higher risk of rippling, a slightly firmer feel, and an increased risk of symptomatic deflation should the implant ultimately fail.

References

1. Brandon H J, Young V L, Jerina K L, Wolf C J: Variability in the properties of silicone gel breast implants. Plast Reconstr Surg 2001;108(3):647–655

2. Young VL, Watson ME: Breast implant research: where we have been, where we are, where we need to go. Clin Plast Surg 2001;28(3):451–483

3. Elliott LF: Breast augmentation with round, smooth saline or gel implants. The pros and cons. Clin Plast Surg 2001;28(3):523–529

4. Dowden RV: Saline breast implant fill issues. Clin Plast Surg 2001;28(3):445–450

5. Drever JM: Cohesive gel implants for breast augmentation. Aesth Surg 2003;23(5):405–409

6. Raj J, Wojtanowski MH: Spontaneous deflation in saline solution-filled breast implants. Aesthet Surg 1999;19(1):24–26

7. Stevens WG, Hirsch EM, Stoker DA, Cohen R: A comparison of 500 prefilled textured saline breast implants versus 500 standard textured saline breast implants: is there a difference in deflation rates? Plast Reconstr Surg 2006;117(7):2175–2178

8. Gutowski KA, Mesna GT, Cunningham BL: Saline-filled breast implants: a Plastic Surgery Educational Foundation Multicenter Outcomes Study. Plast Reconstr Surg 1997;100(4):1019–1027

9. Al-Sabounchi S, De Mey AM, Eder, H: Textured saline-filled breast implants for augmentation mammaplasty: does overfilling prevent deflation? A long-term follow-up. Plast Reconstr Surg 2006;118(1):215–222

10. Lanieri LA, Roudot-Thoraval F, Collins ED, Raulo Y, Baruch JP: Influence of underfilling on breast implant deflation. Plast Reconstr Surg 1997;100(7):1740–1744

11. Spear SL, Mardini S: Alternative filler materials and new implant designs. What's available and what's on the horizon? Clin Plast Surg 2001;28(3):435–443

12. Cederna JP: Valve design as a cause of saline-filled implant deflation (correspondence and brief communication). Plast Reconstr Surg 2002;109(6):2166

13. Kirkpatrick WN, Healy C: Fibrous ring pulls plug on saline-filled implant (correspondence and brief communication). Plast Reconstr Surg 2001;108(1):268–269

14. Rapaport DP, Stadelmann WK. Greenwald DP: Incidence and natural history of saline-filled breast implant deflations: comparison of blunt-tipped versus cutting and tapered needles. Plast Reconstr Surg 1997;100(4):1028–1032

15. Wiener TC: The role of Betadine irrigation in breast augmentation. Plast Reconstr Surg 2007;119(1):12–15

16. Becker JH, Becker CD: The effect of Betadine on silicone implants (correspondence and brief communication). Plast Reconstr Surg 2000;105(4):1570

17. Adams WP Jr, Conner WC, Barton FE, Rohrich RJ: Optimizing breast-pocket irrigation: the post-Betadine era. Plast Reconstr Surg 2001;107(6):1596–1601

18. Dowden RV: Dispelling the myths and misconceptions about transumbilical breast augmentation. Plast Reconstr Surg 2000;106(1):190–194

19. Dowden R: Keeping the transumbilical breast augmentation procedure safe. Plast Reconstr Surg 2001;108(5):1389–1400

20. Baccari ME: Dispelling the myths and misconceptions about transumbilical breast augmentation (discussion). Plast Reconstr Surg 2000;106(1):195

21. Pound EC III, Pound EC Jr: Transumbilical breast augmentation (TUBA). Patient selection, technique, and clinical experience. Clin Plast Surg 2001;28(3):597–605

22. Hedén P, Jernbeck J, Hober M: Breast augmentation with anatomical cohesive gel implants. The world's largest current experience. Clin Plast Surg 2001;28(3):531–552

23. Robinson OG, Benos DJ: Spontaneous autoinflation of saline mammary implants. Ann Plast Surg 1997;39(2):114–118

24. Tuncali D, Ozgar F: Spontaneous autoinflation of saline-filled mammary implants: postoperative volume determination by magnetic resonance imaging. Aesthetic Plast Surg 1999;23(6):437–442

25. Feng LJ, Amini SB: Analysis of risk factors associated with rupture of silicone gel breast implants. Plast Reconstr Surg 1999;104(4):955–963

26. Reiffel RS, Rees TD, Guy CL, Aston SJ: A comparison of capsule formation following breast augmentation by saline-filled or gel-filled implants. Aesthetic Plast Surg 1983;7:113–116

27. Schnur PL, Weinzweig J, Harris JB, Moyer TP, Petty PM, Nixon D, McConnell JP: Silicon analysis of breast and periprosthetic capsular tissue from patients with saline or silicon gel breast implants. Plast Reconstr Surg 1996;98(5):798–803

28. Weinzweig J, Schnur PL, McConnell JP, Harris JB, Petty PM, Moyer TP, Nixon D: Silicon analysis of breast and capsular tissue from patients with saline or silicone gel breast implants. II. Correlation with connective-tissue disease. Plast Reconstr Surg 1998;101(7):1836–1841

29. Peters W, Smith D, Lugowski S: Silicon assays in women with and without silicone gel breast implants—a review. Ann Plast Surg 1999;43(3):324–330

30. Peters W, Smith D, Lugowski S, McHugh A, Keresteci A, Baines C: Analysis of silicon levels in capsules of gel and saline breast implants and of penile prostheses. Ann Plast Surg 1995;34(6):578–584

31. Lipworth L, Tarone RE, McLaughlin JK: Silicone breast implants and connective tissue disease. Ann Plast Surg 2004;52(6):598–601

32. Peters W, Pritzker K, Smith S, Fornasier V, Holmyard D, Lugowski S, Kamel M, Visram F: Capsular calcification associated with silicone breast implants: incidence, determinants, and characterization. Ann Plast Surg 1998;41(4): 348–360

33. Bondurant S, Ernster VL, Herdman R: Safety of silicone breast implants. Committee on the Safety of Silicone Breast Implants, Division of Health Promotion and Disease Prevention, Institute of Medicine 2000

34. Peters WP, Smith D, Lugowski S, Pritzker K, Holmyard D: Calcification properties of saline-filled breast implants. Plast Reconstr Surg 2001;107(2):356–363

35. U.S. Food and Drug Administration: Breast implant questions and answers. Washington, DC, U.S. Food and Drug Administration 2006

36. Strasser EJ: Results of subglandular versus subpectoral augmentation over time: one surgeon's observations. Aesthet Surg 2006;26(1):45–50

37. Sadove R: Cohesive gel naturally-shaped breast implants. Aesthet Surg 2003;23(1):63–64

38. Atiyeh BS, Al-Amm CA, El-Musa KA: The transverse intra-areolar infra-nipple incision for augmentation mammaplasty. Aesthet Plast Surg 2002;26(2):151–155

39. Saad MN: An extended circumareolar incision for breast augmentation and gynecomastia. Aesth Plast Surg 1983;7(2):127–128

40. Carvajal J, Echeverry A: Alternative technique for breast augmentation in patients with a small nipple–areolar complex diameter. Aesth Surg 2005;25(2):117–125

CHAPTER 18

Choice of Prosthesis Surface: Myth or Necessity?

18

Richard Moufarrège, Alexandre Dionyssopoulos

18.1
Introduction

Many different types of prostheses have become available since their introduction 110 years ago with the inception of breast augmentation. Many modifications and design variations have consistently improved implant materials, yet there is such an abundance of them that a misinformed surgeon can easily become confused and may choose the wrong prosthesis for the job.

18.2
History

The modest beginnings of augmentation mammoplasty were initially marred by a paucity of materials, which were gradually perfected and enhanced with the rapid advancements seen in the technological sectors. This allowed the materials to be refined and adjusted in ways never before seen.

The period preceding World War II was first marked by paraffin injections introduced by Gersuvy in 1899, for which substantial complications (paraffinomas, necrosis, emboli) were documented [1–3]. At the beginning of the 20th century, abdominal or epiploic fat was used for augmentation, with mediocre results [4–8]. By the end of World War II, silicones had been developed as injectable materials in the breast. The complications that ensued with this technique are, unfortunately, all too well known [9–14].

The era of breast prosthesis had truly begun by the midpoint of the last century. This period can be split into two parts. The first one corresponds to the use, by chance, of materials that had a smooth or a rugged surface according to the materials discovered at the time, without consideration of the properties or functional aspects of these surfaces. The second part corresponds to the active development of a textured surface prosthesis by Surgitek in 1983, with the objective to decrease fibrous capsule formation and the associated deformity it often induced.

Taken directly from the first part, the Ivalon, derived from polyvinyl alcohol, was a prosthesis with a textured surface, a property acquired by being carved from a special sponge [15]. The second generation of this prosthesis was formed by an Ivalon center engulfed by a polyurethane bag itself covered with Ivalon. This conferred to the prosthesis a very textured surface. Rangman patented the first breast prosthesis in the United States (patent 2842,775, July 1958). This first attempt was quickly abandoned because of fluid would accumulate between the different layers of the prosthesis.

Soon after came the Polystan, consisting of a grouping of polyethylene bands covered with a smooth envelope. This was also rapidly discarded because of the absence of a hermetic seal.

In 1960 Regneault [16] proposed the use of polymethane, also called Etheron, composed of an even finer meshwork of a smooth nature. This was overshadowed by the silicone prosthesis, which made its appearance in Washington in 1963 through the efforts of Cronin and Gerow.

Cronin's prosthesis was considered a hybrid of sorts, due to a combination of smooth and textured patches of Dacron that ensured an anchoring point on its posterior surface [17–19].

In 1965, Arion [20] presented the inflatable prosthesis with a silicone (smooth) shell, which fell by the wayside when its valve was shown to be incompetent, a problem superseded by a more advanced valve system developed by Heyer-Schulte.

Cronin's prosthesis became quite popular and dominated the market during the 1960s and 1970s until reports of a hardened, fibrous pseudocapsule formation around the prosthesis began to surface.

In 1969, Ashley [21, 22] introduced a newer silicone prosthesis with three compartments in a Y-pattern covered with polyurethane, offering a textured surface that allowed stabilization of the prosthesis in its dissected compartment. Nobody at that time could have predicted that this new envelope could counter the formation of the fibrous capsule responsible for the hardened breast.

In the 1970s, Dow Corning refined Cronin's prosthesis by removing the Dacron patches and using a more liquid-based silicone, thus allowing prosthesis insertion through smaller incisions.

At this time, the practice of augmentation mammaplasty was met with a storm of controversy surrounding its most known and talked-about complication: the fibrous capsule [23–30].

Development of a fibrous capsule is due to several important factors: the surgical dissection, impurities, hematoma, seroma, infection, and various immunological mechanisms [29, 31–36]. No matter what factor induces its formation, one common denominator is usually present at one point in its development: the myofibroblast [37–39]. Different methods have been employed to combat the formation of the fibrous capsule: use of water-filled prostheses, placement of the prosthesis in the retromuscular plane, drainage, antibiotic therapy, and use of a thicker-walled prosthetic to prevent silicone from "bleeding" through its membrane [28, 40–44].

In the midst of this controversy, from 1982 to 1984 a new generation of prosthetics covered in polyurethane—called the Natural Y, the Meme, and the Replicon—appeared on the market. These offered a textured material on the entire surface. The goal of this textured material was to directly reduce the force of contraction exerted by the fibrous capsule. This ushered in a new era of breast implant, called the textured prosthesis, with the sole purpose of combating formation of the fibrous capsule. Initial beliefs were that the polyurethane itself was mostly responsible for lowering the rate of fibrous capsule formation [45–48].

With closer study, it became clear that the implant's physical properties and not its chemical composition played a greater role in this phenomenon. With time, capsule formation around the material that becomes "fatigued" will induce a separation between the silicone and the polyurethane layers and will eliminate any physical effect the material offers against capsule formation. From this observation came the development of other textured prostheses, each bypassing the need for polyurethane: the Biocell (McGhan), the Siltex (Mentor), the MSI (Dow Corning), and the Misti (Bioplasty).

18.3
Definitions

Prosthetic materials that appear smooth are referred to as smooth, and those that appear rugged are referred to as textured. In reality, these prostheses are not universally rugged in the same way. They each offer different degrees of ruggedness, with variations from one prosthetic to the next. This index is a function of the depth of its depression and the average width from this depression midway between the most superficial point and the deepest portion of the implant's wall.

18.4
Variety of Available Prostheses

The different types of prostheses available on the market, without mentioning the manufacturers' names explicitly, are as follows:
1. Round, inflatable, smooth
2. Anatomic, inflatable, textured
3. Round, silicone, smooth
4. Round, silicone, textured
5. Anatomic, inflatable, textured
6. Anatomic, silicone, textured

18.4.1
Physical Properties and Characteristics of Smooth Prostheses

1. Easy gliding
2. Fibrous capsule with well-oriented and parallel structures

18.4.2
Physical Properties and Characteristics of Textured Prostheses

1. Difficult gliding
2. Easy adherence to adjacent tissues
3. Creation of disorganized alignment of myofibroblasts and fibers constituting the main structure of the capsule

18.4.3
Texturization of Prostheses

It is evident that the first generation of textured implants was textured because of the inherent nature of the material used, rather than secondary to any additional manufacturing intervention. This was the case with Ivalon.

The polyurethane that covered Ashley's prosthesis, and later the Natural Y as well as the Replicon, is porous by default and required no manipulation to increase its texture.

In contrast, the newest generation of prostheses, in order to avoid the use of polyurethane, are subject to a texturization that differs from one manufacturer to the next.

Inamed imbues its prostheses in a bed of salt, inducing a macrotexturization. Mentor subjects its implants to an impression left in a sponge-like polyurethane surface of regular cellular caliber to give the macrotexturization. In Europe, Sebbin uses a print on a salt bed, resulting in an intermediary texturization.

Whatever the efforts manufacturers have expended, and whatever expertise they have acquired to develop their own way of texturizing, nobody has ever been able to establish the superiority of one kind of texturization over the others. The degree of rugosity does not seem to be of any importance compared to whether a prosthesis is smooth or textured.

18.5
Effect of Texturization and Smoothness on Augmentation Mammaplasty

The smooth prosthesis slides more easily. Whether the prosthesis is inflatable or filled with silicone, its smooth shell allows easier gliding. This property can be advantageous but is not without weaknesses.

18.5.1
Advantages of Smooth Prosthetic Gliding

The ease of introduction is certainly one of its high points. Not only can the prosthesis be introduced through a very small incision (3 cm is enough for an inflatable prosthesis through a submammary incision), but it also facilitates certain less direct approaches (periareolar, axillary, umbilical, abdominal combined with abdominoplasty) [49, 50].

The mobility of a smooth prosthesis in a pocket larger than its base surface gives a certain natural effect to the augmented breast, especially in the horizontal position.

18.5.2
Disadvantages of Smooth Prosthetic Gliding

Undesirable gliding in this prosthesis usually occurs in two ways:
1. Migration upwards, medially, or laterally, but mostly inferiorly: This type of gliding is a weakness seen only in smooth-textured prostheses and in certain conditions relating to the patient, the shape of the thorax, the quality of the surrounding tissues, etc.
2. Rotary migration: This rotation may be clockwise or counterclockwise and has no consequence with round prostheses. On the other hand, anatomic prostheses will often produce undesirable, deform-

ing results after undergoing any rotational displacement (Fig. 18.1) [46].

Prosthetic manufacturers have quickly grasped the importance of avoiding this complication and no longer produce smooth-textured anatomic prostheses. Readjustments needed for this complication have been done since the inception of the prosthesis.

18.6
Effect of Smooth-Textured Prostheses on Augmentation Mammaplasty Surgery

Although trying to avoid the debate surrounding fibrous capsules, it remains useful to mention the effect of a smooth surface on fibrous capsule formation. It is well established that the dynamic element of fibrous contraction relates to the myofibroblast, which is directly implicated in the structure of the fibrous capsule. This cell, which has contractile properties not unlike those of muscle cells (as its name implies), has a contractile effect on the prosthesis or the capsule envelope. This effect can vary depending on the axis in which the contraction is taking place.

In the case of the smooth-textured prosthesis, the structural elements of the capsule are linear and entirely flat, thus acting in a two-dimensional plane. This will induce a tightening of the capsule over a certain area, which, when translated to the entire surface, can produce significant hardening or even deformation of the prosthesis.

The surface of the rugged-textured implant prevents the myofibroblasts and other elements of the capsule from orienting themselves along the same plane, caus-

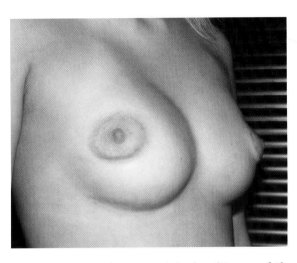

Fig. 18.1 Rotation with an anatomic implant. (Courtesy of Alexander Dionyssopoulos)

ing them to pull in different directions instead. The contraction effect is disorganized and inefficient. This leads us to conclude that smooth-walled prostheses have a naturally higher rate of capsular contraction than their textured counterparts [51–61].

Evidently—and without getting into the subject of fibrous capsules too exhaustively—other factors exist that will increase or decrease capsular contraction. These factors include the retromuscular or premuscular placement of the prosthesis, "bleeding" of silicone across the implant wall, hematomas, seromas, infections, and others.

Following the silicone moratorium of the 1990s, the use of inflatable prostheses has eliminated two of these important factors:

1. The prosthesis using a physiological solution is less likely to produce an aggressive fibrous capsule compared with a prosthesis using silicone.
2. The prosthesis filled with water is being placed more often in the retromuscular plane. We now know that the retromuscular plane has a natural protective effect against development of an aggressive fibrous capsule around a prosthesis.

The moratorium encouraged manufacturers to create cohesive-type silicone prostheses that do not leak and, to this day, have no evidence of transmural bleed. Therefore, these prostheses seem to also exhibit less fibrous capsule formation compared with the traditional silicone models.

18.7
Effect of Textured Prostheses on Augmentation Mammaplasty

Textured prostheses glide with difficulty. This has different consequences:

1. Obligatory extensive incision: The incision used for introducing a textured prosthesis must be longer than one used for a smooth prosthesis. Especially with cohesive gel silicone, these incisions can extend up to 6–7 cm in length.
2. Effect of texturization on indirect introduction: Because of their increased resistance to gliding, it is much more difficult, or even impossible, to introduce these prostheses through incisions other than submammary (axillary, umbilical, areolar, etc.)
3. The Velcro effect: Texturization may, in certain unfavorable conditions, adhere to the puckering that may develop at the surface of the prosthesis and freeze it permanently. Correction of this defect becomes extremely difficult without a radical capsulectomy and replacement of the involved prosthesis (Figs. 18.2, 18.3) [46].

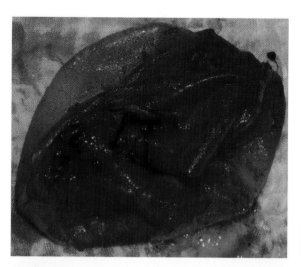

Fig. 18.2 The "Velcro" effect. (Courtesy of Alexander Dionyssopoulos)

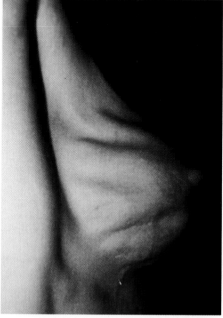

Fig. 18.3 Permanent puckering (folding into ridges) of prosthesis. (Courtesy of Alexander Dionyssopoulos)

18.8
Adherence of Textured Prostheses (Advantage of Adhesion to Surrounding Tissue)

The phenomenon of prosthetic migration is relatively rare because the texture provides an adhesive surface that fixates the implant into its initial position. This is one of the key reasons why anatomic prostheses are always textured. Another application is breast reconstruction in which the pocket is too large for the prosthesis. Here, the texturization maintains the prosthesis in the position established during surgery.

18.9
Effect of Texture on Capsule Formation

For textured prostheses, myofibroblasts become more disorganized and have difficulty inducing aggressive periprosthetic contractions.

18.10
Conclusions

Are all these different types of implants necessary? Do they each have precise applications? Would two experienced surgeons working in different centers in a given situation choose the same prosthesis among all those available; moreover, would they obtain the same results? Or is the goal of having such a massive selection of implants to aid the surgeon in individualizing the needed implant to each patient according to the situation at hand?

From all of this controversy, the author can extrapolate several solid conclusions:

1. The smooth-walled prosthesis induces more capsule formation than textured ones do.
2. The saline-filled prosthesis leads to less fibrous capsule formation than the traditional silicone gel counterpart does.
3. Placing an implant in the retromuscular plane induces less capsule formation compared with placement in front of the muscle. This is a reconciling factor for the continued use of smooth-walled prostheses.
4. The anatomic implants are always textured and must remain this way.
5. Smooth-walled prostheses are easier to insert, require a shorter incision, and allow the use of longer and more indirect introduction methods.
6. Textured implants allow better adhesion to adjacent tissues, all the while preventing migration and rotation.

References

1. Höllander F: Berliner Gesellschaft für Chirurgie Münch. Med Wochenschr 1912; 59:2842 (abstract)
2. Lagarde M: Les injections de paraffine. Paris, Jules Rousset 1903
3. Morestin H: Inconvénients et abus des injections de paraffine. Bull Soc Chir, Paris 1908 ;34:2689–2698
4. Bames HO: Augmentation mammaplasty by lipotransplant. Plast Reconstr Surg 1953;11:404–412
5. Bartlett W: An anatomic substitute for the female breast. Ann Surg 1917;66:208–211
6. Berson M: Derma-fat transplants used in building up the breasts. Surgery 1945;15:451–456
7. Thorek M: Plastic Surgery of the Breast and Abdominal Wall. Amastia, Hypomastia and Inequality of the Breast. Springfield, Charles Thomas 1942
8. Zavaleta De, Marino E: Hipoplasia mamaria unilateral. Ralleno mamario con epiplon mayor transplantado. Prensa Med Argent 1963;50:639–641
9. Chaplin C: Loss of both breasts from injection of silicone. Plast Reconstr Surg 1969;44(5):447–450
10. Conway H, Goulian DJ: Experience with an injectable silastic RTV as a subcutaneous prosthetic material. Plast Reconstr Surg 1963;32:294–302
11. Conway H, Dietz GH: Augmentation mammaplasty. Surg Gynec Obstet 1962;114:373–379
12. Maliniac JW: Breast deformities and their repair. New York, Grune and Stratton 1950
13. Marzoni FA, Upchurch SE, Lambert CI: An experimental study of silicone as a soft tissue substitute. Plastic Reconstr Surg 1959;24:600–608
14. Ortiz Monasterio F, Trigos J: Management of patients with complications from injections of foreign materials in the breasts. Plast Reconstr Surg 1972;50(1):42–47
15. Pangman JJ 2nd, Wallace RM, Hills B: The use of plastic prosthesis in breast or other soft tissue surgery. West J Surg Obstet Gynecol 1955;63(8):503–512
16. Regnault P: One hundred cases of retromammary implantations of Etheron. Transactions of the Third Congress of Plastic Reconstructive Surgery, Washington 1963
17. Cronin TD, Gerow FJ: Augmentation mammaplasty, a new natural feel prosthesis. Transaction of the Third International Congress of Plastic and Reconstructive Surgery. Excerpta Medica 1963:41–49
18. Cronin TD, Brauer RO: Augmentation mammaplasty. Surg Clin North Amer 1971:51(2):441–452
19. Goldwyn RM: An unusual complication of the use of the Cronin implant for augmentation mammaplasty. Br J Plast Surg 1969;22(2):167–168
20. Arion HG: Présentation d'une prothèse rétromammaire. CR Soc Française Gynécol 1965;35:427–431
21. Ashley FL: A new type of breast prosthesis. Preliminary report. Plast Reconstr Surg 1970;45(5):421–424

22. Ashley F: Further studies on the naturally prosthesis. Plast Reconstr Surg 1972;49:414–419

23. Baker JL: Classification of spherical contracture. Aesthetic Breast Symposium, Scottsdale, AZ,1975

24. Baker JL, Bartels SRJ, Doglas WM: Closed compression technique for rupturing a contracted capsule around a breast implant. Plast Reconstr Surg 1976;58(2):137–141

25. Baker JL, LeVier RR, Spielvogel DE: Positive identification of silicone in human mammary capsular tissue. Plast Reconstr Surg 1982;69(1):56–60

26. Biggs TM, Cukier J, Worthing LF: Augmentation mammaplasty, a review of 18 years. Plast Reconstr Surg 1982;69(3):445–452

27. Caffee HH: The influence of silicone bleed on capsule contracture. Ann Plast Surg 1986;17(4):284–287

28. Freeman BS: Successful treatment of some fibrous envelope contracture around breast implants. Plast Reconstr Surg 1972;50(2):107–113

29. Moufarrège R, Beauregard G, Bossé JP, Papillon J, Perras C: Outcome of breast capsulotomies. Ann Plast Surg 1987;19(1):62–64

30. Vinnik CA: Spherical contracture of fibrous capsules around breast implants. Prevention and treatment. Plast Reconstr Surg 1976;58(5):555–560

31. Biggs TM, Yarish RC: Augmentation mammaplasty. Retropectoral versus retromammary implantation. Clin Plast Surg 1988;15(4):549–555

32. Dempsey WC, Latham WD: Subpectoral implants in augmentation mammaplasty. Preliminary report. Plast Reconstr Surg 1968;42(6):515–521

33. Lesesne CB: Textured surface silicone breast implants: histology in the human. Aesthetic Plast Surg 1997;21(2):93–96

34. Glicenstein J: Faut-il interdire les silicones? Ann Chir Plast Estet 1986;31(4):398

35. McKinney P, Tresley G: Long term comparison of patients with gel and saline mammary implants. Plast Reconstr Surg 1983;72(1):27–31

36. Sanders GB: Use of the pectoralis muscle in augmentation mammaplasty. Ann Surg 1968;34(3):236–237

37. Danino A, Rocher F, Blanchet-Bardon C, Revol M, Servant JM: Etude au microscope électronique à balayage des surfaces des implants mammaires à texturation poreuse et de leurs capsules. Description de l'effet « velcro »des prothèses à texturation poreuse. Ann Chir Plast Esthét 2001;46(1):23–30

38. Muller GH: Chimie des silicones. In: Les implants mammaires. Rapport du XXXVIe congrès de la SOFCPRE. Octobre 1991:19–29

39. Wyatt LE, Sinow JD, Wollmann JS, Sami DA, Miller TA: The influence of time on human breast capsule histology: smooth and textured silicone-surfaced implants. Plast Reconstr Surg 1998;102(6):1922–1931

40. Burkhardt BR, Eades E: The effect of Biocell texturing and povidone iodine irrigation on capsular contracture around saline-inflatable breast implants. Plast Reconstr Surg 1995;96(6):1317–1325

41. Elliott LF: Breast augmentation with round, smooth saline or gel implants. Augmentation mammaplasty. Ann Plast Surg 2001;28(3):523–529

42. Muller GH: Les applications cliniques de la chimie des silicones. Ann Chir Plast Esthét 1994;38(6):660–666

43. Muller GH: Les prothèses remplies d'hydrogel. Ann Chir Plast Esthét 1994;38(6):721–725

44. Sitbon E: Manufacturing of mammary implants: a manufacturing of high technology. Ann Chir Plast Esthét 2005;50(5):394–407

45. Capozzi A, Pennisi VR: Clinical experience with polyurethane covered gel filled mammaplasty prosthesis. Plast Reconstr Surg 1981;68(4):512–520

46. Dionyssopoulos A: The non-perfect results of breast implants. Ann Chir Plast Esthét. 2005;50(5):534–543

47. Hester TR, Nahai F, Bostwick J, Cukic J: A 5-year experience with polyurethane-covered mammary prosthesis for treatment of capsular contracture, primary augmentation mammaplasty, and breast reconstruction. Clin Plast Surg 1988;15(4):569–585

48. Herman S: The Meme implants. Plast Reconstr Surg1984;73(3):411–414

49. Kompatscher P, Schuler C, Beer GM: The transareolar incision for augmentation mammaplasty revisited. Aesthetic Plast Surg 2004;28(2):70–74

50. Troques R. Implantation des prothèses mammaires par voie axillaire. Nouv Presse Med 1972;1(36):2409–2410

51. Asplund O, Gylbert L, Jurell G, Ward C: Textured or smooth implants for submuscular breast augmentation: a controlled study. Plast Reconstr Surg 1996;97(6):1200–1206

52. Collis N, Coleman D, Foo ITH, Sharpe DT: Ten-year review of a prospective randomized controlled trail of textured versus smooth subglandular silicone gel breast implants. Plast Reconstr Surg 2000;106(4):786–791

53. Fagrell D, Berggren A, Tarpila E: Capsular contracture around saline-filled fine textured and smooth mammary implants: a prospective 7.5 –year follow-up. Plast Reconstr Surg 2001;108(7):2108–2112

54. Flageul G, Elbaz JS: Les prothèses mammaires textures. Ann Chir Plast Esthét 1994;38(6):711–720

55. Hakelius L, Ohlsen L: A clinical comparison of the tendency to capsular contracture between smooth and textured gel-filled silicone mammary implants. Plast Reconstr Surg 1992;90(2):247–254

56. Hakelius L, Ohlsen L: Tendency to capsular contracture around smooth and textured gel-filled silicone mammary implants: a 5-year follow-up. Plast Reconstr Surg 1997;100(6):1566–1569

57. Heymans O: Smooth or textured implants: what to select? Ann Chir Plast Esthét 2005;50(5):494–498

58. Maxwell GP, Hammond DC: Breast implants: smooth vs. textured. Adv Plast Reconstr Surg 1993;9:209–220

59. Malata CM, Feldberg L, Coleman DJ, Foo IT, Sharpe DT: Textured or smooth implants for breast augmentation? Three year follow-up of a prospective randomized controlled trial. Br J Plast Surg 1997;50(2):99–105

60. McCurdy JA: Relationships between spherical fibrous capsular contracture and mammary prosthesis type: a comparison of smooth and textured implants. Am J Cosm Surg 1990;7:235–238

61. Spear SL, Elmaraghy M, Hess C: Textured surface saline-filled silicone breast implants for augmentation mammaplasty. Plast Reconstr Surg 2000;105(4):1542–1552

CHAPTER 19

Enhanced Projection: Adjustable Gel Implants   19

Hilton Becker, Luis A. Picard-Ami, Jr.

19.1
Introduction

Silicone breast implants were first used in 1962. Saline implants were developed a few years later. The main goal in developing saline implants was to enable the surgeon to place the implant through a smaller incision.

The original silicone gel implants were made of a very thick gel, necessitating a large incision for insertion. A new type of silicone gel implant was later developed, containing a softer, more liquid silicone gel that could be placed through a smaller incision, similar to that of a saline-filled implant. Although the silicone gel implant had a softer, more natural feel, it was more prone to rupture; and if it did rupture, the liquid silicone was more prone to flow out of the implant, often an unpleasant sight at the time of removal. It was those silicone gel implants that fueled the silicone scare of the 1990s.

Good to excellent results may be obtained with saline implants; however, compared with silicone gel implants, they are more likely to have cosmetic problems associated with them. Such problems include rippling and wrinkling, resulting in an abnormal shape and feel, particularly in women with very little breast tissue. Furthermore, the leakage rate of saline implants is higher than for that of silicone gel implants, largely due to shell failure.

Most plastic surgeons feel that silicone gel implants are the superior device. Since the silicone gel moratorium following the silicone scare of the 1990s, saline-filled implants have been the most commonly used implants in the United States; however, saline-filled implants are rarely used in other countries because of the high complication rate.

19.2
Saline Implants

Because of the problems related to saline implants, several improvements were instituted in an attempt to decrease these complications. One approach was to texture the shell, which would, theoretically, decrease the incidence of capsular contracture (hardening around the implant). It was found, however, that texturing actually led to additional rippling and a higher incidence of implant rupture. The thicker shell also made the implant more palpable.

Another advance in the area of saline implants was the introduction of adjustable saline implants. These implants offer many advantages over the standard saline-filled implant. Because the implant can be filled after surgery, the patient has input into the final size. In addition, size can be adjusted accurately in cases of breast asymmetry. Small breasts can also be expanded to improve the shape. Most importantly, rippling can be decreased by adjusting the volume of the implant postoperatively. The spectrum™ valve (used in adjustable saline implants) has a decreased leakage rate compared with the standard diaphragm valve.

After reviewing case studies, it also became evident that the incidence of leakage could be reduced by mildly overfilling the implant. Overfilling did not cause firmness, thus enabling the implant to function well over a wider volume range.

The adjustable saline implant is particularly useful in treating breast implant complications, such as scarring, asymmetry, and capsular contracture. Adjustable saline implants paved the way for wide acceptance of immediate breast reconstruction. The implant can be placed underfilled at the time of mastectomy, thus greatly decreasing the risk of wound breakdown due to excessive pressure on the raised skin flap. Once healed, the tissues can then be safely expanded. Upon completion of the expansion, the injection dome is removed, leaving the implant in position and thereby avoiding an unnecessary two-stage procedure.

Volume adjustability of adjustable saline implants also makes them safer to use for patients in whom radiation will or has been used.

19.3
Silicone Implants

While saline implants continue to be improved, improvements are also being made with silicone gel implants. One of these improvements is the increased viscosity of the gel. The new "fifth-generation" or cohesive gel implant has been shown to have a far lower incidence of rupture. Also, if for some reason the shell does rupture, the gel remains cohesive and in its original form.

Texturing was also applied to gel implants to decrease the incidence of capsular contracture. A consensus of opinion remains regarding the advantages and disadvantages of texturing. Textured implants are more difficult to insert and position. The introduction of anatomical, or shaped, implants was a further innovation. Texturing is necessary in these implants to prevent rotation.

Newer anatomical implants have been developed with enhanced projection ability. The first attempt at an enhanced-projection implant consisted of a double-lumen device with a denser gel in the inner lumen. Although excellent results were initially obtained, a high incidence of rupture occurred where the two shells were joined. The heavier gel, having a different viscoselastic property to the surrounding gel, caused unanticipated shearing forces, which resulted in eventual rupture. An improved version of this enhanced-projection implant, having two different gels within the same shell, has shown encouraging results.

19.4
Double-Lumen Adjustable Implants

To combine the advantages of saline implants with the advantages of gel implants, double-lumen adjustable implants were introduced. These implants function in a similar way to adjustable saline implants with the added advantage of having silicone in the outer chamber, resulting in a better look and feel. The currently available adjustable double-lumen implant has either 25% or 50% gel in the outer chamber, and they are known as the 25/75 and the 50/50, respectively.

Texturing was also added to the adjustable double-lumen implants; however, the thicker shell necessitated by the textured surface decreased the elastic properties, rendering the device less effective as a tissue expander.

The anatomical textured adjustable gel saline implant has been used outside the United States, but it is currently still not approved by the U.S. Food and Drug Administration.

19.5
Enhanced Projection: Adjustable Gel Implant

In choosing a breast implant today, it is no longer simply a matter of volume. The surgeon must consider a wide variety of measurements and factors, including the following:
- Base diameter
- Height
- Projection
- Nipple-to-inframammary distance
- Volume
- Breast asymmetry
- Rib cage projection
- Ptosis
- Other factors stemming from previous surgeries

Adjustable implants have been proven very effective in managing these discrepancies. Today, however, adjustable implants are more like saline implants, with a coating of silicone. Subareolar projection is often deficient. Therefore, a new generation of implant has been developed to address these deficiencies (Figs. 19.1–19.4).

The implant is essentially a gel implant, with a centrally placed small inner lumen to which saline can be added as desired. Should no further projection be desired, the saline chamber can be left completely empty. The degree of enhanced projection can be determined with the implant in position. Alternatively, the fill tube can be attached to an injection dome and buried or exteriorized.

The inner chamber is filled, preferably to a point to where it becomes taut. Projection is greatly enhanced, without firmness, due to the cushioning effect of the surrounding gel. Another advantage of the small inner lumen is that the volume of the implant can be increased without altering the base diameter (that is, with a specific base diameter, the volume and projection can be selected by the surgeon and modified by the patient postoperatively).

The adjustable gel implant known as the Spectra has recently been introduced in Europe, with both a smooth and textured surface. The anatomical version will be released later.

The adjustable gel implant decreases the need for the vast array of shapes and sizes that a surgeon must select from when using fixed volume anatomical implants. Postoperative adjustability will be most beneficial in cases of asymmetry and for patients desiring enhanced projection.

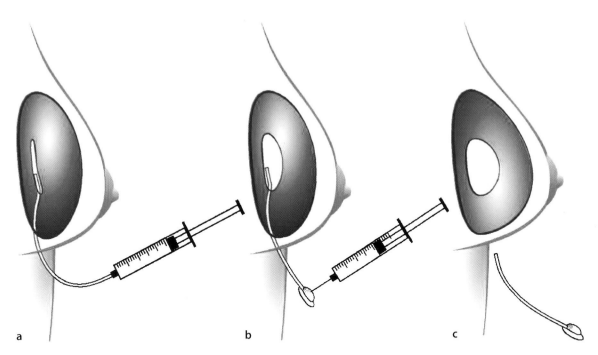

Fig. 19.1 a Implant in position without saline added. Saline may be added on the operating table or after surgery. **b** Saline added postoperatively via dome injection. Saline may be removed at any stage. **c** Implant filled to enhance projection; fill tube has been removed

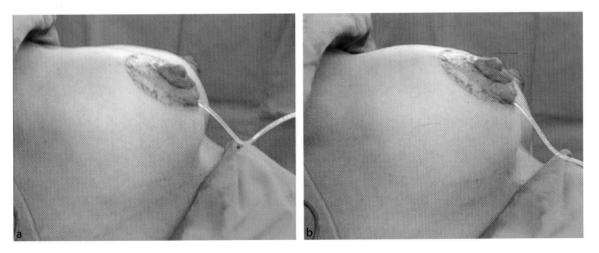

Fig. 19.2 a Breast augmentation with Spectra implant. **b** Volume adjusted before removing fill tube

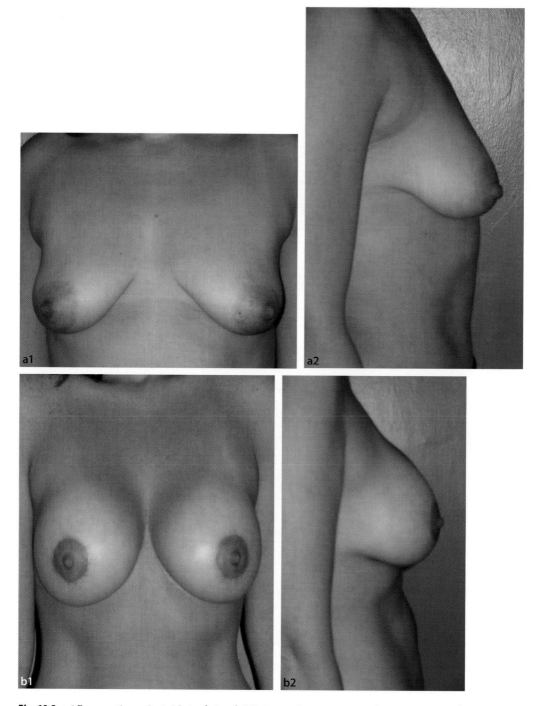

Fig. 19.3 **a** *1* Preoperative patient. *2* Lateral view. **b** *1* Postoperative mastopexy and augmentation with Spectra implants. *2* Lateral view

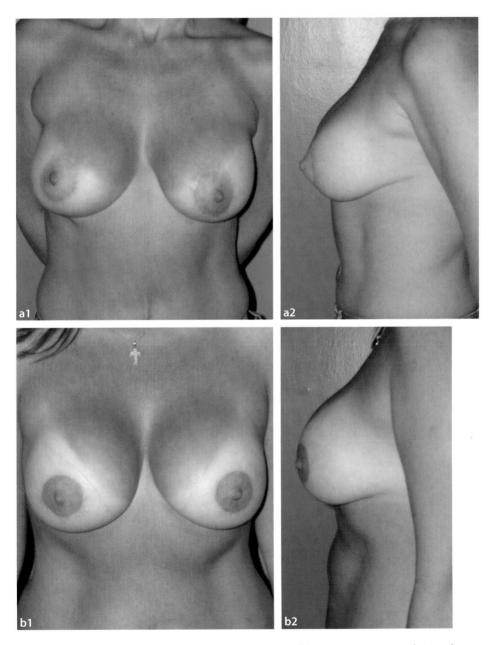

Fig. 19.4 a *1* Preoperative patient with previous mastopexy and breast augmentation with 225-ml implants. *2* Lateral view. **b** Postoperative following circumareolar mastopexy and replacement of prostheses with 275-ml Spectra implants filled to 285 ml on right side and 305 ml on left. *2* Lateral view

CHAPTER 20

Betadine and Breast Implants

Melvin A. Shiffman

20.1
Introduction

Since Becker and Becker's letter to the editor [1, 2], there has been much controversy and misunderstanding about the use of Betadine (povidone) in breast augmentation. The effect of Betadine on breast implants is limited to the studies done on segments of fill tubes of silicone that showed weakening of the fill tubes.

20.2
Study on Betadine

Becker and Becker [1, 2] studied the effects of Betadine on silicone after observing that breast expander implants soaked with Betadine solution for 3 days had fill tubes that turned white. Twelve 2-in segments of fill tube from Spectrum tissue expanders were placed in varying solutions of Betadine (0.1%, 0.5%, 1.0%, 2.0%, 10.0%, and 100%, corresponding to full-strength 10% povidone-iodine) for 2 weeks. The tubes soaked in Betadine for 3 weeks exhibited breaking strengths significantly lower than controls without Betadine soaking.

On analysis of the results, it was established that in heat-cured silicone with a peroxide catalyst, iodine can attack the center methylene group of the trimethylene crosslink, attaching to the center carbon and resulting in a highly unstable crosslink with weakening of the fill tube. Peroxide-cured silicone is found in fill tubes and in portions of the valves in saline-filled breast implants. Implant silicone shells are not made with peroxide-cured silicone. It was suggested that Betadine irrigation of the implant or the implant pocket must also be carefully considered.

Betadine is an excellent antimicrobial irrigant and implant soak except for some damage to the surrounding cells in the pocket. The Betadine in the pocket is usually removed with irrigations during surgery. There are a variety of other antimicrobials that can be used to irrigate the implant pocket and for soaking the implant without weakening the fill tubes or the valves.

20.3
Discussion

Povidone-iodine associated with textured implants may work in a cumulative manner to reduce the early incidence of capsule contracture [3].

Wiener [4] reported that the use of Betadine has no effect on the rate of deflation of saline breast implants. There was also a significant decrease in the rate of capsule contracture with the proper use of Betadine.

20.4
Conclusions

It is within the standard of care to use Betadine as an irrigant for the breast implant pocket and for soaking the implant to prevent infection as long as contact with a fill tube or the valve is not prolonged (3 days to 3 weeks). Betadine should be washed from the implant if soaked prior to implanting, and the pocket should be irrigated with saline if Betadine is used as an antimicrobial in the pocket.

References

1. Becker H, Becker CD: The effect of Betadine on silicone implants. Plast Reconstr Surg 2000;105(4):1570–1571
2. Becker H, Becker CD: The effect of Betadine on silicone implants. Plast Reconstr Surg 2000;106(7):1665
3. Burkhardt BR, Eades E: The effect of Biocell texturing and povidone-iodine irrigation on capsular contraction around saline-inflatable breast implants. Plast Reconstr Surg 1995;96(6):1317–1325
4. Wiener TC: The role of Betadine irrigation in breast augmentation. Plast Reconstr Surg 2007;119(1):12–15

CHAPTER 21

Mechanical Analysis of Explanted Silicone Breast Implants

21

Daniel P. Greenwald, Mark Randolph, James W. May

Data reprinted with permission from Greenwald DP, Randolph M, May JW Jr: Mechanical analysis of explanted silicone breast implants. Plast Reconstr Surg 1996;98(2):269–272, discussion 273–275

21.1
Introduction

Implantable silicone devices have been used for augmentation mammaplasty for the past four decades. Controversy over the fate of liquid silicone in the human body after implant rupture or gel "bleed" resulted in a moratorium on the use of previous generations of gel-filled implants. The modern era has seen large-scale removal of previously placed first- and second-generation implants, either because of health concerns, rupture, or liquid silicone bleed. Of greatest concern is frank rupture of the implant shell with gross spillage of liquid silicone. Of particular interest is how the physical properties of the shells of previous generation silicone implants change in vivo: Do they weaken with time, and if so, to what degree? This study was designed to evaluate how the mechanical properties of previous generation silicone shells change over time in vivo. This information is sought to elucidate structural changes, particularly as they relate to material failure. The authors studied early-generation silicone breast implants that were removed from patients to determine the changes that implant shells have undergone over time and whether these changes resulted in decreased shell integrity. Mechanical testing was performed to determine changes in shell strength, toughness, strain at rupture, and elasticity.

21.2
Materials and Methods

All implants removed from women by a single surgeon (JWM) between May of 1991 and January of 1994 at the Massachusetts General Hospital were labeled and stored in airtight containers at 7°C. All smooth-walled silicone gel implants were entered into the study (25 implants from 15 women). None of the implants was removed because of rupture. Four were found to be ruptured at the time of explantation, and two were ruptured during explantation.

Three pieces of shell material were cut from the periphery of each implant. Specimens measured 1.5×4 cm and were oriented radially (Fig. 21.1). For mechanical analysis, specimens were mounted in nonslip jaws and stretched apart at constant speed (2 cm/min) until failure [1]. Testing was performed by a technician blinded to the age of the specimens tested. Applied force (load) and distance pulled were monitored by a force transducer (Lucas Shaevitz, Pennsauken, NJ, USA; accuracy ± 0.02%) and linear variable differential transformer (LVDT; Lucas Shaevitz, Pennsauken, NJ, USA; accuracy ± 0.01%), respectively. Output signals were amplified, and noise was reduced by a signal conditioner (Omega Engineering, Stamford, CT, USA). Analog data were sampled for digital computer acquisition at 100 Hz (adc488/16; IO Tech, Cleveland, OH, USA). Custom software formatted and analyzed the data. The com-

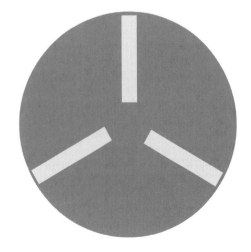

Fig. 21.1 Orientation of radially distributed shell samples

pliance of the machinery was subtracted, and the data were normalized for specimen dimensions (measured by electronic calipers, ±0.001 mm). Instantaneous cross-sectional area was used to calculate stress during loading. Isovolumetric elongation during uniaxial loading was assumed; therefore, a Poisson's ratio of 0.5 was employed [2–4]. Apparent true–stress–true–strain curves were generated; strength was defined as peak stress, and toughness was defined as energy absorbed (calculated as the integral of the stress–strain curve from strain = 0 to strain at maximum stress). Strain = 0 was chosen as the first point in the stretch where load was 5% over background. Strain at rupture was recorded as the natural log of maximum stretched length per initial specimen length. The elastic modulus for each specimen was calculated as the slope of each stress–strain curve taken at 50% strain at maximum stress. Data outside the zone of interest for each specimen's stress–strain curve were eliminated until a least-squares regression of remaining data points yielded a coefficient (r^2) > 0.95 (minimum strain range = 0.1). The zone of interest for each curve is where stress varies almost linearly with strain. The elimination of data from the early and late portions of each curve to a minimum strain range of 0.1% allows the elastic modulus to be measured accurately.

Data from the three specimens from each implant were averaged. To meet the assumption of independence, data from both implants from patients with bilateral explantations were averaged. This yielded 15 data points for analysis.

Regression analysis was performed to examine the relationship between implant age and shell strength,

toughness, strain at rupture, and elastic modulus (Stat-View; Abacus Systems, Berkeley, CA, USA).

21.3
Results

The 25 tested implants had a mean age of implantation of 117 months (minimum 23, maximum 216, SEM 12.9). Data indicate that shells become weaker in vivo. Regression analyses revealed a significant negative correlation between length of time in vivo and mean peak stress (shell strength; $r^2 = 0.391$, $p < 0.05$; Fig. 21.2). Shell toughness (energy absorbed before rupture) also decreased with time ($r^2 = 0.257$, $p < 0.05$; Fig. 21. 3). Not only were shells weakened by their in vivo exposure, but shell elasticity (elastic modulus) decreased with implantation time, resulting in less stiff, more deformable specimens ($r^2 = 0.351$, $p < 0.05$; Fig. 21.4). Strain at rupture did not vary with implant age (mean strain ± SEM = 1.381 ± 0.052; $r^2 = 0.078$, $p = 0.31$).

21.4
Discussion

The degree to which breast implants elicit host responses continues to be a subject of intense interest and debate. While shell material is mechanically more stable than less completely polymerized liquid, it is able to elicit host responses, some of which are able to alter the physical properties of the shell material [3, 5]. The mechani-

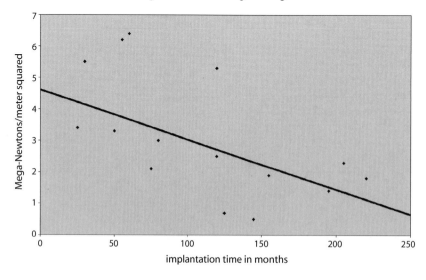

Fig. 21.2 Regression analysis of shell strength versus implant age. Shell strength decreases with time in vivo ($p < 0.05$)

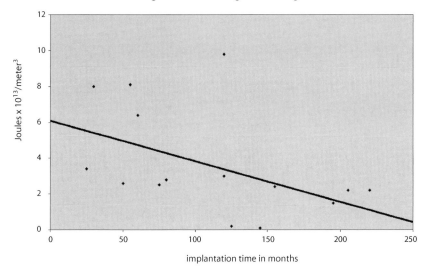

Regression Plot: Toughness vs. Age

Fig. 21.3 Regression analysis of shell toughness versus implant age. Shell toughness decreases with time in vivo ($p < 0.05$)

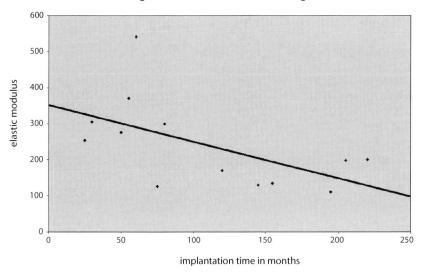

Regression Plot: Elastic Modulus vs. Age

Fig. 21.4 Regression analysis of shell elastic modulus versus implant age. Elasticity decreases with time in vivo ($p < 0.05$)

cal data presented demonstrate that the human body is able to alter the material properties of silicone shells to the point that they become weaker and more compliant over time. Whether this is due solely to primary effects of the body on the shell or whether the slow diffusion of liquid through the shell also contributes to mechanical degradation cannot be determined from the date presented. Modification of so-called inert materials in the in-vivo milieu is not a new observation: As early as 1958, Harrison [6] catalogued the tensile strength of several synthetic vascular prostheses after in-vivo implantation. Teflon, the least reactive material, demonstrated the

least reduction in strength: 1.7% after 1 year. Nylon, the most reaction-inducing material, demonstrated an 85% reduction in tensile strength after 175 days.

In a study comparing the tensile strength of 11 different types of suture materials after 6 weeks of in-vivo exposure, significant changes in the mechanical properties of nylon, polypropylene, and polyester were demonstrated [4]. Clearly, as materials induce tissue reaction, so does tissue reaction induce changes in the physical properties of the materials.

The observation that breast implant shells are sensitive to degradation in the body has been demonstrated by Robinson et al. [7]. They examined a large series of explanted specimens and found a significant correlation between length of time of implantation and incidence of rupture. They studied 592 implants removed from 300 patients and found a significant correlation ($p < 0.5$) between number of years since implantation and rupture rate. Almost all implants older than 10 years were ruptured. The authors concluded, on the basis of clinical findings at explantation, that implant shells weaken over time in vivo.

While matched in-vitro implants would add significantly to the currently presented data set as "on-the-shelf" controls for biologic activity, these controls are not available. Nonetheless, the data developed in the current study support the conclusion, through vigorous mechanical analysis, that the shells of previous generations of smooth-walled silicone breast implants lose structural integrity with time in vivo. Robinson et al. [7] stated that implants should be removed prophylactically after 8 or 10 years of implantation because of significant incidence of rupture. Although the issue of prophylactic implant removal remains controversial pending definitive evaluation of the health risks of free silicone, the weakening of silicone implant shells over time in vivo now seems fairly clear.

The current generation of silicone implants, available since November 2006, are markedly different compared with their predecessors: A trilaminar shell composition functions as a barrier to gel bleed (phenyl groups are substituted for methyl groups to aid in barrier impermeability), and liquid silicone filler material has been replaced with a more cross-linked polymer that provides a cohesive gel consistency that does not "flow" and can maintain shape memory.

References

1. Greenwald D, Mass D, Tuel R: Biomechanical analysis of intrinsic tendon healing and the effects of vitamins A and E. Plast Reconstr Surg 1991;87(5):925–930
2. Vincent J: Structural Biomaterials. Princeton, NJ, Princeton University Press 1990
3. Fung YC: Biomechanics: Mechanical Properties of Living Tissue. New York, Springer-Verlag 1981
4. Wainwright SA, Biggs WD, Currey JD, Gosline JM: Mechanical Design in Organisms. Princeton, NJ, Princeton University Press 1976
5. Kossovsky N, Heggers JP, Parsons RW, Robson MC: Analysis of the surface morphology of recovered silicone mammary prostheses. Plast Reconstr Surg 1983;71(6):795–804
6. Harrison JH: Synthetic materials as vascular prostheses. II. A comparative study of nylon, Dacron, orlon, ivalon sponge and Teflon in large blood vessels with tensile strength studies. Am J Surg 1958;95(1):16–24
7. Robinson OG Jr, Bradley EL, Wilson DS: Analysis of explanted silicone implants: a report of 300 patients. Ann Plast Surg 1995;34:1

CHAPTER 22

Cohesive Gel Silicone Implants

22

Ângelo Rebelo

22.1
Introduction

There are many approaches to perform breast augmentation, which is one of the most popular surgeries nowadays. The approach (areolar, inframammary, axillary, or endoscopic), type of anesthesia (general, local, local tumescent), placement of the implant (retroglandular, retropectoral), and type of implant (silicone, saline, hydrogel) all have to be considered. Opinions and procedures vary considerably.

The author describes the procedure that he believes is safer, with fewer complications and better results, and reports a series of 1674 breast augmentations, 700 done under tumescent local anesthesia and 974 done under tumescent local anesthesia with sedation, from February 1997 until July 2008.

22.2
Patient Selection

The main indications for this procedure are mild to severe hypoplasia and mild to moderate ptosis in women seeking to improve their appearance and enlarge their breasts. Good results can be achieved with minimal scarring with a first-time surgery.

Patients who wished to exchange implants (saline, hydrogel, soybean oil, normal silicone gel), wanted to change size, or had capsular contracture were selected for this procedure. Neither the woman's age nor nulliparous condition was an important factor. Patients with breast disorders were not selected.

22.3
Preoperative Routine Examination

All patients should have a complete clinical history, preoperative routine examinations including mammography and/or echography, and preoperative (and postoperative) photos. Local tumescent anesthesia is used in a high percentage of patients with intravenous sedation.

22.4
Contraindications

Contraindications include patients with a strong family history of breast cancer or with breast disorders that have no indication to be operated on.

22.5
Anesthesia

22.5.1
Local Tumescent Anesthesia

Oral medication is administered 30–60 min before surgery with lorazepam (2.5 mg), lysine clonixinate (250 mg), and hydroxyzine (50 mg). All patients are monitored during surgery, and nowadays all undergo intravenous sedation with propofol and midazolam unless contraindicated.

A modified Klein's formula is used, and infiltration is done with a Byron infiltration canula (Fig. 22.1).

22.5.2
Anesthetic Solution

To each 500 ml of 9% saline solution warmed up to 37 °C, add the following:
1. One ampule of adrenaline 1 mg/ml
2. 600 mg of lidocaine 2% without adrenaline
3. 10 ml sodium bicarbonate

22.6
Technique

The author's first choice is the inferior circumareolar approach because there is no risk of hypertrophic or keloid scaring, and it does not disturb the normal breast anatomy and physiology. The areola should be at least 1.5 cm in diameter. However, an areola expander effect occurs as a result of the tumescent local anesthesia. This makes it possible to use this approach even for smaller areolas.

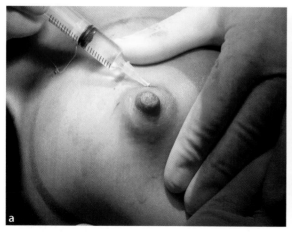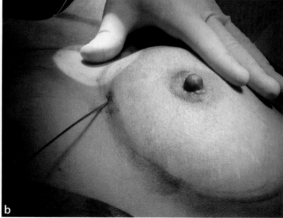

Fig. 22.1 a Local anesthesia. **b** Local tumescent anesthesia

The incision must be made 2–3 mm inside the areola. To avoid the risk of hypertrophic scars or keloids, one should never injure the skin.

This surgery does not disturb breastfeeding, and no infections have ever been reported as a result of ductal transection. As a matter of fact, the use of tumescent local anesthesia is a good way to prevent infections because of the highly bactericidal effect of lidocaine.

If an areolar incision is not possible or if the areola is hypoplastic with a small diameter or is atrophic, the approach should be inframammary with a 4–5–cm incision in the inframammary fold.

Retroglandular placement is the author's first choice. This positioning is preferable because it gives a more natural appearance; there is no discomfort for the patient as occurs in the retropectoral position and no problem with dislocation of the implant. Only in very special situations—such as prosthesis substitution, rare cases of severe breast hypoplasia or aplasia, or severe rippling—is the retropectoral position considered. There is no other reason to put implants in the retropectoral position in normal procedures; one of the principles of plastic surgery is to imitate nature, and that means the mammary gland is not placed under the pectoral muscle.

22.6.1
Implant Choice

The implants used since 1997 are the cohesive gel silicone implants, which are preferable because they are safer and have excellent quality. Silicone gel is the safest and most effective material for breast implants, and silicone implants are the oldest and the most reliable implants worldwide. They have all the silicone charac-

teristics plus the advantage of no bleeding or migration because of the highly cohesive gel, trilaminar shell, microtextured surface, and soft feel.

Reviews of several studies worldwide indicate that the only "problem" with the silicone is the controversy in the United States. Various problems are associated with alternative implants, especially saline and Trilucent implants; many patients have had to be reoperated on to exchange these types of implants for silicone one. The Trilucent implants were even withdrawn in Europe.

22.6.2
Surgical Technique

The incision and breast transection is usually made using the Ellman radiofrequency tool (Ellman, Oceanside, NY, USA; Fig. 22.2), and undermining is then used to make a pocket at least 2–3 cm larger than the prosthesis diameter. Careful hemostasis is necessary, and the implants are placed in the retroglandular position (Fig. 22.3). The wound is closed internally by layers of 2/0 and 3/0 low-absorption suture, and subcuticular tissues are closed with 4/0 fast-absorption suture, with Steri-Strips placed on the skin (Fig. 22.4). A closed vacuum drainage system is routinely applied in the breasts in the majority of cases. Small dressings and a bra are used (Fig. 22.5).

22.7
Postoperative Care

The patients leave the facility 1–2 h after the surgery and return to the clinic the next day for routine follow-up. Drains are removed after 24–48 h.

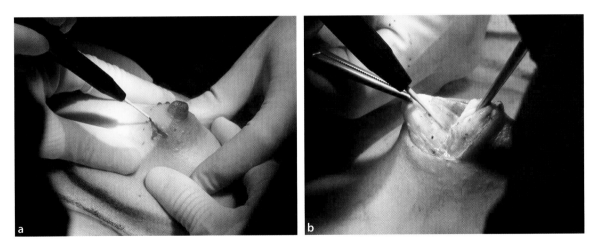

Fig. 22.2 a Skin incision with Ellman. **b** Transection of the breast tissues with the Ellman

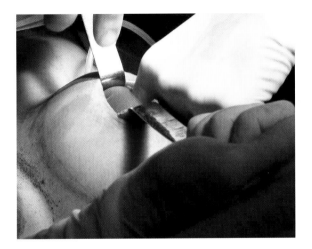

Fig. 22.3 The implant is placed in the subglandular pocket

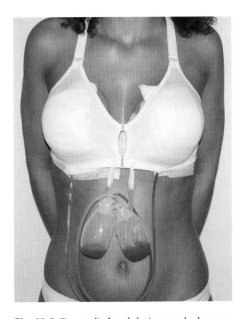

Fig. 22.5 Bra applied and drains attached to reservoir

22.8
Results

Over the past 11 years, using cohesive gel silicone implants with the areolar approach, retroglandular placement, and tumescent local anesthesia, the author has been getting very good results in shape, size, and symmetry. The patients recover quickly with few complications.

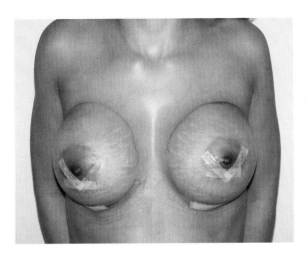

Fig. 22.4 Skin closed with Steri-Strips

22.9
Complications

Out of 837 patients, there have been five cases of unilateral capsular contracture, Becker grade II/III, that were resolved with capsulotomy, and two cases of small superficial hematoma that were drained. All of those cases were resolved successfully and without sequelae.

Temporary diminution of nipple sensibility was observed in a few patients. There were no infections, seromas, skin necrosis, or hypertrophic scars. A few patients showed lack of pigmentation of the scar, which was resolved with scar revision, laser abrasion, or dermopigmentation.

22.10
Conclusions

After many years of experience, study, investigation, and participation in discussions in congresses and workshops, the preference is for breast augmentation with cohesive gel silicone implants, the areolar approach, retroglandular placement, and local tumescent anesthesia with intravenous sedation. The advantages of tumescent local anesthesia are less bleeding, better recovery, an ambulatory patient, less expensive surgery, and an areola expander effect.

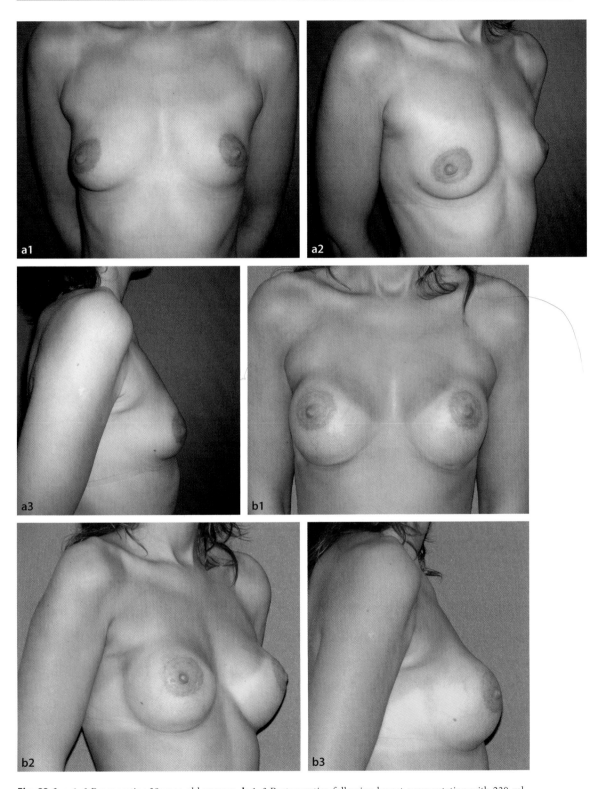

Fig. 22.6 a *1–3* Preoperative 29-year-old woman. **b** *1–3* Postoperative following breast augmentation with 230-ml cohesive gel silicone implants from Perthese

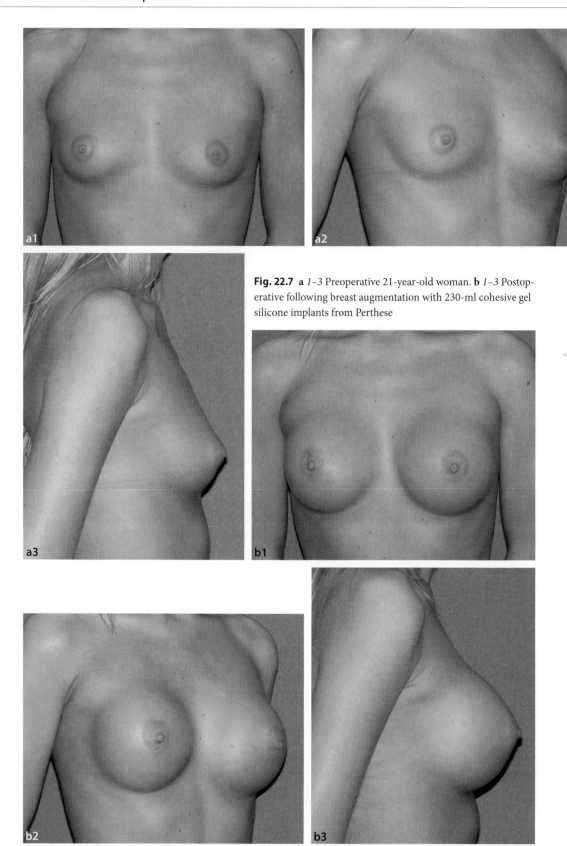

Fig. 22.7 a *1–3* Preoperative 21-year-old woman. **b** *1–3* Postoperative following breast augmentation with 230-ml cohesive gel silicone implants from Perthese

Part IV
Surgical Approaches

CHAPTER 23

Principles of Breast Augmentation Surgery   **23**

Melvin A. Shiffman

23.1
Introduction

Breast augmentation surgery may appear simple to some surgeons, but it has many potential complications. The surgeon should help the patient select the incision site, the implant type (saline or gel, high profile or medium profile, round or anatomic), the implant size, and the implant placement in relationship to the breast and muscle.

23.2
Principles

Following certain principles in performing the surgery may help avoid future problems. These principles are based on 42 years of experience in breast augmentation surgery. They should be guidelines for the student in cosmetic surgery as well as for the experienced breast augmentation surgeon.

1. The implant size should fit the patient's body according to her height and weight.
   a. The patient, however, has the right to choose the size that she feels she wants.
   b. It helps to use one of the methods to determine size, such as placing baggies filled with saline or other substance such as peas or beans or placing filled gel implants in the bra. This can give an approximation of implant size for the surgeon that is satisfactory to the patient.
   c. Make sure that the size decided upon is not influenced by the spouse or boyfriend. The surgery is to please the patient and not others.
   d. The surgeon should question the patient's decision to have a very large breast implant (over 500 ml).
   e. It is questionable when a surgeon has most patients with an average size of implants at 500 ml or more. Usually this is from the surgeon instilling his or her own idea of very large implants as being more "beautiful."
2. Avoid the chronic smoker who will not stop smoking.
   Necrosis can occur.

3. The new inframammary fold should be well developed in the pocket.
   It is better to be too low than too high because a low fold is easier to correct by a well-fitted bra and tape around the inferior portion of the bra around the chest at the new inframammary fold. If it is too high, surgery may be the only choice for correction.
4. The implant should be centrally placed behind the nipple.
   a. The limitation of having significant cleavage must be explained to the patient when the nipple–areola complex is lateral in position prior to surgery.
   b. A bra that lifts is better than nipples pointing outward and the implants bulging medially.
5. The muscular attachments to the ribs and sternum in submuscular implants may need to be completely transected or avulsed in order to fit the implant. This will allow an adequate pocket size.
6.
   Bleeding in the pocket should be carefully controlled.
   Blood is a known cause of capsule contracture.
7. Postoperatively, it is better to fix the implants in proper position for a few days with a bra and wrappings.
   a. The bra should have a well-fitting band at the bottom across the chest that may have to be taped to keep tight and maintain the inframammary fold.
   b. A compression Ace wrap or other device should be placed in the upper half of the breast and taped in place for a few days.
   c. This pushes the implant inferiorly and allows the inframammary fold to remain in proper position.
8. Breast augmentation should not be performed when the patient is lactating (during pregnancy or breast-feeding).
   There should be a delay of at least 3–6 months after completion of lactation.
9. Never use closed compression capsulotomy.
   The dangers of hematoma and/or implant disruption are too great.

10. Delay corrective procedures on the breast augmentation patient for at least 6 months after surgery, if possible.
    a. This delay is to allow the scar to mature and the deformity to be complete so that the corrective procedure corrects all of the deformity.
    b. The exception might be grade IV capsule contracture with severe pain.
11. Know when to stop performing corrective procedures.
    a. More than a few (three or four) procedures to correct deformities or capsule contracture significantly increases the risks of complications and more deformity because of excess scar (and the percentages can catch up with the patient).
    b. Beware of the patient who desires minimal correction. "Perfection is the enemy of good."
12. Sterile technique with the use of some antimicrobial solution to wash the implant and possibly the pocket is essential.

23.3
Controversies of Certain Methods

Surgeons should be aware that there are different techniques and different opinions for performing mastopexy. There may be controversy, but that does not necessarily mean one view is wrong and the other is right.

23.3.1
Visualized Dissection Versus Blind Dissection

Dissection while visualizing the pocket can be done with an endoscope. This requires somewhat expensive equipment and increases surgery time. If an inframammary or periareolar incision is used, the endoscope is usually not necessary. Sometimes, in the axillary and umbilical approaches as well as the subfascial pocket formation, the endoscope is used only to check the position of the implant pocket (below or above the muscle) after a blind dissection is completed. This is used as a learning method by those who have not performed very many breast augmentations, but as experience increases, the blind dissection is usually preferred.

Blind dissection is more rapid and has no greater incidence of postoperative bleeding or capsule contracture. A variety of instruments are available for blind dissection. Neither method, visualized or blind, is below the standard of care.

23.3.2
Electrocautery

Transection of the pectoralis major muscle attachments to the ribs and sternum can be performed with an electrocautery tool. This may leave a thickened edge of the muscle that may be palpable after surgery. The tissue around the area electrocauterized is damaged from the heat increasing the scarring and may lead to seroma formation.

The method of infiltrating a tumescent solution, usually saline with epinephrine (1 mg/1,000 ml) and possibly Lidocaine (250–500 mg/1,000 ml), helps make blunt dissection with the finger or instrument easier, and there is very little likelihood of bleeding. The tearing of the pectoralis major muscle fibers from the ribs and sternum occurs randomly, so there is no ledge or thickened area that would be palpable.

23.3.3
Position of Arms During Surgery

It has been assumed that if the patient's arms are kept at the sides of her body during surgery, there is less tension on the pectoralis major muscle and this would allow an easier dissection in the subpectoral pocket. This would also prevent stretching of the brachial plexus that might cause neurologic injury.

If the arms are kept out from the body, best at 80–85°, there is little chance of neurologic injury except in the case of axillary approach. At 90° or more, there is the possibility of stretching the brachial plexus, especially if the head is turned to the side.

23.3.4
Postoperative Manipulation of the Implants

Postoperative manipulation or massage of the implants to maintain pocket size has been criticized without good reason. There is no harm in manipulating the prosthesis starting 4 days after surgery if this may reduce the incidence of capsule contracture. No adequate study has decided whether manipulation affects the incidence of capsule contracture.

23.4
Conclusions

The principles of breast augmentation are a proposed safeguard for performing the procedure. These may change with more research and as new methods are developed.

CHAPTER 24

Intraoperative Assessment of Breast Prosthesis Volume Using a Set of Graduated Expanders

Beniamino Palmieri, Pierangelo Bosio, Melvin A. Shiffman

24.1
Introduction

One of the most puzzling decisions in augmentation mammaplasty for aesthetic purposes or following mammary gland removal is related to adequacy of the volume of the prosthesis to be inserted [1–10]. Several theoretic methods exist to calculate the final prosthesis volume on the basis of anthropometric measurements of the chest and/or contralateral breast. Nevertheless, in clinical practice such assessments often prove to be inadequate and do not correlate with the patient's actual needs or expectations. Most surgeons use a graduated gauge to measure the surface between the inframammary groove, the supramammary margin, the costoclavicular line, and the anterior axillary line.

A very practical method to assess the patient's expectations has been suggested by Brody [11]. The patient is invited to buy a brassiere of desired size and volume and fill it with cotton wool or other filling material to compensate for mammary gland lack. After the patient has worn the bra for several days or weeks and has found it aesthetically pleasant, the nurse in the plastic surgeon's office measures the lacking volume, replacing the bulk material with small plastic bags filled with a defined amount water. In measuring the likely prosthesis volume by such a gross method, the author observed an average underrating by 50–100 ml on the basis of breast inspection alone.

Another preoperative measure created by Schultz and refined by Tezel [12] includes applying the principle of Archimedes. The breast is inserted into a graduated cylinder filled with water, the spillover of which will correspond to the gland volume in terms of cubic centimeters. This method, initially carried out with direct contact of the water with the breast skin, was then improved using polyethylene bags that were prefilled within the measuring cylinder. The patient was then invited to wear a bra having a size adequate to the new postprosthesis status to anticipate the final result.

Pechter [13] suggests a preoperative assessment based on breast girth, which is measured from the lateral to the median breast fold. An A cup would correspond to 17.78 cm (7 in), a B cup to 20.32 cm (8 in), a C cup to 22.86 cm (9 in), and so on, with a cup increase or decrease by 2.54 cm (1 in). According to the author, such a method may be very accurate on a preoperative basis. Obviously, the physician–patient relationship, while being highly introspective and able to perfectly identify the current needs, cannot result in a thorough interpretation because of the low quality of the measurements that have been carried out. During surgery it is possible to measure the subglandular or retropectoral pocket with traditional cutaneous expanders, which, however, are neither graduated nor shaped according to the exact size of the permanent prostheses, giving rather approximate clues since they never represent the final actual breast projection once the operation is completed.

The authors deemed it necessary to plan the production of a set of expanders, or "phantoms," that are completely identical to permanent prostheses in shape and volume. They are connected to a valved tube that can be filled with sterile physiologic solution, permitting expansion of the breast to reproduce the exact desired shape and size. The expanders are provided within a kit containing low-, high-, and medium-profile round and anatomic shapes. When the volume and type of prosthesis is chosen, the inflatable expander is rapidly deflated and extracted from the mammary cavity to be replaced with the definitive prosthesis.

24.2
Technique

The patients are told that during the operation the surgeon will carry out a technical trial of volume expansion, finally choosing on his or her own responsibility the prosthesis that most suits the patient's desire and the anatomic conformation of the mammary region.

The operation is performed under general anesthesia, with midazolam premedication and propofol induction.

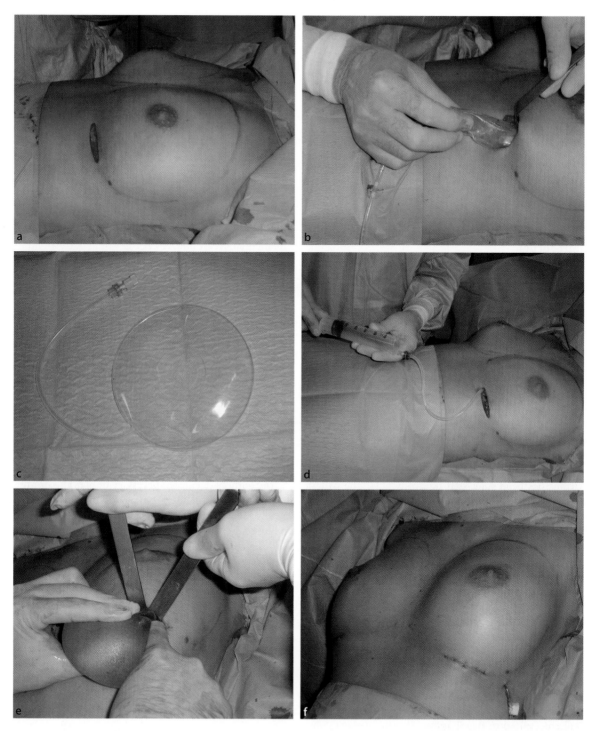

Fig. 24.1 Intraoperative steps. **a** Inframammary incision. **b** Phantom introduction. **c** Phantom inflated through a valved tube. **d** Water filling of phantom in place to foresee the final cosmetic outcome. **e** Introduction of the definite breast prosthesis. **f** Final results at the end of the operation

The periareolar or inframammary cutaneous incision with a perfectly symmetrical 3-cm-wide base is followed by a retroglandular blunt dissection under the control of a light-carrying retractor (Fig. 24.1). Thorough hemostasis is done in each quadrant.

After determining the ideal space for the creation of a suitable pocket in which the prosthesis will be placed, the inflatable prosthesis models are bilaterally inserted. These have various volumes (from 100 ml to 800 ml, with high and low profiles and anatomic and round shapes). The expander is equipped with a tube having an antireflux valve, which can be connected to a 50 ml syringe provided with a 3-way stopcock, thereby permitting the surgeon to rapidly inflate and deflate the

simulators without any liquid loss (Fig. 24.1c). After the phantom is inflated with saline to the desired volume, the expected results are reviewed, observing the breast remodeling in the various profiles (Fig. 24.1d).

Following the indication obtained by the phantom's use, all patients studied had the prosthesis volume changed in eight cases and the shape changed in four cases. The volumes that were introduced varied between 180 ml and 350 ml.

The operation is completed by improving the shape and margins of the retroglandular pocket to obtain a perfect positioning without wrinkling or folding of the prosthetic membrane. In particular, after the extraction of the phantoms, thorough examination and hemosta-

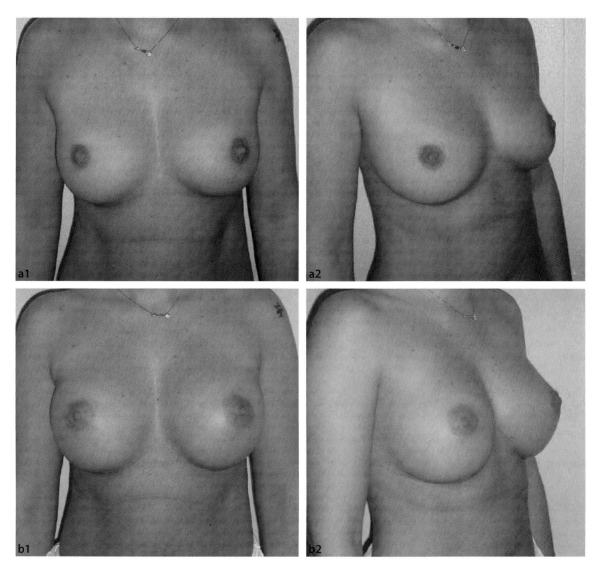

Fig. 24.2 Clinical presentation of a woman implanted using the phantom implant technique. **a** *1,2* Preoperative. **b** *1,2* Postoperative

sis of the dissociated tissues are carried out. Following wide irrigation with saline and diluted Betadine, the definitive prostheses are inserted (Fig. 24.1e), and a two-layer absorbable suture along the cutaneous incision is placed, with a closed-circuit sump drain maintained for 24 h (Fig. 24.1f). The patients are bandaged with elasto-compressive wrap and discharged 24 h later.

At follow-up visits our patients registered their satisfaction on a form which obtained a consensus on outcome in 100% of the 50 cases, which was also reconfirmed in short-term and long term follow-up checks at 3 months and 6 months (Fig. 24.2).

24.3
Discussion

The cases included in this study definitively outline the opportunity to do realistic intraoperative measurements of prosthetic size and shape. In fact, defining the desired volume and profile according to chest morphology in the preliminary assessment of a patient's breast evaluation is a difficult task. The adjustment of the body image of the woman who undergoes augmentation mammaplasty must be aesthetically improved by confirmation, on an intraoperative basis, of the patient's expectations. The surgeon therefore has the opportunity to extemporarily choose the most suitable prosthesis in a very easy and accurate manner during general anesthesia. Without tissue tumescence, intraoperative observation is truly objective. Phantoms are not only useful as confirmation of the potential self-image expectations of the patient, but also of taking care of surgical details such as the final pocket definition, symmetry, and hemostasis control after contact with the phantom silicone environment.

In the authors' experience, the operation planning time when using the phantoms is increased between 10 and 15 min. In fact, the phantoms can be easily deflated and rapidly inflated, allowing the surgeon to do repeated observations of different volumes in rapid sequence.

24.4
Conclusions

Planning with phantom implants is a practical aid to appropriately and consistently select the final breast conformation in augmentation mammaplasty. This is an especially important step to be included in the informed consent, in which the description of the use of the intraoperative phantom, aimed to obtain permission for use, represents a further warranty of accuracy.

Moreover, the satisfaction of all patients with the final outcome of augmentation mammaplasty in this study greatly gratifies the surgeons. Sometimes there is a gap between the expected aesthetic result and the definitive outcome [14–15].

The authors recommend widespread use of the phantom implant, particularly for young plastic and general surgeons in the first stages of the learning curve. A patient's frustration after cosmetic prosthesis surgery can be not only related to a surgeon's lack of experience but also a potential source of medicolegal liability.

References

1.   Bouman FG: Volumetric measurement of the human breast and breast tissue before and during mammaplasty. Br J Plast Surg 1970;23(3):263–264
2.   Kirianoff TG: Volume measurements of unequal breasts. Plast Reconstr Surg 1974;54(5):616
3.   Snyder GB: Planning on augmentation mammaplasty. Plast Reconstr Surg 1974;54(2):312–341
4.   Ellenbogen R: A new device to assist in sizing breasts. Ann Plast Surg 1978;1(3):333–335
5.   Tegtmeier RE: A quick, accurate mammometer. Ann Plast Surg 1978;1(6):625–626
6.   Tegtmeier RE: A convenient, effective mammary sizer. Aesthetic Plast Surg 1979;3:227–229
7.   Ramselaar JM: Precision in breast reduction. Plast Reconstr Surg 1988;82(4):631–643
8.   Godfrey PM, Godfrey NV, Romita MC: Restoring the breast to match the normal side. Ann Plast Surg 1993;31(5):392–397
9.   Edsander-Nord A, Wickman M, Jurell G: Measurement of breast volume with thermoplastic casts. Scand J Plast Reconstr Surg Hand Surg 1996;30(2):129–132
10. Hamas RS: The comparative dimensions of round and anatomic saline-filled implants. J Aesthetic Surg 2000;20:281–283
11. Brody G: Breast implant size selection and patient satisfaction. Plast Reconstr Surg 1981;68(4):611–613
12. Tezel E, Numanoglu A: Practical do-it-yourself device for accurate volume measurement of the breast. Plast Reconstr Surg 2000;105(3):1019–1023
13. Pechter EA: A new method to determinate bra size and predicting postaugmentation breast size. Plast Reconstr Surg 1998;102(4):1259–1265
14. Young VL, Nemecek JR, Nemecek DA: The efficacy of breast augmentation: breast size increase, patient satisfaction, and psychological effects. Plast Reconstr Surg 1994;94(7):958–969
15. Young VL: The efficacy of breast augmentation: breast size increase, patient satisfaction, and psychological effects. (Response) Plast Reconstr Surg 1995;96:1237–1238

CHAPTER 25

Breast Augmentation: Intraareolar Approach

25

Melvin A. Shiffman

25.1
Introduction

The intraareolar approach to breast augmentation results in a scar that is almost always thin and barely noticeable. The complete pocket can be easily visualized above or beneath the pectoralis major muscle. Repeat surgeries can be performed through the same scar.

25.2
Preoperative

The preoperative discussion with the patient should concern the procedure, the possible alternatives, and possible risks and complications of each. All questions should be answered.

The patient preselects the implant size by using baggies filled with water or, in the office, by the use of various sized silicone gel implants placed in the bra. She then looks at her profile while wearing a sweater or T-shirt to decide on the size. Some surgeons prefer rice grains in the baggie so that water leakage is not a problem during the selection.

25.3
Technique

25.3.1
Markings

A Sharpie (Newell Rubbermaid, Atlanta, GA, USA) permanent marker is used with a ruler to mark the midline. The breast template (KMI, Corona, CA, USA) for the preselected size of implant is placed with the highest point of the template centered over the nipple (Fig. 25.1). A mark is drawn around the template and then the same done on the opposite side, making sure that the most medial part of the mark is equidistant from the midline to the opposite side.

The planned inferior intraareolar incision site is

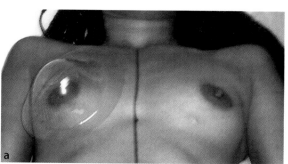
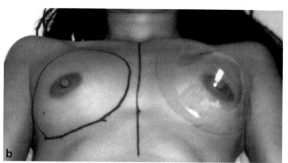
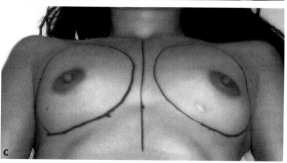

Fig. 25.1 Marking. **a** Midline marked and template placed over right breast, centering the nipple under the highest point of the template. **b** Marking of opposite side. **c** The surgeon should make sure that the medial edge of the template mark on each side is equidistant to the midline

marked with either a curved infra-areolar line 1–2 mm inside the areola skin junction or, with a small areola, an undulating line in the areola (Fig. 25.2).

25.3.2
Incision

The curved intraareolar incision inside the areola skin junction is performed with a #15 scalpel blade. If the areola is small, an undulating incision is used that will allow the tissues to spread wider. The surgeon should stay inferior to the horizontal midline of the areola both medially and laterally.

25.3.3
Dissection

Once through the skin and into the subareolar fat, the tissues are lifted on each side of the incision, and either scissors, scalpel, or electrocoagulation is used to dissect to the breast tissue. At this time the breast itself can be incised or electrocoagulated straight down to the pectoralis major fascia, or dissection can proceed inferiorly, going superficially around the breast and then superiorly beneath the breast.

A pocket is formed in the submammary position by blunt and, if necessary, sharp dissection to conform to the preoperative markings. A submuscular pocket can be performed by incising the muscular fascia and then splitting the muscle in the direction of the fibers, starting over a rib to prevent pneumothorax. Most of the superior portion of the pocket can be formed by blunt finger dissection. The pectoralis major muscle fibers attached to the 4th, 5th, and 6th ribs and medially along the sternum can be bluntly dissected free if tumescent fluid with 1,000 cc lactated Ringer's solution containing 1 mg epinephrine and 250 mg Lidocaine is first

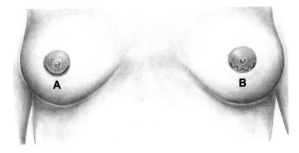

Fig. 25.2 Intraareolar markings. If the areola is of adequate size, the mark can be made 1–2 mm inside the junction of the areola and the skin (*A*). If the areola is small, an undulating line is drawn in the areola (*B*)

injected with a blunt cannula into the muscle. Usually 100–200 cc of fluid on each breast is adequate.

The pocket on each side is checked by finger palpation for adequate size consistent with the preoperative markings. The wounds are irrigated with antibiotic solution consisting of 1,000 cc saline with 1 g Ancef. The areas of dissection are carefully examined by direct vision for any fibrous attachments and oozing or bleeding.

25.3.4
Implants

The preoperatively selected implants are soaked in the Ancef solution and then placed into the pocket. With saline implants, a posterior valve is used with a tube in place that is filled to the desired amount. Holding the wound closed while the patient is place in a sitting position is utilized to check for symmetry and inframammary fold position.

25.3.5
Closure

With the patient in a supine position, the wounds are then closed with two layers of interrupted 2-0 chromic suture in the breast that has been incised and one layer of interrupted 4-0 chromic suture in the subcuticular tissues. The skin is held together with Steri-Strips.

Gentamicin ointment is placed on the wound and a sterile 4 × 4 dressing applied. After the skin is cleansed of blood, the bra is put on, and an Ace bandage is applied firmly over the upper half of the breasts and taped in place. The bra is checked to make sure that the lower band around the chest is at the new inframammary line.

25.4
Postoperative Care

The patient is examined on the 1st postoperative day to check for excessive pain, erythema, or swelling as well as symmetry and inframammary fold position. The bra is readjusted to hold the implants in proper position, and the Ace bandage is reapplied. Compression exercises, pushing the implants superiorly and medially with the contralateral hand, are begun on the 4th postoperative day. This is performed four to five times daily with five compressions each time. While in the office, the patient is shown how much compression to use. The Ace bandage is removed on this visit and the breasts checked again for excessive swelling, symmetry, and inframammary fold position. The patient is seen on the 7th postoperative day, the Steri-Strips are removed, and, if no problems occur, she is seen again at 1 month postoperatively.

25.5
Discussion

The results with the intraareola approach are almost always satisfying to both the patient and the surgeon (Figs. 25.3, 25.4). The scar is usually well hidden in the areola. Occasionally there may be slight loss of pigment around the incision site, usually from using a textured implant that rubs the wound edges when being inserted. However, no patient has desired tattooing to replace the loss when it has been discussed. One patient developed a slight thickening of the scar on one side (Fig. 25.5) but did not want revision.

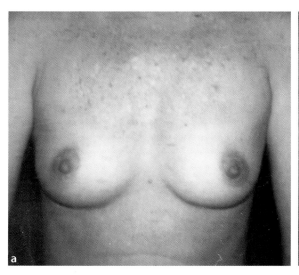
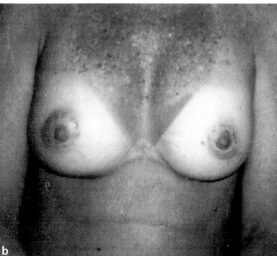

Fig. 25.3 A 5'5," 126-lb patient. **a** Preoperative with small, nicely shaped breasts. **b** Postoperative after 285-cc silicone gel submuscular implants

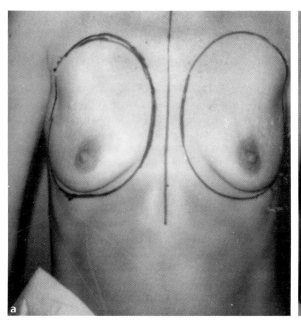
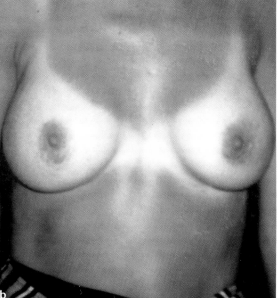

Fig. 25.4 **a** Preoperative patient with very flat breasts and grade 1 ptosis. **b** Postoperative

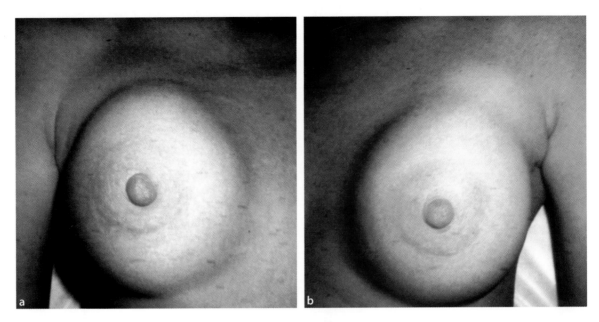

Fig. 25.5 Slightly thickened areolar scars that are still barely visible. **a** Right side. **b** Left side

CHAPTER 26

Breast Augmentation Using the Periareolar Approach

Asuman Sevin, Kutlu Sevin

26.1
Introduction

Four types of incision are commonly employed in breast augmentation: transaxillary, inframammary, periareolar, and transumbilical. After selecting the implant type, the patient and surgeon should decide which incision to use after the options, risks, and benefits of each choice have been explained in detail. The surgeon should offer only the techniques that he or she can apply comfortably. The inframammary incision permits complete exposure of the subpectoral or suprapectoral pocket. However, the technique leaves a visible scar within the inframammary fold. Silicone gel implants often require incisions up to 5.5 cm in length.

The transaxillary incision avoids any scarring on the breast; however, precise implant placement can be more difficult. Transumbilical breast augmentation has the obvious advantage of a single, well-hidden, remote incision. However, it can be used only with saline implants, and precise pocket dissection requires experience. The pocket is dissected bluntly, and hemostasis can be difficult from remote. The periareolar incision is placed at the areolar–cutaneous juncture and generally leaves an invisible scar. The incision allows easy adjustment of the inframammary fold. Disadvantages include transection of the parenchymal ducts, increased risk of nipple sensitivity changes, and visible scarring on the breast mound. This technique should not be used for patients with an areolar diameter less than 30 mm.

The selection of pocket place depends on tissue thickness. In theory, the best position is the subglandular plane to produce a natural shape and form. The reasons for placing implants in the subpectoral plane are to minimize the risk of capsular contracture and to minimize the implant's visibility and palpability. In patients with a pinch test result of more than 2 cm, the implant can safely be placed in the subglandular plane. Subglandular placement may increase the risk of capsular contracture, especially with smooth gel implants. Pockets for these implants must be made larger, and steroid pocket irrigation may also be applied.

Subpectoral augmentation using the periareolar approach was first presented by Gruber and Friedman in 1981 [1]. The operation of periareolar subpectoral augmentation mammaplasty grew out of frustration with the high incidence and unpredictability of capsular contracture, breast scars, and inadequate subpectoral visualization [2].

Submuscular relocation of the implant was also very helpful for those patients who had developed capsular contracture after subcutaneous mastectomy. Therefore, many authors, including Biggs [3] and Mahler and Hauben [4], began to put the implant under the muscle. The scar that had been used for the inframammary approach to a subpectoral implant placement was reasonable but often not as satisfactory as a periareolar scar [5]. The periareolar approach was considered because of its potential for a good scar.

The indications for periareolar approach include virtually every patient who is a candidate for augmentation mammaplasty. One exception would be a patient with an unusually small areola. However, in some cases of small areola, a slight extension lateral to the infraareolar incision can be made so that a larger opening is possible for the implant insertion. Where a mild to moderate degree of ptosis occurs, patients are considered for periareolar subpectoral augmentation. When the ptosis is moderate to severe and the patient refuses mastopexy, she is best treated with suprapectoral rather than subpectoral augmentation because the subpectoral implant can lead to a double-bubble phenomenon.

Other indications for the use of the periareolar subpectoral procedure include complications following suprapectoral augmentation. The most common example is capsular contracture following a subglandular augmentation.

26.2
Technique

The patient is placed on a table that can be tilted to 40–45°; this is needed to be able to evaluate the breasts in a simulated upright position. The patient's arms are left at her sides on arm boards for evaluation of the true position of the breasts. More important, the pectoral muscle is looser and easier to elevate with a retractor during dissection, and it is also easier to insert a larger implant in this position.

The type of anesthesia has almost always been general. The markings are made when the patient is in a seated or standing position. The sternal midline is marked as reference. The existing inframammary fold is marked, and the incision is marked from the 3 o'clock to the 9 o'clock positions in the inferior half of the areola along the junction of the areola and the breast skin. The dissection goes directly vertically toward the pectoral muscle after the parenchyma is adequately released. Bleeding is controlled with an insulated electrocoagulator aided by a headlight. Alternatively, fiber optic retractor illumination can also be used.

For subglandular implant placement, dissection is carried out on top of the pectoralis major and serratus anterior fasciae. The dissection is carried out to the extent of the preoperative markings. If the inferior pole of the breast is constricted, radial scoring of the gland in the inferior pole can allow proper redraping of the soft tissue over the implant. Medial dissection should avoid extensive injury to the medial internal mammary perforators. Lateral dissection should avoid injury to the lateral intercostals nerve bundles. The size of the pocket should be significantly larger than the implant. If the pocket is not of sufficient size, the edges of the implant will be visible through the skin. A pocket that is too large, especially laterally and inferiorly, may result in the implant shifting off the breast meridian postoperatively.

For subpectoral implant placement, the dissection is carried down through the breast tissue in an oblique fashion angled inferiorly until the pectoralis fascia is reached. Then the dissection is continued laterally to identify the lateral border of the muscle. The submuscular dissection is done under direct vision with the use of electrocautery from the lateral to the medial direction. The end point of the dissection is at the sternal border. Attention must be paid to hemostasis at this point because there are bleeders within the muscle. A frequent problem is inadequate splitting of the pectoral muscle to minimize bleeding, resulting in inadequate preparation of the pocket.

After the pectoralis muscle is split to the length desired, blunt dissection is done in the superolateral quadrant where the pectoralis minor is located. Every attempt should be made not to enter the pectoralis minor muscle; doing so would cause a great deal of bleeding and prevent adequate dissection of the pocket in the inferolateral quadrant. After the superolateral aspect of the pocket is developed, dissection is continued toward the inferolateral quadrant using blunt dissection. Then the dissection proceeds medially toward the sternum by transecting muscle fibers that arise from the ribs. When the dissection of the inferior portion of the cavity is complete, 1–2 cm of the superiormost aspect of the rectus fascia is seen. The surgeon may alter the level of the inferior dissection to avoid nipple malposition, whereas the lateral dissection of the cavity is limited by the location of the nerves.

The sternal component of the pectoral muscle can be continuously released toward the midline of the chest. This should be done with care; obviously, it would not be desirable to continue too far because the cavities on both sides may be merged to create a tenting effect. Therefore, dissection should be stopped approximately 1 cm from the midline. Release of the pectoralis proceeds superiorly up to the level of the nipple. Very little dissection is required in the superomedial quadrant. Injury to the medial internal mammary and lateral intercostal vascular and nerve bundles should be avoided. The size of the pocket should be significantly larger than the implant to be inserted.

After both pockets are completed, sizers are used to evaluate the dissection and to determine the final prosthesis to be implanted. Also, the degree of symmetry is checked, meticulous hemostasis is done, and the cavities are irrigated with an antibiotic solution. By applying upward traction, the implants are inserted. If the pocket is tight, further blunt dissection should be performed. The pockets should be roughly symmetrical in size to allow postoperative symmetry. The patient should be placed in the upright position on the operating table with her arms at her sides to make certain of the end result.

Wound closure consists of absorbable suture such as 3-0 and 4-0 polyglycolic acid for the parenchyma. The skin is closed with deep everting dermal sutures and a running subcuticular 5-0 nylon suture. If the pockets have been properly created and the implants are of appropriate size, they should seat properly and symmetrically. The patient is placed in a light gauze dressing and comfortable stretch brassiere upon leaving the operating room. Postoperative medications include oral antibiotics for 5 days.

26.3
Results

The results were evaluated during a study in which 314 patients underwent augmentation mammaplasty with periareolar incision. In 126 patients (40%) the implant placement was subglandular and in 188 (60%) was subpectoral (Table 26.1). The follow-up period ranged from 5 to 10 years (average 7 years). Silicone gel round

Table 26.1 Complications of periareolar augmentation mammaplasty in a study of 314 cases

Complication	Subglandular implant 126 cases (%)	Subpectoral implant 188 cases (%)	Total (%)
Capsular contracture Baker II	9 (7.1)	5 (2.7)	14 (4.5)
Capsular contracture Baker III	4 (3.2)	2 (1.1)	6 (1.9)
Capsular contracture Baker IV	0 (0)	0 (0)	0 (0)
Scar hypertrophy	2 (1.6)	1 (0.5)	3 (1)
Hematoma	0 (0)	2 (1.1)	2 (0.6)
Implant rupture	1 (0.8)	1 (0.5)	2 (0.6)
Infection	0 (0)	0 (0)	0 (0)

textured implants made by McGhan (Inamed, County Wicklow, Ireland) were used in all cases. In general, natural-looking breasts were obtained, and the periareolar scar was inconspicuous. In all cases, the periareolar diameter was longer than 30 mm. For various reasons, such as capsular contracture or implant rupture, the prostheses were renewed once in eight patients (2.5%). In terms of satisfaction, the patients reported that they were extremely satisfied or very satisfied (Fig. 26.1). A total of 13 patients were dissatisfied (4.1%). A total of 37 patients were extremely satisfied (11.8%), and 264 were satisfied (84.1%). Of the 314 cases, four (1.3%) had diminished areolar sensation postoperatively as interpreted by the patient. Hematoma occurred in two patients (0.6%). Three patients required surgical correction of the periareolar scar. No case of implant displacement was seen. No infection was noted.

Twelve patients (3.8%) responded that they had implant folds or edges they could feel but that it was not a major concern for them. Capsular contracture was an indication for six of the revision surgeries for the cases, graded as Baker III (1.9%). Baker II capsular contracture occurred in 14 patients (4.4%). Implant rupture was diagnosed in two cases (0.6%) by magnetic resonance imaging (MRI).

26.4 Discussion

The choice of breast augmentation procedure is determined almost entirely by three variables: the selection of incision location, the pocket plane for implant placement, and the appropriate implant [6]. Implant-related variables include size, shape, shell texture, filler substance, and final implant fill volume in the case of saline implants [7]. Although no clear evidence exists to support the superiority of one combination of

choices over another, cases may be best treated with a specific combination of options. In all cases, we used silicone gel round textured implants. Heden et al. [8] reported satisfactory results with such implants in 823 women. In addition, Bogetti et al. [9] noted that augmentations with silicone gel-filled prostheses were excellent. The authors used textured implants because they have caused less capsular contracture. Asplund et al. [10] found lower rate of firm capsules with textured implants. Studies on saline-filled implants have shown conflicting results. Burkhardt and Demas [11] reported that saline-filled implants caused Baker III capsules in 2% and Baker IV capsules in 40% of their cases. In contrast, Tarpila et al. [12] found no difference in the rate of capsular contracture between saline-filled textured and smooth implants.

The most popular surgical approach for breast augmentation is by the inframammary route. However, a significant drawback of this technique is scarring on the aesthetic unit of the breast [13]. To retain the virginity of the breast, the transaxillary approach has been suggested. But this technique was criticized by Hoehler [14] for its questionable lack of intraoperative visualization and higher rate of complications. The transaxillary approach does not lend itself to extensive and controlled muscle release and therefore does not lend itself to exact placement of the implant of the desired size. Theoretically, there is some concern about the fact that the branches of the nerves to the nipple are more likely to be damaged or injured in a blind technique using the transaxillary approach. The periareolar approach provides a central point of access for creating the implant pocket, which allows easy and accurate dissection in all directions [15]. The implant can be placed subglandularly or submuscularly. Among the advantages of submuscular implantation are less risk of nipple sensitivity loss and less palpability of the implant edges [16]. The decision of subglandular or subpectoral implant place-

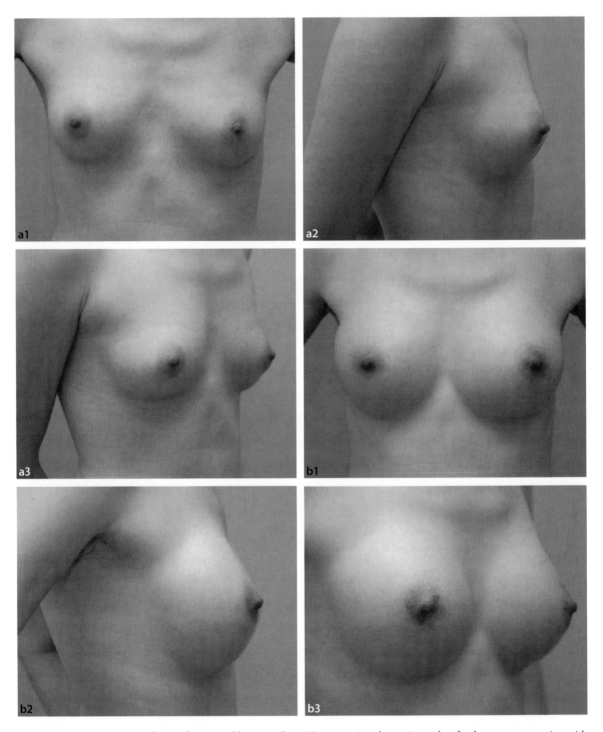

Fig. 26.1 **a** *1–3* Preoperative photos of 22-year-old woman. **b** *1–3* Postoperative photos 6 months after breast augmentation with subpectoral implants using an inferior periareolar incision

ment depends on tissue thickness. For patients with a pinch test result of less than 2 cm, the implant must be placed in the subpectoral plane.

The choice of implant placement has been and will continue to be a topic of debate, but it is generally considered the surgeon's choice. With submuscular placement, some disadvantages may occur. The lower third or half of the implant is not covered by the pectoralis major muscle. Also, submuscular placement of the implant may cause the prosthesis to reside in a more lateral position because of the sternal origins of the muscle.

Complications in augmentation mammaplasty are relatively infrequent but can include hematoma, infection, periareolar paresthesias, asymmetries, implant displacement, capsular contracture, and implant rupture. If a hematoma forms postoperatively, immediate attention must obviously be given to this matter. Capsular contracture has decreased markedly since the introduction of the textured implant. The use of drains has largely been abandoned by most surgeons; it may cause irritation of the implant and ingress of bacteria. In the presented study, no wound infection was observed. The rate of implant rupture was 0.6% (Table 26.1). On the basis of Baker's classification, capsular contracture of grade II was found in 4.5% of the cases [17]. Capsular contracture was found at higher percentages in subglandular breast augmentation cases compared with subpectoral implant cases (Table 26.1).

Periareolar subpectoral augmentation can also be used to improve the difficult problems seen in a thin-skinned patient in whom a suprapectoral augmentation has been performed: When the sternal skin is thin, the implant edges can be seen, and the patient may also complain of wrinkling of the breast. This type of distortion is correctable by any submuscular approach. Although it is a fact that even after adequate release, contraction of the pectoralis will flatten the breast and distort its shape to some degree, the distortion is seen only under unusual circumstances.

The authors believe that the instructions issued by Tebbetts [16] should be strictly followed. For this purpose, bleeding should be checked, the periosteum and perichondrium should not be touched, and the dissection should be performed under direct vision.

26.5
Conclusions

Periareolar subpectoral augmentation has proved to be highly effective, especially in reducing the incidence of capsular contracture. Moreover, the scar in the pe-

riareolar area has been more than satisfactory in most cases. The ability to visualize the nerves to the nipple and avoid them is easiest through the periareolar approach, as is the ability to obtain complete hemostasis. The periareolar incision does not usually limit the size of the implant that can be inserted. Finally, the periareolar approach is ideal for correcting the problems associated with complications following other approaches, including distortion problems or capsular contracture due to a suprapectoral approach.

References

1. Gruber RP, Friedman GD: Periareolar subpectoral augmentation mammaplasty. Plast Reconstr Surg 1981;67(4): 453–557
2. Gruber RP, Friedman GD: Augmentation mammaplasty. In: Georgiade NG (ed). Aesthetic Surgery of the Breast. Philadelphia, WB Saunders 1990, pp 83–100
3. Biggs TM: Augmentation mammaplasty. In: Georgiade NG (ed). Aesthetic Breast Surgery. Baltimore, Williams & Wilkins 1990, pp 65–73
4. Mahler D, Hauben DJ: Retromammary versus retropectoral augmentation: a comparative study. Ann Plast Surg 1982;8(5):370–374
5. Regnault D, Daniel RK: Breast augmetnation. In: Regnault P, Daniel RK (eds). Aesthetic Plastic Surgery. Boston, Little, Brown 1984, pp 559–568
6. Hidalgo DA: Breast augmentation: choosing the optimal incision, implant, and pocket plane. Plast Reconstr Surg 2000;105(6):2202–2216
7. Sevin A, Sevin K, Senen D, Deren O, Adanali G, Erdogan B.: Augmentation mammaplasty: retrospective analysis of 210 cases. Aesthetic Plast Surg 2006;30(6):651–654
8. Heden P, Jernbeck J, Hober M: Breast augmentation with anatomical cohesive gel implants: the world's largest current experience. Clin Plast Surg 2001;28(3):531–552
9. Bogetti P, Boltri M, Balocco P, Spagnoli G: Augmentation mammaplasty with a new cohesive gel prosthesis. Aesth Plast Surg 2000;24(6):440–444
10. Asplund O, Gylbert L, Jurell G, Ward C: Textured or smooth implants for submuscular breast augmentation: a controlled study. Plast Reconstr Surg 1996;97(6):1200–1206
11. Burkhardt BR, Demas CP: The effect of Siltex texturing and povidone-iodine irrigation on capsular contracture around saline inflatable breast implants. Plast Reconstr Surg 1994;93(1):123–128
12. Tarpila E, Ghassemifar R, Fagrell D, Berggren A: Capsular contracture with texturd versus smooth saline-filled implants for breast augmentation: a prospective clinical study. Plast Recontr Surg 1997;99(7):1934–1939

13. Momeni A, Padron NT, FohnM, Bannasch H, Borges J, Ryu SM, Stark GB: Safety, complications, and satisfaction of patients undergoing submuscular breast augmentation via the inframammary and endoscopic transaxillary approach. Aesth Plast Surg 2005;29(6):558–564

14. Hoehler H: Breast augmentation: The axillary approach. Br J Plast Surg 1973;26(4):373–376

15. Biggs TM, Cukier J, Worthing JF: Augmentation mammaplasty: a review of 18 years. Plast Reconstr Surg 1982;69(3):445–452

16. Tebbetts JB: Breast augmentation with full-height anatomic saline implants: the pros and cons. Clin Plast Surg 2001;28(3):567–577

17. Baker JL Jr: The effectiveness of alpha-tocopherol (vitamin E) in reducing the incidence of spherical contracture around breast implants. Plast Reconstr Surg 1981;68(5):696–699

Inframammary Approach to Subglandular Breast Augmentation

Anthony Erian, Amal Dass

27.1
Introduction

Breast augmentation is the most popular cosmetic surgical procedure in both the United States and the United Kingdom today. In 2005 alone, there were approximately 279,000 such procedures performed in the United States [1] and a year-over-year increase of 51% in the number of women having breast augmentation in the UK [2].

Attempts at surgical enhancement of the breasts are not new. From paraffin injections in the early 20th century to liquid silicone injections in the 1950s and 1960s [3], various foreign materials were used in early efforts to augment the breasts. These ranged from petroleum jelly to solid materials such as rubber, polyurethane, Teflon, and various plastic sponges [4], but were all either rejected as a foreign body or failed to produce a favorable aesthetic result. Autologous tissue augmentation was also attempted in the form of dermal fat grafts but failed due to fat resorption [5].

It was the introduction of the silicone gel prosthesis in 1963 by Cronin and Gerow [6] that ushered in the current era of breast augmentation. Through myriad changes and refinements since then in both the implants and surgical techniques, breast augmentation is today performed with minimal morbidity and with an expectation of a reasonable aesthetic result.

The breast is a complex symbol that relates to a woman's femininity, sexuality, and role as a woman and mother. Her attachment to her breasts physically and psychologically is much more than regarding them as a secondary sexual characteristic [7]. Although not every woman with small breasts seeks augmentation, the ones who do are invariably psychologically and socially uncomfortable with them [8]. These concerns seem to be well addressed by breast augmentation. The vast majority of women who have undergone breast augmentations are pleased that they did so, even if the results were less than ideal or were accompanied by complications [9]. The popularity and success of breast augmentation is thought to result from the predictability and success of the procedure.

27.2
Breast Implants and Subglandular Breast Augmentation

The choice of approach and placement of implants has been historically influenced more by implant constraints than aesthetic ideals. Subglandular breast augmentation requires the placement of current-generation silicone implants for the best aesthetic results. These implants are considered by many to have the most natural feel while providing the best aesthetic outcome with a favorable safety profile and complication rate [10].

The hangover from the days of their moratorium, however, will ensure that cosmetic surgeons will still be faced with many questions regarding the use and safety of silicone implants, especially in the United States. Knowledge of the critical issues that have shaped our perspectives on breast implants and their use in breast augmentation is thus vital.

27.2.1
Capsular Contracture

Capsular contracture remains the single most important factor in influencing the techniques of breast augmentation. The very first silicone gel implants were thick silicone-shelled implants that were filled with viscous silicone gel and had a Dacron fixation patch on the base [6]. Unfortunately, they became associated with a very high incidence of capsular contracture, up to 40–60% [11–13].

To address this problem, thin-shelled smooth silicone gel implants without Dacron patches were introduced. Though they may have decreased the capsular contracture rate somewhat, they suffered from a higher incidence of implant rupture and silicone bleed [14], in which particles of silicone extravasate out of the capsule. Silicone bleed has been postulated to increase the incidence of capsular contracture [15].

The next generation of implants was the first to have a double lumen—two layers of high-performance elastomer with a thin fluorosilicone barrier in between to solve the problem of implant rupture and bleeding. There has been some evidence that this feature enhanced shell life and improved capsular contracture rates [15].

The emphasis then changed to submuscular placement of implants after a lower rate of capsular contracture was found in a study that reconstructed the breast submuscularly after subcutaneous mastectomy [12, 16]. This lower rate was validated by numerous other studies [17, 18]. In fact, the incidence of capsular contracture was found to decrease even further after insertion of a saline implant submuscularly [12]. Capsular contracture rates had now decreased from 40–60% to less than 10%, a rate that was considered acceptable.

Saline implants were first introduced in the 1960s, not to reduce capsular contracture rates but to minimize the size of the incisions used in their insertion [15]. Only subsequently were they found to be associated with a lower rate of capsular contracture [12, 17–19]. Although the major problems of deflation [20] and valve failure [21] have been addressed in newer generations of saline implants, they still suffer from significant disadvantages such as wrinkling and folding if left underfilled and a hard spherical appearance if overfilled [10], especially when used in a subglandular pocket. However, they are still popular due to both the low capsular contracture rates and the previous U.S. Food and Drug Administration (FDA) moratorium on silicone implants.

27.2.2
Texturization

Texturing implant surfaces came to the fore in the 1990s. Lower capsular contracture rates with polyurethane-covered silicone implants were attributed not only to delamination of the polyurethane surface but also to its surface texture [12, 16]. These have been since been withdrawn because of concerns over the breakdown products of polyurethane [22].

The importance of texturization to subglandular breast augmentation was not recognized immediately [10]. This was due to several factors. First, the capsular contracture rates for submuscular breast augmentation were already low. Texturing showed significant benefits primarily in the subglandular position, reducing capsular contracture to rates comparable to those with submuscular insertion [6, 23]. Second, the degree of texturing varies between manufacturers [16, 24]. Finally, animal models actually showed an increase in the capsular contracture rate with texturization [25]. However, this has not been upheld in a 10-year prospective randomized clinical trial that showed capsular contracture rates of 11% with textured implants compared with 65% with smooth implants [23].

Thus evolved the current 5th-generation silicone implant—the double-lumen form-stable cohesive gel silicone implant. These are available in smooth or textured surfaces, round or anatomic shapes, and a variety

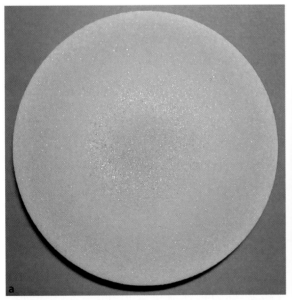
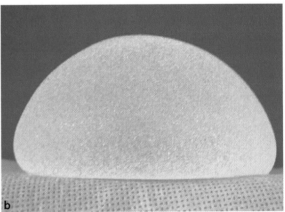

Fig. 27.1 a Fifth-generation double-lumen cohesive gel silicone implants: Eurosilicone (MediCor), very high profile (**b**), round, textured

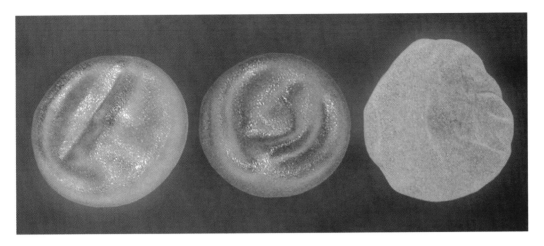

Fig. 27.2 *Left to right*: Silicone gel, Trilucent, and hydrogel implants

of profiles (i.e., implant heights). Subsequent enhancements to this version include a textured surface, shown to reduce the incidence of capsular contracture, and a cohesive silicone gel that has superior consistency and form stability; that is, it does not leak when ruptured (Fig. 27.1) [15].

A host of other implants have been tested and brought to market over the years. Among the more popular were the Surgitek polyurethane-covered silicone implants, the Trilucent soybean-oil-filled implant, and the hydrogel implants, which were filled with an organic polymer (Fig. 27.2). They have all been withdrawn [26, 27] because of viability and safety concerns, leaving silicone or saline implants as the only viable options available to the cosmetic surgeon today.

27.2.3
Safety Issues with Silicone Implants

In November 2006, the FDA lifted a 14-year ban on the use of silicone gel implants outside of clinical studies. This ban was initially enforced in 1992 by the FDA commissioner against the recommendations of the advisory panel, noting that although breast implants were not unsafe, more data were required to establish their safety [28]. This message was interpreted by the media and public to mean that breast implants were not safe. The subsequent media frenzy that followed and several lay jury decisions that found silicone implants to be responsible for common pathological conditions culminated in a class-action lawsuit involving more than 400,000 women, a $4 billion out-of-court settlement, and the withdrawal of major implant makers from the market.

Silicone implants were thus implicated in causing a higher risk of connective tissue disorders and an increased risk of breast cancer. The evidence, however, contradicted or failed to confirm either of these allegations. The Independent Expert Advisory Group set up by the UK Department of Health stated in a report published in 1993 that there was "no evidence of an increased incidence of connective tissue disease associated with silicone gel breast implants" [29].

Similar reviews were conducted in Canada (Canadian Expert Advisory Committee review, 1992), France (ANDEM, 1996), the United States (U.S. National Science Panel, 1997–1998, and Institute of Medicine, 1999), and the European Parliament (STOA report), out of which a clear consensus emerged that no appreciable link existed between silicone gel breast implants and connective tissue diseases. By the late 1990s, more than 20 studies had upheld this conclusion.

The risk of tumors in patients implanted with silicone gel breast implants was also considered by the Independent Review Group (IRG) that was commissioned by the Chief Medical Officer UK. Their 1998 report [30] stated that "analyses of large groups of women both with and without breast implants have shown there is a slightly reduced incidence of breast cancer in women with breast implants. Studies looking at the incidence of other cancers have failed to demonstrate a statistically significant increase among women with breast implants." Moreover, the IRG also concluded that silicone gel breast implants posed no greater risk than any other surgical implant and that they induce a conventional biological response rather than a toxic one.

It must be noted that silicone has been used in medical practice for decades as a coating for hypodermic needles and in various prostheses. It is an inert substance that has become highly purified with technological advances.

It is ironic that perspectives on breast augmentation have been driven not by aesthetic ideals but rather by implant constraints. For years, American surgeons were prevented from using silicone implants for nonreconstructive work. Across the Atlantic, though, cosmetic surgeons have had the option of using either silicone or saline implants even through the 1990s. The popularity of silicone implants, with over 80% of implants used in the UK being silicone based [29], bears out the authors' view that the current generation of silicone gel breast implants provides the best aesthetic result with a low complication rate and an excellent safety profile. With the removal of restrictions on their use in the United States, a marked increase in preference for silicone gel breast implants and for the subglandular approach for their placement is expected.

27.2.4
Subglandular Breast Augmentation via an Inframammary Approach

The authors' current preference is for a subglandular approach using a double-lumen textured round silicone gel implant. Breast augmentation via a subglandular approach is at least in theory an anatomically correct approach: We seek augmentation of the breasts, not the pectoral muscles. The ideal breast has a teardrop shape, a well-defined inframammary fold, good volume, and adequate projection. With subpectoral augmentation, the breast assumes a hemispherical shape, especially when viewed laterally, because of pectoral muscle cover and its compression of the implant [10]. This fullness of the superior pole is also contributed to by contraction of the muscle, which has a tendency to push the implant upward. It has been noted that patients have a preference for the shape of the breast after subglandular augmentation compared with submuscular placement [31]. Many surgeons who prefer subglandular breast augmentation also have difficulty in justifying the division of the inferior medial fibers of the pectoralis major muscle during submuscular placement for an aesthetic procedure [10].

The inframammary fold anchors the breast to the chest wall [24] and is important to the eventual aesthetic result of breast augmentation. Submuscular placement of the implant frequently blunts the inframammary fold. Destruction of the inframammary fold or placement of the implant inferior to it, as has been suggested by a few authors [13, 32], frequently leads to

migration of the implant beneath it, creating a "double-bubble" phenomenon

The inframammary approach also gives better control over the inframammary fold, which may need to be lowered with inferior quadrant hypomastia. It also permits complete visualization of the pocket, enabling an easier dissection. The scar can be fashioned such that it is hidden by the lower pole of the augmented breast. The inframammary approach can also accommodate larger implants, unlike the periareolar or transumbilical approaches. The transaxillary approach is most likely to lead to asymmetric pocket dissection and a double-bubble phenomenon [32]. It is interesting that Tebbetts [33], one of the early proponents of the transaxillary approach, now prefers the inframammary approach.

Implant sizes are frequently 20–50 cc smaller in subglandular augmentations to achieve the same volume and projection as in subpectoral augmentations, due to the added muscle coverage over the implant.

27.2.5
Contraindications to Subglandular Augmentation

There are only a few absolute contraindications to subglandular breast augmentation:
1. Deficient skin cover/breast parenchyma (skin pinch test <2 cm)
2. Irradiated breast

Thin skin/thin tissue cover is seen in hypomastia or post partum. Implant placement subglandularly will lead to visible implant edges and, more than likely, rippling.

Interference with the blood supply in radiated breasts makes subglandular implant placement the safer and more sensible choice.

Ptosis is only a relative contraindication. Subglandular breast augmentation in women with glandular ptosis or grade I ptosis can produce excellent results [32]. In greater degrees of ptosis, the patient may benefit from a concomitant mastopexy. Detection of breast pathology and interference with mammography used to be another argument for placing implants submuscularly The advent of magnetic resonance imaging of the breast as the most specific and sensitive modality in detecting breast cancer, even in subglandularly implanted breasts, has mitigated that argument somewhat [34].

With 5th-generation textured cohesive gel silicone implants, the issues of capsular contracture, implant bleed, rupture, and migration are no longer the problems they once were. With proper patient selection, subglandular augmentation produces an excellent and

Table 27.1 Advantages and disadvantages of subglandular breast augmentation (adapted from Tebbetts [36])

Trade-offs	Potential benefits
Increased risk of edge visibility or palpability	Increased control of breast shape
Increased risk of rippling	Usually a more rapid postoperative recovery
Possible increased incidence of capsular contracture[a]	Minimal or no distortion with pectoralis contraction
Possible increased interference with mammography[b]	Increased control of inframammary fold position and shape

[a]The incidence of capsular contracture has decreased dramatically with the evolution of implant texturization. Capsular contracture rates of textured implants in the subglandular position are comparable to those seen with submuscular placement [23]

[b]Mammograms are more difficult to perform in subglandularly augmented patients, and there is a risk of rupturing the implants due to breast compression to obtain adequate views. There is also a risk that some of the breast tissue may be obscured by the implants. However, the advent of magnetic resonance imaging of the breast has now presented patients with an imaging modality that is much more sensitive and specific, albeit more expensive [34]

predictable aesthetic result with significantly lower morbidity (Fig. 27.3, Table 27.1).

27.3
Patient Evaluation

The patient is ultimately the judge of the success of any cosmetic surgery. Complication-free surgery does not guarantee an acceptable result to the patient. It is no different with breast augmentation.

Up to 40% of claims relating to cosmetic surgery arise from breast operations, with breast augmentations accounting for almost half of these [35]. Patient evaluation is thus a critical step in determining the successful outcome of the operation. Any consultation needs to cover in detail any past medical history, including psychiatric history. Red flags are raised in patients with a psychiatric history, depression, body dysmorphia, or a recent change in psychiatric medication. In these cases, psychiatric evaluation is advised even when the patient appears to exhibit normal orientation and behavior.

The motivation for surgery is always sought. In our experience, the typical patient presenting for breast augmentation is in her 20s to 40s with congenital hypomastia or loss of volume after pregnancy and has been

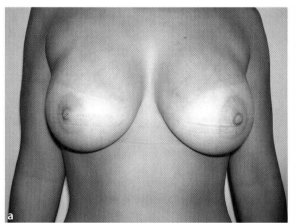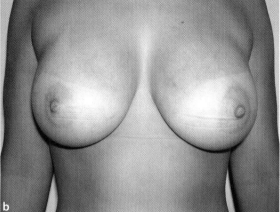

Fig. 27.3 a Preoperative grade I ptosis. **b** Subglandular breast augmentation via an inframammary approach. The breasts look aesthetically pleasing with volume restoration, projection, camouflage of scars, and lack of implant visibility

considering the procedure for some time. It is always important to elicit any history of recent separation, divorce, bereavement, or any other psychological trauma. Patients who elect to have breast augmentation at the behest of their partners or to alleviate their psychological trauma seldom make the best candidates. The patient's expectations are also discussed to make sure they are realistic.

Informed consent implies more than a legally worded, signed document explaining the procedure and risks. The patient must be an adult capable of understanding the facts and coming to a rational decision about the surgery. The patient must be provided with adequate information about the procedure, risks, benefits, and alternatives in order to make a choice to proceed with the surgery. The discussion should always be conducted by the surgeon who will perform the procedure. A second consultation before surgery is preferred. Consent also needs to be obtained for preoperative and postoperative photography, which should be considered part of the mandatory documentation.

27.4
Patient Examination

The evaluation of the breast and chest wall is used to determine the approach and suitability for the procedure. The examination should always start with an evaluation of the patient's chest and thorax. This includes noting if the patient has a short or long thorax and assessing the bony and muscular component of the chest wall and any deformities of the chest wall, such as pectus excavatum or carinatum. Next, the skin envelope is assessed. Factors to note include skin elasticity and laxity. The appearance of stretch marks must be noted.

The pinch test is then performed. This involves gathering both the skin and breast parenchyma in the superior pole of the breast with the thumb and index finger. The distance between the two is measured. A pinch test of less than 2 cm may preclude subglandular augmentation because of implant visibility and palpability through a deficient skin and glandular cover.

Next, the breast is characterized. This includes describing the quantity and quality of breast parenchyma. The shape of the breasts is noted. Tuberous breasts, ptosis, pseudoptosis, and any nipple–areolar complex abnormalities or asymmetries are noted. The correction of these deformities is beyond the scope of this chapter; however, the surgeon can determine whether these will be corrected concomitantly or as separate procedures.

Precise measurements are taken with the patient standing (Fig. 27.4). These include suprasternal notch to nipple, nipple to inframammary line, breast width or diameter, and distance from midline to medial edge

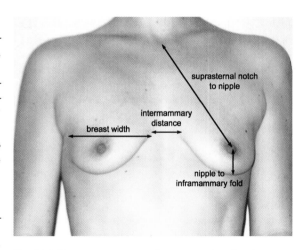

Fig. 27.4 Breast measurements for preoperative planning

of breast. A prospective implant size can then be determined by using the breast diameter, the base width of the projected implant, and the patient's desired cup size. The incision and approach can then be decided upon.

The breast diameter describes the width of the base of the breast. This extends from the medial edge of the breast to the anterior axillary fold and determines the size of the pocket that can be created for the implant. The patient's expectations must be matched to the size of the implant that can be fitted given the existing breast dimensions.

27.5
Operative Technique

The patient is cleaned and draped under general anesthesia in the supine position with her arms placed by her sides. All preoperative markings are rechecked.

27.5.1
Incision

The incision is placed in the projected inframammary crease. The true inframammary crease may need to be lowered in cases of hypomastia of the inferior pole to give the projected crease. This usually corresponds to a distance of 6 cm from the nipple.

A vertical line is drawn from the nipple down to the inframammary crease. One-third of the incision should be placed medial to this point, with the rest extending laterally along the crease. The incision is usually between 4.5 cm and 6 cm in length, depending on the size of the implant. Fashioning the incision in this manner hides the scar in the resulting inframammary crease and avoids the weight of the implant riding on the bulk of the scar. The sternal region and medial chest wall are also avoided because these are the areas most prone to hypertrophic and keloid scarring.

27.5.2
Dissection: Inframammary Approach

The supine patient is cleaned and draped under general anesthesia with her arms at right angles to the thorax. The incision sites are infiltrated with 2–3 ml of 1% lidocaine with 1:1,000 epinephrine to aid hemostasis. This infiltration is extended via a long 22-gauge needle into the subglandular fascial component, where approximately 120 ml of the same solution is infiltrated under the breast tissue directly above the pectoralis muscle on each side.

The incision is made and dissection continued through Scarpa's fascia until the prepectoral fascia is identified (Fig. 27.5). Dissection is then continued using fiber optic light retractors. Meticulous hemostasis is mandatory while creating a precise pocket that conforms to the preoperative markings to accommodate the implant (Fig. 27.6). Medial dissection must be especially cautious due to some medial perforating vessels and thinning breast parenchyma in this area.

Exact sizers are introduced to check the pockets and to evaluate the eventual results (Fig. 27.7). Any asym-

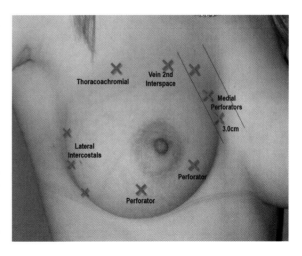

Fig. 27.6 Commonly encountered vessels during subglandular dissection

metry or undissected areas are corrected. The implants and the dissected pockets are then prepared by irrigation with an antibiotic solution (50,000 units of bacitracin, 1 g cefazolin, and 80 mg gentamicin in 500 ml of normal saline).

After further checking of the pockets to ensure hemostasis, the implants are introduced via a no-touch technique and the final result checked. If satisfactory, a

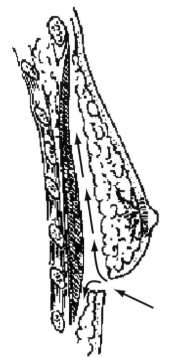

Fig. 27.5 Inframammary approach to subglandular breast augmentation

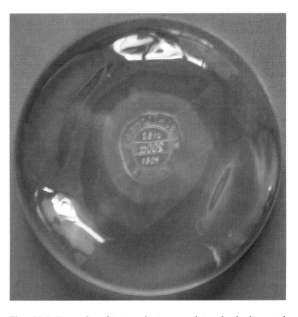

Fig. 27.7 Example of internal sizer used to check dissected pocket and verify final implant size and volume

multilayer closure is performed with absorbable Vicryl sutures. The most important step with this is to close the implant pocket meticulously as one layer before proceeding with the rest. The skin edges are approximated with subcuticular Vicryl to the skin. Once complete, the wound is dressed with Steri-Strips and dressings applied. No drains are used.

The authors' preference is not to strap the chest with figure-8 bandages but to place a well-fitting sports bra instead to provide support postoperatively.

27.6
Postoperative Care

Patients are usually kept for overnight observation after breast augmentation, although many surgeons perform breast augmentation as an outpatient procedure.

The patient is discharged the next day with oral analgesics and a 7-day course of a 1st-generation cephalosporin. Vigorous activity and lifting are not permitted for 3–4 weeks.

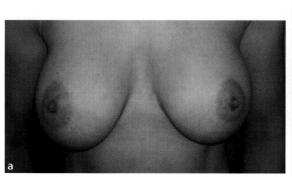
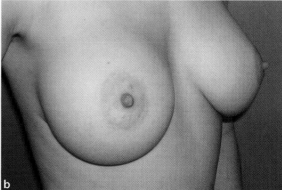

Fig. 27.8 a Subglandular breast augmentation 6 weeks postoperatively. **b** 280-cc medium-profile round cohesive gel Eurosilicone (style ES 802) implants were placed bilaterally in subglandular pockets

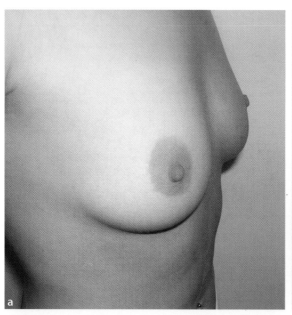
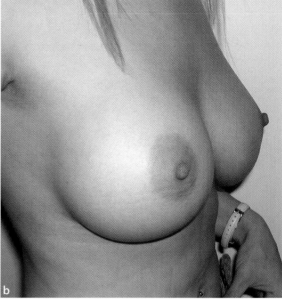

Fig. 27.9 a Preoperative. **b** Six weeks after subglandular breast augmentation via an inframammary approach; 240-cc medium-profile round cohesive gel Eurosilicone (style ES 802) implants were placed bilaterally in subglandular pockets

The patient is seen at 1 week and 6 weeks postoperatively. If free from complications, she is discharged from care with advice to continue with surveillance of the breast for lumps and to have the implants checked every 5 years or so.

27.7
Complications

The complications of breast augmentation are covered in detail in Part IV.

Briefly, the more commonly described complications of subglandular breast augmentation are infection, hematoma, seroma, nipple paresthesia or hypersensitivity, capsular contracture, asymmetry, rippling, implant migration, and herniation.

Implant deflation or rupture, valve failure, rippling, and fold failure are much less commonly seen in the enhanced cohesive silicone gel implants and are problems that have been largely avoided in our practice because of their use.

References

1. American Society of Plastic Surgeons: 2005 quick facts, cosmetic and plastic surgery trends. American Society of Plastic Surgeons, 2006
2. British Association of Aesthetic Plastic Surgeons: Over 22,000 surgical procedures in the UK in 2005. British Association of Aesthetic Plastic Surgeons, 2006
3. Ellenbogen R, Ellenbogen R, Rubin L: Injectable fluid silicone therapy. JAMA 1975;234(3):308–309
4. Gonzales-Ulloa M: Correction of hypotrophy of the breast by means of exogenous material. Plast Reconstr Surg 1965;25:15
5. Conway H, Smith J Jr: Breast plastic surgery: reduction mammaplasty, mastopexy, augmentation mammaplasty and mammary construction; analysis of two hundred forty-five cases. Plast Reconstr Surg 1958;21(1):8–19
6. Cronin T, Gerow F: Augmentation Mammaplasty; a new natural feel prosthesis. Transactions of the Third International Congress of Plastic Surgery. Amsterdam, Excerpta Medica Foundation 1964, p 41

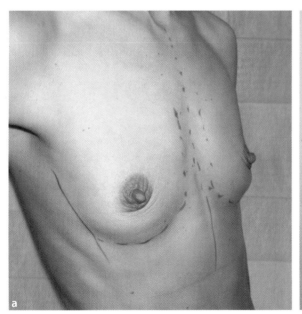
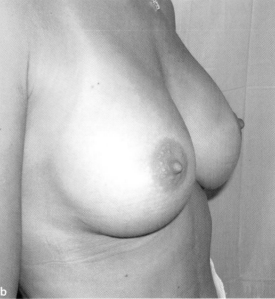

Fig. 27.10 **a** Preoperative. **b** Six weeks after subglandular breast augmentation via an inframammary approach; 260-cc high-profile round cohesive gel Eurosilicone (style ES 81) implants were placed bilaterally in subglandular pockets

7.   Beale S, Lisper H, Palm B: A psychological study of patients seeking augmentation mammaplasty. Br J Psych 1980;136:133

8.   Sarwer DB, LaRossa D, Bartlett SP, Low DW, Bucky LP, Whitaker LA: Body image concerns of breast augmentation patients. Plast Reconstr Surg 2003 Jul;112(1):83–90

9.   Park AJ, Chetty U, Watson AC: Patient satisfaction after insertion of silicone breast implants. Br J Plast Surg 1996;49(8):515–518

10. Hudson DA: Submuscle saline breast augmentation: are we making sense in the new millennium? Aesthet Plast Surg 2002;26(4):287–290

11. Biggs TM, Yarish RS: Augmentation mammaplasty: retropectoral versus retromammary implantation. Clin Plast Surg 1988;15(4):549–555

12. Burkhardt BR: Capsular contracture: hard breasts, soft data. Clin Plast Surg 1988;15(4):521–532

13. Hidalgo DA: Breast augmentation: choosing the optimal incision, implant, and pocket plane. Plast Reconstr Surg 2000;105(6):2202–2216; discussion 2217–2218

14. Feng LJ, Amini SB: Analysis of risk factors associated with rupture of silicone breast implants. Plast Reconstr Surg 1999;104(4):955–963

15. Maxwell PG, Hartley WR: Breast augmentation. In: Mathes SJ (ed). Plastic Surgery, 2nd edn. Philadelphia, Elsevier Saunders 2006, pp 1–33

16. Spear SL, Elmaraghy M, Hess C: Textured-surface saline-filled silicone breast implants for augmentation mammaplasty. Plast Reconstr Surg. 2000;105(4):1542–1552 discussion 1553–1554

17. Burkhardt BR, Dempsey PD, Schnur PL, Tofield JJ: Capsular contracture: a prospective study of the effect of local antibacterial agents. Plast Reconstr Surg 1986;77(6):919–932

18. Puckett CL, Croll GH, Reichel CA, Concannon MJ: A critical look at capsule contracture in subglandular versus subpectoral mammary augmentation. Aesthetic Plast Surg 1987;11(1):23–28

19. Gylbert L, Asplund O, Jurell G: Capsular contracture after breast reconstruction with silicone-gel and saline-filled implants: a 6-year follow-up. Plast Reconstr Surg 1990;85(3):373–377

20. Gutowski KA, Mesna GT, Cunningham BL: Saline-filled breast implants: a Plastic Surgery Educational Foundation multicenter outcomes study. Plast Reconstr Surg 1997;100(4):1019–1027

21. Cederna JP: Valve design as a cause of saline-filled implant deflation. Plast Reconstr Surg 2002;109(6):2166

22. Hester TR Jr, Tebbetts JB, Maxwell GP: The polyurethane-covered mammary prosthesis: facts and fiction (II): a look back and a "peek" ahead. Clin Plast Surg 2001;28(3):579–586

23. Collis N, Coleman D, Foo IT, Sharpe DT: Ten-year review of a prospective randomized controlled trial of textured versus smooth subglandular silicone gel breast implants. Plast Reconstr Surg 2000;106(4):786–791

24. Muntan CD, Sundine M, Rink RD, Acland RD: Inframammary fold: a histologic reappraisal. Plast Reconstr Surg 2000;105(2):549–556 discussion 557

25. Caffee HH: Textured silicone and capsule contracture. Ann Plast Surg 1990;24(3):197–199

26. Gherardini G, Zaccheddu R, Basoccu G: Trilucent breast implants: voluntary removal following the Medical Device Agency recommendation. Report on 115 consecutive patients. Plast Reconstr Surg 2004;113(3):1024–1027

27. MHRA UK: Medical Device Alert DA 2000(07) Breast Implants—PIP Hydrogel, December 2000

28. Kessler DA: The basis of the FDA's decision on breast implants. N Engl J Med 1992;326(25):1713–1715

29. Tinkler JJB, Campbell HJ, Senior JM, Ludgate SM: Evidence for an association between the implantation of silicones and connective tissue disease. MDD Report MDD/92/42. London, UK Department of Health 1993

30. Report of the Independent Review Group Silicone Gel Breast Implants, July 1998:25–26

31. Baker JL: Augmentation mammaplasty: general considerations. In: Spear SL (ed). Breast Principles and Art. Philadelphia, Lippincott Raven 1998

32. Tebbetts JB: Transaxillary subpectoral augmentation mammaplasty: long-term follow-up and refinements. Plast Reconstr Surg 1984;74(5):636–649

33. Tebbetts JB: A surgical perspective from two decades of breast augmentation: toward state of the art in 2001. Clin Plast Surg. 2001;28(3):425–434

34. Ahn CY, DeBruhl ND, Gorcyzca DP, Shaw WW, Bassett LW: Comparative silicone breast implant evaluation using mammography, sonography, and magnetic resonance imaging: experience with 59 implants. Plast Reconstr Surg 1994;94(5):620–627

35. Gorney M: Preventing litigation in breast augmentation. Clin Plast Surg 2001;28(3):607–615

36. Tebbetts JB: Dual plane breast augmentation: optimizing implant-soft-tissue relationships in a wide range of breast types. Plast Reconstr Surg 2001;107(5):1255–1272

CHAPTER 28

Breast Augmentation: Axillary Approach

28

George John Bitar

28.1
Introduction

Breast augmentation has become a very popular procedure with a variety of techniques with which it is performed. The literature describes the evolution of various techniques of breast implant placement in the submuscular versus the subglandular plane; silicone versus saline implants; and transaxillary versus transumbilical, inframammary, or periareolar placement of the incision [1–3]. Within each technique itself is a myriad of nuances and variations among surgeons. As with everything in cosmetic surgery, a surgeon has to choose an operation that works well in his or her hands, makes the patient happy, and has a relatively low complication rate. There is no such thing as the perfect breast augmentation technique; thus, opinions differ, and debates are heated among plastic surgeons as to the best way to perform a breast augmentation. The author believes that the transaxillary breast augmentation with saline implants via a blind dissection technique—i.e., without an endoscope—is a simple procedure with a high level of satisfaction and a low rate of complications. This chapter will focus on this particular procedure and how the surgeon can avoid pitfalls.

28.2
Initial Consultation

An initial consultation is set up to discuss the breast augmentation procedure and to decide whether the prospective patient is a good candidate for the surgery. The medical history is reviewed, a physical exam is performed, and the patient is asked to get medical clearance from her own physician as well as basic labs to ensure that she will undergo the procedure safely. The patient has the opportunity to discuss the procedure with an experienced nurse and the plastic surgeon who will perform the procedure, and she is given the opportunity to talk to patients who have had the same procedure performed by the same surgeon.

It is important for a patient to understand what a breast augmentation will accomplish for her. Limitations, risks, benefits, and postoperative expectations should be discussed in detail. Because a patient will have a long-term prosthesis in her breast, it is even more important to discuss long-term consequences.

In the initial consult, the patient is asked to place known-size silicone breast implants in her bra and wear a shirt that will reveal her silhouette clearly. The patient tries on different sizes of implants until she finds the size she likes. Patients are offered the option to try sizes again on their second consultation. Usually they pick either the same size or a very close size to the one chosen at the initial consultation. Patients are encouraged to choose implants in the range of 150–400 ml, with exceptions in certain situations.

28.2.1
Silicone or Saline Breast Implants

The choice of implant type affects the type of surgery to be performed. It is difficult to perform a silicone breast augmentation through an axillary approach. The incision has to be 5 cm with a silicone implant [4] instead of 2 cm with a saline implant. The technique discussed in this chapter is limited to saline implants inserted through an axillary incision.

Silicone implants are advantageous in certain situations. They feel more natural than saline implants when a woman has had many breast procedures and has very little breast tissue or muscle remaining in the breast. Silicone implants may also be preferable when a woman is very thin, in which case the silicone implants may feel more natural. In these two situations, the patients are offered silicone breast augmentations.

If a woman's breasts are a small B-cup or bigger and the saline implants are submuscular, the feel of the breast is very natural, so the argument that "silicone implants feel more natural" is not a valid reason to have silicone implants.

28.2.2
Saline Versus Silicone Gel Implants

1. Safety: Saline implants are safer. If they rupture, saline is spilled as opposed to silicone, which may

cause local silicone granulomas, egg-shell-like calcification, or hardening of the breast.

2. Scar location: Saline implants are more easily inserted from the transaxillary incision.
3. Scar length: The scar is about 2 cm for saline implants, whereas a silicone implant scar is about 5 cm.
4. Cost: Silicone implants are significantly more expensive in the short and long term than saline implants.
5. Long-term follow-up: There is no need for biannual magnetic resonant imaging (MRI) scans to determine whether there is a silicone rupture, as the U.S. Food and Drug Administration (FDA) recommends with silicone implants. MRI costs $2,000–$3,000.

28.3
Indications for Breast Augmentation

The main indication for a breast augmentation is hypomastia or breast asymmetry. A woman's decision to have a breast augmentation should be explored in the initial consultation. A question as simple and as seemingly obvious as "Why do you want to have a breast augmentation?" can be very telling. Reasons that have been stated have ranged from pleasing someone else, to getting a job promotion, to competing with another woman with larger breasts. The best reason to accept a patient for breast augmentation is so the woman will feel better about herself through a decision that was well thought out and arrived at without external forces. Typically, a woman with this mindset will have the highest likelihood of success and happiness with the operation. Furthermore, she will be in the best position to handle a complication appropriately should there be one.

28.4
Preoperative Work-Up

A patient should get a routine medical clearance and a psychiatric clearance when needed. Medications that can interfere with a good outcome, such as those that increase the likelihood of bleeding, should be stopped before surgery. A pregnancy test should be ordered preoperatively, and a complete blood count and international normalized ratio (INR) give a general idea of the patient's hematological state. A urinalysis is important because a positive test may indicate that treatment is warranted before inserting a prosthesis into a patient with an ongoing infection. A mammogram should be obtained in women at higher risk for breast cancer, based on the recommendations of the American Cancer Society. Patients should also stop smoking for at least 2 weeks prior to the operation and 2 weeks after the operation to improve the surgical outcome.

Two specific circumstances are worth mentioning. If a woman seeking breast augmentation is planning on getting pregnant shortly after the procedure, the prospective patient should understand that pregnancy can create changes in breast shape and size. Also, there is a very small chance that a breast augmentation operation may have complications that can render a woman unable to breastfeed. A future operation, either to change the size of the breast implant, remove it, or perform a mastopexy, may be warranted, and a patient should be well aware of these possibilities. Another situation that is important to address is the history of breast cancer in the woman seeking a breast augmentation or in her family. Whether silicone or saline implants are placed, submuscular or subglandular, the issue of breast cancer detection should be discussed with the patient.

28.5
Augmentation, Mastopexy, or Both?

The decision to have a breast augmentation, mastopexy, or mastopexy-augmentation may not be as straightforward as would seem. Every plastic surgeon handles the situation a little differently. One way to address it is by asking the patient what bothers her about her breasts. If it is clearly the fact that the size is small, then an augmentation is sufficient. If she is not happy with the ptosis but is happy with the size, then a mastopexy is appropriate. If she is happy neither with the ptosis nor the size, then both a mastopexy and augmentation are in order.

Sometimes the lines are not clearly drawn. If a patient has mild ptosis but her main complaint is hypomastia, then it is a judgment call whether to perform a mastopexy with the augmentation or to wait a year and see if the breast will settle nicely, thereby avoiding a mastopexy. If a patient has ptosis and a decent size of breast, then she may be happy with just a mastopexy as opposed to a mastopexy and an implant. These options and the likelihood of requiring a second operation in the future should be discussed thoroughly with the patient.

28.6
Technique

28.6.1
Surgical Marking

The patient is marked while standing (Fig. 28.1). The inframammary folds are marked, the superior border of where the implant should lie is marked, and the midline is marked. A 2-cm line is drawn at the lower aspect of the hair-bearing area of the axilla.

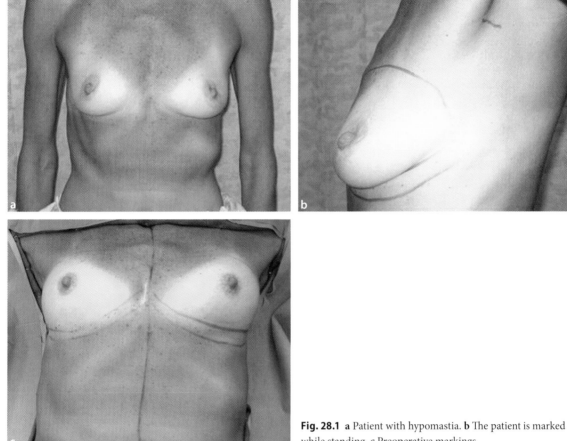

Fig. 28.1 a Patient with hypomastia. **b** The patient is marked while standing. **c** Preoperative markings

28.6.2
Surgical Prep

The patient is initially given prophylactic antibiotics and deep vein thrombosis prophylaxis. She is then intubated with general anesthesia, laryngeal mask anesthesia, or intravenous sedation given as the surgeon's choice. The patient's arms are at right angles to her body and wrapped around the armrest. The breasts are infiltrated in a fashion similar to a liposuction area with about 75–120 ml of tumescent solution on each side for a total of 150–240 ml (500 ml of saline, 50 ml of 1% plain lidocaine, and 1 ampule of epinephrine 1:10,000). The technique with which to inject is important so as to achieve two goals: hydrodissection in the submuscular plane and vasoconstriction of the area to be dissected. A pneumothorax is much less likely if the surgeon lifts the breast with the nondominant hand and injects the tumescent fluid with the dominant hand in a fashion parallel to the rib cage in the submuscular plane (Fig. 28.2). The patient is then prepped in the usual sterile fashion

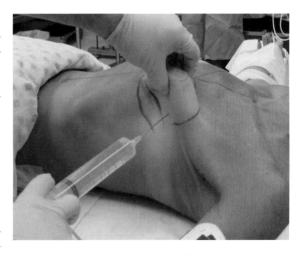

Fig. 28.2 Injection of the tumescent solution in the submuscular plane

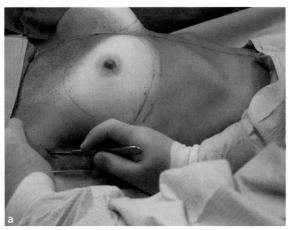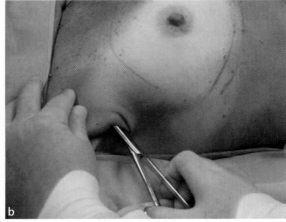

Fig. 28.3 Axillary incision (**a**) followed by dissection with Mayo scissors (**b**)

from the neck to below the umbilicus, including the axilla, while the tumescent fluid is allowed to take effect.

28.6.3
Surgical Technique

After the tumescent solution takes effect, a 2-cm incision is made in the lower pole of the hair-bearing area of the axilla. With a curved Mayo scissors, the pocket is created in the axilla (Fig. 28.3). Next, digital dissection is carried out to establish an intermuscular plane between the pectoralis major and pectoralis minor muscles (Fig. 28.4). Care is given to avoid trauma to vessels and musculature; however, the tumescent solution helps minimize bleeding to the point that electrocautery is seldom used with this technique, since it is almost a bloodless procedure.

When the intermuscular plane has been established, a blunt curved dissector such as a Van Buren or a uterine sound dissector is used to complete the subpectoral pocket (Fig. 28.5). After the submuscular pocket is created, implant sizers are inserted through the axillary incision and are filled to the size on which the patient and surgeon have agreed. The back of the operative table is then elevated so that the patient can be assessed in the sitting position (Fig. 28.6). If the implant pocket needs adjustment, this can be accomplished by either finger dissection or blunt sound dissection until the surgeon is satisfied with the size and shape of the augmented breasts. This is probably the step in which experience helps the most. Medially, the muscle should be elevated enough to create nice cleavage, but not excessively to create symmastia. Inferiorly, insufficient dissection may lead to a "high-riding" implant, and aggressive dissec-

tion may lead to a "double-bubble" sign. Laterally, the breast should have a nice fullness, but if the dissection is too aggressive, then, in the future, the patient will complain that the implant ends up in the axilla when she lies down. Proper dissection of the breast pocket may initially be learned with direct visualization by the endoscopic-guided method, but once a surgeon feels comfortable with the boundaries of the dissection, a blind technique is less costly, more efficient, simpler, and with at least comparable results.

One sizer implant is removed, and the surgeon changes gloves; the axillary incision site is cleaned with Betadine, and the assistant places an Army-Navy retractor to open the pocket for the surgeon. The surgeon empties the air from the saline implant, rolls it, and inserts it through the incision without its touching the skin

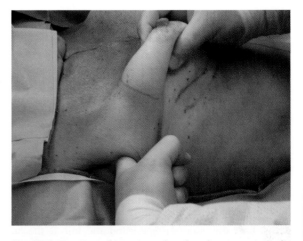

Fig. 28.4 Creation of intermuscular plane between pectoralis major and minor via digital dissection

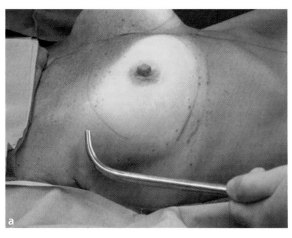
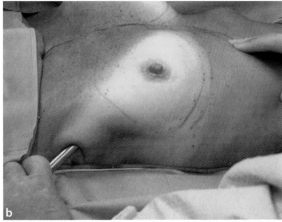

Fig. 28.5 Surgical use of a Van Buren dissector (**a**) to complete the subpectoral pocket (**b**)

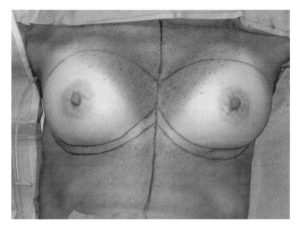

Fig. 28.6 Assessment of the sizers in the sitting position

and with the valve facing anteriorly. When the implant has been completely inserted, it is filled with saline to the desired amount with a one-way stopcock closed system to ensure the sterility of the saline (Fig. 28.7). The sizer in the contralateral breast is kept in place to ensure hemostasis until the time to place the real implant in the contralateral pocket. At that time, the sizer implant is removed, and the saline implant is placed in an identical fashion in the contralateral pocket. Then the implants and general shape of the breast are inspected as the patient is sitting up (Fig. 28.8). When the shape and size are deemed appropriate by the surgeon, the filling tubes are removed. The incisions are then closed with 3-0 Vicryl interrupted sutures for the dermis, and a 4-0 Vicryl subcuticular closure is performed (Fig. 28.9).

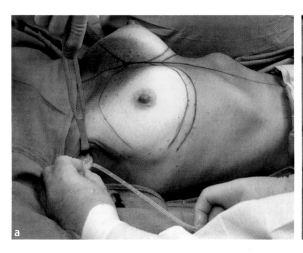
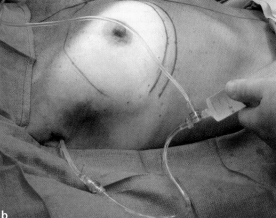

Fig. 28.7 **a** Implant placement. **b** One-way stopcock closed system

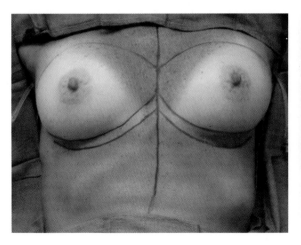

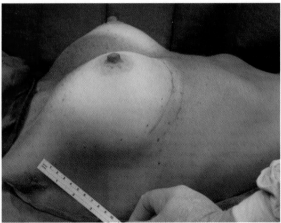

Fig. 28.8 Inspection of the implants with the patient sitting up

Fig. 28.9 Closed 2-cm incision

28.7
Mastopexy and Augmentation Performed Simultaneously:

If a patient wishes to have a mastopexy performed simultaneously with a breast augmentation, there is a simple and practical way to do this procedure. A breast augmentation is performed through an axillary approach, up to the step when the implant sizers are in place. The implant sizers are left in place, and a periareolar or Wise-pattern mastopexy is performed. When the mastopexy is completed, the sizers are removed, and the permanent implants are placed through the axillary incision.

In the author's opinion, the advantages of this technique outweigh traditional insertion of implants through a periareolar or anchor incision. The first advantage is that, with this technique, the pectoralis muscle is left intact, thus decreasing postoperative inflammation and pain as well as preserving intact muscle coverage for the implant in case of an infection of the incision. Second, the option to adjust the implant size based on tension on the nipple–areolar complex exists without difficulty, by inflating or deflating the sizer implants to achieve the desirable volume, before committing to the final implant size. Third, no suturing is done in the vicinity of the implant, so implant exposure and manipulation are minimized, and suturing of the breast incisions can proceed faster without the surgeon having to worry about puncturing the implant. Therefore, precious intraoperative time is saved. The major disadvantage of this approach is an additional axillary scar in addition to the periareolar or anchor incision performed, so the patient has to consent only after a thorough discussion of the available options.

28.8
Postoperative Care

The incisions are covered with Steri-Strips, and foam tape is placed around the breasts to ensure healing in the proper position. The patient is then placed in a bra, and dressings are placed to cover the axillary incisions (Fig. 28.10). The patient is recovered in the ambulatory surgery center or hospital for an hour or two and given antiemetic medicine if needed. She is asked to sleep supine with her head elevated and to take the appropriate antibiotic and analgesic medications.

The patient is seen the following day, and the incisions are inspected as well as the overall appearance of the patient and the breasts. Any early problems are addressed in a timely fashion. Most patients heal uneventfully and have minimal ecchymosis and minimal to moderate edema. The tape is removed after a week, and a breast binder is applied to the breasts to apply pressure and expedite the "settling" of the implants. Daily activity is resumed in a few days, work can be resumed in about a week, and exercise can be resumed after the third week in most cases.

28.9
Results

Patients who have had this procedure in the author's practice have ranged in age from 17 to 66 years old. Some have had simultaneous procedures with their breast augmentations, such as mastopexy, liposuction, abdominoplasty, or facial rejuvenation procedures. The overall satisfaction rate has been very high, with a very low rate of complications.

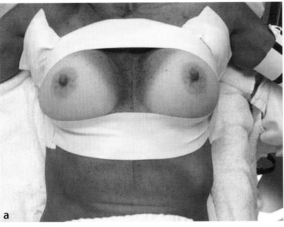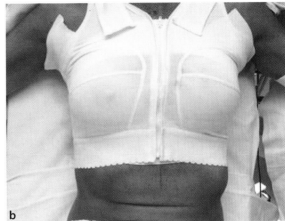

Fig. 28.10 Postoperative placement of the foam tape (**a**) and bra (**b**)

With this technique, pain has been limited to the first few days and controlled with analgesic medications. Return to daily activity has occurred within a week to 10 days. Exercise is usually encouraged after the third week. The complications have been limited to hematomas (less than 1%), capsular contracture (1%), deep vein thrombosis (less than 1%), and implant deflation (less than 1%), and a few patients were dissatisfied for reasons of asymmetry. It is important to note that there were no implant infections, high-riding implants, double-bubble signs, pneumothorax, loss of ability to breastfeed, permanent loss of nipple sensation, major medical complications, or mortality.

28.10
Avoidance of Common Complications

28.10.1
Postoperative Hematoma

A small hematoma may be observed, but if it is significant or is enlarging, then operative drainage is necessary. The rate of hematomas or bleeding after a breast augmentation is reported to be about 2%. In 2006, Handel et al. [5] reported a 1.5–2.89% incidence of hematoma depending on the method of augmentation used. Before surgery, the author's patients are evaluated by their own physicians and blood tests are obtained, including an INR and a complete blood count. The author uses tumescent solution in breast augmentations. The key is to inject the tumescent solution and wait about 7 min to start the operation. This technique plus minimal dissection, gentle handling of the muscle during the pro-

cedure, and creation of an appropriate pocket size for the implant all contribute in keeping the postoperative hematoma rate low, less than 1%.

28.10.2
Infection

Breast implant infections generally occur in about 1–2% of cases. A study from 2005 reported a 2–2.5% incidence [6]. The most important step to avoid infections is to perform the surgery at a first-rate surgical facility where principles of sterility are applied regularly. Patients are given the appropriate intravenous antibiotic coverage throughout the actual surgery. The author changes gloves multiple times during the operation and is the only one who handles the implants in the operating room to ensure total sterility and avoidance of infection. After the procedure, patients are prescribed a 1-week course of antibiotics to minimize infection. There have been no infections with this technique.

28.10.3
Capsular Contracture

Capsular contracture occurs in 10–15% of women with breast implants, depending on which study is quoted. In 2004, the FDA reported a rate of 10–11% at 5 years for augmentation patients [7]. Capsular contractures may be caused by a subclinical infection, by significant bleeding during the operation, or by time and collagen remodeling alone. The rate of capsular contractures in the author's patient population has been less than 1%.

28.10.4
Rippling

Rippling, especially with saline implants, can lead to patient dissatisfaction in up to 10% of breast augmentation patients. Handel et al. [5] reported the rate of rippling to be 5.7–14.15% depending on the technique and type of implant used. Rippling can be avoided or minimized by giving the breast implant maximum coverage with breast tissue and muscle. For that specific reason, rippling is minimized by placing an implant under the pectoralis major muscle and by selecting an implant size that would be covered almost completely by the muscle. As a result, the implant cannot be felt from the lateral edge of the breast. Because of these two guidelines, the rate of rippling among the author's patients is less than 2%.

28.10.5
Deflation or Rupture

It is difficult to quote rates of breast implant rupture or deflation because this is a function of time. The best way to minimize this risk is by paying attention to each step in the patient's preoperative evaluation, the actual surgical procedure, and the follow-up care. If an implant ruptures or deflates, it needs to be exchanged.

28.10.6
High-Riding Implants

The shape and look of the augmented breasts should be very natural. Critics have cited high-riding implants as a result of the technique used by the author [8]. With

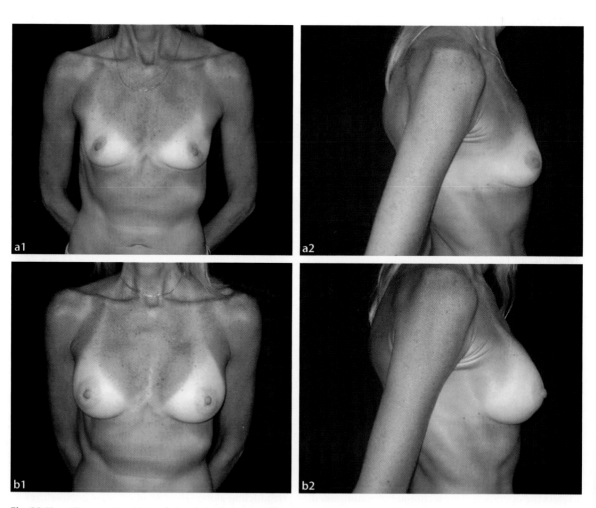

Fig. 28.11 a *1* Preoperative *2* Lateral view. **b** *1* After transaxillary breast augmentation. *2* Lateral view

use of proper surgical technique, good muscle dissection, and a breast binder for pushing the implants down after surgery, this problem has not been clinically significant.

28.11
Discussion

It is critical to address the controversy of performing transaxillary breast augmentations with the "blind approach" instead of the endoscopically-assisted approach. The results of the blind approach are excellent (Figs. 28.11, 28.12). The critics' view that this technique will yield high-riding implants has not been true in the author's breast augmentation patients. The advantages of this technique over the endoscopically-assisted technique is the shorter time in which the operation can be safely performed (the actual surgical time is 25–40 min), which is significantly less than with the endoscopic approach. The second advantage is the lack of reliance on endoscopic equipment, the costs involved, and potential added variables to an operation that is otherwise very simple.

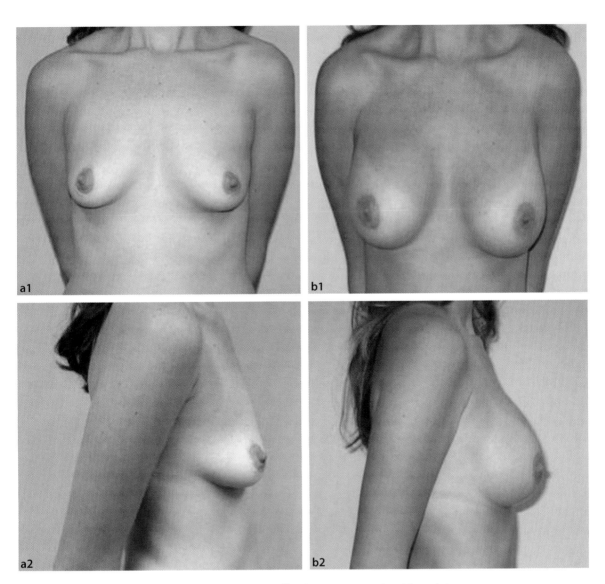

Fig. 28.12 a *1* Preoperative *2* Lateral view. **b** *1* After transaxillary breast augmentation. *2* Lateral view

The axillary incision has certain advantages:

1. The scar is about 2 cm long and heals very inconspicuously, appearing like an axillary crease (Fig. 28.13).
2. The implant can be inserted subpectorally with minimal muscle dissection, so the muscle is minimally manipulated, yielding many advantages: less time needed to perform the surgery, minimal bleeding, less trauma and scarring, less pain, less bruising, and a shorter recovery time with minimal complications.
3. The milk ducts are not manipulated, so the risk of losing the ability to breastfeed after a breast implant with this approach is negligible.
4. The breast tissue is not dissected, so there is no additional scarring that may affect mammogram readings.
5. The scar is relatively distant from the implant, so if there is a superficial scar infection, the implant is well protected.
6. There is a lower probability of injuring the 4th intercostal nerve that supplies sensation to the nipple, thus there is an extremely high probability of normal nipple sensation after the breast augmentation.

Some of the disadvantages include the following:

1. The scar, although small, can be evident in the axilla the first few months before it heals completely and fades, but it will never completely disappear.
2. If a revision is needed in the future, the difficulty in removing an implant from an axillary incision means that another approach may be used at that time.
3. There is a possibility of loss of sensation in a small area of the axilla if the costobrachial nerve is injured.

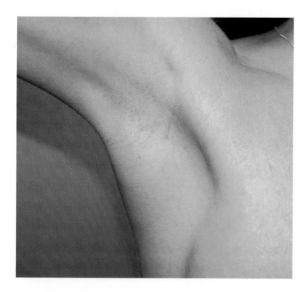

Fig. 28.13 The axillary scar is virtually imperceptible

28.12
Conclusions

The "blind" technique of transaxillary breast augmentation is a safe, effective, and simple way to perform this popular procedure. As with any procedure, a learning curve is always expected, but this is truly an elegant, simple, and highly effective procedure with a minimal rate of complications.

References

1. Momeni A, Padron NT, Fohn M, Bannasch H, Borges J, Ryu SM, Stark GB: Safety, complications, and satisfaction of patients undergoing submuscular breast augmentation via the inframammary and endoscopic transaxillary approach. Aesthetic Plast Surg 2005;29(6):558–564
2. Dowden R: Keeping the transumbilical breast augmentation safe. Plast Reconstr Surg. 2001;108(5):1389–1400, discussion1401–1408
3. Hendricks H: Complete submuscular breast augmentation: 650 cases managed using an alternative surgical technique. Aesthetic Plast Surg 2007;31(2):147–153
4. Serra-Renom J, Garrido MF, Yoon T: Augmentation mammaplasty with anatomic soft, cohesive silicone implant using the transaxillary approach at subfascial level with endoscopic assistance. Plast Reconstr Surg 2005;116(2):640–645
5. Handel N, Cordray T, Gutierrez J, Jensen JA: A long-term study of outcomes, complications, and patient satisfaction with breast implants. Plast Reconstr Surg 2006;117(3):757–67, discussion 768–772
6. Pittet B, Montandon D, Pittet D: Infection in breast implants. Lancet Infect Dis 2005;5(2):94–106
7. U.S. Food and Drug Administration. Breast Implant Consumer Handbook 2004, accessed 30 May 2007. http://www.fda.gov/cdrh/breastimplants/handbook2004/localcomplications.html
8. Troilius C: A ten-year evaluation following corrections of implant ptosis subsequent to transaxillary subpectoral breast augmentation. Plast Reconstr Surg 2004;114(6):1638–1641, discussion 1642–1643

CHAPTER 29

Hydrodissection Axillary Breast Augmentation   **29**

Sid J. Mirrafati, Melvin A. Shiffman

29.1
Introduction

Breast augmentation is a procedure that has been done for many years, but the technique has not advanced. There are four routes by which augmentation can be done: inframammary, periareolar, umbilical, or axillary. The inframammary is the original route that was used when surgeons first began doing breast augmentation . Although it is the most direct route for placing the implant, the scar can be undesirable. The most common approach is the periareolar. Most surgeons and patients choose this route for the ease of implant placement, and the scar is fairly unnoticeable. The periareolar route, however, causes too much damage to the breast tissue and may cause capsular contraction. The umbilical route is too far away from the breast, and there is no manual feeling of the pocket.

The axillary approach is the least damaging to the breast tissue. There is a learning curve to this approach, but once the technique is mastered, it is the fastest to perform and involves the shortest recovery period. The scar can be virtually undetectable. Hydrodissection axillary augmentation is the best way to do a breast augmentation. Tumescent fluid is injected into the pocket under high pressure, which will dissect the pocket, causing less damage to the breast. In turn, this will allow faster recovery with fewer complications. Cautery (Bovie) is not used because it can distribute heat damage to the surrounding breast tissues. The only time a scalpel blade is used is in making the axillary fold incision. The rest of the surgery is done by finger and blunt instrument dissection.

29.2
Preoperative

The patient is prepared starting 3–4 weeks before surgery. The chest size is measured by drawing a line in the middle of the sternum, and at 1.5 cm lateral to this line, the distance to the anterior axillary line is measured. This will determine the diameter of the implant for the largest implant size that the patient can choose; of course, the patient can choose a smaller implant size. All the possible risks and complications of breast augmentation are discussed with the patient. Statistically, there is a 3–5% chance of capsular contraction. All patients are started on vitamin K and vitamin C (2,000–3,000 mg/day) for 7 days before surgery along with Keflex the day before surgery and continuing for 9 days after surgery. The patient is told to shave her armpit on the morning of surgery and to wash her breast and armpit area with a surgical scrub that is given to her.

29.3
Surgical Technique

Marking is done at the anterior axillary line and the midline margin of the breast. The author prefers to lower the inframammary fold line to avoid having the implant placed too high. The axillary fold is marked and extended to 1 in. The patient is placed in a supine position, and after she is placed under general anesthesia, intermittent leg compression garments are applied. The patient's breast and axilla are prepped with Betadine gel. The patient's arms should be at a 65° angle from her body. The axillary marking in the axilla is infiltrated with lidocaine with 1:200,000 epinephrine; 2 ml is injected into each axillary marking.

The incision is then made using a Senn retractor, and the skin is retracted over the pectoralis major muscle. Using Metzenbaum scissors, the incision is expanded down to the pectoralis fascia (Fig. 29.1). When the white glistening of the fascia is seen, the surgeon uses his or her index finger to feel the edge of the pectoralis. If the placement will be subpectoral, then the surgeon rolls the finger under the muscle, pushes through, and provides an opening (Fig. 29.2). If the placement will be subglandular, then the finger stays on top of the muscle and then pushes through the tissue to provide an opening.

The tumescent infiltrating cannula is placed into the opening and pushed through to the inframammary fold and to the lower edge of the marking (Fig. 29.3). The tumescent fluid, consisting of 1 l of saline, 2 ml of 1:1,000 epinephrine, and 500 mg of lidocaine, is infiltrated under high pressure inferiorly, medially, and laterally. About 300–400 ml of tumescent is injected, and the pocket is expanded (Fig. 29.4). The same is done

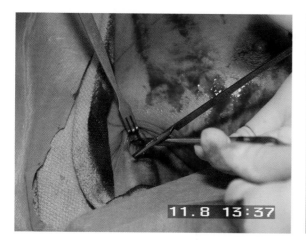

Fig. 29.1 Metzenbaum scissors are used to expand the incision down to the pectoralis fascia

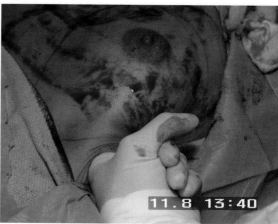

Fig. 29.2 The finger is rolled under the muscle and pushed through to provide an opening

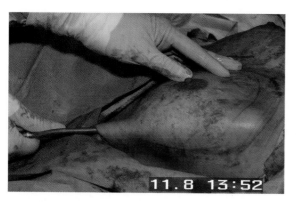

Fig. 29.3 The tumescent infiltrating cannula is placed into the opening and pushed through to the inframammary fold and to the lower edge of the marking

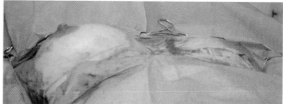

Fig. 29.4 The pocket is expanded with tumescent fluid

to the opposite breast to allow the tumescent fluid to stay in the pocket for at least 10 min. By now, the pocket is literally made by hydrodissection, and the pocket is further expanded by using the iconoclast, paddle, and hockey stick (Fig. 29.5). Antibiotic irrigation is done, and the expander implant is placed in the pocket to check for any retraction and proper pocket formation (Fig. 29.6). Compression can also be applied from outside by the assistant as the surgeon prepares the other breast pocket; this will provide further homeostasis.

The expanders are removed, and the implants are placed in the pockets (Fig. 29.7). The incisions are closed using a 5-0 nylon running mattress suture (Fig. 29.8). A compression dressing is applied (Fig. 29.9).

29.4
Postoperative Care

The patient is seen on the first postoperative day. The compression dressing is removed, and a Band-Aid is applied to the incision. The patient is told to wash the armpit three times a day with alcohol and apply antibiotic ointment. She is shown a set of arm exercises to do, such as rotation of the arm forward and backward. She is also advised to walk as often as possible.

The sutures in the axilla are removed in 6–7 days. At the same time, the patient is told to massage the breast and rotate over the implant in a circular motion for 5 min a day. At first the implant appears to be sitting too

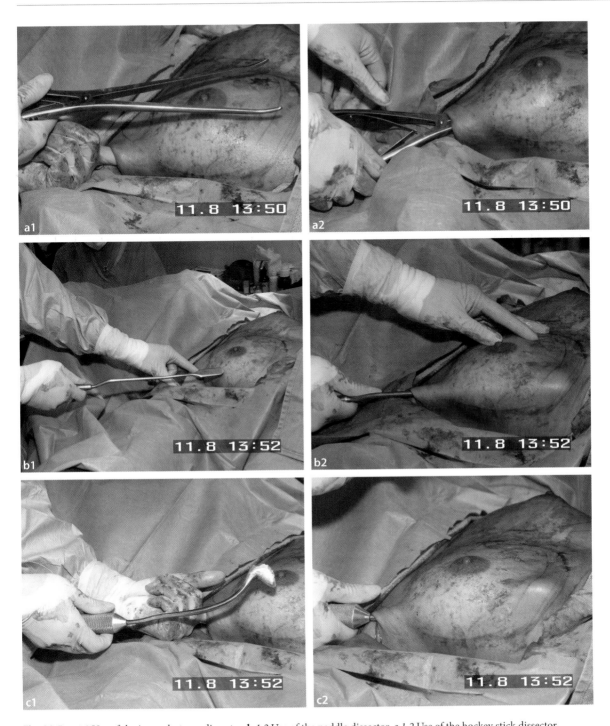

Fig. 29.5 a *1,2* Use of the iconoclast as a dissector. **b** *1,2* Use of the paddle dissector. **c** *1,2* Use of the hockey stick dissector

high, but as the weeks go by, the implant will start to settle and get softer. The patient can start taking showers on the 2nd postoperative day and go back to work on the 3rd postoperative day as long as the work is not too physically strenuous. She can resume normal exercise in 6 weeks.

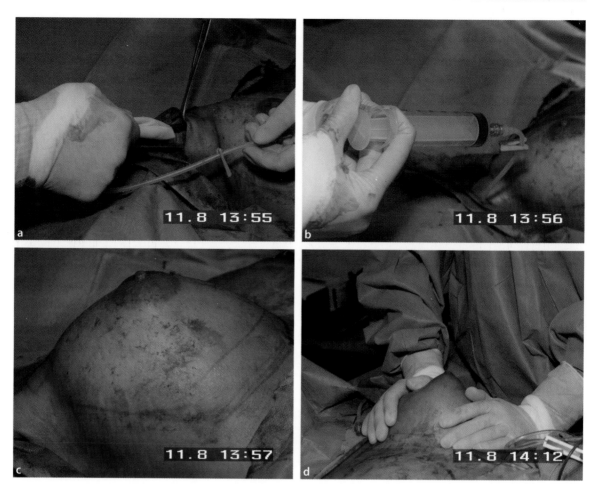

Fig. 29.6 a The expander implant is placed in the pocket. **b** The expander is filled with saline. **c** Expander fully expanded. **d** Compression is applied for hemostasis

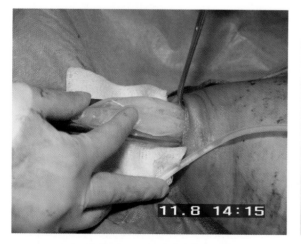

Fig. 29.7 Implant is folded and inserted into pocket

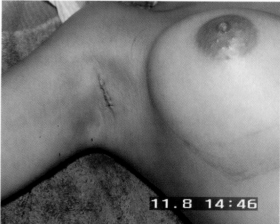

Fig. 29.8 Axillary incision closed with running mattress suture of 5-0 nylon

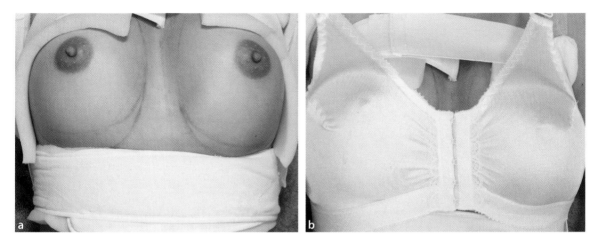

Fig. 29.9 **a** Initial dressings with foam and breast strap.**b** Bra applied

29.5
Complications

This technique of breast augmentation involves a learning curve, but once the technique is mastered, there are very few complications, and recovery is rapid. The patient has less tenderness compared with other augmentation techniques.

We have seen one case of postoperative bleeding; the patient had to be taken back to surgery the 1st postoperative day, at which time the pocket was irrigated, the hematoma was removed, and the incision was closed. There have been no cases of capsular contraction.

29.6
Conclusions

Hydrodissection for axillary breast augmentation is an excellent way to enlarge a patient's breasts (Fig. 29.10). There are fewer complications, recovery is rapid, and the surgery can be performed in less than 40 min.

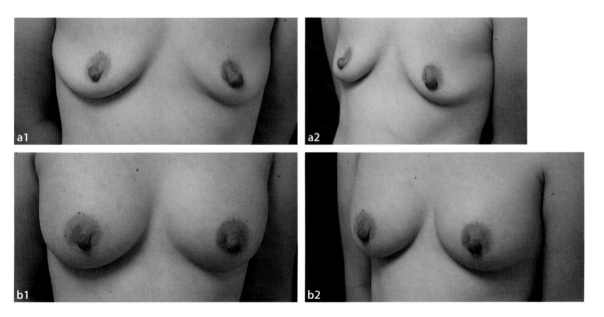

Fig. 29.10 **a** *1,2* Preoperative hypotrophic breasts. **b** *1,2* Postoperative hydrodissection augmentation

Chapter 30

Nipple or Areolar Reduction with Simultaneous Breast Augmentation

30

Richard A. Baxter

30.1
Introduction

Patients seeking breast augmentation may present with large or elongated nipples. Although the incidence has not been determined, and aesthetic ideals for nipples are subjective, requests for nipple reduction are not uncommon in my practice. The pendulous nipple may be more prevalent in women who have breastfed, and it seems to occur with higher frequency in Asians [1]. Asymmetry of areolar diameter is another frequent occurrence [2]. In either case, correction can often be accomplished with the resultant scar very well concealed at the base of the nipple. The elasticity of the areolar skin allows for adequate access for placing a saline implant via the same incision. With proper instrumentation, either a submuscular or subglandular implant pocket can be dissected under direct vision. The technique has proven to be practical and is not associated with sensory changes to the nipple [3].

Scar visibility and location are of increasing concern to patients considering augmentation. The nipple base incision has been previously reported to result in a highly satisfactory and inconspicuous scar [4, 5]. By combining the augmentation with a nipple or areolar reduction when indicated, patients are spared an unnecessary additional scar. Unlike approaches from incisions away from the breast, reoperation for adjustment or implant replacement is not difficult.

30.2
Surgical Technique

The method for nipple reduction involves removing a ring of skin from the base of the nipple, while areolar reduction is accomplished by excising a donut-shaped area whose inner diameter abuts the nipple base. The nipple reduction technique is adapted from Regnault [6], who reported a method involving excision of a band of skin toward the nipple tip. By moving the excision to the base instead, scar camouflage is improved,

and access for augmentation is gained. For central areolar reduction, a purse-string closure secures the scar at the junction to the nipple base.

Implant size is selected preoperatively in consultation with the patient and according to dimensional measurements, most importantly the base diameter. Smooth round saline implants with an anterior valve work best with this approach. Markings for implant position are made in the upright position. Nipple reduction is determined intraoperatively, so preoperative markings on the nipple are unnecessary. For areolar reduction, markings are made with the patient either upright or supine.

The nipple base and areolar tissues are infiltrated with lidocaine 1% and 1:100,000 epinephrine. A 4-0 nylon traction suture is double-looped through the nipple, and a circumferential incision is made at the base. For nipple reduction, a second incision circumscribes the nipple at a level corresponding to the degree of desired reduction, usually about 5 mm or 6 mm above the base. A full-thickness excision is then done (Fig. 30.1).

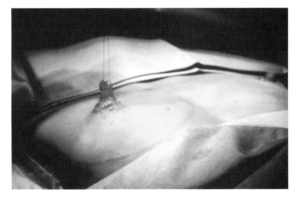

Fig. 30.1 A 4-0 nylon traction suture is double-looped through the nipple, and a circumferential incision is made at the base. For nipple reduction, a second incision circumscribes the nipple at a level corresponding to the degree of desired reduction, usually about 5 mm or 6 mm above the base. A full-thickness excision is then done

For areolar reduction, the donut ring of skin is removed. If this is a unilateral reduction, the distance between the outer edge of skin removal and the areolar margin should equal the distance from the nipple base to the areolar boundary on the opposite side (Fig. 30.2). In either case, after skin removal the areolar skin is undermined with a #15 blade scalpel and/or iris scissors in the superficial plane to the outer margin but not beyond. Skin hooks are used (Fig. 30.3) along with needle-tip monopolar cautery as needed.

At this point a lighted right-angle retractor with a 1-cm-wide, 6-cm-long toothed blade (custom-made by Electro Surgical Instrument, Rochester, NY, USA) can be introduced. The nipple "tucks" into a pocket under the skin in the superior portion of the wound, while dissection proceeds into the deeper subcutaneous plane toward the inframammary fold. A lighted Aufrecht retractor may also be used, but the angle is not optimal. As the exposure improves, a second retractor is inserted. Once the chest wall is encountered, the implant pocket can be made in the subpectoral, subfascial, or subglandular plane as desired.

After pocket irrigation, the implant is rolled tightly around the fill tube and inserted. A closed fill system is used. After the appropriate positioning and orientation of the implant are confirmed, the skin edges are approximated with a 4-0 or 5-0 PDS suture in a purse-string fashion, modified to incorporate bites of the nipple base tissue alternating with the outer skin edge. Further refinement of the closure can be done with interrupted 6-0 fast-absorbing gut suture, but this is not typically necessary. Operating time is typically about 60 min total.

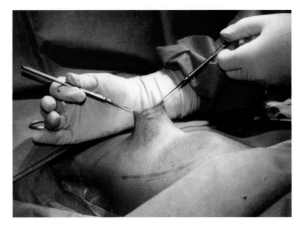

Fig. 30.3 Skin hooks are used along with needle-tip monopolar cautery as needed

For dressings, the nipple is usually loosely wrapped with Xeroform or petrolatum-impregnated gauze, and then cotton gauze pads with a hole cut out for the nipple (to avoid excess pressure) are applied. Dressings are removed at 3–5 days, and antibiotic ointment is recommended.

30.3 Results

Simultaneous breast augmentation via the nipple or areolar reduction approach has yielded consistent results with a high degree of patient satisfaction. I have used smooth round saline implants exclusively with this technique, ranging in size from 240 cc to 475 cc, with fill volumes typically 5–10% above nominal implant size.

Figure 30.4 shows a representative case. This patient presented with postpartum involution and ptotic nipples following pregnancy, requesting augmentation with saline implants. The nipple-base excision technique was employed. Figure 30.5 shows close-up views of a different patient, with 1-year follow-up, confirming that results are stable over time.

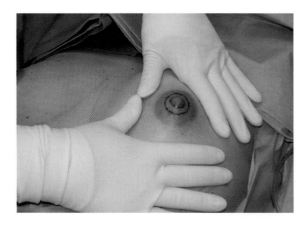

Fig. 30.2 For areolar reduction, the donut ring of skin is removed. If this is a unilateral reduction, the distance between the outer edge of skin removal and the areolar margin should equal the distance from the nipple base to the areolar boundary on the opposite side

30.4 Complications

One patient in my series developed a capsular contracture approximately 6 months postoperatively. While this is theoretically attributable to bacterial contamination resulting from dissection in the vicinity of milk ducts close to the nipple, this process remains speculative. The

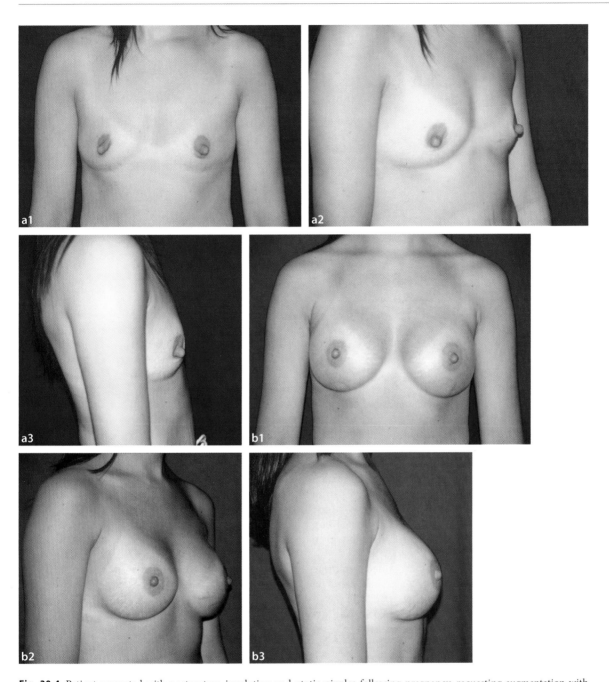

Fig. 30.4 Patient presented with postpartum involution and ptotic nipples following pregnancy, requesting augmentation with saline implants. **a** *1–3* Preoperative photos. **b** *1–3* Postoperative photos after nipple-base excision technique was employed

author's usual incision is periareolar, and overall contracture rates are in the range of 1–2%. This patient was reoperated on for an open capsulotomy, utilizing the same nipple-base approach with satisfactory outcome.

I have seen two unfavorable scars since I first reported this technique. These were successfully revised under local anesthesia. No patient has experienced sensory nipple changes.

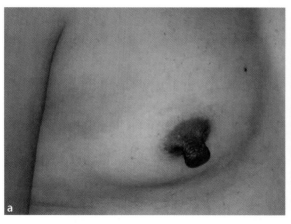 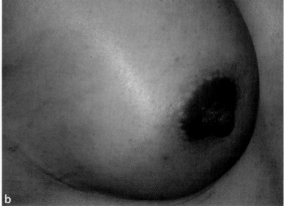

Fig. 30.5 a Preoperative. **b** One year postoperatively, confirming that results are stable over time

30.5
Discussion

The contribution of the nipple–areolar complex to overall breast aesthetics may be receiving increasing attention from breast augmentation patients. They have ready access to a massive Internet database, allowing for greater scrutiny and comparison. There may be practical considerations as well, with the potential for chafing from pedunculated or overly large nipples. However, nipple reduction remains a relatively uncommon procedure for a variety of reasons, including patient ignorance of their options and hesitancy on the part of plastic surgeons to recommend it. The latter may be due to concerns about possible sensory loss with incision and dissection on the nipple, though this has not been manifest.

Although the access is somewhat limited, a satisfactory implant pocket can be dissected under direct vision in whatever plane is desired, with appropriate instrumentation. I have not found the need to consider endoscopic assistance. If exposure is ever felt to be inadequate, there is the option of extending the incision radially within the areola, although I have not had to do this. However, that would be preferable to placing excessive stretch trauma on the wound edges.

30.6
Conclusions

For patients requesting nipple reduction and breast augmentation with saline-filled implants, this tech-

nique provides a useful option. Areolar reduction of up to 1 cm overall diameter can be readily accomplished as well. Because a certain percentage of breast implant patients will require reoperation, consideration of future surgery and scars is worthwhile. Although this procedure allows comparatively less access than some others, reentry is not difficult should that become necessary. Potential risks, especially sensory changes, have not been an issue.

References

1. Cheng MH, Smartt JM, Rodriguez ED, Ulusal BG: Nipple reduction using the modified top hat flap. Plast Reconstr Surg 2006;118(7):1517–1525
2. Rohrich RJ, Hartley W, Brown S: Incidence of breast and chest wall asymmetry in breast augmentation: a retrospective analysis of 100 patients. Plast Reconstr Surg 2003;111(4):1513–1519
3. Baxter RA: Nipple or areola reduction with simultaneous breast augmentation. Plast Reconstr Surg 2003;112(7):1918–1921
4. Becker H: The intra-areolar incision for breast augmentation. Ann Plast Surg 1999;42(1):103–106
5. Lai YL, Weng CJ, Chen YR, Noordhoff MS: Circumnipple-incision, longitudinal-breast dissection augmentation mammaplasty. Aesth Plast Surg 2001;25(3):194–197
6. Regnault P: Nipple hypertrophy. A physiologic reduction by circumcision. Clin Plast Surg 1975;2(3):391–396

CHAPTER 31

Classification of Breast Ptosis

31

Melvin A. Shiffman

31.1
Introduction

Ptosis classification is a means for following patients, informing consultants, and informing future surgeons. Multiple classifications are in use, and it is important for the physician to distinguish which classification is being used.

The determination of whether to augment a breast, perform mastopexy, or do a combination of both involves the physician discussing the pros and cons of each procedure with the patient and the patient deciding what is to be done.

31.2
Lalardrie–Jouglard Classification

According to the Lalardrie–Jouglard classification [1] (1973), ptosis occurs as the thoracomammary angle decreases and falls below 90° and is accompanied by a change in the form of segment II (Fig. 31.1), which is normally convex but becomes straight and then concave.

31.2.1
Glandular Ptosis

Glandular ptosis is due to a decrease in the volume of the normal or hypertrophic breast. There is a decrease in anterior projection, with the nipple–areola complex falling back toward the thoracic plane (Fig. 31.2).

31.2.2
Skin Ptosis

Involvement of the skin envelope predominates and is evidenced by elongation of segments II and III. This is due to physiologic aging of the skin envelope. The skin overdevelopment relative to glandular size results

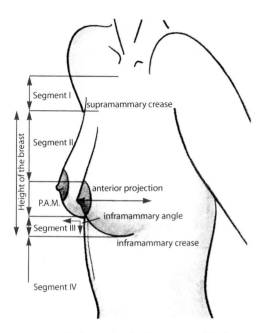

Fig. 31.1 Lalardrie and Juglard: segments of the breast

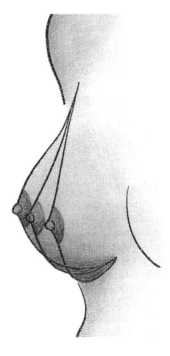

Fig. 31.2 Lalardrie and Juglard glandular ptosis. Segments II are not elongated, and the nipple has fallen back

in segment II being relatively much longer than segment III, with the areola directed downward and situated in a dependent position at the lower pole of the breast (Fig. 31.3).

31.3
Regnault Classification of Breast Ptosis

The standard classification for breast ptosis has been that of Regnault [2] (1976; Fig. 31.4):

- First degree (minor ptosis): The nipple lies at the level of the submammary fold, above the lower contour of the gland and skin brassiere.
- Second degree (moderate ptosis): The nipple lies below the level of the fold but remains above the lower contour of the breast and skin brassiere.
- Third degree (major ptosis): The nipple lies below the fold level and at the lower contour of the breast and skin brassiere.
- Pseudoptosis: The nipple lies above the submammary fold level. The breast is not ptotic.

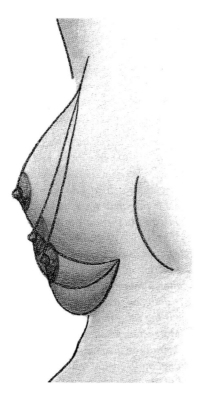

Fig. 31.3 Lalardrie and Juglard cutaneous ptosis. Segments II and III are elongated, and the nipple has descended more than it has fallen back

Partial ptosis: The gland and skin brassiere follow the influence of gravity, while the nipple remains above the level of the fold because the upper portion of the skin brassiere has not changed whereas the lower one has elongated.

31.4
Lewis Classification

The Lewis classification [3] (1983) concerns surgical classification of mammary ptosis:

1. Mildly ptotic breasts of adequate size, without hypertrophy or atrophy
2. Mildly ptotic breast with atrophy
3. Mild to moderate ptosis with mild to moderate hypertrophy
4. Markedly ptotic breast with marked hypertrophy
5. Moderate or markedly ptotic breasts with adequate total breast bulk
6. Moderately or markedly ptotic breasts with inadequate breast bulk
7. Mildly or moderately ptotic breasts with chronic cystic mastopathy
8. Breasts with marked ptosis or marked hypertrophy with cystic mastopathy
9. Asymmetry of the breasts (of significant degree)

31.5
Brink Classification

The Brink classification [4] (1990) is as follows:

- True ptosis: The nipple–areola complex's relation to the fold when the gland, skin, and nipple descend
- First-degree (minor) ptosis: Nipple–areola complex at the fold and above the breast contour (gland behind the nipple–areola complex)
- Second-degree (moderate) ptosis: Nipple–areola complex below the fold but above the breast contour (gland behind the nipple–areola complex)
- Third-degree (major) ptosis: Nipple–areola complex below the fold and below the breast contour (gland above the nipple–areola complex)

31.6
Brink Procedural Specifics
for Forms of Breast Ptosis

Brink's 1993 classification [5] attempted to distinguish between true ptosis, glandular ptosis, parenchymal maldistribution, and pseudoptosis (see Table 31.1).

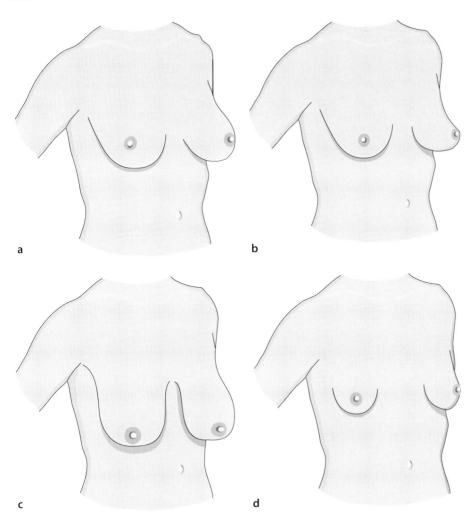

Fig. 31.4 a Regnault first-degree (minor ptosis). **b** Regnault second-degree (moderate ptosis). **c** Regnault third-degree (major ptosis). **d** Regnault pseudoptosis

Table 31.1 Procedural specifics for forms of breast ptosis

	Inframammary fold position	Parenchymal position	Nipple–areolar position	Nipple-to-fold distance	Clavicle to nipple	Clavicle to fold
True ptosis	Fixed normal	Fixed rotated	Low downwardpointing	Unchanged	Elongated	Elongated
Glandular ptosis						
Common	Mobile descending	Mobile descending	Low forward-pointing	Elongated	Elongated	Elongated
Uncommon	Fixed normal	Mobile descending	Low relative to fold	Elongated	Normal to elongated	Unchanged
Parenchymal maldistribution	Fixed, high	Fixed, high	Normal downwardpointing	Short	Normal	Short
Pseudoptosis	Variable, usually low	Mobile, redescending	Surgically, fixed	Elongated, fixed	Surgically elongated	Variable, usually

31.7
LaTrenta and Hoffman Classification

In 1994 LaTrenta and Hoffman [6] added to the Regnault classification actual measurements in centimeters from the nipple to the inframammary fold to determine the grade of ptosis (Fig. 31.5), although stating that the classification was from Regnault's 1976 paper:

- First-degree ptosis (minor ptosis): The nipple is within 1 cm of the level of the inframammary fold above the lower contour of the gland and skin envelope.
- Second-degree ptosis (moderate ptosis): The nipple is 1–3 cm below the level of the inframammary fold and above the lower contour of the gland and skin envelope.

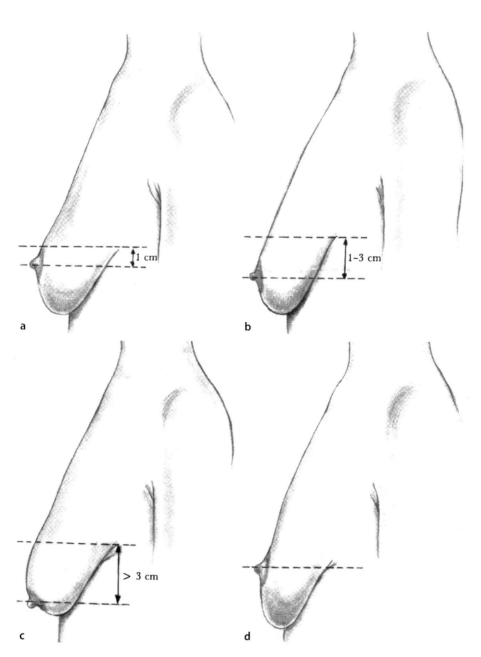

Fig. 31.5 a LaTrenta first-degree ptosis (minor ptosis). **b** LaTrenta second-degree ptosis (moderate ptosis). **c** LaTrenta third-degree ptosis (severe ptosis). **d** LaTrenta pseudoptosis

– Third-degree ptosis (severe ptosis): The nipple is greater than 3 cm below the level of the inframammary fold and below the lower contour of the breast and skin envelope.

– Pseudoptosis: The nipple is above or at the level of the inframammary fold with a loose, "saggy" skin brassiere, giving the impression of true ptosis.

31.8
De la Torre and Vasconez Classification

The de la Torre and Vasconez classification [7] (2007) is as follows:

Grade 1: Mild ptosis—nipple just below inframammary fold but still above lower pole of breast

Grade 2: Moderate ptosis—nipple further below inframammary fold but still with some lower pole tissue below nipple

Grade 3: Severe ptosis—nipple well below inframammary fold and no lower pole tissue below nipple; "Snoopy nose" appearance

Pseudoptosis: Inferior pole ptosis with nipple at or above inframammary fold; usually observed in postpartum breast atrophy

31.9
Conclusions

The classification of ptosis helps determine the type of surgery for mastopexy. The patient has to be the one to decide on the type of mastopexy surgery considering the position of the scars.

References

1. Lalardrie JP, Jouglard JP: Chirurgie Plastique du Sein. Paris , Masson 1973

2. Regnault P: Breast ptosis: definition and treatment. Clin Plast Surg 1976;34(2):193–203

3. Lewis JR Jr.: Mammary ptosis. In: Georgiade NG (ed). Aesthetic Breast Surgery. Baltimore, Williams & Wilkins 1983, pp 130–145

4. Brink RR: Evaluating breast parenchymal maldistribution with regards to mastopexy and augmentation mammaplasty. Plast Reconstr Surg 1990;84:715–719

5. Brink RB: Management of true ptosis of the breast. Plast Reconstr Surg 1993;91(4):657-662

6. LaTrenta GS, Hoffman LA: Breast reduction. In: Rees TD, LaTrenta GS (eds). Aesthetic Plastic Surgery, 2nd edn. Philadelphia, WB Saunders 1994, pp 971, 975

7. de la Torre J, Vasconez LO: Breast mastopexy. 2007. http://www.emedicine.com/plastic/topic128.htm

CHAPTER 32

Breast Augmentation with Mastopexy

Myron M. Persoff

32.1
Introduction

The breast has been synonymous with femininity since the dawn of time and has assumed various roles in female beauty ever since. If one were to infer from art and statuary of women over the ages, size was not an important feature of femininity until the mid-20th century when media began dictating the tenets of beauty, which became increasingly associated with youth. The ideal breast assumed a more youthful posture, and size has become increasingly more important. Mastopexy responded to the "need" created by a fallen breast (the word "ptosis" in Greek means "falling").

The early surgical procedures to correct ptosis were not especially sensitive to the scarring produced. However, toward the end of the 20th century, interest in minimal-scar techniques such as crescent mastopexy [1], the Benelli procedure [2], the vertical lift of Lejour [3], and other techniques [4, 5] arose in response to patients' dislike of excessive breast scarring. Reports of procedures for breast lifts appeared as early as the 1950s [6]; however, no reliable method of breast augmentation was available until Cronin and Gerow [7], with the help of Dow Corning Corporation, brought the silicone gel breast implant to the medical marketplace in 1963. The early reports of combinations of these two operations appeared in the mid-1960s [8–11]. The major problems posed by performing these two procedures simultaneously were eloquently summarized by Hammond [12]: "Augmentation mastopexy has proven to be one of the most difficult breast procedures plastic surgeons currently performed. There are several reasons for this. First is the fact that nearly every variable that determines the ultimate shape of the breast is being manipulated to some degree, including breast position, inframammary fold location, breast skin envelope surface area, position of the nipple–areola complex (NAC), and breast volume. All of this is performed through the most limited scar pattern possible, and it must all be done so as to create the same result on each side, despite the fact that more often than not there was preoperative asymmetry to start with. Second is that the procedure

is an aesthetic operation, and patient expectations are generally exceedingly high and tolerance for complications low. Lastly, the procedure involves the use of breast implants in all their various sizes, shapes, compositions, and textures, and all of the potential complications associated with the use of breast implants come into play."

32.2
Definition of Ptosis

In general, the term "ptosis" refers to drooping of the nipple–areola and breast skin and/or gland due to elongation of the connective tissue reticular network from stretching, atrophy, or loss of elasticity in a significant way compared with the adolescent breast. While ptosis can be developmental, occurring with early breast growth, most often it occurs over time because of gravity, hormonal changes, weight loss, pregnancy, or glandular regression due to menopause.

32.2.1
Pseudoptosis

If the nipple is in a normal position—that is, no more than 21 cm from the sternal notch in the "average" woman—and the inframammary crease (IMC) is higher than the nipple level, there is glandular ptosis and what has been referred to as pseudoptosis. This condition normally does not require mastopexy because an augmentation will usually suffice, along with lowering of the IMC by 1–2 cm (Fig. 32.1).

32.2.2
Minor Ptosis

In the classification of Bostwick [13], if the nipple is at or 1–2 cm lower than a "normal" IMC (21–23 cm), then minor ptosis exists, and some combination of lowering of the crease with a small elevation of the NAC will suffice (Fig. 32.2).

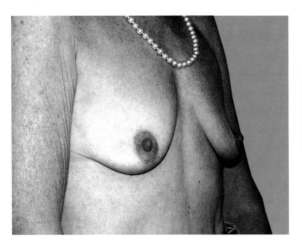

Fig. 32.1 A 58-year-old woman with postmenopausal atrophy of breasts. Nipple at 21 cm from sternal notch and inframammary crease is slightly higher

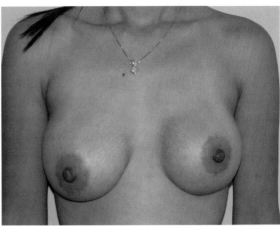

Fig. 32.2 A 28-year-old woman with asymmetry. The right nipple is minimally ptotic, with the nipple just below the level of the inframammary crease

32.2.3
Moderate Ptosis

When the nipple is 2–3 cm lower than the IMC, then moderate ptosis is said to exist. This can be treated by a Benelli lift, a vertical lift, or an anchor lift, depending on the preferences of the surgeon and patient (Fig. 32.3).

32.2.4
Major Ptosis

In major ptosis, the nipple is greater than 3 cm from the IMC, and, usually, the operation of choice would be the anchor lift, or a vertical lift. The greater the ptosis, a more a vertical lift will usually require a wedge resection of skin and gland at the IMC, either as a primary or a secondary procedure (Fig. 32.4).

Spear and others [12, 14–19] have written of complications encountered due to combining the two procedures of breast augmentation and mastopexy; these include nipple–areolar necrosis, implant malposition, contour deformities, poor scarring, and implant infections. Many plastic surgeons have advised against performing these two procedures simultaneously. However, when they are done as a single procedure, excellent results can be obtained, and this practice is preferred by patients as being less expensive and less inconvenient than staged procedures. An understanding of the problems and their etiology is in order:

1) Nipple–areolar necrosis: As we know from anatomy, the various pedicles used to elevate the nipple–areola have a random, not axial, blood supply, and the

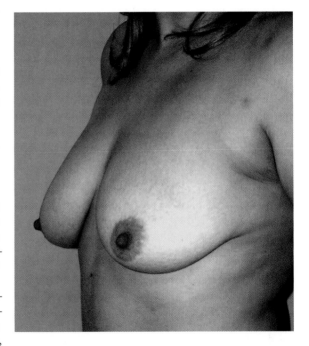

Fig. 32.3 A 30-year-old woman with breasts moderately ptotic. The nipple is 2–3 cm below the level of the inframammary crease

longer the pedicle, the more vulnerable it is to hypoperfusion. This disaster can occur during a routine breast reduction or mastopexy, but when excess skin tension occurs because of the presence of an implant, whether above or below the pectoralis muscle, it becomes more likely, even though the submuscular approach may be less damaging to the blood supply of the breast and nipple–areola. Planning the procedure with a small implant and moderate skin resection may help but may also limit the aesthetics of the final result.

2) Implant malposition: This problem is most often associated with the submuscular placement of the implant for several reasons:
   a. Inadvertent high positioning of the pocket for the implant
   b. Postoperative muscular spasm
   c. Inadequate pocket size and shape
   d. Fibrous capsular contracture

3) Contour deformities: When the breast tissue remaining after mastopexy is significantly heavy (large B cup or greater) with a submuscular implant, in time (usually 4–6 months) the breast tissue will rotate downward and create a "Snoopy dog" deformity. Additionally, if the gland is not carefully "trimmed" during a vertical mastopexy, or if the vertical incision is too long, lower-pole ptosis can occur.

4) Poor scarring can be caused by a number of conditions, including excessive wound tension, poor surgical technique, and adverse wound healing due to individual patient characteristics.

Breast reduction and mastopexy are essentially the same procedure, differing mainly in the amount of breast tissue removed. When performing a mastopexy or reduction, the surgeon should attempt to minimize the scars, obtain the best possible shape, and fulfill the patient's expectations with regard to size. Often, the use of an implant in a mastopexy or reduction will do as much to improve the shape as to increase the size. In fact, with proper planning, the implant can add longevity to the early result. Choosing the proper technique can be daunting to the novice.

32.3 Types of Mastopexy

Mastopexy is a continuum of procedures directly related to the amount of breast drooping. The normal breast is at one end of the spectrum, needing only volumetric enhancement, with various procedures being appropriate as the breast and nipple–areola descends. The procedures should be chosen not only to attempt to minimize scarring but primarily to address the degree of skin or glandular atrophy, glandular type, asymmetry, and degree of ptosis. While asymmetry may exist preoperatively in any patient, the author prefers to use the same technique on both breasts so as not to produce additional asymmetry because of the differences between techniques.

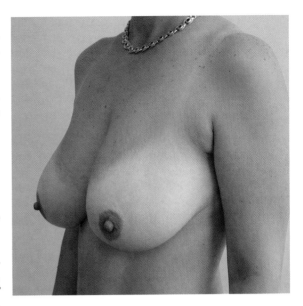

Fig. 32.4 Major ptosis is noted in this 26-year-old woman. The nipples are 3 or more centimeters below the inframammary crease

1) Crescent mastopexy: This involves removing a crescent of skin from 9 o'clock to 3 o'clock to elevate only the nipple point between 1 cm and 2 cm. This technique does not affect the shape of the breast but can be useful for very minimal lifts in cases of nipple asymmetry. This is not usually used for a reduction. With this technique, an implant can be placed either submuscularly or subglandularly with a superior nipple–areolar entry point. In a unilateral case, if an implant is to be used, I will make an upper areolar incision on the opposite side in order to have the same scars on both sides.

2) Circumareolar (Benelli) mastopexy: This is done completely around the nipple–areola and involves removing an inferior wedge of breast tissue and using a "round block" [2, 20, 21] nonabsorbable suture to close the larger (outside) diameter against the smaller (inside) diameter and to hold the position. This is a deceptively difficult procedure to perform and has a very long learning curve. Often, the nipples end up stretched with unsightly scars, and the shape is only marginally improved. It has been my experience that the ptosis recurs in less than a year and that the maximal "lift" is about 3–4 cm. This technique can be used for reductions as well. An implant can be placed in either the submuscular or subglandular space, but extreme care should be taken not to overaugment to prevent avascular necrosis of the NAC.

3) Vertical mastopexy: Also called the lollipop lift, this is a minimal-scar technique that affords excellent shape and longevity to the result and can be done

with or without implants. It is an extension of the circumareolar technique, whereby a vertical inferior wedge of skin and gland is removed and reshaped to improve the nipple–areolar size and breast shape. It is a very useful technique for reductions. However, depending on the skin quality and the length of the nipple–areolar pedicle, a persistent "dog ear" may form at the breast base along with some lower pole excess that may require later or simultaneous wedge excision, resulting in a small "inverted T" scar. The nipple pedicle is either vertical or medial, and an implant can be placed submuscularly or subglandularly.

4) Wise pattern [22] (anchor lift or inverted T): This can be used for virtually any size of breast, but it has several drawbacks:
    a. The horizontal scar is very often hypertrophic at the medial and lateral extremes.
    b. The technique relies on the skin brassiere for the lift, but this often fails over time.
    c. Although the shape is initially excellent, lower-pole ptosis can occur later.

This technique can be performed with almost any nipple pedicle, parenchymal resection, or implant location. However, the author prefers to extend the vertical technique and remove a medial and lateral horizontal wedge of skin and gland, thus converting to a limited inverted T, keeping the horizontal limbs as short as possible. The vertical technique using glandular reshaping gives the best long-term shape to the breast.

32.4
Estimating Volume

Understanding how to estimate the volume of the implant and the final breast size is key to the mastopexy-augmentation procedure. To estimate the patient's current breast size, measurements should be taken with the patient wearing a soft, nonpadded bra. The following measurements are required:
1) Sternal notch to nipple (in centimeters)
2) Nipple to nipple (in centimeters)
3) Sternal notch to IMC (in centimeters)
4) IMC to nipple (in centimeters)
5) Breast width (in centimeters) directly on the breast with calipers
6) Chest width from lateral breast edge to opposite lateral breast edge (divide this by one-half and subtract 1 cm to get the maximum base width of the implant)

Measurements 1–5 are not for volume but for evaluating symmetry, ptosis, nipple position, and base width.

7) Chest circumference at the IMC (in inches)
8) Chest circumference at nipple level (in inches)

In the average case, every cup size for a brassiere is an increment of 200 ml of implant or grams of breast tissue, so an A cup would be 200 g, a B cup 400 g, a C cup 600 g, and so on. To estimate the cup size, use measurements 7 and 8 as follows:
1) The "strap" size is determined by adding 5 in to the chest circumference at the IMC; i.e., if the measurement is 29 in, the strap size would be 29+5=34.
2) The "cup" size is the difference between the chest measurement at the nipple level and at the IMC, with a difference of 5 in equal to an A cup and each additional inch another cup. A difference of 4 in would be a AA cup, and a difference of 3 in a AAA cup. If the IMC measurement is 29 in and the nipple level circumference is 36 in, this would be 36–29=7, or a C cup. When less than 5 in, divide the A cup by 2 for a AA cup (100 g) or by 3 for a AAA cup (80 g).

Use these measurements to plan the size and base diameter of the implant as simple addition. If no breast tissue is to be removed, this is very simple. A patient with an A cup (200 ml) desiring to be enlarged to a C cup (600 ml) will require a 600–200=400-ml implant. However, when doing either a breast reduction or mastopexy, tissue will be removed, and, of course, this will affect the final breast volume. The surgeon must estimate the amount of breast to be removed, and this is not an easy task. However, one can usually guess within a half cup size (100 g) and add this to the implant size. Using a postoperatively adjustable implant (Mentor Spectrum) makes this much easier and safer [24, 25, 26].

The decision regarding implant placement, submuscular versus subglandular, also must be made. Of course, in a very thin woman with small atrophic and ptotic breasts, submuscular placement is favored, and in a woman with a ptotic "B" cup, the subglandular route could be more appropriate. However, the author prefers to use a "totally submuscular" pocket because if the musculofascial attachments are maintained, the implant will not "bottom out" over time. To minimize the descent of the breast over the muscle, one should maximize the breast tissue removed so that the remaining breast (without an implant) would be reduced to 200–300 g (A/B cup). By way of example, a woman with a discoid ptotic C cup who wishes to have her breasts lifted but to remain a C cup could have a 300-g reduction, leaving her with 300 g, and then have a 300-cc totally submuscular implant to end up with a C cup, half of which would be from the implant and half of which would be her own tissue.

As a rule, a totally submuscular implant should never be larger than around 350 ml without the use of the postoperatively adjustable implant or the use of "tailor-tacking" [12–27].

32.5
Technique

32.5.1
Crescent Mastopexy-Augmentation

Normally, crescent mastopexy-augmentation (Fig. 32.5) is useful for no more than a 2-cm elevation of the nipple. As previously stated, it does not contribute to breast shape. The planning involves drawing a semicircle from 9 o'clock to 3 o'clock, starting and ending as a tangent to the outer edge of the areola, and going about 2 cm above the nipple's upper edge at the 12 o'clock position. Then measure above this point the desired elevation of the nipple, not exceeding 2 cm, and draw the upper part of the ellipse, which is next deepithelialized (Fig. 32.2). Leaving about 2 mm of dermis on the upper edge, incise through the dermis and create a thin subcutaneous pocket (with some fat on the skin) into which the dermal flap will be placed on closure. At this point, spread the upper breast ducts down to the reflection of the pectoralis fascia and incise the fascia parallel to the pectoral fibers and open into the submuscular space.

Create the pocket by blunt and electrocautery dissection to the following limits: superiorly to about 2–3 cm from the clavicle, laterally to the anterior axillary line, medially to within 1 cm of the midline, and inferiorly to the position of the existing IMC line marked on the skin

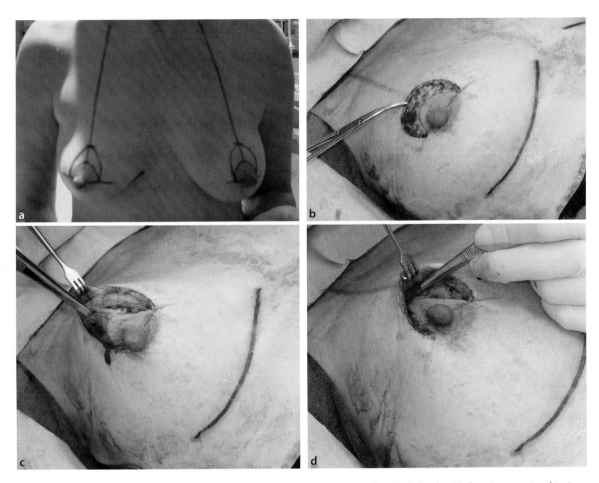

Fig. 32.5 a Preoperative markings in minimal ptosis for crescent mastopexy. Arc of crescent is placed from 9 o'clock to 3 o'clock from 1 cm to 2 cm above 12 o'clock position of areola. **b** Crescent is deepithelialized. **c** Undermine superior skin 2 cm cephalad. **d** Position to which dermal flap will later be sutured

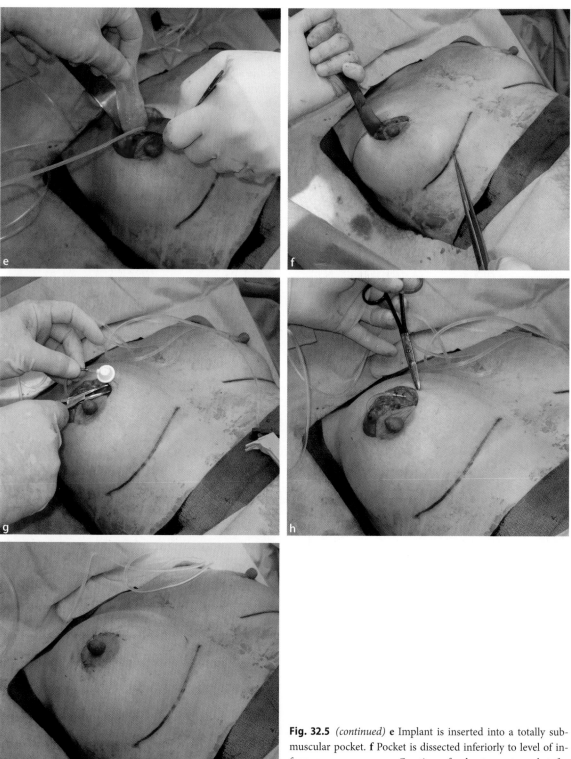

Fig. 32.5 *(continued)* **e** Implant is inserted into a totally submuscular pocket. **f** Pocket is dissected inferiorly to level of inframammary crease. **g** Creation of subcutaneous pocket for microreservoir near the incision. **h** Position of microreservoir sutured to the soft tissue to minimize movement. **i** Completed procedure

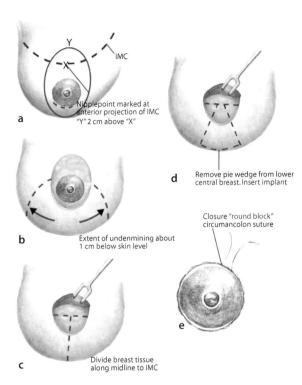

Fig. 32.6 **a** Mark the nipple point at the anterior projection of the inframammary crease (IMC). Point *A* is 2 cm above the nipple point (*X*). **b** Perform deepithelialization and circumcision of nipple. Note extent of peripheral undermining. Inferior circumareolar incision. **c** Divide breast down to pectoralis and to IMC level and undermine peripherally. **d** Remove pie-wedge from lower breast and insert implant submuscularly. **e** Close with "round block" circumareolar suture

NAC (2 cm higher than the nipple point) down to the bottom of the current NAC, which is then circumcised to a diameter of 3–4 cm, leaving the area in between the two circles to be deepithelialized. If a postoperatively adjustable implant is not used, the deepithelialization should be done only after the implant is inserted and the surgeon has determined by tailor-tacking [12, 27] the skin that the closure will not be too tight. The lower incision is made full thickness at the lower border of the areola, leaving a rim of dermis on the outer ellipse. The skin is then undermined for several centimeters from 8 o'clock to 4 o'clock and down to the IMC. The lower breast tissue is divided from the center of the inferior areolar incision, and an inferior central wedge of breast tissue is removed down to the pectoralis muscle. The muscle is then opened along the direction of its fibers and a completely submuscular space created, into which the implant is placed. The central wedge is closed (similar to the vertical technique below).

Central to the use of this technique is the use of a heavy-caliber deep circumareolar suture called the "round block" suture, which is usually nonabsorbable. The purpose of this suture is to close a larger outer diameter of the breast skin around the smaller diameter areolar skin, and in so doing, elevate the nipple point. The vector forces are from the base of the breast, 180° and upward toward the nipple, which results in downward pressure toward the center of the breast and/or implant, which tends to flatten the breast and create an abnormal bulge above the NAC (Fig. 32.7). In addition,

preoperatively. It is difficult to insert an implant larger than 250–300 ml through this upper incision, so a saline or a postoperatively adjustable implant is advised. When closing the dermal flap, suture the upper edge of the dermis to the dermis of the skin above with interrupted absorbable sutures, and then the upper edge of the areola to the dermal strip of the upper skin edge with a running intradermal suture.

32.5.2
Circumareolar (Benelli) Technique

The circumareolar (Benelli) technique (Fig. 32.6) employs a circumareolar incision and is advocated to elevate the NAC from 2 cm to 5 cm. The breast meridian and IMC are marked on the patient while she is standing. The new nipple position is marked in the breast meridian at the anterior projection of the IMC. A vertical ellipse is drawn from the intended new upper edge of the

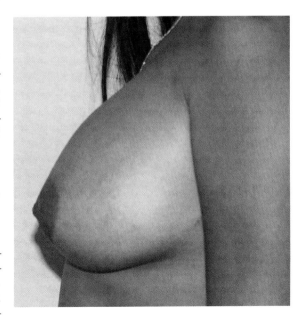

Fig. 32.7 Postoperative, showing abnormal bulge above nipple-areolar complex on left breast

there is usually considerable wrinkling of the periareolar skin, which later can create a stellate scar.

Although results with this technique can be very good (Fig. 32.8), the poor results from a well-done Benelli are overwhelmingly greater. The author has occasionally had to convert a good number of Benelli procedures to vertical lifts by removing an inferior wedge of skin and breast tissue, and uses this technique sparingly, if at all.

32.5.3
Vertical Technique

For ptosis greater than 2–12 cm, the author prefers the vertical technique (Fig. 32.9). The nipple is elevated in relation to the anterior projection of the inframammary line. Then, using any standard nipple–areola keyhole marker, an "opened circumference" the same size as the circumcised areola is used to mark the circle around the upper edge of the new areolar position and a "keyhole" of about 5 cm to create a 5-cm superior pedicle for the NAC. If the pedicle length is greater than 10–12 cm, the surgeon can alternatively use the medial pedicle as described by Hall-Findley [4] to shorten the distance by 2–3 cm. Then, as originally described by Lejour [3], by pushing the breast to either side of the midline, the outline of the vertical ellipse is marked from the open ends of the keyhole inferiorly to a point 3 cm above the existing inframammary line.

At this point, the areola is circumcised and the tissue within the NAC circumference keyhole is deepithelialized, creating the vertical dermoglandular pedicle. If a postoperatively adjustable implant is not used, the vertical incisions should not be made until after inserting the implant. Then the surgeon tailor-tacks the proposed vertical closure until he or she is certain that there is adequate skin for closure. A full-thickness incision is

then made around the circumcised areola upward into the deepithelialized keyhole for about 1 cm on each side, and then the dermoglandular pedicle is cut, leaving at least 1 cm of breast tissue under the NAC, beveling the dissection both cephalad and downward to the pectoralis muscle. Then a full-thickness incision is made on the vertical limbs down to the inferior apex 3 cm above the IMC. This incision goes about 0.5–1 cm into the breast tissue and then undermines the skin peripherally for about 2 cm, leaving a shield-shaped island of skin attached to the inferior gland. This shield is divided sharply down to the pectoralis fascia, creating a medial and a lateral column. It is at this point that the pectoralis should be opened along the direction of its fibers and the totally submuscular space created down to the level of the IMC, laterally to the anterior axillary line, superiorly to about 2 cm from the clavicle, and, finally, medially to within 1 cm of the midline. The muscular opening should be about 4–5 cm. If a silicone or fixed saline implant is to be used, the size should be no greater than 300 ml, and the vertical incision lines should be narrowed by about 1 cm on each side to account for the increased volume, or the tailor-tack method can be used as above. If a larger size is required, a Spectrum implant should be used to prevent overstretching the skin, and it should be initially filled to 300 ml or less as dictated by the skin tension. The fill tube is brought through the muscular incision, and the incision is closed with a 3-0 absorbable suture. Then the medial column is pulled laterally and divided at the breast meridian, and the lateral column is pulled medially and similarly divided. The total length of the columns should be no more than 8–9 cm, and the inframammary area should be defatted along the IMC down to the fascia.

The two columns are then closed with a large-caliber absorbable suture, such as PDS or Monocryl, with a running posterior layer from above to below and then

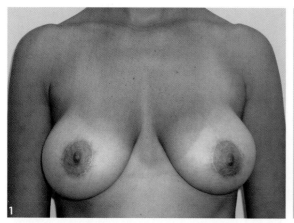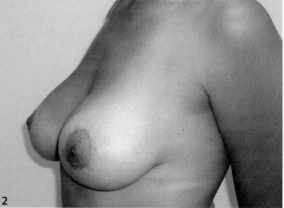

Fig. 32.8 *1* Good results from Benelli lift. *2* Lateral view

an anterior layer from below to above, with the fill tube coming out at the midpoint of the columns. It is at this point that 60 cc or more of the 300 cc placed into the implant should be withdrawn to release tension, the fill tube clamped and divided, and the microreservoir attached. The skin should now be closed in multiple layers, the last of which should be a running intradermal (PDS) from the inferior apex to the 6 o'clock position of the keyhole, pleating the skin along the way to shorten the length of the incision. If there is too much tissue at the apex of the incision and a large "dog ear" is noted, a short horizontal ellipse can be done either at this point or later as a secondary procedure under local anesthe-

sia. At about the midpoint of the closure, the microreservoir should be placed into a subcutaneous pocket and a few sutures placed into the rim of the reservoir and the breast tissue to prevent it from moving or flipping over later. If the surgeon feels the skin tension is too great, additional fluid can be removed using a 23-gauge butterfly percutaneously into the microreservoir. The areola is sutured into the keyhole with a two-layer closure, and the wounds are dressed with Steri-Strips or Tegaderm.

If the Spectrum implant is used, it can be filled starting on the 2nd postoperative week to the desired volume for symmetry and size.

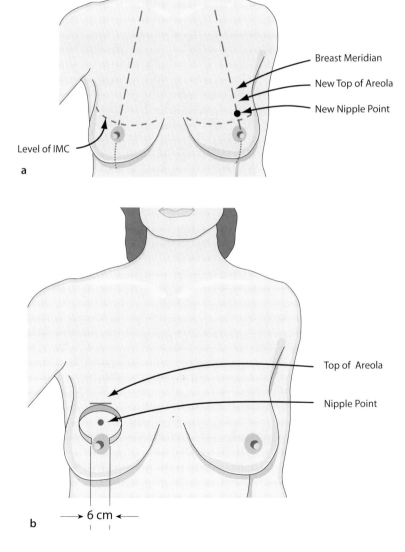

Breast Meridian

New Top of Areola

New Nipple Point

Level of IMC

a

Top of Areola

Nipple Point

6 cm

b

Fig. 32.9 a Placing the preoperative markings. **b** Marking the nipple–areolar complex (NAC)

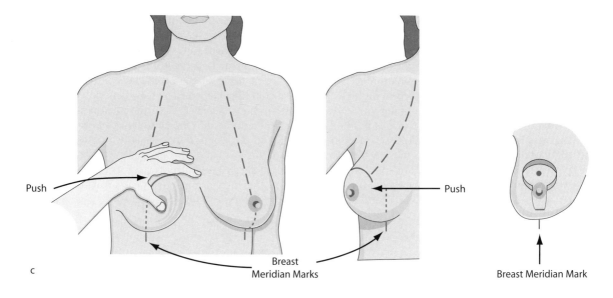

Push   Push

Breast
Meridian Marks

Breast Meridian Mark

c

Fig. 32.9 *(continued)* **c** Estimating the skin resection by pushing the breast medial and then lateral, marking the skin in reference to the breast meridian line at the inframammary crease (IMC), marking from above and down. Start at either end of the areolar arc and end at a point 3 cm above the IMC. **d** Nipple–areolar marker and cookie cutter. **e** The nipple is circumcised to the same circumference as the areolar arc, and a 1-cm rim is drawn around the new areolar circumference, which is deepithelialized along with the keyhole position for the NAC

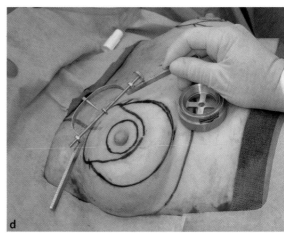

d

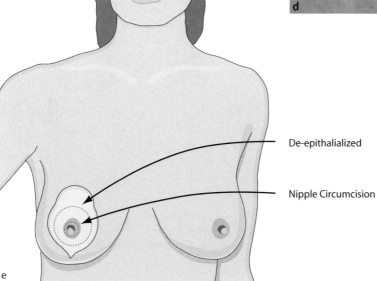

De-epithalialized

Nipple Circumcision

e

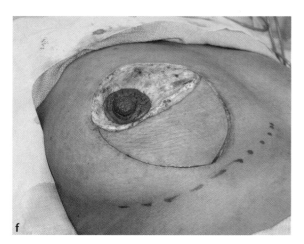

f

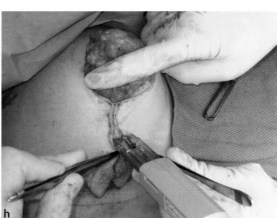

Fig. 32.9 *(continued)* **f** Deepithelialization of keyhole and nipple–areolar circumcision. **g** The nipple pedicle is divided inferiorly and dissected down to the pectoralis fascia, going cephalad to debulk the undersurface of the areolar pedicle. If using a postoperatively adjustable implant, the vertical incisions can be made with 1–2 cm lateral undermining. Then the lower breast tissue can be divided, creating medial and lateral breast columns. **h** If a nonadjustable implant is used, the lateral incisions should be made after implant insertion and "tailor-tacking" are done to determine the safe amount of skin excision. **i** Pectoralis muscle with cephalad undermining of the superior NAC pedicle and Senn rake on lower breast flap. **j** Lower breast flap being divided in the midline down to the pectoralis fascia, creating the medial and lateral columns of breast tissue

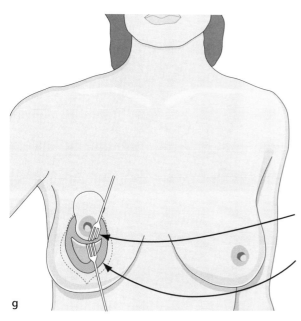

g

h

Lower Division
of Nipple Pedicle

Area of
Undermining

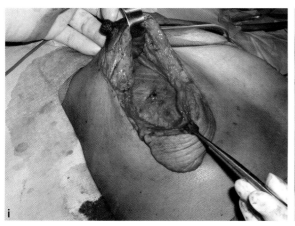

i

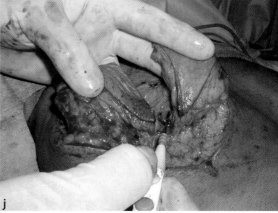

j

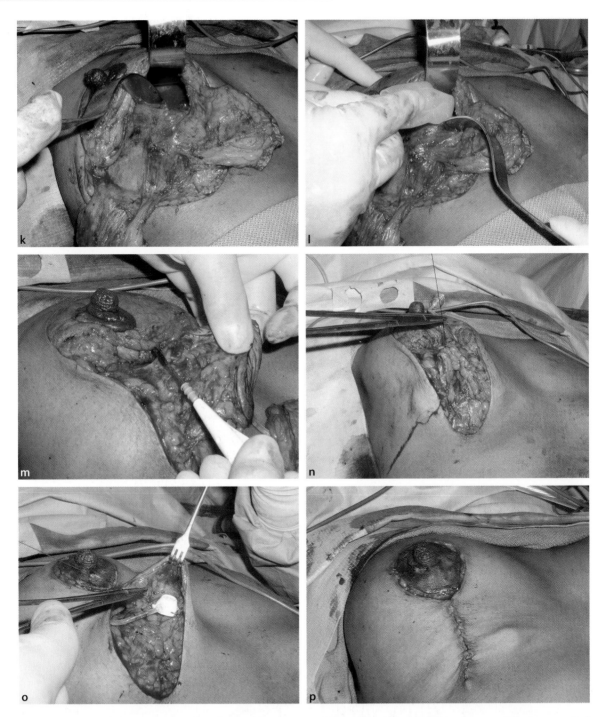

Fig. 32.9 *(continued)* **k** Opening into the submuscular space. Note medial and lateral columns. The pectoralis fascia is opened at the level of the NAC along the direction of the fibers. **l** The implant is inserted, and the muscle incision is closed. **m** The columns are pulled to the midline and divided with the electrocautery. They are then sutured together with a two-layer closure of heavy, long-term absorbable suture (0-PDS). The vertical length of the columns should not exceed 9 cm. Defat the IMC and lower breast flap just below the apex of the lower vertical incision. **n** Closure of the two columns. **o** Insertion of the microreservoir into a subcutaneous pocket. It should be sutured to the surrounding tissue to prevent later movement. **p** Vertical closure of the skin in two layers with pleating of the skin to shorten the vertical length. Note the position of the reservoir. Also notice how the IMC has moved upward about 3 cm to the base of the incision

32.5.4
Wise Pattern

The most widely used breast reduction or mastopexy technique, the Wise pattern involves the anchor or inverted-T incision, although many different pedicles have been proposed, including central mound [28], Skoog [29], superior [30], lateral [31], superoinferior [32], and inferior [33] techniques. All of these different pedicle techniques employ similar skin incisions, and Dr. Wise "reverse-engineered" a brassiere pattern to create a template for these various procedures. As with all reductive techniques, the longer the nipple–areolar pattern, the more at risk is the NAC circulation, thus the plethora of pedicle designs. Also, the horizontal scar, if too lateral or too medial, tends to become hypertrophic (Fig. 32.10).

For the purpose of reduction or mastopexy with augmentation, the author prefers the superior pedicle because of its easy access to the pectoral muscle for submuscular placement of the implant, as well as the lack of excessive inferior bulk of pedicle and breast. The vertical technique is preferred, so if there is significant doubt at the end of the procedure about whether the lower skin will shrink enough, by using the tailor-tack method, the central inferior dog-ear can be trimmed out laterally just above the IMC, and the vertical procedure can be converted to an anchor procedure. The decision to cut this excess can be delayed and done months later if shrinkage does not occur.

32.6
Case Examples

32.6.1
Pseudoptosis with Augmentation

This 58-year-old patient has atrophy of her breasts associated with menopause (Fig. 32.11). She is currently a 34AAA cup and wishes to be enlarged to a full B cup. The following measurements were taken:

1. Sternal notch to nipple, 21 cm bilateral
2. Sternal notch to IMC, 20 cm bilateral
3. Chest circumference at IMC, 29 in
4. Chest circumference at nipple, 32 in

The measurements show that the nipple is in the appropriate position, although the IMC is just above the nipple. Her size is 29 + 5 = 34 strap, and the cup is 32 − 29 = 3, with A = 5-in difference, AA = 4-in difference, and AAA = 3-in difference. Her request was to

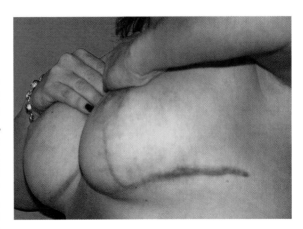

Fig. 32.10 Inverted T, where the horizontal scar often becomes hypertrophic

have a full B cup, so an increase in the range of 400 ml is required. An implant along with lowering the IMC by 1 cm will rotate the nipple up and fill the empty breast without a mastopexy.

The patient received a completely submuscular Spectrum implant 375–450 ml, overfilled to 500 ml for 6 weeks. The final volume was 425 ml.

32.6.2
Crescent Mastopexy with Augmentation

The patient is a 42-year-old woman who has had two prior pregnancies (Fig. 32.12). She wishes to be "natural" but enlarged from her current 36A+ to a B or C cup. Her breasts show minimal ptosis, with the following measurements:

1. Sternal notch to nipple, 22 cm bilateral
2. Sternal notch to IMC, 21 cm bilateral
3. Chest dimension at IMC, 32 in
4. Chest dimension at nipple level, 36 in

The measurements show that the nipple is just below the IMC (minimal ptosis) and that she should wear a 36 (32 + 5 = 37, but bras come only in even strap sizes) AA bra (36 − 32 is 4, which is a AA size).

With such minor ptosis, a crescent mastopexy will suffice, and the superior-areolar incision will be used for the augmentation, using a Spectrum implant. Because she is a AA cup (half of an A cup = 100 g) and wishes to be a full B/C cup, she will need an augmentation of around 400 ml, so a postoperatively adjustable implant is used with a range of 325–390 ml. The IMC will be intentionally lowered about 1 cm.

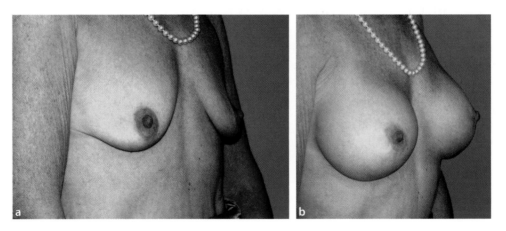

Fig. 32.11 **a** Preoperative pseudoptosis. **b** Postoperative with Spectrum implants filled to 425 cc final volume, submuscular. Note the apparent upward nipple rotation

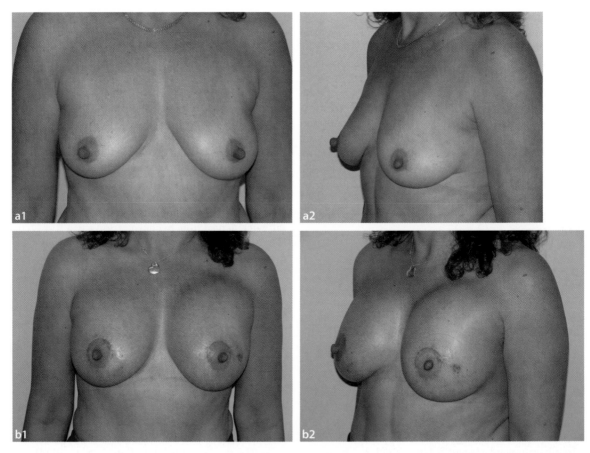

Fig. 32.12 **a** *1* Preoperatively, nipples are just below the infra-mammary crease (minor ptosis). *2* Lateral view. **b** *1* Two months postoperative. *2* Both Spectrum implants were filled to 500 cc for 6 weeks. Then 150 cc was removed from the right side, for final volume of 350 cc on the right side and overfilled volume of 500 cc on the left

32.6.3
Circumareolar (Benelli) Mastopexy-Augmentation

This patient is 28 years old and has significant deflation after a prior pregnancy (Fig. 32.13). Additionally, she has a mild pectus colorectal and marked upper-pole emptiness. She wears a 32A cup bra and wishes to be enlarged to a full C cup. Because of the minimal to moderate ptosis, a submuscular augmentation with circumareolar (Benelli) mastopexy was planned. Her preoperative measurements are as follows:

1. Sternal notch to nipple, right 24 cm, left 25 cm
2. Sternal notch to IMC, right 22 cm, left 22 cm
3. Chest diameter at IMC, 28 in
4. Chest diameter at nipple level, 33 in

An A cup is approximately 200 g, and with the mastopexy, perhaps 50 g of breast tissue will be removed from each side, leaving approximately 150 g per side. Because the patient wishes to be a full C cup, she will need 600 ml–150 cc (g) =450 ml. This would require a 425–550 ml smooth-walled Spectrum implant because the proper fill is within the range of the implant.

A circumareolar mastopexy-augmentation was done and the implants temporarily filled to 600 cc on each side for 6 weeks and then reduced to 500 ml on each side.

32.6.4
Vertical Mastopexy-Augmentation

The patient is 31 years old, multiparous, and has breast-fed (Fig. 32.14). Her breasts have deflated and dropped since breastfeeding, and she is now a 34B cup with major ptosis and asymmetry. She wishes to have her breasts lifted and enlarged to a full C cup. Her preoperative measurements are as follows:

1. Sternal notch to nipple, 26 cm right and 24 cm left
2. Sternal notch to IMC, 22 cm bilateral
3. Chest circumference at IMC, 29 in
4. Chest circumference at nipple level, 35 in

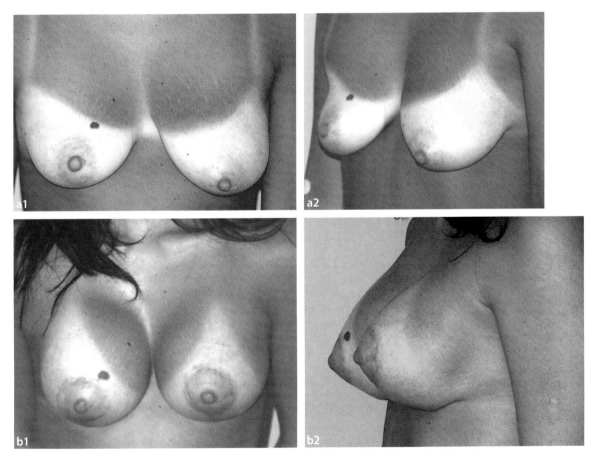

Fig. 32.13 a *1* Preoperative. *2* Patient has A-cup size and moderate ptosis. **b** *1* Postoperatively, the patient has a C cup with Spectrum final volume of 500 cc bilaterally. *2* Lateral view

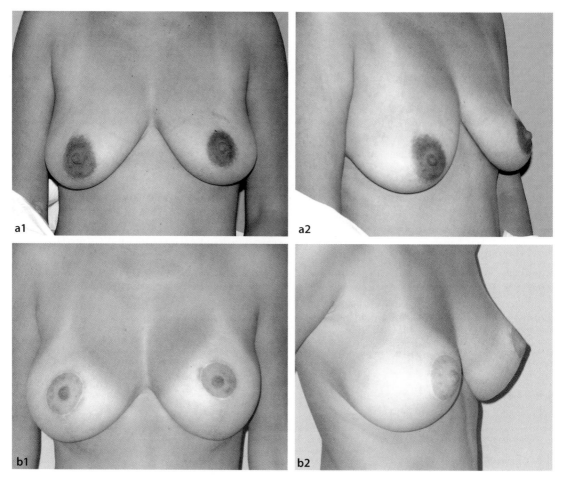

Fig. 32.14 a *1* Preoperative. *2* Patient has B-cup size and moderate to severe ptosis. **b** *1* Two years postoperative after removing 125 g on the right side and 95 g on the left. A postoperatively adjustable implant was used, initially filled to 240 cc and then later reaching a total volume of 375 cc on the right and 390 cc on the left. *2* Lateral view

This patient wishes to be enlarged from a B cup to a C cup, an increase of 200 g. However, with the mastopexy, at least 100 g will be removed; therefore, a postoperatively adjustable implant with a 325–390-ml range will be used. (Note: Always use a slightly larger implant range than calculated because the majority of patients will opt to be "a little larger" at the end of the process.)

32.6.5
Anchor Mastopexy Augmentation

This patient is a 28-year-old woman who has had two prior pregnancies and breastfed each child about 4 months each (Fig. 32.15a). She experienced significant drooping and asymmetry in her breasts. Her prior size was a 36C cup, but she is shown preoperatively as a

36A/B cup, with the left breast lower and larger than the right. Her preoperative measurements are as follows:
1. Sternal notch to nipple, right 24 cm, left 26 cm
2. Sternal notch to IMC, right 22 cm, left 22 cm
3. Chest diameter at IMC, 31 in
4. Chest diameter at nipple level, 37 in

Because of her asymmetry, her "average" breast size would be $31 + 5 = 36$ strap size and $37 - 31 = 6$ in (with 5= A, 6= B, 7= C), so because the left breast is visibly larger than the right, the "best guess" is that the left is less than a B cup and the right is more. So with 200 g per cup, the arbitrary volume is 300 g on the right and 500 g on the left.

The patient desired a C cup, which would have been a total of 600 g. However, with the mastopexy, 50 g of breast tissue was removed from the right side, leaving

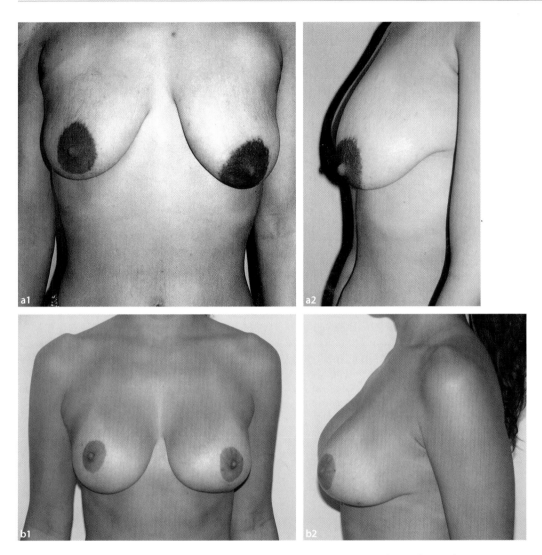

Fig. 32.15 a *1* Preoperative with extreme atrophy, ptosis, and asymmetry. *2* Lateral view. **b** *1* Twelve years postoperative after removal of approximately 300 g per side and placement of a 300-cc smooth-walled silicone gel implant submuscularly. *2* Lateral view

250 g, and 200 g was removed from the left side, leaving 300 g. A 300-ml smooth-walled silicone gel implant (moderate profile) Mentor was used.

32.7
Conclusions

Ptosis and atrophy of the breast occur along a continuum, from the youthful ("perky") appearance to an atrophic, hanging, aged-appearing breast (Fig. 32.16). Lifting and augmentation of the breast can be done with an implant alone in the case of pseudoptosis, and with a spectrum of techniques, from nipple lifting (only) to circumareolar, circumvertical, and, finally, the inverted-T techniques, each method also employing an implant. When the two procedures are combined, the complications can increase dramatically. These may include hematoma; infection; implant malposition; skin, breast, or nipple–areolar necrosis; poor incisional scarring; and fibrous capsular contracture. The most important consideration is that one must prepare for the advent of removing too much skin to allow for a safe closure after inserting the implant. If a nonadjustable implant is to be used, probably no more than 350 ml should be used, and the tailor-tack method of adjusting the pro-

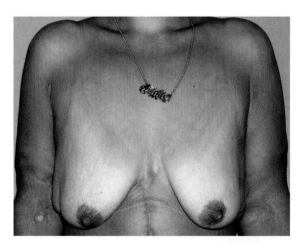

Fig. 32.16 Patient with extremely discoid, atrophic, and ptotic breasts after massive weight loss

posed incision lines before cutting is preferred. The author would recommend, however, the use of the postoperatively adjustable implant (Spectrum) in a "totally submuscular" pocket. Although there are potentially many pitfalls with the combination of augmentation and mastopexy, it remains a very satisfying procedure for the patient and is well worth the few additional risks if the surgeon uses these techniques.

References

1. Goulian D Jr: Dermal mastopexy. Plast Reconstr Surg 1971;47(2):105–110
2. Benelli L: A new periareolar mammaplasty: the "round block" technique. Aesthet Plast Surg 1990;14(2):93–100
3. Lejour M: Vertical mammaplasty and liposuction of the breast. Plast Reconstr Surg 1994;94(1):100–114
4. Hall-Findley EJ: Vertical breast reduction using the superomedial pedicle. In: Spear SL (ed). Surgery of the Breast: Principles and Art, 2nd edn. Philadelphia, Lippincott Williams & Wilkins 2006
5. Lassus C: A 30-year experience with vertical mammaplasty. Plast Reconstr Surg 1996;97(2):373–380
6. Gillies H, Marino H: The Periwinkle shell principle in the treatment of the small ptotic breast. Plast Reconstr Surg 1958;21(1):1–7
7. Cronin TD, Gerow F: Augmentation mammaplasty—a new "natural feel" prosthesis. In: Transactions of the 3rd International Congress of Plastic Surgeons. Amsterdam, Exerpta Medica 1964
8. Regnault P: The hypoplastic and ptotic breast: a combined operation with prosthetic augmentation. Plast Reconstr Surg 1966;37(1):31–37
9. Hinderer UT: Cirugia plastica mamaria de aumento y reduccion. Ann Acad Med. Quarterly Exp 1965;50:3
10. Courtiss EH (ed). Aesthetic Surgery: Trouble—How To Avoid It and How To Treat It. St. Louis, Mosby 1974
11. Owsley JQ: Simultaneous mastopexy and augmentation for correction of the small, ptotic breast. Ann Plast Surg 1975;2:195
12. Hammond DC: Augmentation mastopexy: general considerations. In: Spear SL (ed). Surgery of the Breast: Principles and Art, vol. 2, 2nd edn. Philadelphia, Lippincott Williams & Wilkins 2006, pp 1403–1416
13. Bostwick J: Correction of breast ptosis. In: Bostwick J (ed). Aesthetic and Reconstructive Breast Surgery. St. Louis, Mosby 1983, pp 209–250
14. Spear SL, Boehmler JH IV, Clemens MW: Augmentation/ mastopexy: a 3-year review of a single surgeon's practice. Plast Reconstr. Surg; 2006;118(7 suppl):136S–147S
15. Spear SL, Venturi ML: Augmentation with periareolar mastopexy. In: Spear SL (ed). Surgery of the Breast: Principles and Art, vol. 2, 2nd edn. Philadelphia, Lippincott Williams & Wilkins 2006, pp 1393–1402
16. Spear SL, Pelletierre CV, Menon N: One-stage augmentation combined with mastopexy: aesthetic results and patient satisfaction. Aesthet Plast Surg 2004;28(5):259–267
17. Spear SL, Giese SY: Simultaneous breast augmentation and mastopexy. Aesthet Surg J 2000;20:155
18. Spear SL: Augmentation/mastopexy: "Surgeon, beware." Plast Reconstr Surg 2003;112(3):905–906
19. Rohrich RJ, Gosman AA, Brown SA, Reisch J: Mastopexy preferences: a survey of board-certified plastic surgeons. Plast Reconstr Surg 2006;118(7):1631–1638
20. Goes J: Peri-areolar mammaplasty: double skin technique with application of polyglactin 910 mesh. Rev Soc Bras Cir Plast 1992;7:1–3
21. Elliott LF: Circumareolar mastopexy with augmentation. Clin Plast Surg 2002;29(3):337–347
22. Wise RJ: A preliminary report on a method of planning the mammaplasty. Plast Reconstr Surg 1956;17(5):367–375
23. Persoff MM: Expansion-augmentation of the breast. Plast Reconstr Surg 1993;91(3):393–403
24. Persoff MM: Use of the adjustable Spectrum implant in aesthetic breast surgery. In: Innovations in Plastic Surgery 2005;1(1):64, QMP Clinical Series
25. Persoff MM: Expansion-augmentation of the breast. Aesthetic Surg J 2000:20(3):208–212
26. Persoff M: Vertical mastopexy with expansion-augmentation. Aesthet Plastic Surg 2003;27(1):13–19
27. Whidden PG: The tailor-tack mastopexy. Plast Reconstr Surg 1978;62(3):347–354
28. Balch CR: The central mound technique for reduction mammaplasty. Plast Reconstr Surg 1981;67(3):305–311
29. Skoog T: A technique of breast reduction: transpositions of the nipple on a cutaneous vascular pedicle. Acta Chir Scand 1963;126:453 –465

30. Weiner DL, Aiache AI, Silver L, Tittiranonda T: A single dermal pedicle for nipple transposition in subcutaneous mastectomy, or mastopexy. Plast Reconstr Surg 1973;51(2):115–120

31. Nicolle FV: Reduction mammoplasty and mastopexy: a personal technique. Aesth Plast Surg 1984;8(1):43–50

32. McKissock PK: Reduction mammaplasty with a vertical dermal flap. Plast Reconstr Surg 1972;49(3):245–252

33. Ribeiro L: A new technique for reduction mammaplasty. Plast Reconstr Surg 1975;55(3):330–334

CHAPTER 33

Crescent Mastopexy with Augmentation

André Auersvald, Luiz Augusto Auersvald

33.1
Introduction

Mastopexy associated with augmentation for small volume and mild ptotic breasts has historically challenged plastic surgeons' creativity. The perfect balance between breast volume, scar, shape, and long-lasting results has been the main focus of the work of many authors.

Circumareolar, periareolar, and donut mastopexy are different names for a common approach to patients with a ptotic breast. The technique, introduced in the mid-1970s, is based on resecting skin from the entire periphery of the areola as a way to lift the breast [1–7]. The crescent mastopexy was later conceived as a modification of this approach in which the skin resection (in a crescent shape) is restricted to the segment adjacent to the upper half of the areola [8–11]. Although limited in its indications, this technique is an important surgical strategy for patients with borderline ptotic breasts.

33.2
Indications

Understanding the parameters for circumareolar mastopexy with augmentation is crucial for selecting the ideal patient for crescent mastopexy with augmentation, since the latter technique derives from the first.

33.2.1
Ptosis Grading

In 1976, Regnault [3] established three different levels for breast ptosis (Table 33.1, Fig. 33.1). Patients with grade 1 (nipple at the inframammary fold level) are best suited for either the crescent or the circumareolar mastopexy with augmentation [5]. Grade 2 patients are borderline regarding indication for crescent mastopexy and are generally accepted as good candidates for the circumareolar approach. On the other hand, the crescent technique is viewed as contraindicated for grade 3 patients because a lift of more than 3–4 cm is very difficult to achieve by simply excising skin adjacent to the upper half of the areola [9, 12].

Another important issue when considering crescent mastopexy with augmentation is the distance between the nipple–areola complex and the inframammary fold. In patients presenting with glandular ptosis and pseudoptosis (nipple at the inframammary fold level but with loose skin brassiere), this distance tends to be greater than what one would find in grade 1 ptosis (Fig. 33.2). This scenario is considered a poor indication for a circumareolar approach and a strong contraindication for the crescent mastopexy with augmentation because the excess skin and gland in these situations are not addressed adequately by crescent skin removal. A vertical, L-shaped, or inverted T should be considered here instead [13, 14].

Table 33.1 Regnault's classification of breast ptosis

Grade	Description
1st-degree (minor) ptosis	Nipple is at the inframammary fold
2nd-degree (moderate) ptosis	Nipple below the inframammary fold but still located on the anterior projection of the breast mound
3rd-degree (major) ptosis	Nipple below the inframammary fold and on the dependent position of inferior convexity of the breast mound
Glandular ptosis	Nipple above the fold, but the breast hangs below the fold
Pseudoptosis	Nipple above the fold, but the breast is hypoplastic and hangs below the fold

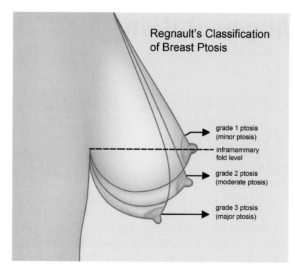

Fig. 33.1 Regnault's classification of breast ptosis

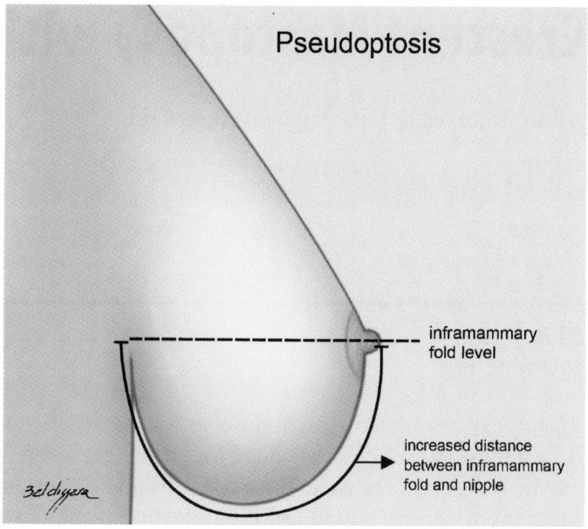

Fig. 33.2 Pseudoptosis according to Regnault

33.2.2
Nipple–Areolar Complex Diameter

Both crescent and circumareolar mastopexy with augmentation are best indicated in patients with a nipple–areolar complex diameter greater than 35–40 mm. Spear et al. [12, 15] suggested a mathematical method to guide the planning of circumareolar mastopexy. This method is based on rules that determine the amount of skin removed in an attempt to prevent tension on closure and to avoid hypertrophic scarring and areolar spreading. According to their guidelines, the outer incision should be less than three times the diameter of the inner circle and is generally less than 10 cm total.

Crescent mastopexy with augmentation is also well indicated in patients with a nipple–areolar complex diameter greater than 35–40 mm who need a lift of no more than 25–30 mm [14]. However, because the skin is not excised in the entire periphery of the areola, this technique should be indicated with care in patients with larger areolas (diameter greater than 8 cm, in the authors' experience).

33.2.3
Skin Characteristics

Thicker and pigmented skins tend to have worse healing when crescent and circumareolar mastopexy with augmentation are performed. Unsightly scarring and areolar enlargement may also occur in a patient with a small and well-delineated nipple–areolar complex [12].

33.3
Technique

Markings should be done before the anesthetic procedure with the patient in a sitting position. At this time, if not done previously, eventual asymmetries should be considered and discussed with the patient, preferably in front of a mirror. It is important to highlight that thoracic asymmetries may not only be of soft tissue origin (skin, gland, and muscle) but also of bone structure, and that the latter are not addressed in the surgery and will persist after the procedure.

The higher point of the nipple–areolar complex is marked and the new point established on an imaginary vertical line 1–3 cm above the original point. The crescent can then be drawn with two almost parallel curves starting at 9 o'clock, passing through the higher points (the original and the new) and going down to the 3 o'clock point (Fig. 33.3) [7].

Local or epidural blockage associated with sedation or general anesthesia are chosen according to the surgeon's and the anesthesiologist's preferences. Infiltrating the skin and the plane to be dissected with adrenaline (1:500,000) may help reduce bleeding.

Incision with a #15 blade scalpel and subsequent deepithelialization is performed. Dissection through the gland should be perpendicular to the thoracic plane and may be performed with electrocautery or with a #22 blade scalpel. If using the scalpel, one should be careful in splitting the gland in only one plane. Thorough hemostasis and placement of a tubular suction drain (if such a device is used) should be done before introducing the implant.

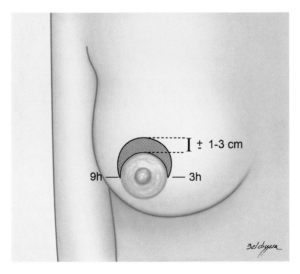

Fig. 33.3 Markings of the crescent mastopexy and augmentation

Closure should follow three planes: glandular, subdermal, and intradermal levels. In all of them, the authors' preference is for poliglecaprone (Monocryl, Ethicon): 3-0 interrupted sutures for the glandular and subdermal planes and 4-0 for the intradermal suture.

In 2006, Gruber et al. [14] proposed a variant approach to the technique described above, the so-called extended crescent mastopexy with augmentation. The objective, according to these authors, is to minimize skin tension by gland removal under the crescent, thereby reducing the potential for nipple–areolar complex spreading and scar hypertrophy.

33.4
Case Results

Case 1: This 31-year-old patient came seeking treatment for her hypomastia and grade 1 ptotic breasts (Fig. 33.4). She underwent bilateral crescent mastopexy with augmentation. A 250-ml silicone implant (anatomic profile) was used.

Case 2: This 29-year-old sought treatment for her small-volume breasts and the asymmetry of her nipple–areolar complex position (Fig. 33.5). On the right side she presented a grade 1 ptosis, and on the left side, no ptosis. A crescent mastopexy with augmentation of her right breast was planned; on the left side, the implant was placed through the upper half of the areola, but no skin was removed. Both implants were of silicone gel and anatomic profile (275 ml). She underwent simultaneous liposuction.

33.5
Complications

Complications of crescent mastopexy with augmentation are not well documented in the literature. However, as mentioned in the beginning of this chapter, crescent

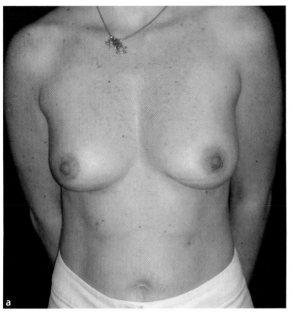
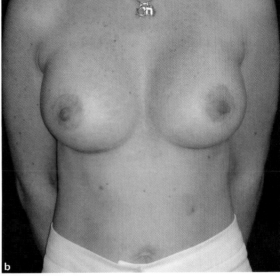

Fig. 33.4 Case 1. **a** Preoperative. **b** One year postaugmentation

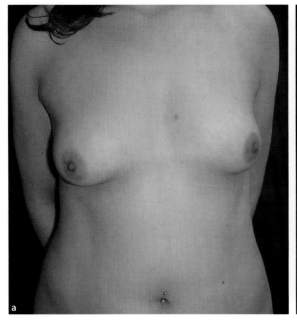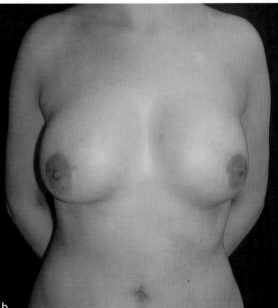

Fig. 33.5 Case 2. **a** Preoperative. **b** Two years postaugmentation

and circumareolar mastopexy are intrinsically analog, and therefore one can extract from the latter potential complications for the former.

Although no specific incidence is reported in the literature, infection, partial and transient loss of nipple–areolar complex sensitivity, and hematoma are listed as possible early complications. Higher bleeding rates are generally expected when approaching the submuscular plane through the upper quadrant [3]. Skin pleats tend to accommodate in the first few months; revision is rarely required for this reason. Globular-shaped and flat

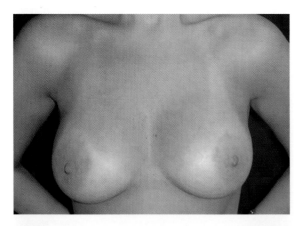

Fig. 33.6 Bilateral areolar spreading 2 years after crescent mastopexy with augmentation

breasts can eventually be found after surgery and may persist as late complications [4].

Areolar spreading and distortion are also among the complications (Fig. 33.6) [16]. When analyzing long-term results in a series of 26 patients who received crescent mastopexy with augmentation, Puckett et al. [9] reported 12 cases of areolar spreading greater than 5 mm and five individuals with oval areolas.

Another important complication of this technique that is poorly indicated in the literature is early and late recurrence of ptosis. Because no gland work is performed, this complication depends greatly on the quality of the patient's skin. Thicker skin tends to keep the result for a longer period than thinner skin.

33.6
Discussion

Balancing shape, volume, and scar with a low recurrence rate is the main goal when considering lifting and augmenting the breast. Although the use of crescent mastopexy and augmentation is restricted to few patients [17], it can be of great help for women with grade 1 or borderline grade 2 ptosis with a normal or near-normal distance between the nipple–areolar complex and the inframammary fold [14].

Other important factors also have to be considered when choosing a good candidate for this technique.

Those with lighter and thinner skins and with areolar diameters greater than 35–40 mm and less than 80 mm tend to heal better.

Upper-pole fullness is among the priorities of women from many cultures when breast augmentation and lift are considered. Therefore, one of the mandatory issues to be discussed with the patient prior to surgery is the recurrence of breast ptosis, a possible late complication of this procedure. In the crescent technique, the blood supply is interrupted on the upper half of the nipple–areolar complex; therefore, a secondary mastopexy using a vertical, inverted T, or L-shaped incision may be precluded—at least for the first few years—for concerns with the areolar skin viability [13].

One of the approaches used by the authors to overcome this problem is to combine the crescent mastopexy with augmentation via the inframammary fold or the axilla. Because the implant is not introduced through the areola, the deepithelialization of the skin (crescent) spares the periareolar dermal and subdermal plexuses. If a vertical, inverted T, or L-shaped mastopexy is needed in the near future, these intact plexuses will provide the blood supply to the areola.

This alternative method (crescent skin excision only and introduction of the implant through the inframammary fold or through the axilla) may be very helpful in patients with asymmetric breasts in which the desired lift is slightly different for each side. For instance, patients with no ptosis on one side but with grade 1 or 2 ptosis on the other side may benefit from this approach (case 2).

33.7
Conclusions

Crescent mastopexy with augmentation is a technique used for patients with a small grade of ptosis in which the desired lift of the nipple–areolar complex does not exceed 3 cm. Thick- and light-skinned patients tend to have better results compared with those with thin or dark skin. Areolar distortion and spreading and early or late recurrence are possible complications (Fig. 33.6). When appropriately indicated, this approach may lead to a good balance between shape, scar, and long-lasting results.

References

1. Rees TD, Aston SJ: The tuberous breast. Clin Plast Surg 1976;3(2):339–347
2. Bartels RJ, Strickland DM, Douglas WM: A new mastopexy operation for mild or moderate breast ptosis. Plast Reconstr Surg 1976;57(6):687–691
3. Regnault P: Breast ptosis: definition and treatment. Clin Plast Surg 1976;3(2):193–203
4. Benelli L: A new periareolar mammaplasty: the "round block" technique. Aesth Plast Surg 1990;14(2):93–100
5. de la Fuente A, Martin del Yerro JL: Periareolar mastopexy with mammary implants. Aesth Plast Surg 1992;16(4):337–341
6. Dinner MI, Artz JS, Foglietti MA: Application and modification of the circular skin excision and purse-string procedures. Aesth Plast Surg 1993;17(4):301–309
7. Elliot LF: Circumareolar mastopexy with augmentation. Clin Plast Surg 2002;29(3):337–347
8. Seitchik MW: Augmentation of the minimally ptotic breast. Ann Plast Surg 1980;5(6):460–463
9. Puckett CL, Meyer VH, Reinisch JF: Crescent mastopexy and augmentation. Plast Reconstr Surg 1985;75(4):533–543
10. Nigro DM: Crescent mastopexy and augmentation. Plast Reconstr Surg 1985;76(5):802–803
11. Karnes J, Morrison W, Salisbury M, Schaeferle M, Beckham P, Ersek RA: Simultaneous breast augmentation and lift. Aesth Plast Surg. 2000;24(2):148–154
12. Spear SL, Giese SY, Ducic I: Concentric mastopexy revisited. Plast Reconstr Surg 2001;107(5):1294–1299
13. Auersvald A, Auersvald LA: Extended crescent mastopexy with augmentation (discussion). Aesth Plast Surg 2006;30(3):275–276
14. Gruber R, Denkler K, Hvistendahl Y: Extended crescent mastopexy with augmentation. Aesthetic Plast Surg 2006;30(3):269–274, discussion 275–276
15. Spear SL, Kassan M, Little JW: Guidelines in concentric mastopexy. Plast Reconstr Surg 1990;85(6):961–966
16. Baran CN, Peker F Ortak Sensoz TO, Baran NK: Unsatisfactory results of periareolar mastopexy with or without augmentation and reduction mammaplasty: enlarged areola with flattened nipples. Aesth Plast Surg 2001;25(4):286–289
17. Regnault P: Crescent mastopexy and augmentation: discussion. Plast Reconstr Surg 1985;75(4):540

CHAPTER 34

Breast Augmentation with Periareolar Mastopexy

34

Steven P. Davison, Mark W. Clemens

34.1
Introduction

Augmentation with mastopexy is one of the most satisfying but challenging operations in breast surgery. Fundamentally, it is a reconstructive operation of an involved breast held to cosmetic standards both by patients and in legal claims. The goals of augmentation and mastopexy are diametrically opposed—volume enhancement with skin envelope reduction—yet they must be combined to yield the best results when breast augmentation alone will not suffice. Multiple variables such as volume, skin amount, nipple position and inframammary distance, must all be accounted for, requiring meticulous planning, staging, and execution.

34.2
Indications

Careful planning is paramount in augmentation mastopexy. The surgeon must decide whether the patient's primary goal is augmentation of volume, a breast lift, or both. By combining the two operations, one reduces the need for excessively large implants to correct ptosis.

34.3
Augmentation Alone

Mastopexy may not be necessary when 1) the nipple is above the inframammary fold, 2) the areola is above the lower border of the inframammary fold with unpigmented skin visible below it, and 3) no more than 3 cm of breast overhangs the inframammary fold.

34.4
Staging

Augmentation mastopexy can be an immediate or a delayed two-stage operation, the latter being more predictable and less risky with few variables. The goal is to tailor the skin while maximizing breast volume. It is not advisable and potentially disastrous to reduce the skin envelope beyond the limits required to close over an implant.

34.5
History

Gonzalez-Ulloa (1960) [1] and Regnault (1976) [2] originally contributed to the development of augmentation mastopexy by describing the correction of the hypoplastic breast with alloplastic augmentation mastopexy.

Persoff [3] defined the goals of augmentation with simultaneous mastopexy as 1) elevation of the mound, 2) elevation of the nipple–areolar complex, 3) conversion from a ptotic breast to a clinical breast, 4) enlargement of volume, and 5) improved breast symmetry.

The concept of a donut and vertical mastopexy was introduced by Gruber and Jones in 1980 [4], but a widened scar limited the acceptance. In an effort to address this, Benelli [5] described the technique of using round-block sutures. Most recently, Hammond et al. [6] detailed an interlocking periareolar suture to reduce tissue tension and distortion. This has been described as a wagon-wheel suture.

34.6
Preoperative Planning

34.6.1
Ptosis Staging

Most of the current classifications for ptosis staging were described by Regnault [7] as the following (see also Fig. 34.1):

Grade 1 ptosis: Nipple lying at the fold

Grade 2 ptosis: Nipple below the fold but still on the anterior portion of the breast

Grade 3 ptosis: Nipple at the most inferior portion of the breast

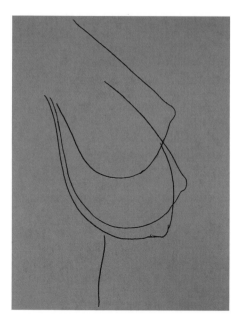

Fig. 34.1 Degrees of ptosis. *Superior*: pseudoptosis. *Middle*: grade 2 ptosis. *Inferior*: grade 3 ptosis. Note that the position of the nipple should be evaluated in relation to the inframammary fold and its position on the breast mound

> Glandular ptosis: An important component is to determine how much breast is below the inframammary fold

34.6.2
Implant Size

The size of the implant is influenced by several factors. The surgeon should consider the following:

1. Note whether a large-sized ptotic breast involutes the breast walls, such as during breastfeeding. This suggests the size of the skin envelope and skin redundancy.
2. What size does the patient want the final breast to be?
3. Measure the base width of the breast to determine what size of implant the chest wall can accommodate. This can be manipulated by using a high-profile implant with less base width to volume size.
4. Inframammary fold distance. A short distance can accommodate a large implant by releasing the inframammary fold to prevent distortion. Approximate inframammary fold lengths correspond to cup sizes as follows: C cup =6 cm and D cup =7 cm (estimates).

34.6.3
Skin Excision

As with reduction patterns, a progressive number of skin excisions may be performed. Among them are the following:

1. Periareolar or donut mastopexy: This is attractive because it limits scars while lifting the nipple. Problems occur when it is pushed to accommodate too large an implant. The surgeon should note that the widened scars and nipple distortion offset the benefit.
2. Lollipop or short-scar vertical limb: This procedure removes more skin in the horizontal direction while maintaining the inframammary fold distance. The vertical limb improves projection at the expense of a scar.
3. Wise pattern and/or short horizontal scar: A truly excessive skin envelope requires more excision, and a Wise skin pattern may be needed. This reduces the envelope horizontally and vertically with the inframammary fold scar. With this type of augmentation mastopexy, it is preferable, and may be necessary, to stage the operation. Note the following indications for Wise pattern and/or short horizontal scar:
   a. The nipple is more than 2 cm below the inframammary fold.
   b. No skin lies below the areola, which is at the inferior cup of the breast.
   c. The nipple-to-fold distance is greater than 9 cm.
   d. Severe breast ptosis is observed when the breast overhangs the inframammary fold by 4 cm or more.

34.6.4
Markings

The patient is marked while she is standing. Standard breast marking includes noting the chest midline from the sternal notch to xyphoid, inframammary fold, and breast median. Next, the median of the breast is drawn from the clavicle down through the mound and should not be influenced by the position of the nipple–areolar complex, which may be offset. A mastopexy can be designed with asymmetrical excision patterns to help centralize nipple positions. The marked median is used to help define the ideal new position of the nipple as opposed to the nipple's being used to determine the correct position of the median.

Setting the nipple height is paramount because this position is determined by multiple factors, including the final breast volume, the patient's height, inframammary fold position, and body habitus. As opposed to nipple placement in breast reductions, the nipple–areolar complex should always end up above the inframammary fold. The most common error is inadequate elevation of the nipple. However, an excessively high nipple is a serious complication and very difficult to correct. If it occurs, it looks unnatural and exacerbates glandular ptosis.

The nipple height should be at or up to a few centimeters above the inframammary fold. At the peak of the anticipated breast mound, the new nipple position is marked by an X (Fig. 34.2). The new margin of the areola, A, is marked 2 cm above X. The future scar is taken into account when drawing the anticipated new nipple diameter, usually between 38 mm and 42 mm. The amount of skin to leave from the inferior edge of the areola to the inframammary fold depends on the desired final breast volume. A large breast, C or B , may require 7 cm and a small breast 5 cm. The inferior margin of the resection is marked by point B.

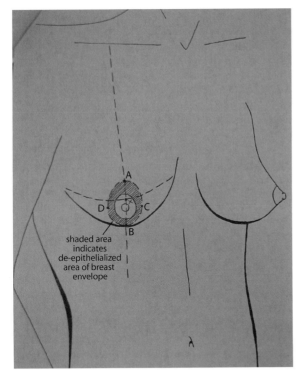

Fig. 34.2 Preoperative markings. The point of intersection between the inframammary fold and the breast meridian is marked with an X. The breast meridian (from the middle of the clavicle) is used to determine medial and lateral nipple position. Point A is marked approximately 2 cm above point X. The oval resection is made asymmetric to avoid excessive flattening of the nipple. Points C and D can be adjusted medially or laterally to correct any asymmetry

shaded area indicates de-epithelialized area of breast envelope

The skin excision more often than not is oval, reflecting greater vertical skin excess than horizontal. The amount of skin to lift medially, point C, and laterally, point D, is assessed. Mediolateral movement of the nipple–areolar complex is achieved by eccentric placement of the periareolar markings. If none is needed, point D is often more or less equidistant to the median as the median is from point C.

To complete the marking, the anticipated pocket dissection is outlined, and the periareolar excision is marked from 4 o'clock to 8 o'clock at the inferior margin of the existing nipple–areolar complex.

34.6.5
Circumvertical Marking

The initial markings and establishment of the nipple–areolar complex position are the same as in the previous section. Superomedial and superolateral traction is applied to the breast, and vertical lines from the inframammary fold and the meridian to the areola are marked. This wedge or V from the circumareolar excision stops above the fold.

The skin is then pinched or tailor-tacked to make sure closure will be possible after augmentation. The surgeon should be confident that the skin excess is sufficient to allow for tension-free closure. The excess incision for the implant pocket is marked in the vertical limb, which will help preserve nipple blood supply.

34.7
Operative Technique

A circle 38–45 mm in diameter is marked on the nipple within the pigmented areola. The diameter is based on personal patient preference, with postpartum diameter being larger than prepartum, and the ultimate dependence is on final breast volume. The augmentation component is always done first. A periareolar incision is made along the inferior of the areola in the vertical limb of the circumvertical mastopexy. Using electrocautery, an oblique dissection is carried down through the breast parenchyma to the pectoral fascia. The inferior flap is left at least 1 cm thick for adequate soft tissue coverage of the inferior pole of the implant figure (Fig. 34.3). The next phase of the operation depends on subglandular or partial subpectoral implant placement.

For a subglandular implant, a precise pocket is dissected using a lighted retractor to enhance direct vision. The pocket is created between the pectoralis major fascia and the gland. The pocket extension is limited to the serratus and the inframammary fold. Medial dissection

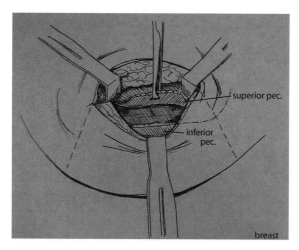

Fig. 34.3 Release of the lower border of the pectoralis major. The periareolar incision is carried obliquely through the breast parenchyma until reaching the pectoralis fascia, creating an inferior flap (shown by *dotted lines*) at least 1 cm thick. The release is carried medially and superiorly (*dotted line*), no higher than the level of the nipple

is carried out to the desired medial border, taking care to avoid overdissection and the risk of symmastia. The superior dissection should be high enough to allow sufficient redraping of the glandular tissue while limiting implant migration.

For a subpectoral implant, a limited subglandular dissection from the inframammary fold to nipple is performed to allow redraping. The pectoralis muscle is grasped with an Alice clamp and then lifted along its inferior border. Electrocautery is used to carefully incise the sternal and medial attachments of the pectoralis muscle. Adequate hemostasis of perforators is extremely important in this area. Medial muscle resection is limited to the lower third of the muscle below the nipple. Lateral subpectoral dissection lifts the pectoralis major off the minor but limits inferolateral dissection to keep the implant off the axilla, a common complaint in excessive pocket dissection.

34.7.1
Implant Position

The decision of whether to place the implant subglandularly or partially subpectorally is influenced by multiple factors. If the implant is placed in the subglandular position, its impact will be greater. This is illustrated when a patient has absolute retraction and the influence on the skin is at its maximum. All patients, by definition, have skin laxity, yet the better the recoil of the skin, the more likely that subglandular implants will be a successful. Soft tissue coverage can be determined by noting at least a 2-cm pinch test, preferably 3 cm, in the upper pole. Otherwise, a partial subpectoral implant will be necessary to disguise the shell (Fig. 34.4). The type of implant, saline versus silicone, further dictates plane and positioning because saline is more likely to ripple, requiring greater tissue coverage.

Postbariatric patients present a special dilemma. Their severe evolution favors subglandular implant position as a consequence of poor soft tissue. The use of simultaneous auto-augmentation can be considered for increasing the amount of soft tissue coverage and allowing the implant to be placed in the subglandular position.

The implant is inserted into the pocket and its accurate position confirmed by sitting the patient up. Adjustments are then made, and the breast parenchyma is closed over the implant with absorbable sutures. A saline implant would be filled to desired capacity at this point. The initial periareolar skin excision is tacked and the patient set upright. The nipple position and degree of ptosis are now critically reassessed. The excessive skin relative to the new volume is calculated and the decision for mastopexy revisited.

For the periareolar mastopexy, the nipple–areolar complex is marked 38–45 mm. The areola and periareolar skin to be excised is deepithelialized. The dermis is incised between the areola and breast, taking care to preserve at least 5 mm of dermis for secure suture closure. Unless there are concerns about nipple viability, the breast skin is undermined circumferentially outward for at least 1 cm to allow tissue redraping. Benelli

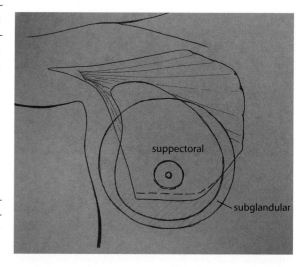

Fig. 34.4 The dual-plane implant pocket. Note that the implant is placed partially subglandularly and partially subpectorally

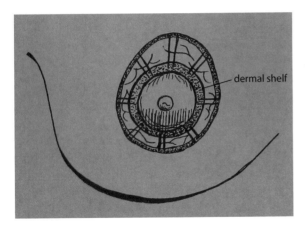

Fig. 34.5 Closure of the periareolar incision. Note interlocking dermal sutures using Gore-Tex on a straight needle. A small dermal shelf is maintained around the areola to anchor the suture

advocated suspending the nipple by dermal anchor sutures at the 12 o'clock position, followed by key dermal vertical sutures to orient the areolar complex. A round, inverted dermal suture is then placed to circle the skin. The authors have previously used a 3-0 Mersilene or Gore-Tex suture. Regardless of the suture, a straight needle serves best to allow the suture to follow the cut dermal edge (Fig. 34.5). It minimizes periareolar scalloping as is often observed when a half needle is used. A recent modification by Hammond suggests a wagon-wheel pattern to reduce tension and better distribute the force surrounding the areola. A 42-mm cookie cutter is used as a guide to size and shape the areola as the suture is tied. Final closure is subcuticular, Monocryl, or cuticular Prolene.

34.7.2
Vertical Component

If the periareolar skin excision is inadequate, a vertical limb or wedge is deepithelialized. This increases access for inserting the implant into the dissected pocket. The vertical wedge is tailor-tacked and adjusted to maximize projection without excessive tension. If the nipple is pushed up and appears "stargazing," the inframammary fold to areolar distance may need to be shortened. A triangle of skin is excised above the inframammary fold, creating a short-scar T-junction. This ensures and shortens the inframammary fold distance. The corners of the triangle are tapered upward to lie in the fold at final closure. This vertical limb shortening with reduction of the base width can increase projection while minimizing glandular ptosis.

34.8
Risks and Complications

All operations have risks, yet combining seemingly opposed surgical procedures intuitively multiplies them. Gorney et al. [8] discussed this as a combination of both cosmetic risk added to breast risk. Spear et al. [9] compared complication rates of augmentation, 1.7%, versus those of primary augmentation mastopexy at 17% and secondary augmentation mastopexy at 23%. Complications were expectedly high at 8.7–16.6% for revision augmentation mastopexy.

Surgeons should keep the following in mind:
1. There is increased risk of skin necrosis because an overly small envelope increases tension.
2. There is increased risk of nipple loss with an implant under the breast mound that relies on peripheral blood supply.
3. The incisions for the mastopexy may decrease peripheral blood supply.
4. Scar stretching is a concern, especially periareolar. Techniques to decrease this phenomenon include the Benelli blocking suture and the Hammond wagon wheel.
5. There is an increased risk of implant extrusion through extra incisions.
6. Nipple herniation is less than an ideal result when too large a nipple–areolar complex is pushed out of its pocket. Careful nipple release and a small nipple–areola complex could help prevent this.
7. Asymmetry and flattening of the breast may occur secondary to excess skin tension.
8. The worst complications of excessive skin excision occur during wide mediolateral dissection. All skin excision should remain within the preoperative markings and be tailor-tacked.
9. Other complications, hematoma (1–2%), or infection (1–4%) are comparable to other breast operations.

34.9
Conclusions

Augmentation mastopexy is an operation with conflicting goals. The augmentation increases the breast volume, which requires expanding the skin envelope. The mastopexy elevates the nipple, tightens the skin, and decreases the skin envelope. The third dimension is that all of these goals must be combined while maintaining nipple blood supply and sensation. Despite these opposing forces, augmentation mastopexy is a valuable combination to address a lack of skin envelope, pseudoglandular ptosis, and 1st-degree or mild 2nd-degree breast ptosis (Figs. 34.5, 34.6).

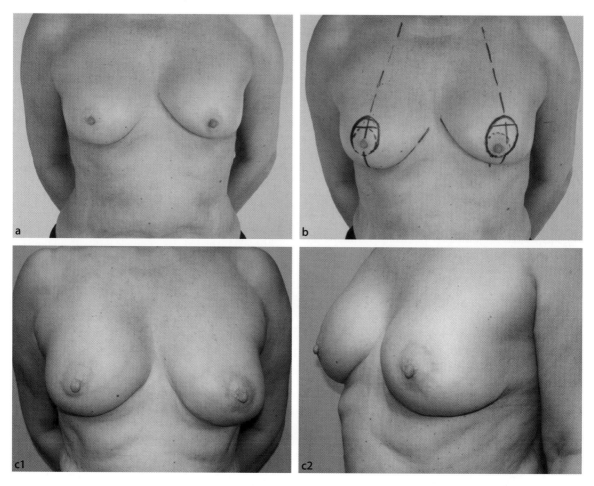

Fig. 34.6 a Preoperative 46-year-old woman with a 36B-cup breast size, ptotic nipples 1 cm below the inframammary line, and marked asymmetry. **b** Asymmetric operative plane. **c** *1* Eight months postoperative after augmentation with 300-ml saline implants and bilateral periareolar mastopexy. *2* Lateral view

Simultaneous augmentation and periareolar mastopexy are effective because enlargement of a breast with an implant helps fill out much of the excess ptotic skin, while the periareolar mastopexy removes the remaining excess and repositions the nipple. If a periareolar skin excess excision is inadequate, the addition of a vertical limb is a good solution. The addition of a permanent suture placed uniformly along the dermal edge reduces irregularities, scalloping, periareolar scar, and the risk of areolar widening. The success of this procedure depends on careful patient selection, planning, and careful surgical technique.

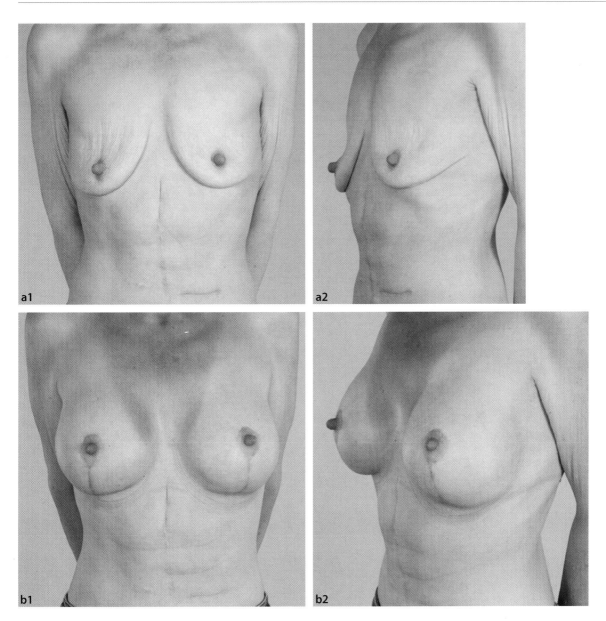

Fig. 34.7 a *1* Preoperative 56-year-old woman with a 34A-cup breast size, ptotic nipples below the inframammary line, and moderate asymmetry. *2* Lateral view. **b** *1* Four months postoperative after augmentation with 300-ml saline implants and bilateral circumvertical mastopexy. *2* Lateral view

References

1. Gonzalez-Ulloa M: Correction of hypotrophy of the breast by means of exogenous material. Plast Reconstr Surg 1960;25:15–26
2. Regnault P: The hypoplastic and ptotic breast: a combined operation with prosthetic augmentation. Plast Reconstr Surg 1966;37(1):31–37
3. Persoff MM: Vertical mastopexy with expansion augmentation. Aesthetic Plast Surg 2003;27(1):13–19
4. Gruber RP, Jones HW Jr: The "donut" mastopexy: indications and complications. Plast Reconstr Surg 1980;65(1):34–38
5. Benelli L: A new periareolar mammaplasty: the "round block" technique. Aesthetic Plast Surg 1990;14(2):93–100
6. Hammond DC, Khuthaila DK, Kim J: The interlocking Gore-Tex suture for control of the areolar diameter and shape. Plast Reconstr Surg 2007;19(3):804–809
7. Regnault P: Breast ptosis. Definition and treatment. Clin Plast Surg 1976;3(2):193–203
8. Gorney M, Maxwell PG, Spear SL: Augmentation mastopexy. Aesthetic Surg J 2005;5(3):275–284
9. Spear SL, Boehmier JH, Clemens MW: Augmentation/mastopexy: a 3-year review of a single surgeon's practice. Plast Reconstr Surg 2006;118(7 suppl):136S–147Svvv

CHAPTER 35

Mastopexy/Reduction and Augmentation Without Vertical Scar

35

Sid J. Mirrafati

35.1
Introduction

Breast lift or reduction is a common procedure frequently performed by a cosmetic breast surgeon. Breast reduction is a very satisfying procedure for the patient because she does not have to carry such a massive weight, and she experiences relief of lower back pain and/or shoulder pain radiating to the arm. The results are so satisfying that patients, for the most part, do not complain about the scarring that is left behind from the breast reduction procedure. In the case of breast lift with augmentation, patients are so happy with the new upright, fuller breast that they are not too concerned about the incisional scar.

But as cosmetic surgeons, we owe it to our patients to always strive for the best results with minimal incisions. Cosmetic surgeons around the world have been introducing new techniques to deliver results with minimal scarring. Several techniques have been introduced for the full breast lift/reduction procedure that entail having a vertical scar running down from the areola to the inframammary fold. The only scars that seem to bother most patients are the vertical scar and the scar on the sides when the inframammary scar is not kept under the breast, such as with the McKissock reduction and the Lejour technique.

The lift/reduction that the author uses avoids the vertical incisional scar and keeps the inframammary incisional scar invisible under the breast. This technique would not work for a woman with extremely large breasts that she would like to be moderately small or for an A-cup size, but it would work for most other instances. If the patient adamantly does not want the vertical scar and there is too much skin or the surface area is too large, then the inferior part of the vertical scar that is mostly hidden by the inferior pole of the breast can be added. This technique would work very well for the ptotic breast that requires a full breast lift and an augmentation.

35.2
Consultation

During the consultation it is important for the surgeon to completely assess the patient and review all the available options, especially for a ptotic breast for which the patient would like to have a moderately large implant. Generally in grade II ptosis, if the patient is willing to place a large implant and if the skin integrity is good with not many stretch marks, the patient can have a crescent lift with augmentation and can avoid the full lift. But in grade III ptosis, the patient would require a full breast lift no matter how big the implant size will be. The chest size is measured from the midline, going 2 cm laterally to the anterior axillary line. One centimeter is reduced from this measurement; this is the diameter of the implant that can be placed.

Even though the vertical scar is not created, the patients are still told about the other scars. They are told that the scar takes 1 year to become less visible. It will first look red, and then turn dark, and eventually will be the color of the skin.

35.3
Surgical Procedure

Preoperative photos are taken in a straightforward position, 45° angle, and 90° angle.

35.3.1
Marking

Preoperative markings are done (Fig. 35.1). The areola is marked with a cookie cutter with a 4-cm diameter. The new nipple position is marked by palpating the inframammary fold and transferring this to the surface of the breast. The new areolar position is marked with a 6-cm cookie cutter. The midclavicular line to the areo-

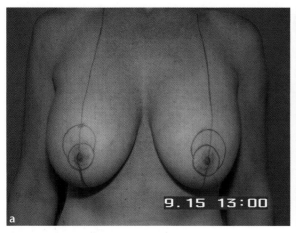 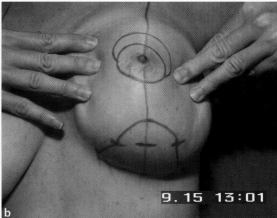

Fig. 35.1 a Marking the breast. **b** The inframammary line is drawn so that the line cannot be seen when the breast is placed in a relaxed position

lar superior pole is measured to be 19 cm, and if implant placement is planned, this measurement should be 20 cm. This precaution should be taken to make sure that the areola does not sit too high and show through the patient's bikini top or bra. The surgeon should be conservative because the areolar position can be made higher at a later time, but once it is pulled too high, it would be very difficult to lower the position. A 5-cm line is drawn from the inferior pole of the new areolar position.

The inframammary line is drawn so that the line cannot be seen when the breast is placed in a relaxed position. The medial and lateral aspects of the infra-mammary breast line are marked and then marked 1 cm further in from each side. This will ensure that the incision will not be visible after surgery. The breast is retracted laterally, and a straight line is drawn from the end of the 5-cm line to the inframammary fold. The breast is then retracted medially, and another line is drawn to the medial mark of the inframammary fold line. This will create a triangle that will be cut later to act as a support and to shape the breast.

The 5-cm vertical line can sometimes be extended if a large implant is planned, depending on the shape of the patient's chest and the size of the implant. The surgeon should double-check again to make sure the inframammary marking is not seen when the patient is standing. Sometimes, if the breast is very ptotic and there is too much skin, the marking is modified to have a vertical scar only on the inferior aspect 2 cm from the inframammary line. This is usually hidden by the lower pole of the breast when the surgery is completed.

35.3.2
Technique

The patient is placed in a supine position, and the breast is prepped with Betadine. If breast reduction, lift, and augmentation are to be performed, the procedure begins with the reduction. Tumescent fluid is injected into the breast until it is moderately firm and full. The tumescent fluid consists of 1 l of saline with 2 ml of 1:1,000 epinephrine and 500 mg of lidocaine. Approximately 500 ml is injected into each breast.

Liposuction may be performed to reduce the breast using a 5-mm open spiral cannula and a 4-mm cannula to fine-tune the area. The superior pole of the breast is usually not liposuctioned so that there will be good projection after surgery. If the breast is to be reduced by 500 g, then 500 ml is liposuctioned from each breast. This will require a lot of palpation to make sure that both breasts feel the same.

An incision is made along the preoperative markings around the areola as well as the new position of the areolar complex (Fig. 35.2). Deepithelialization of the skin is done as well as 1 cm of undermining.

The areola is lifted and anchored to its new position using 4-0 Monocryl. The four quadrants are evenly distributed and sutured to the areola using 4-0 Monocryl. The skin is closed using 5-0 nylon. There will be some pleating when the areola is completely closed. This will usually resolve, and the skin will become evenly retracted. If some pleating persists after 6 weeks, the surgeon should be patient because essentially all such pleating resolves by 6 months. If for some reason it does

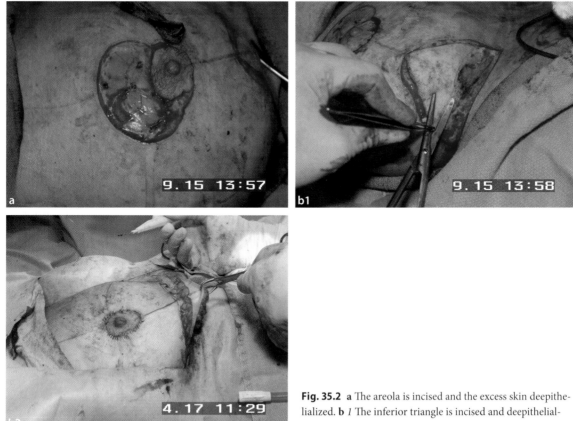

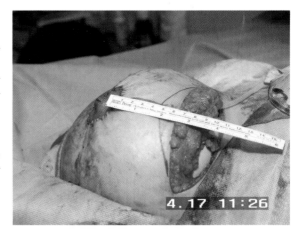

Fig. 35.2 a The areola is incised and the excess skin deepithelialized. **b** *1* The inferior triangle is incised and deepithelialized. *2* It can be resected if breast reduction is to be performed

not resolve after 6 months, revision can be done to even out the pleating.

The inframammary incision is performed and the dissection taken down to the pectoralis fascia. A pocket is developed in the subglandular plane. In reduction mammoplasty, the implant is generally placed in a subglandular plane unless the skin in the medial superior region is thin or the patient requests submuscular placement. In either situation a pocket is developed, and the implant is placed after proper hemostasis and antibiotic irrigation.

The triangle that was preoperatively marked is resected with the breast tissue (Fig. 35.2b). This is where the preoperative marking has to be modified depending on the size of the implant. The 5-cm line can be 6 cm or longer depending on the implant size (Fig. 35.3). The incisions may be modified to include an inferior vertical scar if the skin is too loose (Fig. 35.4). After the triangle is taken out, the incision is closed using 4-0 Monocryl subcutaneously, and the skin is closed using 5-0 nylon suture. A compression dressing is applied.

Fig. 35.3 The line from the lowest aspect of the areola to the superior point of the lower triangle should be 5 cm but can be adjusted to accommodate an implant

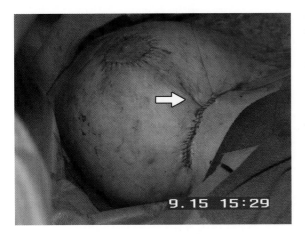

Fig. 35.4 Modify the markings to include an inferior vertical scar 2-cm long if the skin is too loose

toma, and incision healing, and she is told to apply antibiotic ointment to the incision and to change the dressings daily. Patients are given simple arm exercises and can take showers starting 48 h after the surgery. They are told to continue taking Keflex 500 mg twice daily and 2,000–3,000 mg of vitamin C daily.

35.5
Complications

Other than one patient having hypertrophic scarring around the areola, there have been no other complications. Sometimes when the implant size is large, there is an indentation in the center that will stretch out in time. There is always some settling or sometimes "bottoming out" of the lift with time, but this is a problem that can occur with any lift or reduction procedure.

35.4
Postoperative Care

The patient should be seen on the 1st postoperative day. The dressing is changed and the compression dressing left off. In this technique of reduction mammoplasty or mastopexy, there is no real concern about nipple–areolar necrosis because there is no vertical incision. The patient is examined for proper implant position, hema-

35.6
Conclusions

This lift avoids the most unwanted and most obvious scar associated with a breast lift or reduction procedure, the vertical scar (Fig. 35.5). Many different types of lifts have been introduced in textbooks and the literature, but they mostly involve the vertical scar, which this technique avoids. Patient satisfaction is high, and the complication rate is very low.

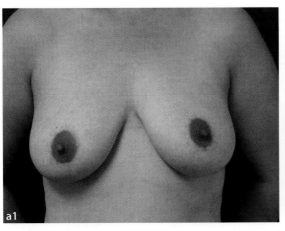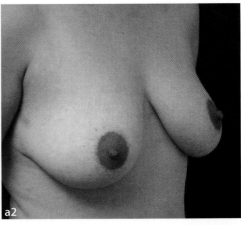

Fig. 35.5 a *1* Preoperative patient. *2* Lateral view

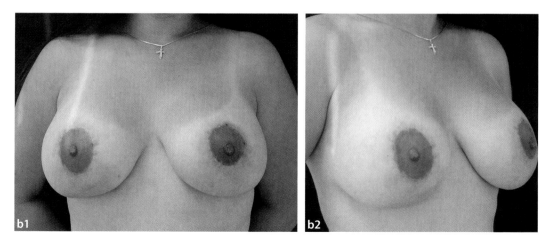

Fig. 35.5 *(continued)* **b** *1* Postoperative. *2* No visible inframammary fold scar, and no vertical scar

CHAPTER 36

Classification of the Tuberous Breast

36

Melvin A. Shiffman

36.1 Introduction

The tuberous breast has multiple variations, and in order to treat the problem, the surgeon must understand these varieties. By identifying the type of classification used, the physician can communicate better with referring physicians and consultants and during litigation.

36.2 Von Heimburg Classification

A modified classification was reported by von Heimburg [1], which varied from the original article published in 1996 [2]. This classification consists of four types (Fig. 36.1):

Type I: Hypoplasia of the lower medial quadrant
Type II: Hypoplasia of the lower medial and lateral quadrants
Type III: Hypoplasia of the lower medial and lateral quadrants with deficiency of the skin in the subareolar region
Type IV: Severe breast constriction with minimal breast base

36.3 Grolleau Classification

Grolleau et al. [3] described three variations in the tuberous breast, which were derived from the von Heimburg classification (Fig. 36.2):

Type I: Hypoplasia of the lower medial quadrant
Type II: Hypoplasia of both lower quadrants
Type III: Hypoplasia of all four quadrants

Grolleau et al. proposed that the cause of the tuberous breast was from anomalies of the fascia superficialis that involve strong adherence between the dermis and the muscular plane, restricting peripheral expansion of the breast during breast development at puberty. Mammaplasty techniques that were used varied according to the type of deformity.

36.4 Discussion

Surgically, each type of tuberous breast deformity is treated differently according to the specific defect.

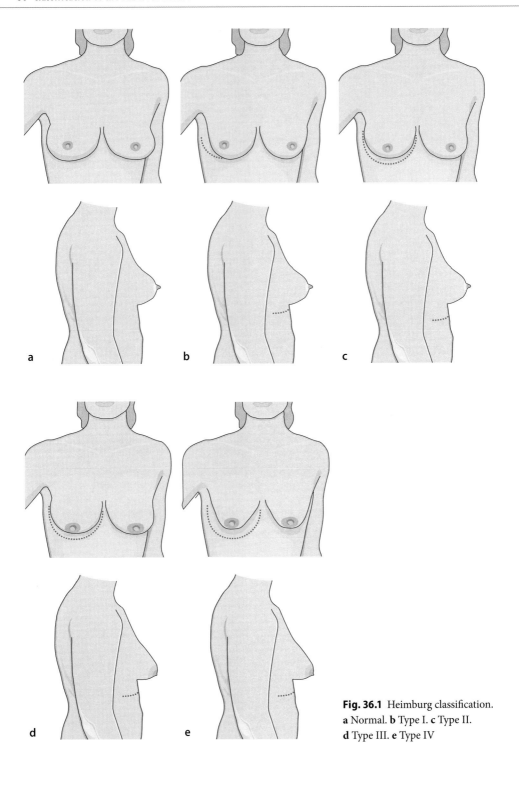

Fig. 36.1 Heimburg classification.
a Normal. **b** Type I. **c** Type II.
d Type III. **e** Type IV

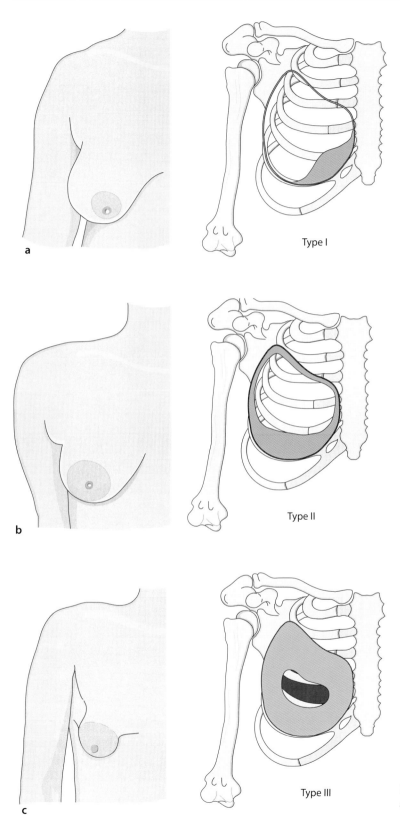

Type I

Type II

Type III

Fig. 36.2 Grolleau et al. classification.
a Type I. **b** Type II. **c** Type III

References

1. von Heimburg D: Refined version of the tuberous breast classification. Plast Reconstr Surg 2000;105(6):2269–2270
2. von Heimburg D, Exner K, Kruft S, Lemperle S: The tuberous breast deformity: classification and treatment. Br J Plast Surg 1996;49(6):339–345
3. Grolleau J-L, Lanfrey E, Lavigne B, Chavoin JP, Costagliola M: Breast base anomalies: treatment strategy for tuberous breasts, minor deformities, and asymmetry. Plast Reconstr Surg 1999;104(7):2040–2048

The Incidence of Tuberous Breast Deformity in Asymmetric and Symmetric Mammaplasty Patients

Danielle DeLuca-Pytell, Rocco C. Piazza, Julie C. Holding, Ned Snyder, Lisa M. Hunsicker, Linda G. Phillips

37.1
Introduction

Tuberous breast deformity is characterized by an aberration of breast shape. Characteristics include a constricted breast base, hypoplastic breast tissue, herniated nipple–areola complex, deficient skin envelope inferiorly, and elevated inframammary fold [1]. Other names for tuberous breast deformity include herniated areola complex, Snoopy deformity, tubular breast, constricted breast, lower-pole hypoplasia, and narrow-based breast [1, 2]. Although many authors have described their approach to the surgical correction for tuberous breast deformity, none have clearly addressed how to identify tuberous deformities and anomalies associated with tuberous breasts in the full spectrum of surgical breast candidates. This is the first study to focus on the incidence and identification of tuberous breast deformity in all patients seeking changes in their breast size, not just those seeking corrections for asymmetry. By applying the classification set forth by Grolleau et al., our definition of tuberous breasts includes a spectrum of deformity ranging from minor to severe (or classic) tuberous breast deformity. This study presents the incidence of tuberous breast deformity among women with symmetric and asymmetric breasts who presented to our clinic over a 10-year period. These results will aid in clearly identifying the deformity before operative management to aid in optimal postsurgical outcomes. Most importantly, this is the first large study to demonstrate that tuberous deformity is strongly associated with asymmetry.

37.2
Technique

A retrospective analysis was performed on standard preoperative photographs of 616 female patients presenting to our plastic surgery clinic desiring augmentation or reduction mammaplasty. Of the 616 patients, 50% (n=308) presented for breast augmentation mammaplasty, 45.3% (n=279) for breast reduction mammaplasty, and 4.7% (n=29) for mastopexy. Women were excluded if they had congenital anomalies, tumors, infection, radiation, chest wall deformities, previous breast surgery, or incomplete chart data. After exclusion, 375 women were included in this study [51.2% (n=192) for breast augmentation mammaplasty, 47.2% (n=160) for breast reduction mammaplasty, and 6.1% (n=23) for mastopexy].

The presence of symmetry versus asymmetry, tuberous deformity, and nipple–areola involvement was evaluated by a minimum of five evaluators, including two medical students, three junior and senior residents, and one senior author. Every case was analyzed by visual inspection of photographs, by volume of implant fill, and by the amount of tissue removed. A minimum of five photographs were viewed for each case and always included the right lateral and oblique, the left lateral and oblique, and anterior–posterior views. Patients were analyzed until a consensus was achieved.

By applying the conclusions set forth by Grolleau et al., we have defined tuberous deformity as a spectrum of deformity ranging from minor to severe (or classic) tuberous deformity. Tuberous deformity classification was assigned using Grolleau's classification system [3] (Table 37.1, Fig. 37.1). Type I tuberous breasts are defined as a lower, medial base constriction that projects

Table 37.1 Tuberous deformity classification

Type I	Lower medial quadrant deficient
Type II	Both lower quadrants deficient
Type III	All four quadrants deficient with constriction of breast base horizontally and vertically

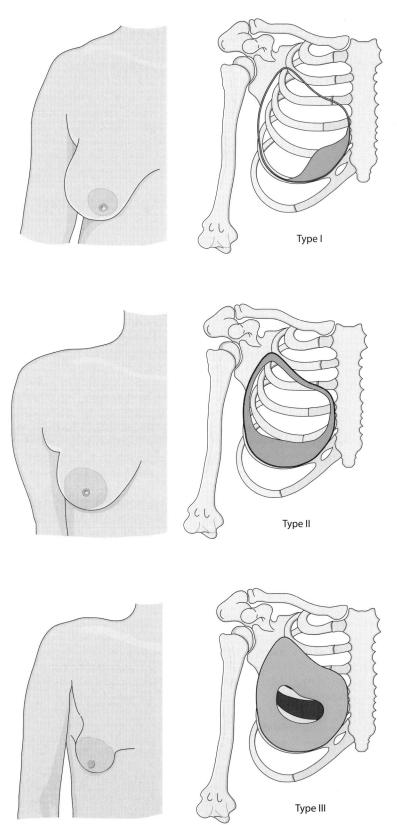

Fig. 37.1 Examples of tuberous deformity using Grolleau's classification system [3]. Consensus by evaluators was achieved in all examples. **a** Type I breasts have a deficiency of breast tissue at the lower medial quadrant. **b** Type II breasts have a deficiency of breast tissue in both the lower medial and lateral quadrants. **c** Type III breasts are deficient in all quadrants, with a constriction of the breast base vertically and horizontally

Table 37.2 Asymmetry classification

Type I	Unilateral micromastia
Type II	Unilateral macromastia
Type III	Micromastia and macromastia
Type IV	Bilateral asymmetric micromastia
Type V	Bilateral asymmetric macromastia

as a deficiency of breast tissue at the lower medial quadrant. Type II breasts are defined as a lower, medial, and lateral base constriction that projects as a deficiency of breast tissue at the lower medial and lateral quadrants. Type III breasts are deficient in all quadrants as a result of constriction of the breast base vertically and horizontally. Determination of the tuberous deformity was made if the deficiency was clearly visible in the breast mound, the nipple–areola complex, or both. Nipple–areola involvement was also noted.

If the patient was asymmetric based on visual assessment, implant fill, or amount of tissue removed, she was assigned to an asymmetry classification using Elsahy's system [4] (Table 37.2, Fig. 37.2). Elsahy categorizes asymmetry as type I patients with unilateral micromastia, type II patients with unilateral macromastia, type III patients with both micromastia and macromastia, type IV patients with bilateral asymmetric micromastia, and type V patients with bilateral asymmetric macromastia.

37.3
Results

Of the 375 consecutive patients analyzed, 304 patients (81.1%) demonstrated breast asymmetry, and 71 (18.9%) presented with breast symmetry (Table 37.3). This includes patients requesting evaluation for breast hypertrophy and patients desiring breast augmentation. The most common asymmetry was type IV (bilateral asymmetric micromastia), occurring in 59.2% of patients (n=180), followed by type V asymmetry (bilateral asymmetric macromastia) in 38.2% (n=116) of the asymmetric patients studied. Types I, II, and III asymmetry were less common, with only 2% of the patients (n=6) presenting with unilateral micromastia or macromastia, and only 0.7% (n=2) of the patients presenting with combined micromastia/macromastia.

Tuberous breast deformity was found in a total of 275 women—in 270 (88.8%) of the 304 patients with asymmetry and five (7%) of the 71 patients who were symmetric. Tuberous deformity was found in a total of 95 (59%) of all breast reductions and 180 of all breast augmentations (84.1%) done at our facility over a 10-year period (Table 37.4). Type III deformities were most common, comprising 60.3% of all tuberous deformity (n=320) in our study. Types I and II were less common, with 15.6% (n=83) and 24.1% (n=125), respectively. Nipple–areola complex involvement was found in 42.2% (n=116) of patients with all types of tuberous breast deformity. Type III deformity was most commonly accompanied by nipple–areola involvement compared with the other tubular deformities, at 87.9% (n=102).

37.4
Discussion

This large series of consecutive patients presented primarily with complaints of micromastia or macromastia. Stringent retrospective analysis reveals an 81.1% frequency of asymmetry. It is the first study using the Grolleau classification of breast base deformities to demonstrate that 88% of asymmetric patients are constricted, resulting in a spectrum of tuberous deformities (Table 37.5).

Our study confirms that most women have some degree of breast asymmetry [5]. This is in contrast to Pitanguy, who found asymmetry in only 4% of 1,400 patients presenting for breast treatment [6]. Smith et al. state in their 1986 study that asymmetry is common, but asymmetry severe enough to warrant plastic surgery is rare [7]. In a review of the literature on asymmetry and tuberous deformity, a variety of findings have been presented from studies of as few as 16 to as many as 76 women [1, 2, 4, 7, 8]. In a study by Meara et al., unilateral tuberous deformity was more commonly seen than bilateral [1]. Von Heimburg et al., however, found bilateral tuberous deformity to be more common [2]. Von Heimburg types II and III, which correspond to Grolleau's tuberous deformity type II, were less common separately but the most common deformity when combined. Our results, however, found only 24.1% of Grolleau's type II deformity and 60.3% to be Grolleau's type III. Von Heimburg noted that the more severe the tuberous deformity, the greater the incidence of areolar involvement. Our results supported this in that 87.9% of our population with tuberous deformity and concurrent nipple–areola complex were classified as the more severe type III tuberous deformity. Von Heimburg also stated that asymmetry is found more commonly with tuberous deformity than with simple micromastia or macromastia [2]. This mirrors our data, which demonstrated an 81.1% prevalence of asymmetry, of which 88.8% of patients were tuberous. Rohrich et al. found

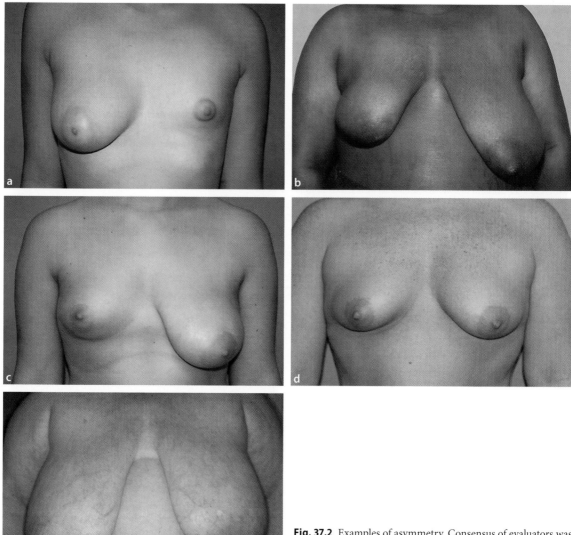

Fig. 37.2 Examples of asymmetry. Consensus of evaluators was achieved in all examples. **a** Unilateral micromastia. **b** Unilateral macromastia. **c** Micromastia and macromastia. **d** Bilateral asymmetric micromastia. **e** Bilateral asymmetric macromastia

an 88% prevalence of some degree of asymmetry in a retrospective analysis of 100 random patients presenting for breast augmentation [9].

The strong relationship between tuberous deformity and breast asymmetry has not previously been demonstrated. Of our 304 patients presenting for mammaplasty, 81.1% demonstrated visible asymmetry, and of those, 88.8% (*n*= 270) exhibited tuberous deformity. We believe that our study underscores the importance of assessing the presence of asymmetry and tuberous deformity in all women who present for mammaplasty. Increased awareness of the spectrum of these breast

anomalies will facilitate planning so that surgical approaches can be optimized preoperatively. Improved breast contour, such as avoidance of the "double bubble" with implant use, can be achieved. Patients may also benefit from increased understanding of their bodies, and may in turn develop more realistic expectations for their postoperative results.

This study has the inherent self-selection bias of women desiring mammaplasty. To decrease this bias, future studies are planned to determine the incidence of asymmetry and tuberous deformity in women presenting for well-woman physical examinations. Our vi-

Table 37.3

Data summary (*NAC* nipple–areola complex)							
		Included	Tubular	Nontubular	Asymmetric	Symmetric	NAC
No. of patients		(%)	(%) (*n*=275)	(%) (*n*=100)	(%) (*n*=304)	(%) (*n*=71)	(%) (*n*=117)
Included	375	100	—	—	—	—	—
Tubular (unilateral or bilateral)	275	73.33	100	—	—	—	—
Nontubular	100	26.67	—	100	—	—	—
Asymmetric	304	81.07	—	—	100	—	—
Symmetric	71	18.93	—	—	—	100	—
NAC	117	31.20	—	—	—	—	100
Tubular and asymmetric	270	72	98.18	—	88.82	—	—
Tubular and symmetric	5	1.33	1.82	—	—	7.04	—
Symmetric nontubular	66	17.60	—	66	—	92.96	—
Asymmetric nontubular	34	9.07	—	34	11.18	—	—
Asymmetric and NAC	117	31.20	—	—	38.49	—	100
Symmetric and NAC	0	0	—	—	—	0	0
Tubular and NAC	116	30.93	42.18	—	—	—	99.15
Nontubular and NAC	1	0.27	—	1	—	—	0.85

Table 37.4 Number of patients for each mammaplasty procedure (*NAC* nipple–areola complex)

Procedures	Total no. of patients	Asymmetric (%)	Symmetric (%)	Tubular (%)	NAC involvement (%)	Asymmetric with tubular (%)	Symmetric with tubular (%)
Augmentations	214	184 (85.98)	30 (14.02)	180 (84.11)	92 (42.99)	178 (83.18)	2 (0.93)
Reductions	161	120 (74.53)	41 (25.47)	95 (59.01)	25 (15.53)	92 (57.14)	3 (1.86)
Mastopexies	23	22 (95.65)	1 (4.35)	22 (95.65)	11 (47.83)	22 (95.65)	

sual assessment of asymmetry and tuberous deformity is also subject to bias; however, in a study by Malata et al. on the measurement of breast symmetry, no significant error was noted for visual assessment of breast symmetry alone when compared with more quantified methods [10].

Asymmetry exists on a continuum, with perfect symmetry on one end and severe asymmetry on the other. By evaluating all women who presented for mammaplasty as opposed to those who self-select by presenting with asymmetry, the authors were able to evaluate

Table 37.5 Breasts with Grolleau tubular deformity classification (*n*=275)

Grolleau class	No. of breasts	Total tubular
1	83	15.6%
2	125	24.1%
3	320	60.3%
Total	531	100%

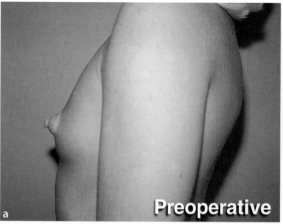
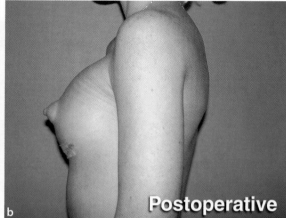

Fig. 37.3 a Preoperative patient with nipple–areola complex herniation before placement of implants. **b** Accentuation of nipple–areola complex herniation after breast augmentation demonstrates the importance of addressing this deformity preoperatively

not only those severe cases but also moderate and mild cases that were previously unrecognized. Tuberous deformity, nipple–areola complex involvement, and breast asymmetry may contribute to a patient's preoperative decision to seek surgical correction, and also, if the problems are not corrected intraoperatively, to postoperative dissatisfaction. It is essential that patients be evaluated for asymmetry and, thus, tuberous deformity so that these breast abnormalities may be identified and addressed during preoperative planning to ensure an optimal outcome for the patient.

37.5
Conclusions

This is the first study to demonstrate that tuberous deformity exists on a spectrum, from minor to severe, and is strongly associated with breast asymmetry in the mammaplasty population. It should be considered in the preoperative planning of all asymmetric women to ensure optimal outcome and patient satisfaction (Fig. 37.3).

In addition, this is also the first study to demonstrate that all of the patients with nipple–areola complex constriction are asymmetric and that 99% of patients with the constriction are tuberous. Of the tuberous nipple–areola complex constricted population, 87.9% had a type III tuberous deformity.

References

1. Meara JG, Kolker A, Bartlett G, Theile R, Mutimer K, Holmes AD: Tuberous breast deformity: principles and practice. Ann Plast Surg 2000;45:607–610
2. von Heimburg D, Exner K, Kruft S, Lemperle G: The tuberous breast deformity: classification and treatment. Br J Plast Surg 1996;49(6):339–345
3. Grolleau JL, Lanfrey E, Lavigne B, Chavoin JP, Costagliola M: Breast base anomalies: treatment strategy for tuberous breast, minor deformities, and asymmetry. Plast Reconstr Surg 1999;104(7):2040–2048
4. Elsahy NI: Correction of asymmetries of the breast. Plast Reconstr Surg 1976;57(6):700–703
5. Bostwick J: Breast asymmetry. In: Bostwick J (ed). Plastic and Reconstructive Breast Surgery, vol 5. St. Louis, Quality Medical Publishing 1999, p 634
6. Elliott RA: Asymmetric breasts. In: Georgiade NG, Georgiade GS, Riefkohl R (eds). Aesthetic Surgery of the Breast. Philadelphia, WB Saunders 1990, p135
7. Smith DJ, Palin WE, Katch V, Bennett JE: Surgical treatment of congenital breast asymmetry. Ann Plast Surg 1986;17(2):92–101
8. Kuzbari R, Deutinger M, Todoroff BP, Schneider B, Freilinger G: Surgical treatment of developmental asymmetry of the breast: long term results. Scand J Plast Reconstr Hand Surg 1993;27(3):203–207
9. Rohrich RJ, Hartley W, Brown S: Incidence of breast and chest wall asymmetry in breast augmentation: a retrospective analysis of 100 patients. Plast Reconstr Surg 2003;111(4):1513–1519
10. Malata CM, Boot JC, Bradbury ARB, Sharpe DT: Congenital breast asymmetry: subjective and objective assessment. Br J Plast Surg 1994;47(2):95–102

CHAPTER 38

Aesthetic Reconstruction of the Tuberous Breast Deformity

Apostolos D. Mandrekas, George J. Zambacos

38.1
Introduction

The tuberous breast deformity is a rare entity affecting teenage women unilaterally or bilaterally [1, 2]. Its exact incidence has not been properly investigated and remains unknown [1, 2]. Nonetheless, this deformity produces much psychological morbidity and presents a reconstructive challenge for the plastic surgeon.

The tuberous breast deformity was first described in 1976 by Rees and Aston [3] and was thus named because "it resembled the shape of a tuberous plant root." Unfortunately, in that same, seminal paper the authors described another "similar," as they said, deformity, the "tubular breast," and since then several papers have been published on the subject, each using its own nomenclature and producing much confusion among plastic surgeons [4].

Tuberous breasts [3, 5], tubular breasts [3, 5, 6], Snoopy breasts [5–9], herniated areolar complex [5, 6, 9, 10], domed nipple [9, 10], nipple breast [9, 11], constricted breast [6], lower-pole hypoplasia [5, 6], and narrow-based breast [5, 6] are some of the names used to describe this deformity or so-called new deformities, which under careful inspection are no different from the original one described by Rees and Aston.

The essence of the matter remains that there is deficiency in the vertical and/or horizontal dimensions of the breast (Fig. 38.1), usually underdevelopment of the breast, and often herniation of breast tissue into the areola with expansion of the areola [1–3, 6, 8–10, 12–14].

38.2
History

Since Rees and Aston's description, several authors have attempted to describe, classify, and correct the problem, using various methods with varying results [1, 2, 4–21].

Rees and Aston [3] described a technique of radial incisions on the posterior aspect of the breast parenchyma to release the constriction and allow the breast to assume a more natural shape. Vecchione, also in 1976 [22], described the donut-type periareolar excision for correcting the "domed nipple." Williams and Hoffman [23] described a technique with periareolar excision, radial incisions on the posterior aspect of the breast parenchyma, and implant placement. Toranto [1] used a two-stage technique, with implant augmentation in the first stage and an Arie–Pitanguy type of skin–areola reduction at a second stage.

Ribeiro at al. [15] recognized the need to release the constricted breast, but they concentrated on a horizontal division of the inferior part of the breast, developing an inferiorly based flap. Puckett developed a similar "unfurling" technique (C. Gasperoni, personal communication, 1998). Dinner and Dowden [12] and Elliott [16] believed the deformity was due to skin shortage in the inferior part of the breast and followed a different

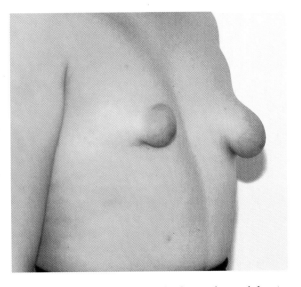

Fig. 38.1 Typical case of bilateral tuberous breast deformity with deficiency in both the vertical and horizontal dimensions of the breast, underdevelopment of the breast, and herniation of breast tissue toward the areola and expansion of the areola on the left side

approach using skin flaps from the inframammary fold. Muti [20] also developed a technique based on inferiorly based glandular flaps coupled with the use of silicone implants.

38.3
Anatomy and Embryology

Embryologically, the breast comes from the mammary ridge that develops in utero from the ectoderm during the 5th week of gestation [24, 25]. Shortly after its formation (7th–8th weeks), most parts of this ridge disappear except for a small portion in the thoracic region that persists and penetrates the underlying mesenchyme (10–14 weeks) [25]. Further differentiation and development of the breast occurs during intrauterine life and is completed by the time of birth, after which essentially no further development occurs until puberty [24].

The next series of steps in the development of the breast is activated at puberty in the female, consisting of growth of the mammary tissue beneath the areola with enlargement of the areola until the age of 15–16, when the breast assumes its familiar shape [24–26].

As a result of the ectodermal origin of the breast and its invagination into the underlying mesenchyme, the breast tissue is contained within a fascial envelope, the superficial fascia [24, 25, 27]. This superficial fascia is continuous with the superficial abdominal fascia of Camper and consists of two layers: the superficial layer of the superficial fascia, which is the outer layer covering the breast parenchyma, and the deep layer of the superficial fascia, which forms the posterior boundary of the breast parenchyma and lies on the deep fascia of the pectoralis major and serratus anterior muscles [24, 25, 27]. The deep layer of the superficial fascia is penetrated by fibrous attachments called the suspensory ligaments of Cooper, joining the two layers of the superficial fascia and extending to the dermis of the overlying skin and the deep pectoral fascia [24, 25, 27].

A critical point in understanding the tuberous breast deformity is the fact that the superficial layer of the superficial fascia is absent in the area underneath the areola, as can easily be demonstrated by the invagination of the mammary bud in the mesenchyme [26].

Clinical experience has shown [2, 15] that in cases of tuberous breasts there is a constricting fibrous ring at the level of the periphery of the nipple–areola complex inhibiting the normal development of the breast. This constricting ring of fibrous tissue is denser at the lower part of the breast and does not allow the developing breast parenchyma to expand during puberty. Histology has confirmed the existence of such dense fibrous

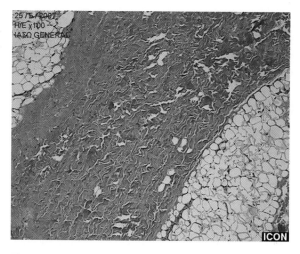

Fig. 38.2 Hematoxyline/eosin staining of tissue taken from the clinically palpable fibrous ring (×100). Dense fibrosis with stromal thickening and large concentrations of collagen and elastic fibers, arranged longitudinally

tissue in the area of this constricting ring. Specimens from two of our patients have been examined, and they showed large concentrations of collagen and elastic fibers, arranged longitudinally (Fig. 38.2). This ring represents a thickening of the superficial fascia. Perhaps the two layers of this fascia join at a higher level than usual, or the suspensory ligaments are thicker and more dense [5].

The result in either case is that the developing breast cannot expand inferiorly [5], and because there is no superficial layer of the superficial fascia under the areola, the breast parenchyma herniates toward the nipple–areola complex. The severity of the deformity depends on the severity of the malformation of the superficial fascia and ranges from slight underdevelopment of the inferior medial quadrant of the breast with near-normal breast volume, to major hypoplasia of all four quadrants with various degrees of herniation of the breast parenchyma toward the areola, as has been described in several classifications submitted over the years [5, 6, 14, 28]. The authors have adopted the classification of Grolleau et al. [5] (Fig. 38.3), according to which the deficiency of the lower medial quadrant is type I, deficiency of both lower quadrants is type II, and deficiency of all four quadrants is type III. Based on this understanding of the anatomical basis of the deformity, the authors were able to develop a protocol for treatment of the tuberous breast deformity that relies on correcting the anatomical malformations.

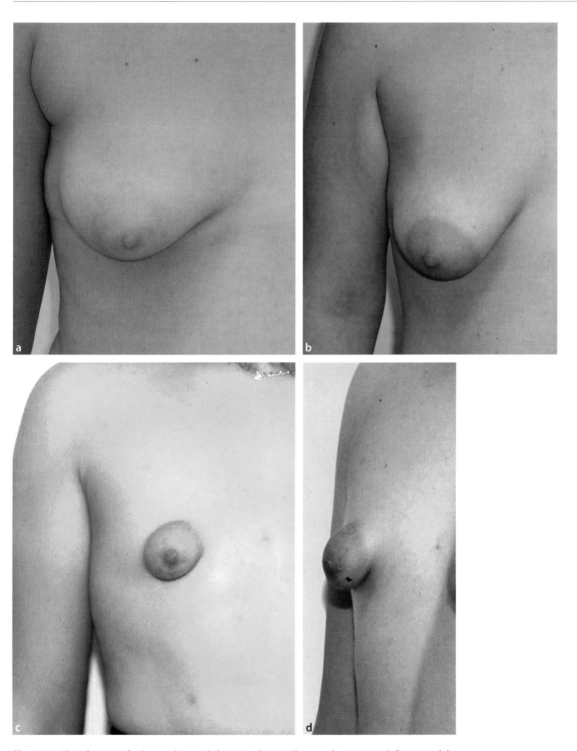

Fig. 38.3 Classification of tuberous breast deformity after Grolleau et al. **a** Type I: deficiency of the lower medial quadrant. **b** Type II: deficiency of both lower quadrants. **c** Type III: deficiency of all four quadrants. **d** Lateral view

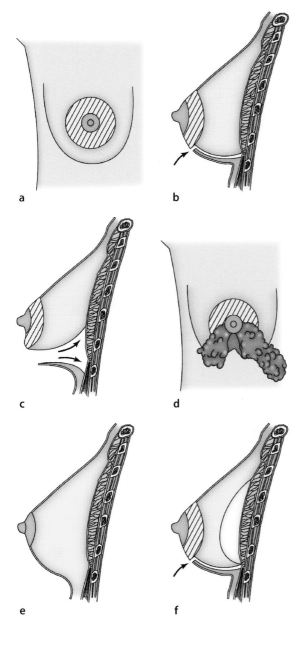

◄ **Fig. 38.4** Operative technique (schematic diagrams). **a** Periareolar donut-type skin deepithelialization. **b** The skin of the inferior half of the breast is undermined down to the pectoralis fascia with sharp dissection. **c** The dissection continues further down toward the new inframammary fold and then upward, behind the breast with blunt dissection. The breast parenchyma is dissected off the deep pectoral fascia, leaving only the superior part of the breast attached. **d** The breast parenchyma is exteriorized through the periareolar opening. The exteriorized inferior half of the breast is transected with a vertical incision along the middle. **e,f** If necessary, a silicone breast implant is used to augment the breast. The implant can be placed in a purely subglandular or a dual-plane position (upper part submuscular, lower part subcutaneous/subglandular), depending on the individual patient's configuration

38.4
Techniques

The procedure begins with the preoperative marking of the new inframammary fold in the standing and supine positions, by projection of the contralateral breast in unilateral cases or by using the 6th rib as a landmark in bilateral cases [8]. The breast is infiltrated with a li-

docaine/epinephrine solution (20 ml of 0.5% lidocaine solution with 1:400,000 epinephrine) [29].

A periareolar donut-type skin deepithelialization is performed to reduce the areola to the desired size, usually 4–4.5 cm in diameter (Figs. 38.4, 38.5). The skin of the inferior half of the breast is undermined down to the pectoralis fascia with sharp dissection (Fig. 38.4). Once the lower border of the breast parenchyma is reached, the dissection continues further down toward the new inframammary fold and then upward, behind the breast, along the natural plane between the deep layer of the superficial fascia and the deep fascia bluntly (Fig. 38.4). The breast parenchyma is dissected off the deep pectoral fascia, leaving only the superior part of the breast attached. The dissection is also extended laterally and medially, and the breast parenchyma is exteriorized through the periareolar opening (Fig. 38.5). The exteriorized inferior half of the breast is transected with a vertical incision along the middle (Figs. 38.4, 38.5). The constricting fibrous ring is thus divided, and two breast pillars are created (Fig. 38.5), which allow the breast parenchyma to redrape, assuming a more natural shape. If the pillars are short, they are simply loosely approximated using absorbable sutures (4/0 Vicryl, Ethicon). If the two pillars are long, then the proximal parts are again approximated using absorbable sutures, and the distal parts are either allowed to redrape freely or are folded over each other like a double-breasted jacket to create added volume in the inferior portion of the breast. On rare occasions, we can secure the lower part of the pillars at the new inframammary fold with bolster-type sutures. This is the case when the pillars are very short and they do not freely reach the new inframammary fold.

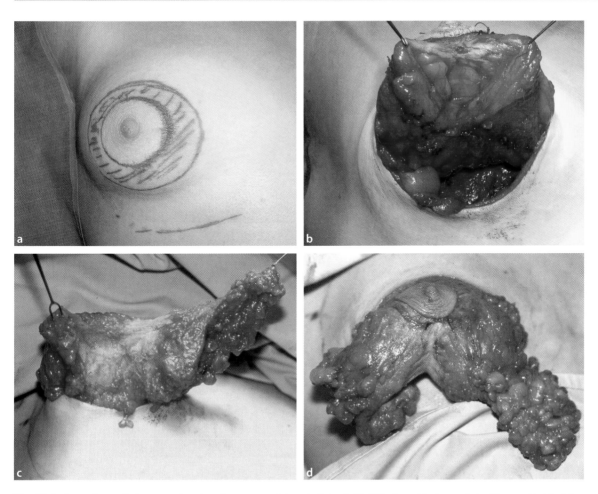

Fig. 38.5 Operative technique, periareolar donut-type skin deepithelialization. **a** Skin markings. **b** The breast parenchyma is exteriorized through the periareolar opening. **c** The exteriorized inferior half of the breast is transected with a vertical incision along the middle. **d** The constricting fibrous ring is divided, and two breast pillars are created

If necessary, a silicone breast implant is used to augment the breast. The implant can be placed in a purely subglandular or a dual-plane position (upper part submuscular, lower part subcutaneous/subglandular), depending on the individual patient's configuration (Fig. 38.4). Care should be taken to ensure that the pillars cover the implant in its entirety. The decision to use a breast implant is usually made at the preoperative consultation at which the physician and patient discuss whether additional volume will be required. Round textured silicone gel implants are usually used. The periareolar incision is sutured in layers with deep subcutaneous and intradermal sutures, using long-lasting dissolvable material (4/0 PDS or Monocryl, Ethicon). So far, with a maximum follow-up of 9 years, we have not had any problems with stretching of the periareolar scar.

The resulting breast has a normal-size areola, a natural shape, a volume matching the contralateral breast, and no evidence of the "double-bubble" deformity (Figs. 38.6–38.9).

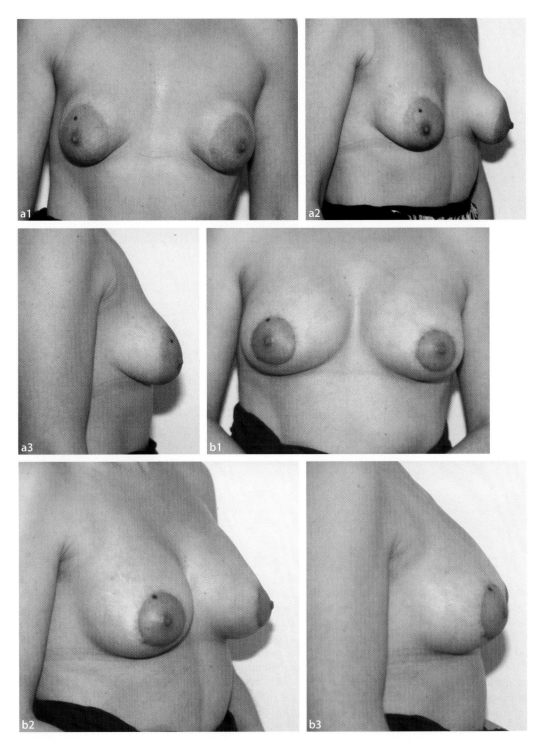

Fig. 38.6 a *1* Preoperative 46-year-old woman with a previous failed attempt to reconstruct a bilateral type II tuberous breast deformity with subglandular placement of 110-ml silicone breast implants. *2* Both breasts are constricted in both the vertical and horizontal axes, with herniation of the breast parenchyma toward the nipple–areola complex and increased size of the areola. *3* Lateral view. **b** Four months after periareolar donut-type deepithelialization was followed by removal of the implants, capsulectomy, dissection of the breast parenchyma, division of the fibrous ring with development of two pillars, and placement of 275-ml implants in the same subglandular pocket. *2,3* Lateral views

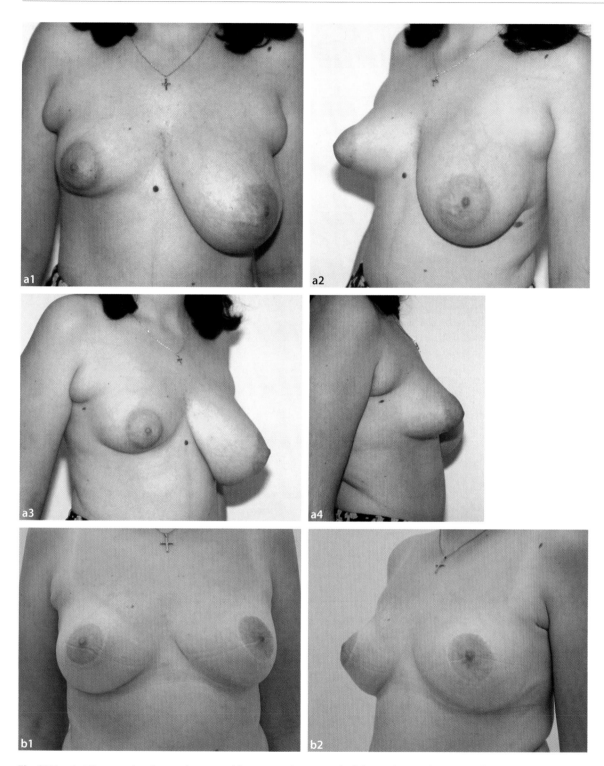

Fig. 38.7 **a** *1–4* Preoperative photos of 23-year-old patient with type II right tuberous breast deformity with hypoplasia of the inferior pole, herniation of the breast parenchyma toward the nipple–areola complex, and moderately increased areolar diameter. The left breast is slightly large with Regnault's class A ptosis [31]. **b** *1–4* Photos taken 1 year after the right breast had a periareolar donut-type deepithelialization and readjustment of the breast parenchyma without the use of an implant and the left breast had an inferior pedicle-type breast reduction coupled with excision of the axillary tail of Spence

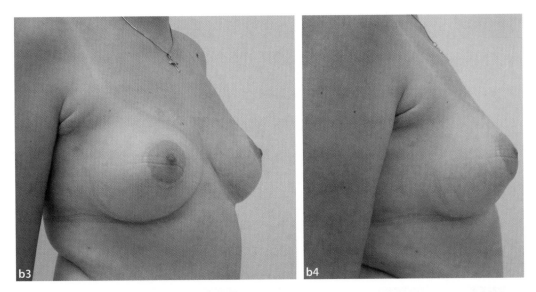

Fig. 38.7 *(continued)* **b** *1–4* Photos taken 1 year after the right breast had a periareolar donut-type deepithelialization and readjustment of the breast parenchyma without the use of an implant and the left breast had an inferior pedicle-type breast reduction coupled with excision of the axillary tail of Spence

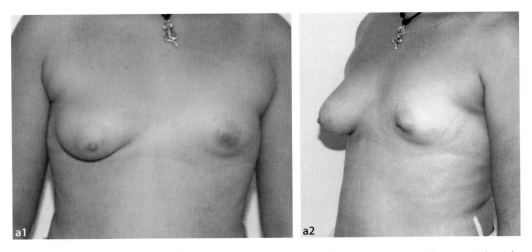

Fig. 38.8 a *1* Preoperative 17-year-old patient with bilateral asymmetrical tuberous breast deformity. *2* The right breast is characterized by underdevelopment of the inferior pole (type II)

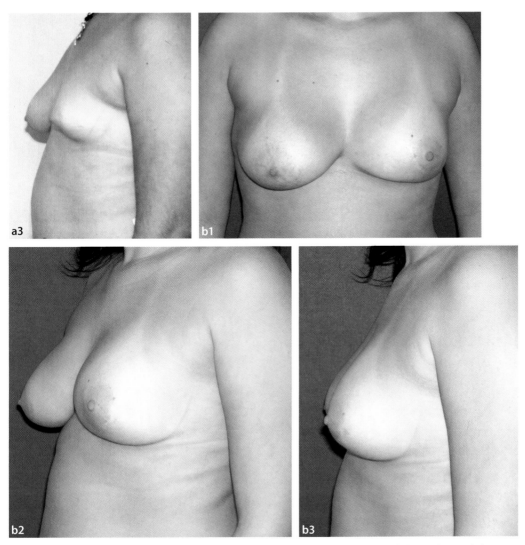

Fig. 38.8 *(continued)* **a** *3* On the patient's left side, there is severe hypoplasia of the whole breast (type III). **b** *1* Four years postoperative. *2* Both breasts were treated with semicircular periareolar incision, readjustment of the breast parenchyma, and subglandular placement of silicone breast implants (right 200 ml, left 300 ml). *3* Lateral view

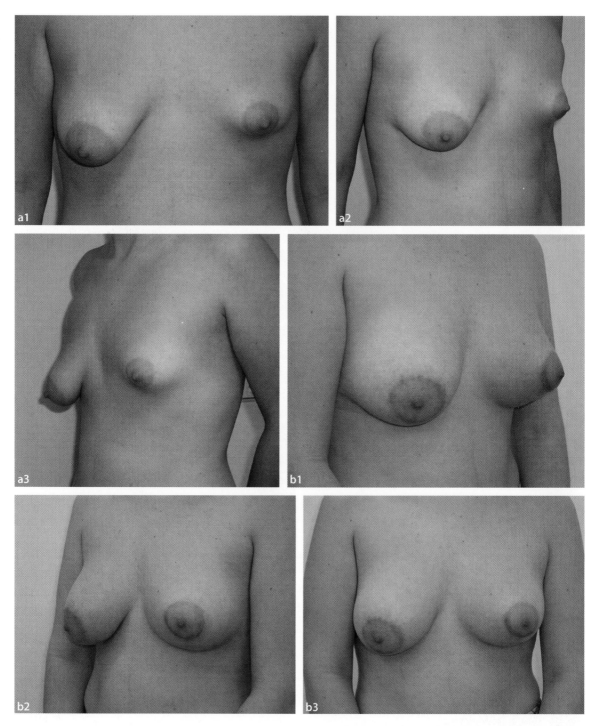

Fig. 38.9 a *1* Preoperative 21-year-old patient with asymmetrical tuberous breast deformity. *2* The right breast is characterized by underdevelopment of the inferior medial quadrant (type I). *3* On the patient's left side, there is severe constriction in both horizontal and vertical axes (type III). **b** *1* Five months postoperative. *2* The right breast was treated with periareolar donut-type deepithelialization and readjustment of the breast parenchyma without the use of an implant. *3* The left breast was treated with a semicircular periareolar incision, readjustment of the breast parenchyma, and subglandular placement of a 225-ml silicone breast implant

38.5
Complications

Bruising and swelling are the most common complications, are considerable, and are almost always to be expected and should be pointed out to the patient beforehand so that she will not be alarmed when she first sees her breasts.

Hematoma formation is probably the next most common complication to be expected, and meticulous hemostasis should be performed. In our series of 20 patients (37 breasts) with a maximum follow-up of 9 years, we have had one case of hematoma on the right breast of a bilateral reconstruction, which had to be evacuated. Nonetheless, we do not use drains routinely.

Another complication that should be avoided by careful technique is skin necrosis in the lower part of the breast. The technique requires subcutaneous dissection in the lower half of the breast, and care should be taken not to make the flaps too thin or to damage the skin by careless use of the electrocautery.

Nipple–areolar sensation could be affected if the subglandular dissection is extended superolaterally, and care should be taken to avoid damaging the 4th and 5th intercostal nerves.

Capsular contracture was recognized in one case in our series (Baker III, in the patient who developed the hematoma and contracture on the side of the hematoma; Fig. 38.10); the risk, however, should be equal to that of breast augmentation patients if an implant has been used.

38.6
Discussion

The tuberous breast deformity was first described in 1976 by Rees and Aston [3]. Since then several authors have attempted to describe, classify, and correct the problem, using various methods with varying results [1, 2, 4–21]. The large number of papers published on the subject demonstrates the psychological morbidity the deformity has on patients as well as the difficulty in developing a satisfactory surgical solution to the problem.

The authors have been dealing with this problem for 10 years, and the initial unsatisfactory results using conventional methods led us back to the basics to find the answers we needed. The study of the breast's anatomy and embryology enabled us to understand the nature of the deformity and formulate a surgical approach capable of restoring normal breast aesthetics.

Other authors have also referred to the embryology of breast development, but the theories put forward are far from satisfactory. Von Heiberg et al. (1996) [6] stated that Glaesmer (1930) suggested a phylogenetic relapse and that Pers (1968) postulated that tissue differentiation fails in a limited zone of the fetal thorax. Pers's theory might be suitable to explain deformities in the line of amastia and Poland's syndrome, but as far as the tuberous breast deformity is concerned, the authors believe that things are much simpler than what both theories suggest and that the only aberration is a thickening of the superficial fascia [5], as has already been explained in detail.

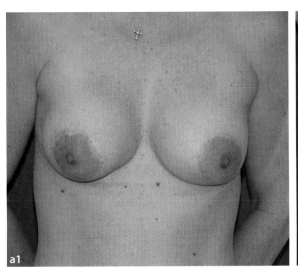 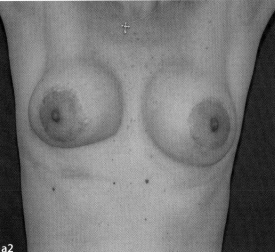

Fig. 38.10 *1* Postoperatively the patient developed a hematoma in the right breast that had to be evacuated. *2* The patient later developed Baker III capsular contracture on the side of the hematoma (shown 6 years postoperatively)

The authors' own understanding of the development of the deformity is as follows: During the 10th–14th weeks, the developing breast, which is ectodermal in origin, starts pushing inward into the underlying mesenchyme. As a result, the breast is enclosed within a fascial envelope, with the only point not covered by this fascia being the point of entry, which subsequently develops to become the nipple–areola complex.

The absence of the superficial layer of the superficial fascia underneath the areola [24, 26] coupled with the constricting ring [2] formed by the thickening of the superficial fascia [5], especially in the lower pole of the breast, inhibits the expansion of the developing breast and leads to a herniation of the breast parenchyma toward the nipple–areola complex. As already mentioned, the severity of the deformity ranges from mild hypoplasia of the inferior medial quadrant of the breast to major hypoplasia of all four quadrants, with varying degrees of herniation and areola enlargement [5, 6, 14, 28].

Many scientists have addressed the issue of this constricting ring [15, 24, 30], but nobody has actually looked into its nature until very recently, when we performed histological studies of the involved tissues of two of our most recent patients. Histology confirmed the existence of a band of dense connective tissue in the area (Fig. 38.2).

A recent study by Pacifico and Kang [31] also looked at the etiology of tuberous breasts, discarding the theory of the constricting ring and concentrating on the thickness of the skin in the nipple–areola region. They suggested that there is transient decreased thickness of the skin in the nipple–areola region due to hormonal imbalance during puberty, and that this caused the herniation of the breast parenchyma. Unfortunately, this theory is based on pure speculation with no anatomical or histological evidence to substantiate it.

Most authors acknowledge that merely placing an implant behind the deformed breast accentuates the deformity instead of correcting it [3, 5, 10, 13, 32]. Some authors advocate that there is skin deficiency in the inferior part of the breast [2, 12, 14, 16], with the inframammary fold being situated much higher than normal. But if one carefully examines the affected breast, the skin in the inferior part of the breast is lax, and the constriction lies deep within the subcutaneous tissue [2, 15].

Failure to address this problem is the main reason why the results yielded by most methods are far from satisfactory. There are, however, some authors who have focused on this point and have tried to rearrange the breast parenchyma to mold a more natural-looking breast.

Rees and Aston were the first to talk about radial incisions on the back of the breast to expand its base [3], but their technique did not actually transect the constricting ring. Dinner and Dowden realized that there was something constricting the breast in its inferior pole, but they thought it was the skin that was responsible for this constriction and used a full-thickness incision through skin, subcutaneous tissue, and breast to release it, followed by transposition of a skin and subcutaneous tissue flap [12]. Other authors have tried to rearrange the inferior pole of the breast, transecting the breast parenchyma horizontally and then unfolding the flap inward or outward [5, 15, 33], but the results have not always been aesthetically satisfactory.

The technique developed by Ribeiro and colleagues [15, 31, 34], which in principle is very similar to the authors', recognizes the existence of the constricting ring that needs to be transected in order to allow the breast to reshape. Ribeiro transects the ring in a horizontal axis and then develops a flap from the inferior portion of the breast to enhance the projection of the hypoplastic breast, doing away with implants because his patients are not particularly concerned with large breast volumes.

The authors' approach is slightly different. The constricting ring is transected at the 6 o'clock semi-axis of the breast, thus creating two pillars in the inferior part of the breast. The pillars are then either simply loosely reapproximated using absorbable sutures or are folded over each other in the fashion of a double-breasted jacket to add volume in the inferior portion of the breast, with the optional addition of a breast implant underneath the breast or the pectoralis major muscle to correct any volume deficiency.

This technique is simple, technically easy, and yields consistently good results. The scars are confined to the periareolar margin and most of the time are virtually invisible, and there is the additional advantage of not disturbing the lactiferous ducts, thus allowing normal breast function (provided that adequate breast parenchyma was present before the procedure).

References

1. Toranto IR: Two-stage correction of tuberous breast. Plast Reconstr Surg 1981;67(5):642–646
2. Atiyeh BS, Hashim HA, El-Douaihy Y, Kayle DI: Perinipple round-block technique for correction of tuberous/tubular breast deformity. Aesth Plast Surg 1998;22(4):284–288
3. Rees TD, Aston SJ: The tuberous breast. Clin Plast Surg 1976;3(2):339–347
4. Williams JE: Two-stage correction of tuberous breast. Discussion. Plast Reconstr Surg 1981;67(5):647
5. Grolleau JL, Lanfrey E, Lavigne B, Chavoin JP, Costagliola M: Breast base anomalies: treatment strategy for tuberous breasts, minor deformities, and asymmetry. Plast Reconstr Surg 1999;104(7):2040–2048

6. von Heimburg D, Exner K, Kruft S, Lemperle G: The tuberous breast deformity: classification and treatment. Br J Plast Surg 1996;49(6):339–345

7. Gruber RP, Jines HW Jr: The "donut" mastopexy: indications and complications. Plast Reconstr Surg 1980;65(1):34–38

8. Panettiere P, Del Gaudio GA, Marchetti L, Accorsi D, Del Gaudio A: The tuberous breast syndrome. Aesthetic Plast Surg 2000;24(6):445–249

9. Gasperoni C, Salgarello M, Gargani G: Tubular breast deformity: a new surgical approach. Eur J Plast Surg 1987;9:141

10. Teimourian B, Adham MN: Surgical correction of the tuberous breast. Ann Plast Surg 1983;10(3):190–193

11. Bruck HG: Hypoplasia of the lower medial quadrant of the breast. Aesthetic Plast Surg 1992;16(4):283–286

12. Dinner MI, Dowden RV: The tubular/tuberous breast syndrome. Ann Plast Surg 1987;19(5):414–420

13. Scheepers JH, Quaba AA: Tissue expansion in the treatment of tubular breast deformity. Br J Plast Surg 1992;45(7):529–532

14. Meara JG, Kolker A, Bartlett G, Theile R, Mutimer K, Holmes AD: Tuberous breast deformity: principles and practice. Ann Plast Surg 2000;45(6):607–611

15. Ribeiro L, Canzi W, Buss A, Accorsi A Jr: Tuberous breast: a new approach. Plast Reconstr Surg 1998;101(1):42–50

16. Elliott MP: A musculocutaneous transposition flap mammaplasty for correction of the tuberous breast. Ann Plast Surg 1988;20(2):153–157

17. Wilkinson TS: Mammaplasty for the tuberous breast. Ann Plast Surg 1988;21(3):294–296

18. Marchioni EE: Surgical treatment of tuberous breasts with bilateral mega-areola with a periareolar scar technique. Ann Plast Surg 1993;30(4):363–366

19. Kneafsey B, Crawford DS, Khoo CT, Saad MN: Correction of developmental breast abnormalities with a permanent expander/implant. Br J Plast Surg 1996;49(5):302–306

20. Muti E: Personal approach to surgical correction of the extremely hypoplastic tuberous breast. Aesthetic Plast Surg 1996;20(5):385–390

21. Argenta LC, VanderKolk C, Friedman RJ, Marks M: Refinements in reconstruction of congenital breast deformities. Plast Reconstr Surg 1985;76(1):73–82

22. Vecchione TR: A method of recontouring the domed nipple. Plast Reconstr Surg 1976;57(1):30–32

23. Williams G, Hoffman S: Mammaplasty for tubular breast. Aesthetic Plast Surg 1981;5(1):51–56

24. Hughes LE, Mansel RE, Webster DJT: Breast anatomy and physiology. In: Hughes LE, Mansel RE, Webster DJT (eds). Benign Disorders and Diseases of the Breast: Concepts and Clinical Management. London, Bailliere Tindal 1989, pp 5–13

25. Osborne MP: Breast development and anatomy. In: Harris JR, Hellman S, Henderson IC, Kinne DW (eds). Breast Diseases, 2nd edn. Philadelphia, Lippincott 1991, pp 1–13

26. Moore KL: The integumentary system. In: Moore KL (ed). The Developing Human. Clinically Oriented Embryology, 4th edn. Philadelphia, WB Saunders 1988, pp 426–428

27. Bostwick J III. Anatomy and physiology. In: Bostwick J III (ed). Plastic and Reconstructive Breast Surgery, 2nd edn. St. Louis, Quality Medical Publishing 2000, pp 89–93

28. von Heimburg D: Refined version of the tuberous breast classification. Plast Reconstr Surg 2000;105(6):2269–2270

29. Mandrekas AD, Zambacos GJ: Preoperative infiltration with lidocaine and epinephrine for breast reduction. Plast Reconstr Surg 1999;103(7):2087

30. Ribeiro L, Accorsi A Jr, Buss A, Pessja MC: Short scar correction of the tuberous breast. Clin Plast Surg 2002;29(3):423–431

31. Pacifico MD, Kang NV: The tuberous breast revisited. J Plast Reconstr Aesth Surg 2007;60(5):455–464

32. de la Fuente A, Martin del Yerro JL: Periareolar mastopexy with mammary implants. Aesthetic Plast Surg 1992;16(4):337–341

33. Puckett CL, Concannon MJ: Augmenting the narrow-based breast: the unfurling technique to prevent the double-bubble deformity. Aesthetic Plast Surg 1990;14(1):15–19

34. Regnault P: Breast ptosis: definition and treatment. Clin Plast Surg 1976;3(2):193–203

CHAPTER 39

Periareolar Technique for Correction and Augmentation of the Tuberous Breast

39

Bobby Arun Kumar, Darryl J. Hodgkinson

39.1
Introduction

Tuberous breast is an uncommon, if not rare, entity; it is generally a sporadic developmental disorder recognized in young women, occurring soon after puberty with breast development presenting from the ages of 12 or 13 years [1, 2].

The various anomalies of tuberous breast deformity have resulted in its being referred to as "Snoopy" breast, tubular breast, herniated areolar complex, nipple breast, constricted breast, lower pole hypoplasia, narrow-based breast[1–4], and domed breast [1].

The tuberous breast is an asymmetrical breast shape, and the deformity is defined anatomically by a constricting ring at the base of the breast, resulting in a deficient and narrow horizontal and vertical breast base [1, 2, 3, 5]. As a result, there is a concomitant deficiency or hypoplasia of the horizontal and vertical development of the breast parenchyma with or without resultant herniation of the breast parenchyma toward the nipple–areolar complex [1–3, 5]. The aberrant breast shape also includes a deficient inferior skin envelope, an elevated inframammary fold, and an enlarged areola [1–3].

Dinner and Dowden [6] describe the tuberous breast deformity as a skin envelope deficiency (always present), hypoplasia of portions of the breast (usually present), reduced vertical extension of the breast (usually present), ptosis (usually present), and hypertrophy of the areola (often present).

The incidence of tuberous breast deformity is not firmly established. In 2004 Deluca-Pytell et al. [3] attempted to define the incidence of tuberous breast by a retrospective analysis of 375 consecutive female patients who presented for mammoplasty during a 10-year period. They concluded that of the 375 patients, approximately 73% had tuberous deformity [3].

Mandrekas and colleagues [2, 7] suggested that, in their own experience, the incidence remains unknown and is considerably much lower than was found by Deluca-Pytell et al., and that given the small size of clinical series, it still suggests an incidence of less than 3% of patients presenting for breast enhancement.

39.2
Anatomy

The anatomical etiological cause for tuberous breast deformity is best understood by reviewing the embryological development of the breast. Breast development of the fetus occurs during week 5 of gestation in utero from the mammary ridge and arises from the ectoderm [1, 8, 9]. The majority of the mammary ridge disappears around weeks 7–8, although a small portion remains in the thoracic region and subsequently penetrates the underlying mesenchyme at 10–14 weeks [1, 9].

Breast development in the form of primary and secondary mammary buds continues during intrauterine life. Following birth, breast development ceases until puberty, when in females breast tissue develops below the nipple–areolar complex and enlargement of the areola occurs; this process continues until 15–16 years of age [1, 8]. As a consequence of the previous events in utero, the invagination of the ectoderm into the mesenchyme results in a fascial layer covering the breast tissue [1].

The relevant anatomy of the breast demonstrates that the superficial fascia of the breast is contiguous with Camper's fascia of the abdomen [1]. The superficial fascia of the breast parenchyma consists of two layers: a superficial layer, which is the outer layer, and a deep layer, which overlies the deep fascia of the pectoralis major and serratus anterior muscles [1, 8].

Fibrous attachments extend from the deep muscle fascia and the deep fascia of the superficial fascia of the breast through the breast parenchyma and eventually join the outer superficial fascia and the dermis of the skin. These fibrous attachments are known as the suspensory ligaments of Cooper [1, 8].

Tuberous breast deformity is postulated to be due to a constricting ring of the superficial fascia, restricting the radial growth of the breast parenchyma in one or all directions [1, 8]. The superficial fascia is absent under the nipple–areolar complex, and there is a constricting ring at the periphery of the nipple–areolar complex with denser fibrous tissue of the inferior breast [1, 8].

The severity of the developmental disorder in the tuberous breast varies from hypoplasia of the inferior medial quadrant of the breast, with relatively normal breast volume, to hypoplasia of all four quadrants of the breast parenchyma as well as degrees of herniation of breast tissue through the nipple–areolar complex [1, 4, 7, 8]. Because the condition is sporadic, there is no evidence related to genetic or other environmental causes during intrauterine growth or puberty.

Several authors have offered classification schema for tuberous breast deformity. Grolleau et al. [4] classify tuberous breast (Table 39.1) as follows: In type I, the lower medial quadrant is deficient; in type II there is lower medial and lateral base constriction with associated deficiency of breast tissue of the quadrants; and the type III breast is deficient in all four quadrants, with the breast base constricted both horizontally and vertically.

Elsahy's system relates to tuberous breast asymmetry when assessing visually for implant fill or a given volume of parenchyma to be removed [3]. In Elsahy's categories (Table 39.2), type I patients have unilateral micromastia, type II patients have unilateral macromastia, type III patients have both micromastia and macromastia, type IV patients have asymmetrical breasts and bilateral micromastia, and type V patients have asymmetry and bilateral macromastia.

In 2000 Von Heimburg [10] refined his previous version for classification of tuberous breasts published in 1996. The classification scheme is applicable to the treatment of tuberous breast (Table 39.3). Type I is hypoplasia of the lower medial quadrant; type II is hypoplasia of

Table 39.1 Grolleau tuberous breast deformity classification

Type I:	Lower medial quadrant deficient
Type II:	Lower medial and lateral base constriction with associated deficiency of breast tissue of the quadrants
Type III:	Breast deficient in all four quadrants, and the breast base is constricted both horizontally and vertically

Table 39.2 Elsahy's asymmetry deformity classification

Type I:	Unilateral micromastia
Type II:	Unilateral macromastia
Type III:	Micromastia and macromastia
Type IV:	Asymmetrical breasts and bilateral micromastia
Type V:	Asymmetrical breasts and bilateral macromastia

Table 39.3 Von Heimburg classification for treatment of tuberous breast

Type I:	Hypoplasia of lower medial quadrant
Type II:	Hypoplasia of medial and lateral quadrant with sufficient skin in subareolar region
Type III:	Hypoplasia of medial and lateral quadrant with deficiency of skin in subareolar region
Type IV:	Severe breast constriction and minimal breast base

the lower medial and lateral quadrants, with sufficient skin in the subareolar region; type III is hypoplasia of the lower medial and lateral quadrants and deficiency of skin in the subareolar region; and type IV is severe breast constriction and a minimal breast base [2, 10].

39.3 Surgical Treatment

Historically, Rees and Aston [11] initially described the tuberous breast disorder in 1976; it was so named because the breast resembles "tuberous plant roots" [1, 4, 5]. Rees and Aston were also first to describe radial incisions to the back of the breast to expand the base [7]; however, their technique did not transect the constricting ring.

Surgical techniques to enlarge the mammary base were described by Longacre in 1954 [5, 12] and Goulian in 1971 [5, 13]. Other authors also embarked on and described their own experiences for correcting tuberous breast deformity, including Williams and Hoffman [5, 14], who performed augmentation mammaplasty via an inframammary fold incision, and Vecchione [5, 15] in 1976, who described repair of the "domed nipple." In 1991 Versaci and Rozelle [16] advocated the use of a tissue expander and augmentation via several staged operative procedures.

A technique describing surgical correction with a particular emphasis on the herniation of the breast parenchyma through the nipple–areolar complex was authored by Bass [5, 17] in 1978. In 1981, Toranto [5, 18] described a two-stage operation, and in 1993, Temourian and Adhan [5, 19] achieved aesthetic results with a technique using two incisions, the areolar and the submammary, in addition to the use of a prosthesis.

In 1987 Dinner and colleagues [1, 5, 6] described the use of flaps from the submammary fold. They surmised that there was something constricting the inferior breast, incorrectly believing this to be the skin.

The tuberous breast presents as a variety of abnormal anatomy as reflected by the previous classifications. As a result, treatment of the tuberous breast may have multiple surgical solutions and techniques that aim to provide adequate correction of the deficient horizontal and vertical hypoplasia, the herniated breast parenchyma through the enlarged nipple–areolar complex, and a high inframammary fold.

The periareolar approach for correcting the tuberous breast has been advocated by Sampaio Goes [20], Muti [21], Ribeiro et al. [5], Mandrekas et al. [1], Hodgkinson [22], and Puckett and Concannon [23] in an attempt to correct all aspects of the tuberous breast deformity.

39.3.1
Glandular Flaps and Shaping Technique

Ribeiro's [5] technique is as follows: The patient is placed in a semi-Fowler's position following general anesthesia. A new areola is outlined, usually 4–5 cm in diameter, and the circumareolar region is deepithelialized. This is followed by dividing the new nipple–areolar complex into superior and inferior poles, with the line of division below the areola.

An incision divides the inferior pole down to the muscular level, with extensive undermining of the deficient inferior skin envelope also down to the pectoralis fascia. The inferior glandular pedicle is resected into the medial and lateral projections, disrupting the constricting fibrous ring and preserving perforating intercostal vessels. In the final stage of the reconstruction, the inferior glandular pedicle is folded over itself to fill the inferior skin envelope, providing projection of the breast.

Ribeiro et al. [5] avoided the use of prostheses for augmentation because this technique is optimal for small breasts as classified according to Grolleau types II and III tuberous breast deformity [2, 4].

39.3.2
Glandular Flaps, Shaping, and Implant Technique

A variation to this theme was proposed by Mandrekas et al. [1]. Using a periareolar incision, sharp dissection is performed on the inferior skin envelope down to the pectoralis fascia and toward the new inframammary fold. Further dissection occurs in a superior fashion, bluntly dissecting the breast tissue off the deep pectoralis fascia and leaving a superior glandular attachment. The inferior half of the breast tissue is exteriorized through its periareolar opening and is subsequently divided in the middle, vertically toward the new areola. The inferior breast pillars are folded over each other in a double-breasted fashion to create volume and projection of the inferior pole.

Mandrekas et al. [1] discussed the use of round textured silicone gel implants placed in a subglandular position with the inferior pillars covering the implant entirely to avoid the "double bubble," which should also provide additional volume if required. They have suggested successful outcomes using their technique in a small group of patients with typically bilateral Grolleau type II deformity.

Muti [21] and Biggs et al. [24] also use glandular flaps with breast implants through a periareolar incision and a vertical scar if required. Puckett and Concannon [23] employed a surgical technique that is primarily used for severe tuberous breast deformity together with an implant if required.

Puckett's technique follows Ribeiro's [5] approach, with release of the inferior skin envelope from the breast parenchyma, dissecting down to the pectoralis fascia and the new inframammary fold. The glandular component is dissected in a superior direction off the muscular wall, mobilizing half of the inferior breast parenchyma. An inferior based flap is designed by a difficult posterior approach, with division of the glandular pedicle in an anterior direction and toward the subareolar region, thereby maintaining an anterior subareolar pedicle and good vascularization of the glandular flap.

The technique is completed by placing a submuscular implant and reshaping the inferior glandular flap over the implant, thus providing breast volume inferiorly and avoiding a double fold of the inframammary crease. The technique is primarily used for severe tuberous breast deformity, and an implant is used if required. It provides good aesthetic results for Grolleau types II and III [4] tuberous breast deformity.

39.3.3
Glandular Flaps, Shaping, Implant, and Prosthesis Technique

Sampaio Goes [20] described a periareolar mammaplasty technique with application of a polyglactine or mixed mesh to provide repositioning of all components of the breast. His work has been used and modified by Hodgkinson [22] for treating tuberous breast deformity.

Hodgkinson's technique [22] similarly approaches augmentation via a periareolar incision, dissection, and elevation of the deficient inferior skin envelope and reshaping of the breast with glandular flaps. The subsequent breast shape is supported and maintained by a nonabsorbable fine suture mesh that is permanent and thus avoids irregular glandular bulges and surface contours under the skin envelope. Once again, a breast implant can be added to provide inferior pole volume and repositioning of the inframammary fold if required.

39.4
Results and Complications

Given the lack of substantial data regarding periareolar correction and augmentation of the tuberous breast, it is difficult to conclude that a particular technique is superior to all other techniques. The variety of surgical approaches clearly indicates that appropriate techniques exist for correcting different anatomical presentations of the tuberous breast disorders and that each one therefore has a possible successful aesthetic outcome. Each technique aims to result in a normal-size areola, a natural breast shape with matching breast volumes, and an expanded lower segment with a new, lowered inframammary fold.

The significant complications associated with surgical correction and augmentation of the tuberous breast include dilatation or widening of the areola, flattening of the breast, and poor periareolar scars [25]. Also, the failure to release the constricting fibrous bands and the overzealous and wide resection of the skin flaps will result in poor correction of the deficient horizontal and vertical breast base and volume of the inferior pole of the breast, limiting adequate envelope expansion [1, 22].

Augmentation of the tuberous breast by the use of glandular flaps has been shown to cause irregular bulges that can be seen through the skin envelope; this is corrected by the use of an absorbable mixed mesh or permanent fine suture mesh [20, 22].

The other recognized complications have been "double-crease" of the inframammary fold and "double-bubble" formation, recurrence of areola protrusion, and, often, a dystotic areola [4] with the use of a breast implant. Consequent correct placement of the implant with redraping of the glandular flaps avoids these complications.

During dermal and glandular dissection, preservation of vascularity has been recognized as a potential complication, along with postoperative infection, although uncommon, and exposure of the prosthesis through thin skin. Operative techniques that do not adequately correct the primary tuberous breast disorder and require subsequent reoperations and corrections are in themselves a complication.

It is also recognized that it is advisable to avoid doing procedures in active smokers to reduce the potential complication of wound breakdown with the periareolar approach.

39.5
Discussion

The degree of severity of the tuberous breast disorder and the application of an appropriate classification scheme will lead to selection of a technique to reconstruct the deformity (see Figs. 39.1–39.4). As noted by previous authors, satisfactory aesthetic outcomes are not always achieved, and secondary procedures will necessitate revision of the primary procedure.

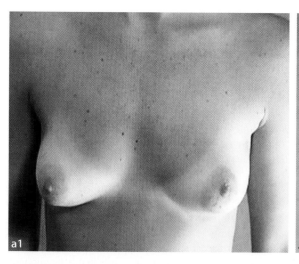 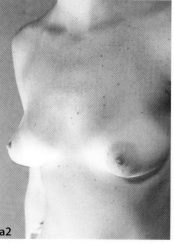

Fig. 39.1 a *1* Preoperative patient with mild tuberous breasts. *2* Lateral view

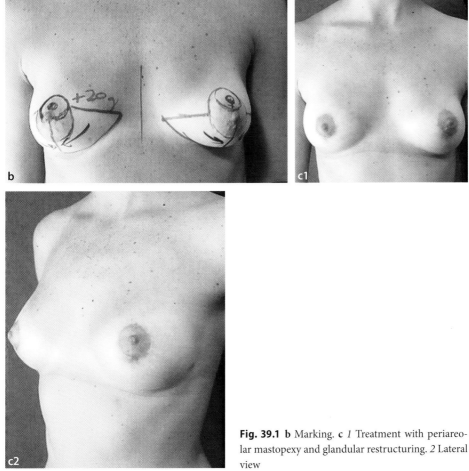

Fig. 39.1 b Marking. **c** *1* Treatment with periareolar mastopexy and glandular restructuring. *2* Lateral view

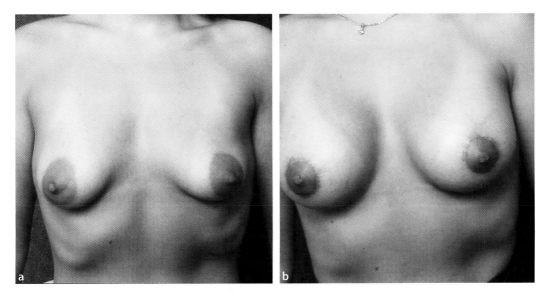

Fig. 39.2 a Preoperative with mild tuberous breast. **b** Treatment with periareolar mastopexy and breast enhancement using partial subpectoral 275-ml smooth saline implants

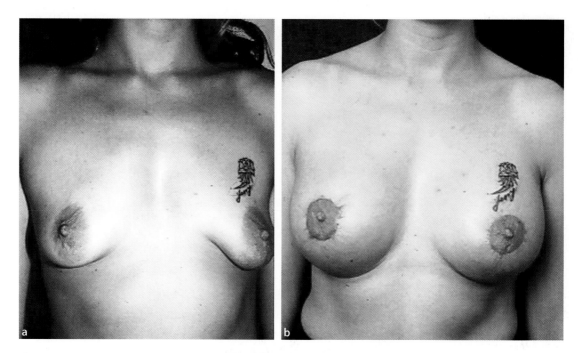

Fig. 39.3 a Preoperative severely tuberous breasts with asymmetry. **b** Corrected with periareolar mastopexy glandular scoring and size 340-ml smooth saline implants in a partial subpectoral pocket

Other surgical approaches have been used, such as the Maillard Z-plasty, the superior pedicle mammaplasty with lateral dermatoglandular flap, the inverted "T" incision of the breast envelope, and insertion of a tissue expander via an inframammary incision [2, 4, 16, 22, 24].

39.6
Conclusions

Selection of an appropriate periareolar surgical technique that is dependent on the severity and nature of the tuberous breast deformity and is a one-stage procedure has been demonstrated to provide better surgical correction and augmentation of the tuberous breast deformity.

►**Fig. 39.4 a** *1* Preoperative breast asymmetry and severe left tuberous breast deformity. *2* Lateral view. **b** Preoperative marking. **c** Intraoperative. **d** *1* Corrected with periareolar approach, glandular reshaping, and mesh support. *2* Right breast enhanced with 220-ml saline implant in a partial subpectoral position

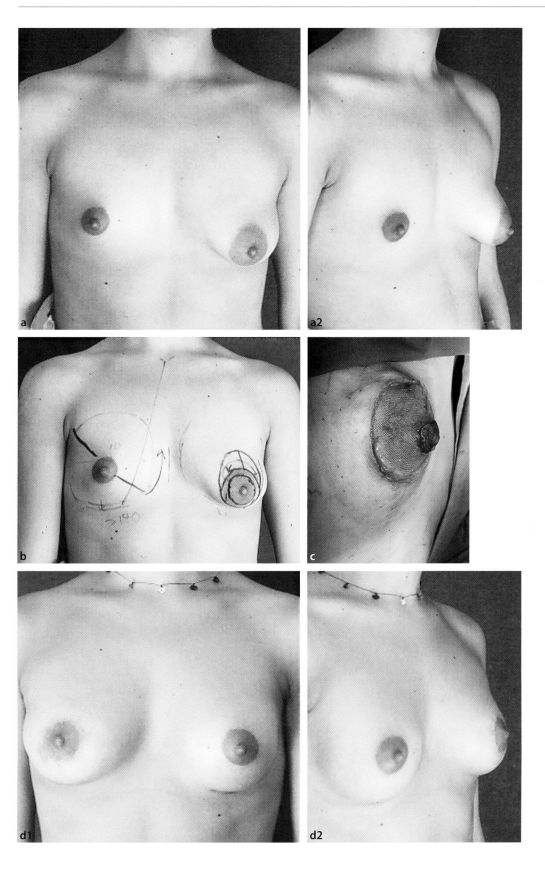

References

1. Mandrekas AD, Zambacos GJ, Anastasopoulos A, Hapsas D, Lambrinaki N, Iolannidou-Mouzaka L: Aesthetic reconstruction of the tuberous breast deformity. Plast Reconstr Surg 2003;112(4):1099–1108

2. Mathes SJ, Seyfer AE, Miranda EP: Plastic Surgery: Trunk and Lower Extremity, vol. 6. Philadelphia, Elsevier 2006, p 513

3. Deluca-Pytell DM, Piazza RC, Holding JC, Snyder N, Hunsicker LM, Phillips LG: The incidence of tuberous breast deformity in asymmetric and symmetric mammaplasty patients. Plast Reconstr Surg: 2005;116(7):1894–1899

4. Grolleau JL, Lanfrey E, Lavigne B, Chavoin JP, Costagliola M: Breast base anomalies: Treatment strategy for tuberous breasts, minor deformities and asymmetry. Plast Reconstr Surg 1999;104(7):2040–2048

5. Ribeiro L, Canz W, Buss A, Accorsi A: Tuberous breast: a new approach. Plast Reconstr Surg: 1998;101(1):42–50

6. Dinner MI, Dowden RV: Tubular breast syndrome. Ann Plast Surg 1987;19(5):414–420

7. Zambacos GJ , Mandrekas AD: The incidence of tuberous breast deformity in asymmetric and symmetric mammaplasty patients. Plast Reconstr Surg 2006;118(7):1667

8. Hanna MK, Nahai F: Applied Anatomy of the Breast: The Art of Aesthetic Surgery: Principles and Techniques. St. Louis, Quality Medical Publishing, 2005, pp 1790–1815

9. Moore KL: The Developing Human: Clinically Orientated Embryology, 3rd edn. Philadelphia, WB Saunders 1982, p 436

10. von Heimburg D: Refined version of the tuberous breast classification. Plast Reconstr Surg: 2000;105(6):2269–2270

11. Rees TD, Aston S: The tuberous breast. Clin Plast Surg 1976;3(2):339–347

12. Longacre TJ: Correction of hypoplastic breast with special references to reconstruction of the "nipple type breast" with local dermoflap. Plast Reconstr Surg 1954;14(6):431–441

13. Goulian D: Dermal mastopexy. Plast Reconstr Surg 1971;47(2):105–110

14. Williams JE, Hoffman S: Mammaplasty for tubular breast. Aesthet Plast Surg 1981;5(1):51–56

15. Vecchione TR: A method of recontouring the domed nipple. Plast Reconstr Surg 1976;57(1):30–32

16. Versaci AD, Rozelle AA: Treatment of tuberous breast utilizing tissue expansion. Aesthet Plast Surg: 1991;15(4):307–312

17. Bass CB: Herniated areola complex. Ann Plast Surg 1978;1(4):402–406

18. Toranto IR: Two stage correction of tuberous breast. Plast Reconstr Surg 1981;67(5):642–646

19. Teimourian B, Adhan NM: Surgical correction of the tuberous breast. Ann Plast Surg 1983;10(3):190–193

20. Sampaio Goes JC: Periareolar mammaplasty: double skin technique with application of polyglactine or mixed mesh. Plast Reconstr Surg 1996;97(5):959–968

21. Muti E: Personal approach to surgical correction of the extremely hypoplastic tuberous breast. Aesth Plast Surg 1996;20(5):385–390

22. Hodgkinson DJ: Tuberous breast deformity: principles and practice. Ann Plast Surg 2001;47(1):97–98

23. Puckett CL, Concannon MJ: Augmenting the narrow based breast: the unfurling technique to prevent the double bubble deformity. Aesth Plast Surg 1990;14(1):15–19

24. Biggs TM, Taneja A, Muti E: The Art of Aesthetic Surgery: Principles and Techniques. St. Louis, Quality Medical Publishing 2005, p 2006

25. Spear SL, Giese SY, Ducic I: Concentric mastopexy revisited. Plast Reconstr Surg 2001;107(5):1294–1299

The Effect of Breast Parenchymal Maldistribution on Augmentation Mammoplasty Decisions

40

Robert R. Brink, Joel B. Beck

Evaluating augmentation mammoplasty candidates with the appearance of breast ptosis can be difficult when breasts fit the classical definition of ptosis but are not really ptotic. This can happen because the definitions of ptosis compare the position of the mammary parenchyma to the inframammary fold (IMF) without accounting for the possibility that the position of the IMF position might be aberrant. Thus, in addition to the classical definitions of breast ptosis, the surgeon must understand that the nipple–areolar complex (NAC) and the IMF are both subject to variable positions that raise concerns to the physician with regard to the most optimal approach to surgery. This requires the surgeon to understand the relationship between the NAC and the IMF, in addition to the NAC with the lower breast contour. As it has been reviewed in the senior author's previous explanation of this topic, the IMF is not fixed and poses a challenge in understanding previous attempts to evaluating breast ptosis (Table 40.1).

The standard definitions of breast ptosis compare the position of the nipple with that of the existing IMF, without considering the possibility that the fold is not in the ideal location (Table 40.1). Because the standard definitions of ptosis are deeply ingrained among surgeons, the breast with an abnormally high IMF is likely to be considered ptotic by unwary practitioners

because it fits the classic definition and appears "ptotic" (Fig. 40.1). Rather than insist that such a breast is not really ptotic, the senior author has come to refer to the

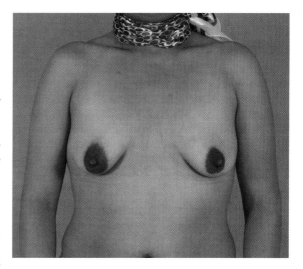

Fig. 40.1 Note that the patient's breasts appear ptotic, yet lowering the inframammary fold would be the operation of choice rather than a mastopexy

Table 40.1 Criteria for evaluating breast ptosis

Degree of ptosis	Characteristics
True ptosis	The nipple–areola complex's relation to the fold when the gland, skin, and nipple descend together
1st-degree (minor) ptosis	Nipple–areola complex at the fold and above the breast contour
2nd-degree (moderate) ptosis	Nipple–areola complex below the fold but above the breast contour
3rd-degree (major) ptosis	Nipple–areola complex below the fold and below the breast contour

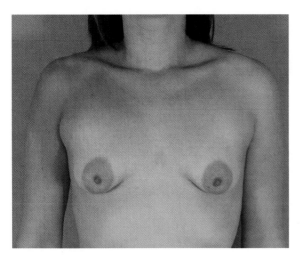

Fig. 40.2 Despite a short sternal-notch-to-nipple distance, this patient's breasts appear ptotic

condition as "false ptosis," because since the NAC is not low, mastopexy would be an inappropriate treatment.

Contrary to what one would think from reading the literature, it is not the position of the NAC that is instrumental in creating the appearance of ptosis, but rather the position of the IMF. In our experience, measurements have shown that breasts have looked ptotic with the nipples located as high as 17 cm from the sternal notch if the IMF was high enough (Fig. 40.2). Conversely, aesthetically acceptable breasts may have the nipples located 25 cm from the sternal notch if the IMF is located low enough (Fig. 40.3).

The solitary high IMF is a variant of the tubular breast deformity that can run a continuum from minor to very severe and is characterized in its full expression by three hallmarks:
1. High IMF
2. Narrow parenchymal distribution
3. Areolar distortion in the form of expansion and distention

In its lesser expressions, the "forme frusta" tubular breast may have, because of parenchymal maldistribution, nothing more than a high IMF. It is this visible characteristic that has led to various descriptions: lower pole hypoplasia, inferior pole hypoplasia, and, more recently, lower hemisphere hypoplasia, to name a few. In any case, the narrow and high distribution of parenchyma results in an abnormally high IMF that gives the breasts a ptotic appearance and fits the definition of ptosis. Thus, lower hemisphere hypoplasia can be confused with breast ptosis if the position of the IMF is not considered. Failure to recognize the lesser expressions of this deformity in a patient who appears to have ptotic breasts, but in fact has an abnormally high IMF, can lead the surgeon to perform a mastopexy when lowering of the IMF is indicated.

Whereas breasts with normal parenchymal distribution respond predictably well to implants of almost any size, placed either subglandularly or subpectorally, this is not the case with parenchymal maldistribution resulting in a high IMF. These patients do best with a prosthesis in the subglandular space because the subglandular dissection releases the gland from the pectoralis fascia and allows it to conform better to the underlying

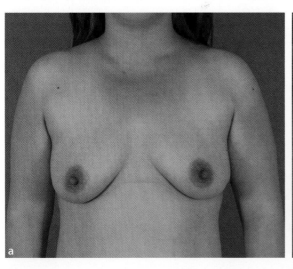

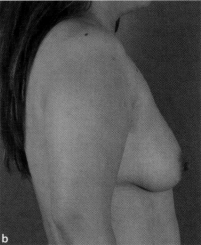

Fig. 40.3 a Note that the patient's breasts are aesthetically acceptable, yet slightly involuted from motherhood. **b** Lateral view

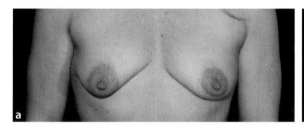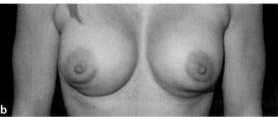

Fig. 40.4 a Preoperative. **b** This patient underwent a transaxillary subpectoral breast augmentation with a smooth round saline 300-ml implant. Note the double inframammary fold appearance. She would have been better served with subglandular placement of the implant with release of the gland from the pectoralis fascia

implant. Subpectoral placement in these patients is associated with a high risk of the double-bubble (double IMF) deformity that arises with increasing implant size and progressively lower implant placement (Fig. 40.4). Although a subglandular parenchymal release can also be done with subpectoral implants in these patients, the dual dissection plane increases morbidity and is associated with its own problems, such as window-shading of the pectoralis when it is released both superficially and from its origins along the sternal margin.

To avoid the visible rippling that bedevils subglandular saline implants without adequate soft tissue cover, the authors used the "forme fruste" tubular breast definition to qualify our patients for gel implants prior to their general reintroduction. With the reintroduction of gel implants, it is no longer necessary to qualify patients for silicone gel implants.

The surgeon should realize that the high IMF reflects a relative tissue deficiency in the lower hemisphere and that the higher the IMF, the larger the implant needed for augmentation. Large implants not only provide the appropriate volume to replace the volume deficit, but they are more effective at lowering the IMF to the appropriate level because they are positioned lower on the chest than smaller implants.

References

1. Brink R: Evaluating breast parenchymal maldistribution with regard to mastopexy and augmentation mammaplasty. Plast Reconstr Surg 1990;86:715–719

2. Brink R: Evaluating breast parenchymal maldistribution with regard to mastopexy and augmentation mammaplasty. Plast Reconstr Surg 2000;106:491–496

3. Papillon J: Pros and cons of subpectoral implantation. Clin Plast Surg 1976;3:321vv

CHAPTER 41

Management of Anterior Chest Wall Deformity in Breast Augmentation

41

Darryl J. Hodgkinson

41.1
Introduction

Chest wall deformities are sometimes detected in patients requesting breast augmentation. The failure to recognize the presence and significance of a deformity, and its contribution to breast asymmetry when present, can lead to a suboptimal result for the patient undergoing breast augmentation if breast prostheses alone are used.

41.2
Types of Deformities

The chest wall deformities most frequently encountered are those of the manubrium, including pectus carinatum, pectus excavatum, and a prominent costosternal junction. Rib torsion, rib rotation, sunken chest deformity, and flaring of the lower costal cartilages are also seen. Poland's syndrome is recognizable not only by a chest wall deformity but by the variable loss of the pectoralis major muscle on the affected side and the possibility of hand and axillary deformities. Breast asymmetry is nearly always present in patients with Poland syndrome along with rib torsion, rib rotation, or sunken chest. Torsional chest wall rotation is associated with spinal scoliosis, and breast asymmetry may accompany this deformity.

In the preoperative assessment of any patient in whom breast asymmetry is detected, one should be suspicious that an underlying chest wall deformity exists. A study by Rohrich et al. [1] found that 9% of patients with breast asymmetry had an associated chest wall deformity. Failure to recognize this deformity can result in a dissatisfied patient postoperatively, when the deformity may first become evident as being uncorrected or even magnified by the breast augmentation procedure.

The presence of a chest wall deformity will impact significantly on the choice and type of implant selected, the placement of the implant, the possible need for a separate chest wall implant in combination with a breast prosthesis, and the final expected result of the breast augmentation.

Major thoracic deformities are likely to be referred to a thoracic surgeon, and after the thoracic deformity is corrected, breast enhancement could be considered if micromastia or asymmetry persists.

41.3
Clinical Evaluation

Clinical examination is most important. The patient's posture together with the prominence of the manubrium, sternum, costochondral junction, and costal flare should be noted. Evaluation of a patient's thorax posteriorly should indicate the presence of any spinal deformities such as kyphosis, scoliosis, or rotation of the chest. In lateral evaluation, the asymmetry and the projection of the anterior chest wall can be accurately assessed. Palpation of the anterior chest wall will demonstrate a discrepancy in the projection of both sides of the chest. The contour of the ribs and development of the muscles in relation to an anterior discrepancy should be assessed.

41.4
Radiographic Evaluation

For the most significant deformities, chest radiography, computed tomographic scanning, magnetic resonance imaging, or stereophotogrammetry can be used to define the chest wall deformity more accurately once diagnosed [2]. The degree of deformity and the possibility of a missing rib can be established and the operative plan prepared before undertaking an operative procedure of breast prosthetic insertion alone. The objectification of the chest wall discrepancy helps the surgeon determine the size and shape of a prefabricated chest wall implant if the surgeon chooses to reconstruct using this option.

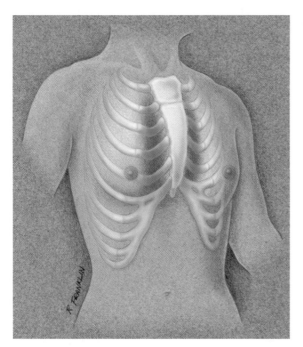

Fig. 41.1 Pectus carinatum with prominence of the manubrium and costochondral junctions

41.5
Manubriosternal Prominence, Pectus Carinatum, and Prominent Costosternal Junction

Manubriosternal prominence and pectus carinatum are not infrequently seen preoperatively (Fig. 41.1). Patients not only request breast augmentation but are also interested in camouflaging the "boniness" of their anterior chest.

Associated with the prominence of the manubriosternal junction is the convexity of the costochondral joints as they bend to insert into the sternum. The usual maneuver chosen to camouflage the "bony" middle chest is to place the breast implants as high and as medial as possible. A wide-based implant is chosen, and placement should be made by dissection in the subglandular space over the medial aspect of the costal cartilages adjacent to the manubriosternal junction. The thin, subcutaneous tissues at the manubriosternal junction and over the medial costal cartilages may limit such a correction. Failure to recognize the presence of this deformity and deal with it by using a lower dissection limits the aesthetic result, which fails to camouflage the boniness. Directing the implant position and volume height toward the manubriosternal junction and over the costosternal joints leads to a camouflage of the boniness (Fig. 41.2).

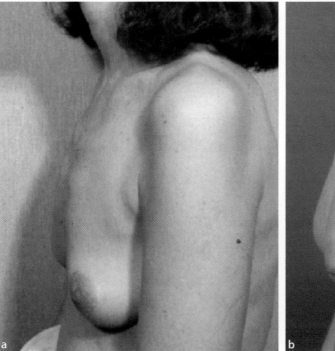
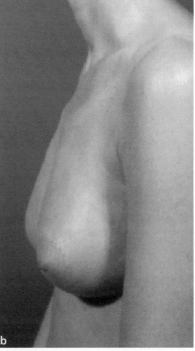

Fig. 41.2 **a** Preoperative. **b** Camouflage of prominent manubrium and bony chest with high placement of subglandular smooth gel 360-ml implants

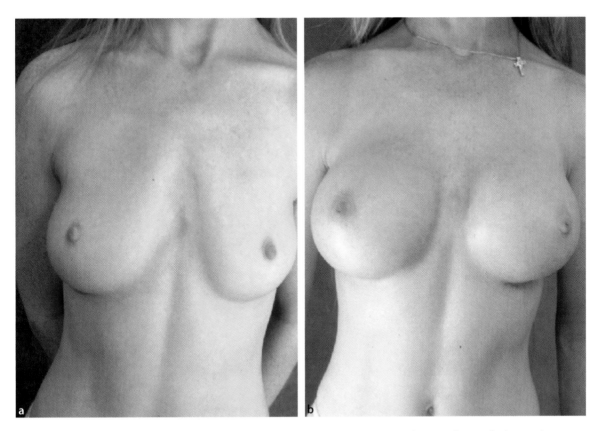

Fig. 41.3 a Preoperative. **b** Camouflage of pectus carinatum with high, partially submuscular, smooth 360-ml saline implants

By choosing an implant with "flow" rather than a cohesive gel type of implant, a more satisfactory placement and manubriosternal camouflage is likely. A smooth-walled gel implant placed in this position will produce the best initial result. The choice of a textured gel or saline implant may depend on a surgeon's preference for placing such an implant in a subglandular or subcutaneous position. A higher "fill" implant is generally preferable.

Figure 41.3 shows a patient with a prominent manubriosternal junction, pectus carinatum, and prominent costochondral joints. These deficiencies were camouflaged by using a smooth-walled, round, 360-ml saline implant of moderate fill and placing it in a partial subpectoral position by a submammary incision.

41.6
Pectus Excavatum

The presence of a moderate pectus excavatum (Fig. 41.4) can at times be advantageous to a patient preoperatively, selectively providing her with a deeper and more prominent cleavage (Fig. 41.5). However, there is a limit

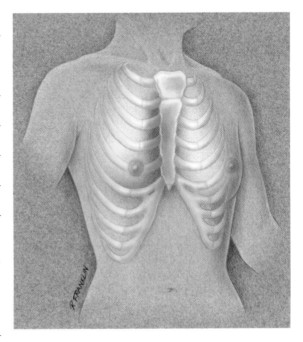

Fig. 41.4 Pectus excavatum with midline depression of manubrium and costal cartilages

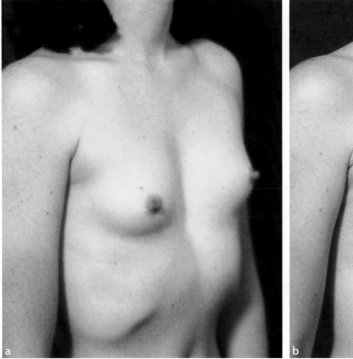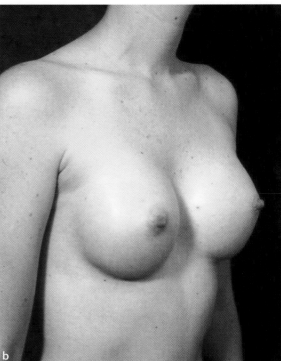

Fig. 41.5 a Preoperative. **b** Partially subpectoral 260-ml smooth gel implants placed adjacent to the excavatum camouflage without accentuating pectus excavatum

to this, and once the depth is greater than 4 cm or the width greater than 8 cm, then the cleavage will be too deep or too flat and needs to be addressed by the use of a possible solid silicone implant to camouflage an unattractive appearance. If the defect is deeper with associated sternal rotation, thoracotomy with rigid fixation of the pectus is indicated [3, 4].

A solid, firm #5 durometer silicone implant can be customized after moulage preparation to insert into the deformity, either as an initial first stage or in a combined procedure with breast augmentation. The decision has to be made whether to place the sternal implant, once manufactured, through the breast augmentation incision or to subsequently perform the augmentation after the sternal implant has been placed by a substernal incision and the implant has settled into place. If sternal implantation is done at the same time as the breast augmentation, there is a danger of coaptation and coalescing of the breast prostheses and sternal implants. The solution to this problem might be to texture the implants so that they do not tend to flow together, although because of the likelihood of seroma from such an approach, two separate procedures would be preferable. Drainage of the sternal pocket is important to prevent seroma accumulation and is advised for all solid chest wall implant surgery. Seroma formation

is possibly reduced by the use of drains and postoperative anti-inflammatory medication [5].

41.7
Poland's Syndrome

Female patients with Poland's syndrome usually present with breast asymmetry, hypomastia, and a smaller nipple–areola complex on the affected side (Fig. 41.6). Further evaluation will ascertain the degree of muscular underdevelopment of the pectoralis major and the associated chest wall deficiency. Torsion of the chest and asymmetry of the cartilages along with manubrial prominence on the unaffected side are often associated with Poland's syndrome.

In dealing with a request for breast symmetry and augmentation in a patient with Poland's syndrome, the contribution of the chest wall and muscular deficiency must be addressed. The lack of pectoral sweep of the pectoralis major is rarely of concern to the patient and is often unnoticed, although previous authors have addressed this problem by using latissimus dorsi muscle transfer. Transfer of the latissimus dorsi, preferably by endoscopic techniques, can certainly reestablish the lateral sweep, although the muscle may be deficient and

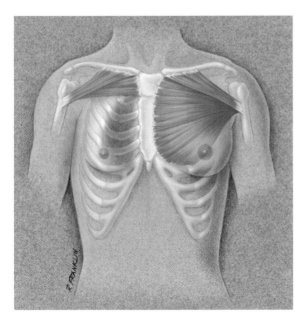

Fig. 41.6 Poland's syndrome with absence of sternocostal pectoralis major muscle and depression of anterior chest wall

is prone to atrophy [6]. The volume of the transferred latissimus muscle is inadequate to provide chest wall projection; for this reason, I prefer to primarily address the lack of chest wall projection rather than the lateral pectoral sweep. If the chest wall projection is greater than 3.0 cm in discrepancy, it is generally dealt with by

using a customized or prefabricated chest wall implant (Fig. 41.7). If the patient has undergone failed procedures in the past or has an absent pectoralis muscle and severe discrepancy, then microvascular free-flap reconstruction might be used as a salvage procedure [6].

41.8
Sunken Chest (Anterior Thoracic Hypoplasia)

Discrepancies in the projection of the anterior chest wall complex are not necessarily associated with Poland's syndrome and occur de novo without any real known cause (Fig. 41.8). This deformity separate from Poland's syndrome was described recently by Spear et al. [7].

The left side of the chest is commonly slightly more protuberant than the right, and this is associated with a flare of the costal cartilages attributable to the presence of the cardiac silhouette on the left side of the chest. Varying degrees of deficiency in a sunken chest are encountered and impact significantly on the potential result of a patient requesting breast augmentation. The use of chest wall implants is indicated when the discrepancy between the two sides is 3 cm or more. It is most unlikely that breast implants alone can adequately address such a discrepancy because the volume/projection ratios are not sufficient enough to overcome the problem of the depressed base or the chest wall itself on which the implant "sits." Careful planning in addition to the preoperative production of a moulage and custom-

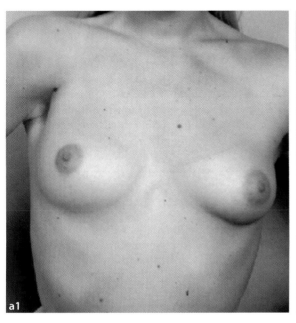

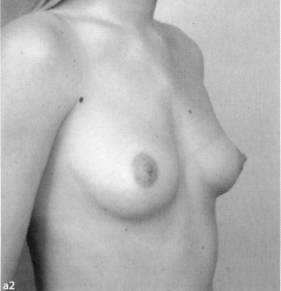

Fig. 41.7 a *1,2* Preoperative patient with Poland's syndrome on her right side

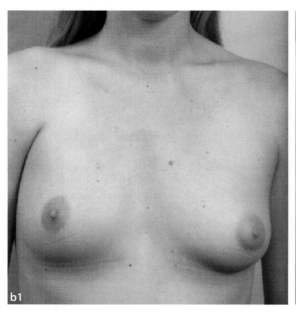
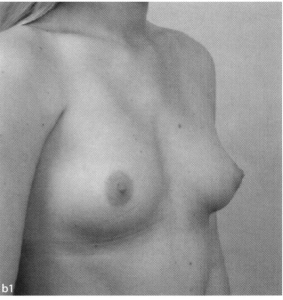

Fig. 41.7 *(continued)* **b** *1,2* Following single chest wall implant, Aiache size 2, via axilla augments the right chest wall

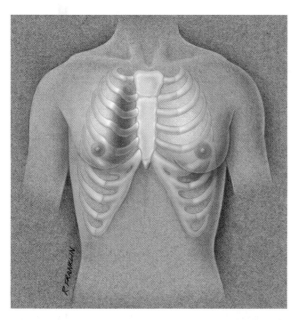

Fig. 41.8 Anterior chest wall hypoplasia with depressed costo-chondral junctions

ized implant are indicated to provide the base on which the breast implant will sit. A customized implant can be inserted by an axillary incision in a total submuscular pocket after detaching the residual sternal origin of the pectoralis major muscle, which allows the chest wall implant to settle along the ribs and costal cartilage. This provides a base on which a subglandular implant can be positioned. It also fills a defect that cannot be satisfactorily addressed by the position, shape, or size of a breast prosthesis (Fig. 41.9).

Usually, a soft #5 durometer silicone chest wall implant with slight texture is chosen so that there will be less implant "show," especially when the patient has thin, subcutaneous tissues or when the percutaneous show of the implant is unavoidable. The softer durometer implant is less likely to be palpable and visible, but it does have a higher risk of capsular contracture and distortion than the firmer #10 durometer implant, and this should be borne in mind whenever choosing the #5 softer implant. In my experience, no capsular contracture has occurred around customized subpectoral chest wall implants for the treatment of sunken chest in either this type of patient or in a patient with Poland's syndrome (Figs. 41.10–41.12).

41.9
Scoliosis

Scoliosis is associated with an axial torsion of the rib cage (Fig. 41.13). This is manifested by one chest wall projecting more than the opposite and, consequently, breast asymmetry. The patient may perceive that one breast is larger than the other, whereas one breast is seated more anteriorly than the other. Attempts to use asymmetric implants will likely fail because the difference in the projection of different implants with differ-

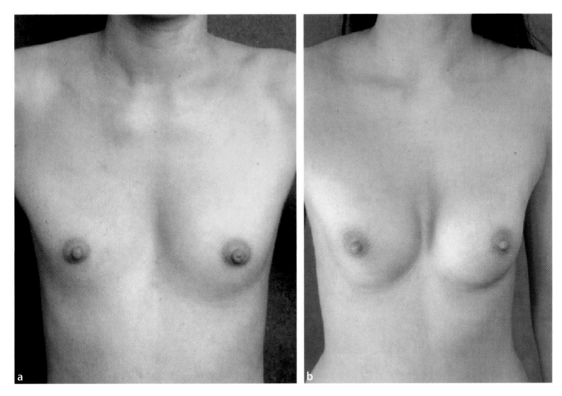

Fig. 41.9 a Preoperative right anterior chest wall depression and hypomastia. **b** Four years after correction via axillary insertion of Aiache size 2 chest wall implant via axilla and 200-ml smooth saline implants via submammary approach

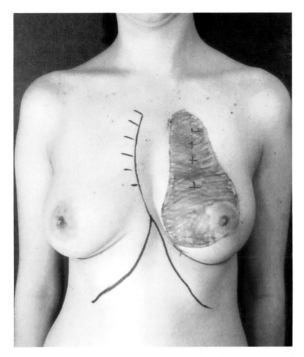

Fig. 41.10 Design for large chest wall implant for correction of left anterior chest wall hypoplasia

ent fills will not make up the discrepancy in projection if the projection approaches a 3-cm difference or more. A prefabricated, modified chest wall implant or a customized solid silicone implant placed subpectorally can assist breast augmentation by providing a suitable base for the breast prosthesis (Figs. 41.14, 41.15).

41.10
Customized Chest Wall Implant: Moulage Preparation

An important prerequisite for successful augmentation of the chest is accurate modelling of the defect using either papier-mâché or plastic modelling clay. The patient should lie supine and comfortable during the modelling process, which may take up to 1 h. The author prefers to use DAS (DAS Pronto; Fila, Pero, Italy), an inexpensive artist's modelling clay that sets firmly and can easily be removed from the patient soon after preparation, rather than papier-mâché, which is required to be on the patient's chest wall for a prolonged period and which, if damp, will lose its curve and contour easily after extrication from the patient.

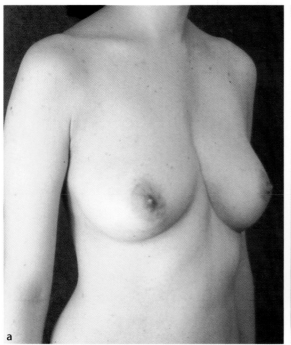
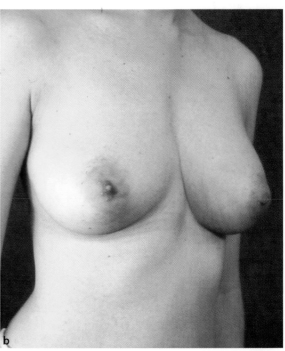

Fig. 41.11 a Preoperative patient with depressed chest wall. **b** Good improvement of depressed chest wall with large cus-tomized #5 durometer textured solid chest wall implant inserted via submammary incision

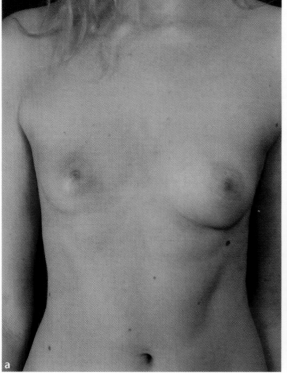
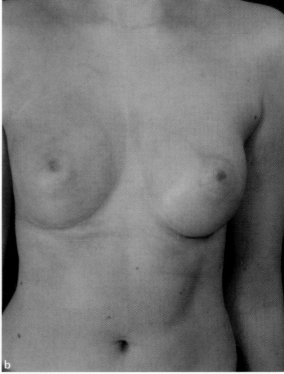

Fig. 41.12 a Breast asymmetry and right anterior chest wall hypoplasia. **b** Following correction with concomitant smooth gel breast implants, 360-ml right, 300-ml left, and right customized solid subpectoral implant

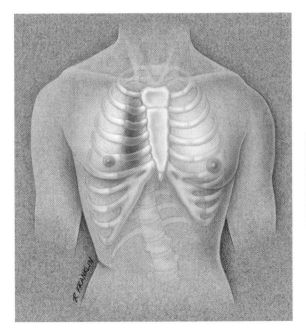

Fig. 41.13 Scoliosis with rotational torsion of anterior chest wall

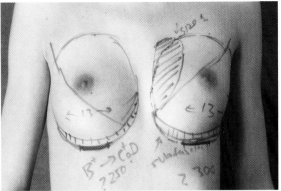

Fig. 41.14 Design of repair and augmentation of patient with scoliosis

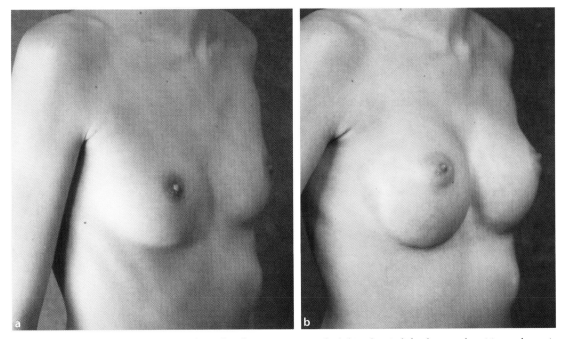

Fig. 41.15 **a** Preoperative patient with scoliosis. **b** Following insertion of solid implant in left subpectoral position and associated subfascial gel augmentation

The moulage preparation should provide an accurate template from which the implant manufacturer will produce a solid implant. In women, a solid implant is best produced in a soft, solid silicone form—specifically, #5 durometer for firmness rather than #10 durometer, which is used for male pectoral implants or for sternal defects. Suture tabs are generally not required, and texture incorporating a smooth surface can be specified. There is always a tendency to make the customized implant too large and too thin on the edges. The surgeon should be prepared to sculpt the implant on the operating table. After moulage preparation, the surgeon may determine that the dimensions are similar to an already available manufactured product that can be modified to suit the defect so that customization of the implant is not necessary.

41.11
Discussion

Although chest wall deformities are present in a small number of patients presenting for breast augmentation, the presence and the degree of deformity, when considered, may alter the technique for optimal correction. The surgeon's comfort level in using chest wall implantation for pectus excavatum, sunken chest, or Poland's syndrome by addressing the problem at the same time as breast augmentation leads to a better aesthetic result for many of these patients. Only a few authors have directed their attention to the role of the chest wall, its evaluation, and correction of deformities in routine breast augmentation [8, 9].

On closer examination, the experienced surgeon notes that in fact many patients have some degree of underlying skeletal deformity and asymmetry that is conferred onto the breasts before and after augmentation mammaplasty. Probably fewer than 2% of patients have skeletomuscular problems significant enough to be taken into account and dealt with separately or together with the breast augmentation to provide an optimal outcome. For patients with a significant skeletomuscular problem, a customized or prefabricated chest wall implant might be the preferred option.

The usual route of chest wall implant insertion is through an axillary approach, or utilizing the same submammary breast augmentation incision. The implant can be rolled into a "roulade" shape and introduced carefully before being unfurled. The softer implants should not be forcibly inserted because of the risk of tearing the implant. A flat "butter knife" instrument or large urethral sound can help when positioning the implant. When breast implants are inserted through a sub-mammary incision, the chest wall implant can also be inserted using a separate submuscular plane from the subglandular or subfascial breast prosthesis plane.

The reconstructive options that have been used for patients with the most severe deformities include tissue expansion, microvascular surgery, and thoracic surgical approaches. In these cases, the primary presentation may be to the thoracic surgeon and not to the plastic surgeon, the former reviewing the most severe cases and performing procedures involving thoracotomy. In these patients, the desire for augmentation may be of secondary importance; the pathologic or gross skeletal deformity probably predominates [10].

41.12
Conclusions

Boniness of the chest caused by prominence of the manubriosternal area can be addressed by high and medial placement of breast prostheses. Customized or prefabricated solid chest wall implants have been used in conjunction with breast prostheses to treat patients presenting for breast enhancement who have significant chest wall deformities. The recognition of associated chest wall deformities in patients who present with breast asymmetry has led to the successful treatment of those asymmetries at the time of breast augmentation. This can be accomplished by using solid chest wall implants to provide a solid base onto which breast prostheses can be seated.

References

1. Rohrich RJ, Hartley W, Brown, S: Incidence of breast and chest wall asymmetry in breast augmentation: a retrospective analysis of 100 patients. Plast Reconstr Surg 2003;111(4):1513–1519
2. Donnelly LF, Taylor CNR, Emery KH, Brody AS: Asymptomatic, palpable anterior chest wall lesions in children: is cross-sectional imaging necessary? Radiology 1997;202(3):829–831
3. Bentz ML, Futrell JW: Improved chest wall fixation for correction of pectus excavatum. Br J Plast Surg 1992;45(5):367–370
4. Nakajima H, Chang H: A new method of reconstruction for pectus excavatum that preserves blood supply and costal cartilage. Plast Reconstr Surg 1999;103(6):1661–1666
5. Hodgkinson DJ: Chest wall implants: their use for pectus excavatum, pectoralis muscle tears, Poland's syndrome and muscular insufficiency. Aesthetic Plast Surg 1997;21(1):7–15

6. Hochberg J, Ardenghy M, Graeber GM, Murray GF: Complex reconstruction of the chest wall and breast utilising a customised silicone implant. Ann Plast Surg 1994;32(5): 524–528

7. Spear SL, Pelletiere CV, Lee ES, Grotting JC: Anterior thoracic hypoplasia: a separate entity from Poland's syndrome. Plast Reconstr Surg 2004;113(1):69–77

8. Hodgkinson DJ: The management of anterior chest wall deformity in patients presenting for breast augmentation. Plast Reconstr Surg 2002;109(5):1714–1723

9. Hoffman S: Augmentation mammaplasty for tuberous breasts and other complex anomalies. In: Spear SL (ed). Surgery of the Breast: Principles and Art. Philadelphia, Lippincott-Raven 1998, pp 907–919

10. Von Rauffer L, Hecht L, Landsleitner B: Mamma-augmentation-plasty after operation for funnel chest deformity. Aesthetic Plast Surg 1980;4:47

CHAPTER 42

Poland's Syndrome

42

Renato da Silva Freitas, André Ricardo Dall'Oglio Tolazzi, Anileda Ribeiro dos Santos, Ruth Maria Graf, Gilvani Azor de Oliveira e Cruz

42.1
Introduction

Poland's syndrome is an uncommon disorder with unknown cause. Although reports of anomalies consistent with Poland's syndrome appeared as early as 1826 [1, 2], the syndrome was first described by Poland in 1841 [3]. Ever since Poland described a group of anomalies with absence of the pectoralis major and minor muscles and syndactyly of the ipsilateral hand, many variations of this condition have been reported in the literature. Thomson, in 1895, added other features, including the absence of ribs, chest wall depression, amastia with or without athelia, the absence of axillary hair, and limited subcutaneous fat. Other authors have described the syndrome by many names, including subclavian artery supply disruption sequence, hand and ipsilateral thorax syndrome, fissura thoracis lateralis, acro-pectoral-renal field defect, pectoral-aplasia-dysdactylia syndrome, and unilateral chest–hand deformity. In 1962, Clarkson [4] gave the credit to Poland for recognizing the syndrome, and since the publication by Baudinne et al. in 1967 [5], the condition has been generally referred to as Poland's syndrome.

Ravitch and Handelsman [6] first reported reconstructive details of the syndrome. During the last decade, large contributing series and literature reviews have been published, elucidating and standardizing several features of the diagnosis and treatment of Poland's syndrome [7–9].

Poland's syndrome is usually, if not always, unilateral, although a single bilateral case has been reported [10]. The general incidence of Poland's syndrome ranges from 1:7,000 to 1:100,000 live births, being more prevalent in males than females (ratio of 2:1 to 3:1) and more frequently (60–70%) affecting the right side of the body. Nevertheless, the incidence and presentation of Poland's syndrome vary with regard to inheritance pattern, gender prevalence, and severity of commitment. Sporadic cases have the same distribution reported above, being more frequent in males and on the right side. However, sporadic female cases show a similar incidence of left and right side, and in familial cases, gender and body-side distribution are almost equal [11–13]. Moreover, the extent and severity of involvement are largely variable, and there is also a lack of correlation among the extent of hand, breast, and thoracic deformities [7, 14–16].

42.2
Etiology

Poland's syndrome is a sporadic, congenital disorder with a low risk (<1%) of reoccurrence in the same family [17, 18]. Familial inheritance is uncommon. It is consistent with delayed mutation of an autosomal dominant gene and is associated with increased parental age (especially paternal) [19–25]. Although there is no substantially increased risk of reoccurrence of the defect in families with only one affected child and no affected parent, genetic counseling is still advisable [19–22, 24, 26]. A thorough examination of the proband's close relatives is recommended and should focus on stigmas such as anomalies of dermatoglyphics and minor shortening of the palm. If they are absent, the prognosis is favorable; if there are minimal manifestations, a risk of up to 50% in the offspring must be foreseen [26].

Several theories have been proposed to explain the etiology of Poland's syndrome, including autosomal dominant inheritance, single gene defects, and intrauterine insults such as trauma, viral infections, teratogenic effects of environmental xenobiotics, and even smoking [27–29]. The most acceptable theory, however, concerns a restrictive vascular phenomenon. At about the end of the 6th week of gestation, an interruption of the embryonic blood supply causes hypoplasia of the ipsilateral subclavian artery or one of its branches. This is supported by data showing evidence of reduction in its diameter and blood flow velocity. Consequently, there is underdevelopment of the ipsilateral mammary gland, local skin, subcutaneous tissue, muscular units, and the upper limb. The extent of commitment depends on the level and branches of the subclavian artery that are affected. Isolated pectoralis major muscle hypoplasia may occur because of internal thoracic artery involvement, while hand malformations are caused by brachial artery hypoplasia [13, 30, 31].

42.3
Clinical Presentations

Although Poland's syndrome is widely variable in its presentation, it is very rare to find all components present in a single patient. Clinical features of Poland's syndrome include the following:

1. Hypoplasia of the breast and nipple–areola complex
2. Scarcity of subcutaneous tissue and thin skin over the pectoral region
3. Absence of the pectoralis major muscle (usually costosternal head)
4. Absence of the pectoralis minor muscle
5. Deficiency of additional chest wall muscles, including the latissimus dorsi, external oblique, and serratus anterior
6. Aplasia or deformity of costal cartilages or ribs
7. Alopecia of the axillary and mammary regions
8. Unilateral brachysyndactyly

The diagnostic criteria of Poland's syndrome should include hypoplasia of the pectoralis major muscle and the ipsilateral breast. This is defined as partial Poland's sequence, and its incidence has been reported as 1:16,500 live births [30, 32]. As we can see, the diagnosis of mild forms of this syndrome may be easily missed in female candidates for breast augmentation who have mild asymmetric bilateral breast hypoplasia. Different forms of commitment may be seen even with familial cases, with only one family member presenting hand deformities associated with pectoral hypoplasia [19, 33].

Since 1998, the authors have treated 20 patients with the diagnosis of Poland's syndrome, comprising 16 females and four males with ages ranging from 2 to 43 years.

42.3.1
Breast and Nipple–Areola Complex

Although Poland's syndrome has a male predominance (3:1), female patients commonly present with marked breast deformities, which cause great psychological stress and make them search for reconstructive procedures more often than men do.

Breast asymmetry is frequently observed in patients with Poland's syndrome, usually due to underdevelopment of the breast during puberty. It ranges from mild hypomastia to complete absence of the breast (amastia) [34]. Not only the mammary glandular tissue is underdeveloped, but also the subcutaneous tissue and overlying skin. Similarly, the nipple–areola complex may also be abnormal, being frequently smaller, hypopigmented, and superiorly sited comparing with the contralateral

developed breast. These findings are easily noticeable in female patients, usually in their teen years.

In our series of 20 patients, among the 16 women treated, breast hypoplasia was found in nine and amastia in seven. The nipple–areola complex on the affected side was always smaller than the normal one. It was elevated in 13 women and all four men and was orthotopic in three women. Fig. 42.1 illustrates variable grades of breast hypoplasia and nipple–areola complex commitment. Even in cases with mild breast commitment, a lack of anterior axillary fold and breast upper-pole hollowness are seen due to major pectoralis muscle hypoplasia.

42.3.2
Trunk Muscles

The most frequent sign in patients with Poland's syndrome is underdevelopment of the sternocostal head of the pectoralis major muscle, which leads to lack of anterior axillary fold. Some authors state that this is the sine qua non or the common denominator of all patients with Poland's syndrome [35]. The clavicular head of the pectoralis major muscle and the pectoralis minor muscle may be absent as well. Other muscles may also be affected, including the latissimus dorsi, external oblique, and serratus anterior. The latissimus dorsi muscle forms part of the posterior axillary fold, which is usually visible by frontal view when the pectoralis major muscle is lacking. Absence of the superior portion of the serratus anterior muscle causes scapula alata (Sprengel's deformity) [13, 36].

These findings are usually seen with physical examination, especially in male patients. Further evaluation using imaging studies may ascertain the degree of muscular underdevelopment and the associated chest wall deficiency. As observed in athletes with Poland's syndrome, its features do not necessarily cause functional impairment [8, 23, 32, 37].

42.3.3
Chest Wall

Similarly to the affected breast, chest wall deformities become more evident during growth periods [14]. The superior portion of the anterior chest wall usually presents variable degrees of depression, not only due to pectoralis muscle hypoplasia but also consequent to costal cartilage and rib cage underdevelopment. Aplasia, hypoplasia, or deformity may be found in about 11–25% of patients, frequently affecting one to three costal cartilages, more often anterior ribs II–IV or III–V [16, 34, 38]. The committed ribs may not fuse to the sternum,

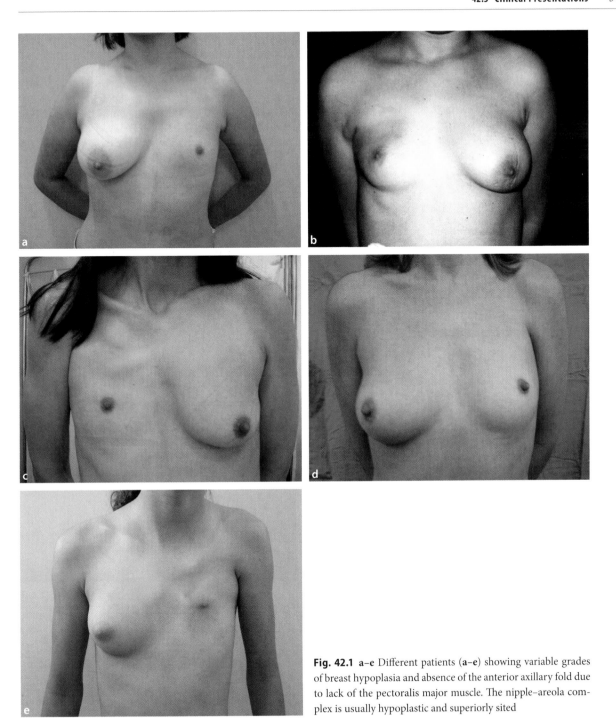

Fig. 42.1 a–e Different patients (**a–e**) showing variable grades of breast hypoplasia and absence of the anterior axillary fold due to lack of the pectoralis major muscle. The nipple–areola complex is usually hypoplastic and superiorly sited

becoming fluctuates. Consequently, the superior portion of the sternum, including the manubrium, rotates internally, leading to asymmetrical contralateral pectus carinatum [16, 23]. Our series included six cases with pectus carinatum, including one man.

42.3.4
Intrathoracic Organs

Even in the most severe forms of Poland's syndrome, pulmonary or cardiac involvement is relatively uncommon. Rib malformations and thoracic depression may cause paradoxical respiratory movements and decrease pulmonary vital capacity. Lung herniation has been reported in 8% of patients [35]. Vital capacity has been shown to be as low as 48%, and it may improve about 20% after surgical correction of the chest wall deformity [39].

The syndrome shows a tendency for the heart to be shifted toward the unaffected side [23]. Thus, left-side syndrome commitment is associated with increased incidence of dextrocardia. Unlike isolated dextrocardia, in Poland's syndrome there is dextroposition without inversion of the cardiovascular structures and without other associated abnormalities. This was reported in 5.6% of a series of 144 patients with Poland's syndrome, in which 9.6% of patients had left-sided disease [13]. Patients of consanguineous parents have an increased incidence of dextrocardia [40, 41].

42.3.5
Upper Limb

Hand anomalies are other common features of Poland's syndrome. Besides commitment of the contralateral hand and lower extremity that has been described [32, 42, 43], it usually involves the ipsilateral limb, with an incidence of 13.5–56% [4, 16, 32, 33]. The characteristic malformation is brachysyndactyly, formed by shortness or absence of the middle phalanges, and interdigital cutaneous webbing. Hypoplasia or aplasia of the middle phalanges is more common in ulnar fingers and is not necessarily confined to the digits involved in syndactyly. The first web space is often moderately shallow, which gives the appearance of a small and malrotated thumb [35, 38, 44].

Among 20 patients being treated in our center, hand malformations were more prevalent in men. Ipsilateral syndactyly involving the 2nd and 3rd fingers was found in only two of 15 women. Two of four male patients had brachysyndactyly, which affected the 3rd and 4th fingers in both cases (Fig. 42.2).

42.3.6
Other Associated Malformations

Poland's syndrome may coexist with several congenital malformations, syndromes, and even acquired diseases. Since the first description in 1973, it has been associated with Moebius syndrome [45–49]. Patients usually present bilateral facial palsy, paralysis of the eye abductors, and variable features of Poland's syndrome. Associated atrial septal defect has also been described [48].

Poland–Moebius syndrome has been found in about 10% of patients with Moebius syndrome, and its etiology has been based on a vascular theory as well [4, 13].

Similarly, Poland's syndrome may be associated with Klippel–Feil syndrome, which is characterized by shortness of the neck. The latter is attributed to fusion of the cervical vertebrae and abnormalities of the brain stem and cerebellum due to a delay in the development of the vertebral arteries [13].

The acro-pectoral-renal malformation is constituted by features of Poland's syndrome associated with urinary malformations, such as renal agenesis or duplication of the urinary collecting system [49, 50]. The renal anomalies may impair renal function or cause renovascular hypertension. Thus, patients with pectoral muscle anomalies should be screened for coexisting renal anomalies.

The syndrome has also been associated with numerous neoplasms, including leukemia, non-Hodgkin's lymphoma, cervical cancer, leiomyosarcoma, and lung cancer [51, 52]. Mammary tissue hypoplasia does not prevent the breast from pathologic processes and in-

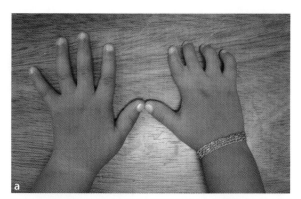

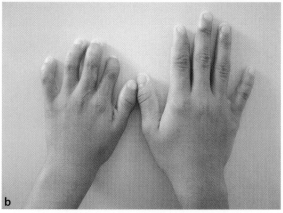

Fig. 42.2 Cases of brachysyndactyly of the 2nd and 3rd fingers. **a** Right hand affected. **b** Left hand affected

vasive ductal carcinomas [35, 53]. Poland's syndrome deformities may also be misdiagnosed as neurological sequelae of trauma [54].

The authors have seen a case of Poland's syndrome associated with hemifacial microsomia, including mandible hypoplasia, ear deformity, and facial palsy.

42.4 Treatment

The goals of surgical repair of these anomalies are twofold: to correct any functional deficits and to create a cosmetically acceptable result. The wide variety of anomalies associated with Poland's syndrome corresponds to a range of reconstructive options. Moreover, indications for surgery also differ depending on the degree of the deformity and the patient's gender and age. The most common indication for surgery is breast asymmetry in females, due to aplasia/hypoplasia of mammary tissue and the pectoralis major muscle. Male patients usually complain about pectoral asymmetry and absence of the anterior axillary fold. Major defects causing chest wall depression, paradoxical respiratory movements, and compromise of intrathoracic organs constitute priorities for surgical correction and demand complex reconstructive procedures. Fortunately, most severe forms of the syndrome, including those with rib involvement, pulmonary commitment, and significant chest wall dysfunction, are rare [55]. Consequently, the great majority of indications for reconstruction are related to aesthetic complaints, with aims to address the adverse psychosocial problems of the deformities.

In both children and adults, severe chest wall deformities should be prioritized for treatment. The rib defect can be reconstructed using split-rib grafts taken subperiostially from the unaffected side, other bony allografts or autografts, mesh-patch, or a combination of several of the above. This form of reconstruction is usually indicated when three or more ribs are absent. To provide stable rib cage reconstruction and to avoid paradoxical respiratory movements and lung herniation, the grafts should be fixed medially to the sternum and laterally to the freshened surface of the ends of the ribs [23]. If synthetic mesh is used, it should be well stretched and sutured to the edges of the defect and to underlying supporting bone grafts. Because the rib grafts may not be effectively stabilized and tend to rotate on their axes, embedding the medial ends of the grafts into a deepened opening in the side of the sternum and suturing the grafts to the prosthetic sheet above is advisable [35]. When only two ribs are absent, a split graft from the adjacent superior and inferior normal ribs may be used, displacing and fixing only the lateral extremity of the graft to

the ends of the aplastic ribs. Fluctuant aplastic ribs that are fused to each other on their anterior ends should be separated and reattached to the sternum [23, 56].

Severe chest wall depression associated with hypoplastic ribs may be corrected by subperichondrial resection and elevation of the costal cartilage segments, with possible mesh reinforcement [23, 57]. Simultaneous sternal inward rotation may be elevated with a high transverse sternotomy and a "reversed" figure-eight wire suture [58]. In children, the scarcity of thoracic soft tissues should usually be addressed after puberty, when the contralateral breast is completely developed. In adults, simultaneous muscle transposition and augmentation mammaplasty may be associated with chest wall stabilization [14, 38, 59].

Breast–pectoralis muscle hypoplasia may be reconstructed with silicone breast implants and muscular or musculocutaneous flaps [8]. In cases with mild breast hypoplasia or minimal infraclavicular hollowness, or if the anterior axillary fold deformity is not prominent, implants alone have been used successfully (Fig. 42.3) [60, 61]. When contralateral breast hypoplasia is also found, bilateral breast implants of different sizes may be used to augment both breasts and to compensate the asymmetry (Fig. 42.4). To obtain enough coverage tissue, patients with scarce skin and subcutaneous tissue will probably need a musculocutaneous flap or local tissue expansion prior to the muscular flap rotation and silicone prosthesis insertion (Fig. 42.5) [14, 38].

The nipple–areola complex is usually involved and can be superiorly sited, hypoplastic, or even absent. Correction of this nipple–areolar complex dystopia is one of the most difficult reconstructive stages. To achieve symmetry, we have made bilateral periareolar incisions with a skin resection on top of the normal nipple–areolar complex and on the bottom of the affected complex. After a round-block suture, the position and size of both complexes are compensated, giving a more symmetric appearance (Fig. 42.6). Moreover, in some cases with a severely hypoplastic nipple–areolar complex, we have used the whole complex to reconstruct the nipple, and a peripheral tattoo was done to achieve areola symmetry (Fig. 42.7).

Over the past two decades, Poland's syndrome reconstruction in female patients has frequently been achieved by performing latissimus dorsi muscle transfer and permanent implant placement [62–67]. The latissimus dorsi muscle partially covers the breast implant, attenuating its superior contour, providing infraclavicular fullness, and recreating the anterior axillary fold, while the implant effectively reconstructs the breast. For men, it has been used to correct the chest concavity and absence of the anterior axillary fold consequent to lack of the pectoralis major muscle.

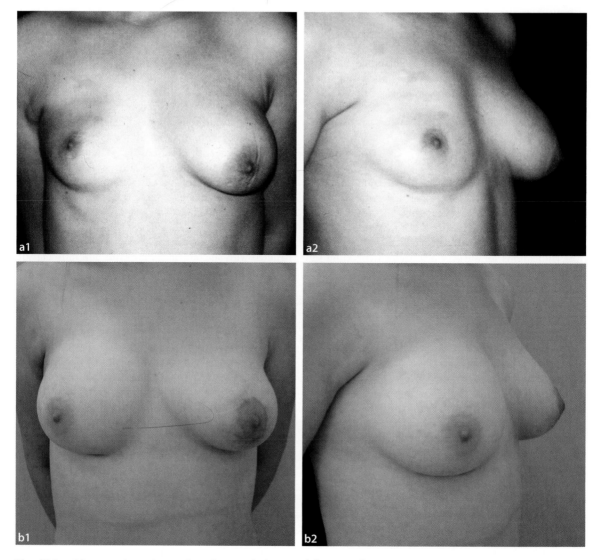

Fig. 42.3 a *1* Preoperative patient with moderate right breast and pectoralis muscle hypoplasia. *2* Lateral view. **b** *1* Postoperative following silicone implantation in right breast (200 ml) and left periareolar mastopexy. *2* Lateral view. (Photos with kind permission of Springer Science and Business Media)

Some authors have stated that the latissimus dorsi muscle flap progressively evolves into atrophy, decreasing the long-term aspect of pectoral fullness and anterior axillary fold reconstruction [62]. The procedure also removes one of the major muscles of the shoulder and arm and leaves another thoracic scar. Because of this, instead of doing a latissimus dorsi flap, some authors prefer prefabricated chest wall implants to recreate pectoral sweep and the anterior axillary fold, especially when large rib defects and significant anterior chest wall depression are present [8, 62, 68]. Nevertheless, if muscle innervation is preserved during surgery and an individualized physiotherapeutic program is instituted postoperatively, some hypertrophy to the transferred muscle flap may be achieved, preserving aesthetic outcomes [23].

Despite the aesthetically pleasing results that can be achieved with this technique, substantial donor-site morbidity exists because of the muscle harvest. In order to minimize nonaesthetic scars and achieve the same reconstructive goals, endoscopically-assisted procedures and reduced-access incisions have been developed for latissimus dorsi muscle harvest and implant placement [69].

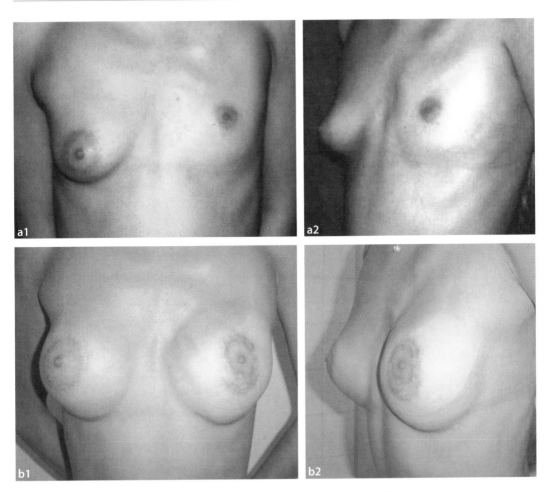

Fig. 42.4 a *1* Preoperative patient with severe hypoplasia of the breast and pectoralis muscle on the right side, associated with mild hypomastia and ptosis on the contralateral side. *2* Lateral view. **b** *1* Postoperative following different-size bilateral silicone breast implantation, rotation of the left latissimus dorsi muscle flap, and reposition of the left nipple–areola complex. *2* Lateral view. (Photos with kind permission of Springer Science and Business Media)

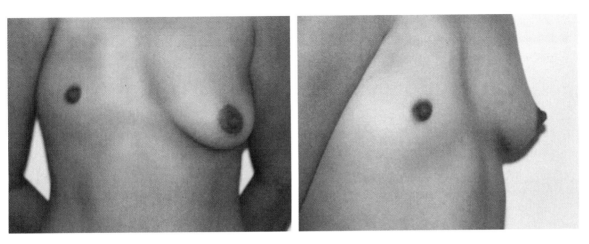

Fig. 42.5 a *1* Preoperative patient with severe hypoplasia of the breast and pectoralis muscle on her right side, associated with mild hypomastia on the contralateral side. *2* Lateral view

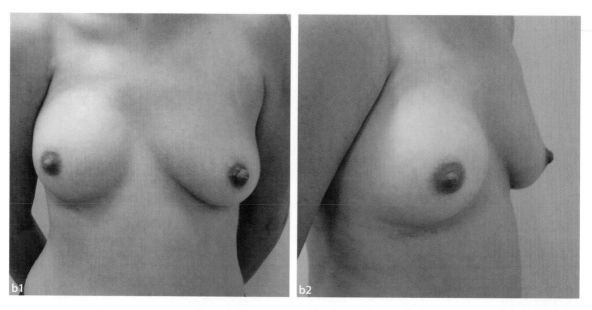

Fig. 42.5 *(continued)* **b** *1* Postoperative following right breast expansion followed by silicone implantation and latissimus dorsi muscle flap coverage. *2* Lateral view. (Photos with kind permission of Springer Science and Business Media)

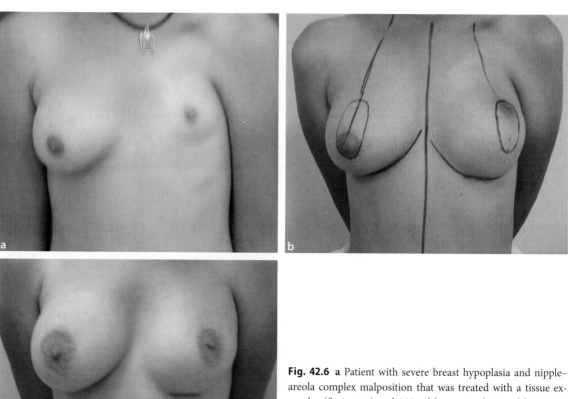

Fig. 42.6 a Patient with severe breast hypoplasia and nipple–areola complex malposition that was treated with a tissue expander (first stage) and 220-ml breast implant and latissimus dorsi flap (second stage). **b** Preoperative markings showing compensating periareolar skin resections. **c** Final result after left breast augmentation and achievement of nipple–areola complex symmetry

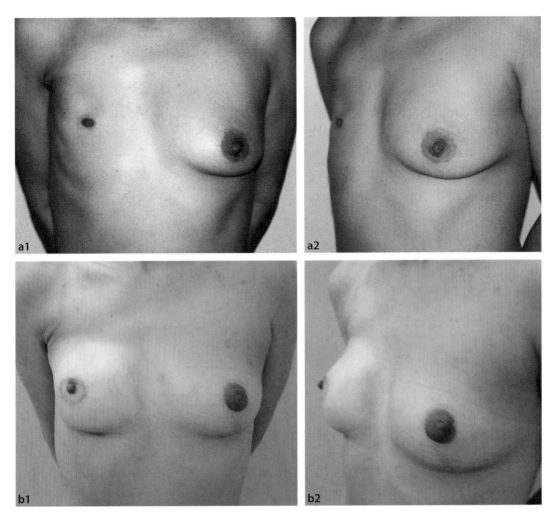

Fig. 42.7 a *1* Preoperative patient with severe hypoplasia of the breast, nipple–areola complex, and pectoralis major muscle on the right side, associated with mild hypomastia on the contralateral side. *2* Lateral view. **b** *1* Postoperative following first-stage right breast expansion, second-stage silicone implantation and latissimus dorsi muscle flap rotation, and third-stage nipple reconstruction using the whole hypoplastic nipple–areola complex. Areola tattooing will be done later on. *2* Lateral view. (Photos with kind permission of Springer Science and Business Media)

The authors' preference is to correct the pectoral breast defect with a latissimus dorsi flap and placement of a breast implant through a single reduced skin access. A 4–6-cm incision is performed longitudinally over the middle axillary line, at the level of the nipple–areola complex, which gives access for both muscle harvest and implant placement (Fig. 42.8). Another option is an S-shaped incision in the axillary fold, dissecting the muscle flap and breast implant space using long light retractors or endoscopic assistance (Fig. 42.9). To achieve better symmetry, sometimes we have also used fat grafting in later stages, especially in the infraclavicular depression.

On the basis of our experience, flowcharts were developed for systematic diagnosis and surgical treatment. The four principal elements evaluated were the affected breast, the contralateral normal breast, the size and position of the nipple–areolar complex, and thoracic deformities (Figs. 42.10–42.12).

Because patients with Poland's syndrome may present latissimus dorsi hypoplasia, other reconstruction options should be considered. Once the posterior axillary fold is formed mainly by the latissimus dorsi and teres major muscles, a normal appearance of the posterior axillary fold may be present even in patients with latissimus dorsi hypoplasia. Based on this, some

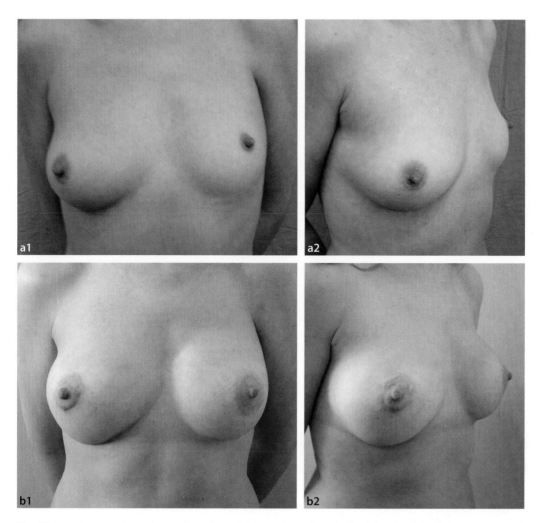

Fig. 42.8 a *1* Preoperative patient with moderate left breast hypoplasia (Poland's) and mild right breast ptosis and hypoplasia. *2* Lateral view. **b** *1* Postoperative following bilateral silicone breast implantation and short scar (4 cm) rotation of the left latissimus dorsi muscle flap, along with fat injection in the infraclavicular area. *2* Lateral view

authors recommend imaging studies (computed tomographic scanning and magnetic resonance imaging) when a latissimus dorsi muscle flap is considered for Poland's syndrome reconstruction [69, 70]. When this first option is not feasible, other pedicle and microsurgical flaps may be indicated, such as a free contralateral latissimus dorsi muscular or musculocutaneous flap, a pedicle or free-TRAM flap, or upper gluteal flaps.

Hand reconstructive surgery ranges depending on the degree of commitment. Syndactylies should be corrected early, preferably in the 1st year of life, before abnormal compensatory function patterns have developed and the deformity has progressed [35]. Despite adequate treatment, the hand will probably retain hypoplastic characteristics.

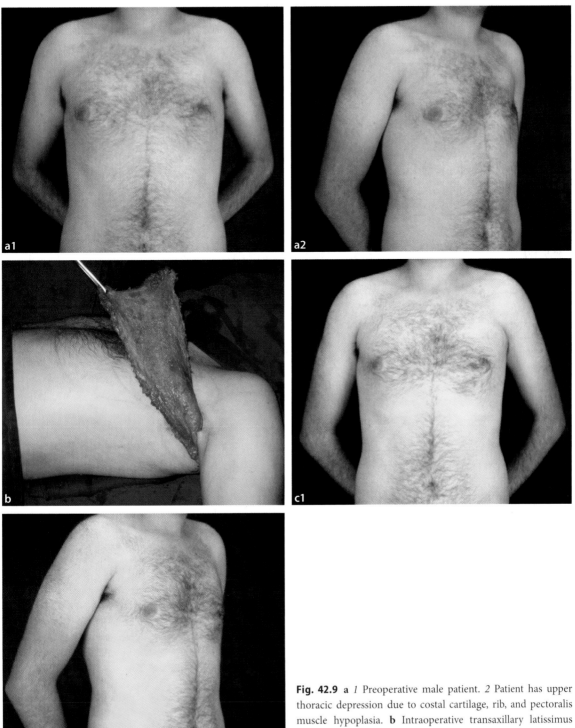

Fig. 42.9 a *1* Preoperative male patient. *2* Patient has upper thoracic depression due to costal cartilage, rib, and pectoralis muscle hypoplasia. **b** Intraoperative transaxillary latissimus dorsi muscle flap rotation. **c** *1,2* Postoperative views showing improvement of the upper thoracic depression

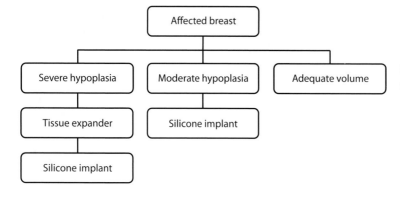

Fig. 42.10 Systematic scheme for treating the affected breast

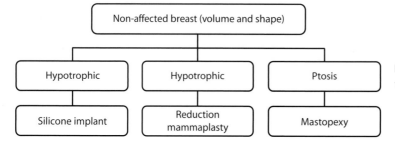

Fig. 42.11 Systematic scheme for treating the unaffected breast

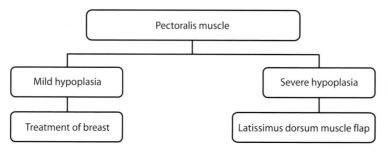

Fig. 42.12 Systematic scheme for treating hypoplastic pectoralis major muscle defect

References

1. Lallemand LM: Absence de trois côtes simulant un enfoncement accidentel. Éphémérides Médicales de Montpelier 1826;1:144–147

2. Froriep R: Beobachtung eines Falles von Mangel der Brustdruse. Notizen aus dem Gebiete der Natur und Heilkinde 1839;10:9–14

3. Poland A: Deficiency of the pectoral muscles. Guy's Hospital Reports 1841;6:191–193

4. Clarkson P: Poland's syndactyly. Guy's Hospital Rep 1962;111:335–346

5. Baudinne P, Bovy GL, Wasterlain A: Un cas de syndrome de Poland. Acta Paediatr Belg 1967;21(5):407–410

6. Ravitch MM, Handelsman JC: Lesions of the thoracic parietes in infants and children. Deformities and tumors of the chest wall, abnormalities of diaphragm. Surg Clin North Am 1952;95(6):1397–1424

7. Urschel HC: Poland's syndrome. Chest Surg Clin N Am 2000;10(2):393–403

8. Glicenstein J: Correction des anomalies thoraciques du syndrome de Poland. Revue générale et a propos de 20 patients. Ann Chir Plast Esthét 2001;466):640–651

9. Da Silva Freitas R, Dall'Oglio Tolazzi AR, Martins VD, Knop BA, Graf RM, de Olivera e Cruz GA: Poland's syndrome: different clinical presentations and surgical reconstructions in 18 cases. Aesthetic Plast Surg. 2007;31(2):140–146

10. Karnak I, Tanyel FC, Tuncbilek E, Unsal M, Buyukpamukcu N: Bilateral Poland anomaly. Am J Med Genet 1998;75(5):505–507

11. Perez Azner JM, Urbano J, Garcia Laborda E, Quevado Moreno P, Ferrer Vergara L: Breast and pectoralis muscle hypoplasia. A mild degree of Poland's syndrome. Acta Radiologica 1996;37(5):759–762

12. Bamforth JS, Fabian C, Machin G, Honore L: Poland anomaly with a limb body wall disruption defect: case report and review. Am J Med Genet 1992;43(5):780–784

13. Bavinck JN, Weaver DD: Subclavian artery supply disruption sequence: hypothesis of a vascular etiology for Poland, Klippel-Feil, and Mobius anomalies. Am J Med Genet 1986; 23:903–918

14. Urschel HC Jr, Byrd HS, Sethi SM, Razzuk MA: Poland's syndrome: improved surgical management. Ann Thorac Surg 1984;37(3):204–211

15. David TJ: The Poland anomaly and allied disorders. Pediatr Res 1981;15(8):1184

16. Shamberger RC, Welch KJ, Upton J III: Surgical treatment of thoracic deformity in Poland's syndrome. J Pediatr Surg 1989;24(8):760–765

17. Gorlin RJ: Risk of recurrence in usually nongenetic malformation syndromes. Birth Defects Orig Artic Ser 1979;15(5C):181–188

18. Stevens DB, Fink BA, Prevel C: Poland's syndrome in one identical twin. J Pediatr Orthop 2000;20(3):392–395

19. Sujansky E, Riccardi VM, Mathew AL: The familial occurrence of Poland syndrome. The National Foundation—Birth Defects: Original Article Series 1977;XIII:117–121

20. David TJ: Familial Poland anomaly. J Med Genet 1982;19(4):293–296

21. Soltan HC, Holmes LB: Familial occurrence of malformations possibly attributable to vascular abnormalities. J Pediatr 1986;108(1):112–114

22. Czeizel A, Vitez M, Lenz W: Letter to the editor: birth prevalence of Poland sequence and proportion of its familial cases. Am J Med Genet 1990;36(4):524

23. Bairov GA, Fokin AA: Surgical treatment of Poland's syndrome in children. Vestn Khir Im II Grek 1994;152(1-2):70–72

24. Samuels TH, Haider MA, Kirkbride P: Poland's syndrome: a mammographic presentation. AJR Am J Roentgenol 1996;166(2):347–348

25. Velez A, Moreno JC: Poland's syndrome and recessive X-linked ichthyosis in two brothers. Clin Exp Dermatol 2000;25(2 pt 1):308–311

26. Kuklik M: Poland–Mobius syndrome and disruption spectrum affecting the face and extremities: a review paper and presentation of five cases. Acta Chir Plast 2000;42(3):95–103

27. Freire-Maia N, Chautard EA, Opitz JM, Freire-Maia A, Quelce-Salgado A: The Poland syndrome—clinical and genealogical data, dermatoglyphic analysis, and incidence. Human Heredity 1973;23(2):97–104

28. David TJ: Nature and etiology of the Poland anomaly. N Engl J Med 1972;287(10):487–489

29. Martinez-Frias ML, Czeizel AE, Rodriguez-Pinilla E, Bermejo E: Smoking during pregnancy and Poland sequence: results of a population-based registry. Teratology 1999;59(1):35–38

30. Merlob P, Schonfeld A, Ovadia Y, Reisner SH: Real-time echo-Doppler duplex scanner in the evaluation of patients with Poland sequence. Eur J Obstet Gynecol Reprod Biol 1989;32(2):103–108

31. Bouvet J-P, Leveque D, Bernetieres F, Gros JJ: Vascular origin of Poland syndrome? A comparative rheographic study of the vascularization of the arms in eight patients. Eur J Pediatr 1978;128(1):17–26

32. Ireland DC, Takayama N, Flatt AE: Poland's syndrome. J Bone Joint Surg 1976;58(1):52–58

33. Al-Qattan MM: Classification of hand anomalies in Poland's syndrome. Br J Plast Surg 2001;54(2):132–136

34. Walker JC Jr, Meijer R, Aranda D: Syndactylism with deformity of the pectoralis muscle—Poland's syndrome. J Ped Surg 1969;4(5):569–572

35. Fokin AA, Robicsek F: Poland's syndrome revisited. Ann Thorac Surg 2002;74(6):2218–2225

36. Hegde HR, Shokeir MH: Posterior shoulder girdle abnormalities with absence of pectoralis major muscle. Am J Med Genet 1982;13(3):285–293

37. Haller JA Jr, Colombani PM, Miller D, Manson P: Early reconstruction of Poland's syndrome using autologous rib grafts combined with latissimus muscle flap. J Pediatr Surg 1984;19(4):423–429

38. Mace JW, Kaplan JM, Schanberger JE, Gotlin RW: Poland's syndrome. Report of seven cases and review of the literature. Clin Pediatr 1972;11(2):98–102

39. Martin LW, Helmsworth JA: The management of congenital deformities of the sternum. J Amer Med Assoc 1962;179:82–84

40. Fraser FC, Teebi AS, Walsh S, Pinsky L: Poland sequence with dextrocardia: which comes first? Am J Med Genet 1997;73(2):194–196

41. Sabry MA, Al Awadi SA, El Alfi A, Gouda SA, Kazi NA, Farag TI: Poland syndrome and associated dextrocardia in Kuwait. Med Principles Pract 1995;4:121–126

42. Powell CV, Coombs RC, David TJ: Poland anomaly with contralateral ulnar ray defect. J Med Genet 1993;30(5):423–424

43. Silengo M, Lerone M, Seri M, Boffi P: Lower extremity counterpart of the Poland syndrome. Clin Genet 1999;55(1):41–43

44. David TJ: Preaxial polydactyly and the Poland complex. J Med Genet 1982;13(3):333–334

45. Koroluk LD, Lanigan DT: Moebius and Poland syndromes. A report of a case. J Can Dent Assoc 1989;55(8):647–648

46. Sugarman GI, Stark HH: Mobius syndrome with Poland's anomaly. J Med Genet 1973;10(2):192–196

47. Rojas-Martinez A, Garcia-Cruz D, Rodriguez-Garcia A, Sanchez- Corona J, Rivas F: Poland–Moebius syndrome in a boy and Poland syndrome in his mother. Clin Genet 1991;40(3):225–228

48. Matsui A, Nakagawa M, Okuno M: Association of atrial septal defect with Poland–Moebius syndrome: vascular disruption can be a common etiologic factor. A case report. Angiology 1997;48(3):269–271

49. Hegde HR, Leung AK: Aplasia of pectoralis major muscle and renal anomalies. Am J Med Genet 1989;32(1):109–111

50. Pranava VM, Rao PSSS, Neelachalam A, Sailendra VH: Poland's syndrome—complicated with renal hypertension. J Assoc Phys India 2000;48(4):452–453

51. Ahn MI, Park SH, Park YH: Poland's syndrome with lung cancer. A case report. Acta Radiologica 2000;41(5):432–434

52. Ravitch MM: Poland's syndrome. In: Wada J, Yokoyama M (eds): Chest Wall Deformities and Their Operative Treatment. Tokyo, AD Printing 1990, pp 209–219

53. Fukushima T, Otake T, Yashima R, Nihei M, Takeuchi S, Kimijima II, Tsuchiya A: Breast cancer in two patients with Poland's syndrome. Breast Cancer 1999;6(2):127–130

54. Higgs SM, Thompson JF: Poland's anomaly: a diagnostic pitfall in upper limb trauma. Injury 2000;31(10):814–815

55. Seyfer AE: Congenital anomalies of the chest wall. In: Cohen M (ed). Mastery of Plastic and Reconstructive Surgery. Boston, Little, Brown 1994

56. Asp K, Sulamaa M: On rare congenital deformities of the thoracic wall. Acta Chir Scandinav 1960;118:392–404

57. Demos NJ: Discussion: Poland's syndrome: improved surgical management. Ann Thorac Surg 1984;37(3):211

58. Robicsek F, Daugherty HK, Mullen DC, Harbold NB Jr, Hall DG, Jackson RD, Masters TN, Sanger PW: Technical consideration in the surgical management of pectus excavatum and carinatum. Ann Thorac Surg 1974;18(6):549–564

59. Haller JA Jr, Colombani PM, Miller D, Manson P: Early reconstruction of Poland's syndrome using autologous rib grafts combined with latissimus muscle flap. J Pediatr Surg 1984;19(4):423–429

60. Gatti JE: Poland's deformity reconstructions with a customized, extrasoft silicone prosthesis. Ann Plast Surg 1997;39(2):122–130

61. Hochberg J, Ardenghy M, Graeber GM, Murray GF: Complex reconstruction of the chest wall and breast utilizing a customized silicone implant. Ann Plast Surg 1994;32(5):524–528

62. Borschel GH, Izenberg PH, Cederna PS: Endoscopically assisted reconstruction of male and female Poland syndrome. Plast Reconstr Surg 2002;109(5):1536–1543

63. Rintala AE, Nordstrom RE: Treatment of severe developmental asymmetry of the female breast. Scand J Plast Reconstr Surg Hand Surg 1989;23(3):231–235

64. Seyfer AE, Icochea R, Graeber GM: Poland's anomaly: natural history and long-term results of chest wall reconstruction in 33 patients. Ann Surg 1988;208(6):776–782

65. Santi P, Berrino P, Galli A: Poland's syndrome: correction of thoracic anomaly through minimal incisions. Plast Reconstr Sur 1985;76(4):639–641

66. Barnett GR, Gianoutsos MP: The latissimus dorsi added fat flap for natural tissue breast reconstruction: report of 15 cases. Plast Reconstr Surg 1996;97(1):63–70

67. Ohjimi Y, Shioya N, Ohjimi H, Kamiishi H: Correction of a chest wall deformity utilizing latissimus dorsi with a turnover procedure. Aesthetic Plast Surg 1989;13(3):199–202

68. Hodgkinson DJ: The management of chest wall deformity in patients presenting for breast augmentation. Plast Reconstr Surg 2002;109(5):1714–1723

69. Borschel GH, Izenberg PH, Cederna PS: Endoscopically assisted reconstruction of male and female Poland syndrome. Plast Reconstr Surg 2002;109(5):1536–1543

70. Beer GM, Kompatscher P, Hergan K: Poland's syndrome and vascular malformations. Br J Plast Surg 1996;49(7):482–484

CHAPTER 43

Breast Augmentation in the Transsexual

43

Nikolas V. Chugay

43.1
Introduction

Breast enlargement is frequently the first serious procedure for males undergoing gender change. The patient's psychological readiness needs to be assessed before performing the procedure; either evaluation by a psychologist or an extensive interview with the plastic surgeon is very important. Some patients already have the physical body that would lend itself well to a gender change and breast enlargement. However, there are other patients who have a male physique to such a degree that breast enlargement would make them look ridiculous. In patients like this, no matter which breast enlargement procedure they would have, they would not look female.

The procedure for breast enlargement in a transsexual patient is very similar to that for female patients.

43.2
Technique

The author prefers the periareolar or axillary approach to the breast in which a pocket is developed under the pectoralis muscle. The inframammary approach is also an excellent one, in which an incision is made in the inframammary fold, dissection is performed and extended underneath the pectoralis muscle, and the pectoralis muscle is split longitudinally to give the breast a pleasing round appearance. The pectoralis in a man is usually thick and provides an excellent covering for the breast prosthesis. Either silicone or saline implants may be used. Silicone implants, if marked encapsulation does not occur, will give the most natural appearance and feel to the breast. With saline prostheses in men, with less fat to cover the breast than in a female patient, ripples from the implants can frequently be seen, and the margin of the prosthesis is more palpable in the inframammary fold region.

An incision is made with a #15 Bard-Parker blade, and then the tissues are dissected by sharp and blunt dissection to the pectoralis fascia. Tissue dissection proceeds inferiorly to the premarked dissection point about 7 cm from the inferior portion of the areola to the inframammary fold. The pectoralis fascia is incised, and the pectoral fibers are spread longitudinally with a curved hemostat. Digital dissection of the plane is established underneath the pectoralis muscle, an Army-Navy retractor is inserted underneath the pectoralis muscle, and the pectoralis muscle is split longitudinally. A Deaver dissector is inserted, and complete dissection is performed underneath the pectoralis muscle. Meticulous hemostasis is then secured, and a silicone gel prosthesis is inserted into the pocket. Then the tissues are repaired in layers, and pressure dressings are applied.

43.3
Discussion

Over the years several patients have desired to remove their breast implants to return to male gender functioning or for religious beliefs. Even if the implant has to be removed 2 or 3 years postoperatively, the skin seems to adapt fairly well and does shrink.

The complications for the procedure would be analogous for any breast enlargement procedure. Infection is a possibility, and all patients are given oral Keflex for 1 week. Bleeding is something that can occur postoperatively. Men tend to bleed more, and again with stress. Patients are requested not to take any aspirin or aspirin products 2 weeks prior to surgery and to stop smoking and drinking alcohol for at least 2 weeks prior to surgery.

Scarring in the areola is not usually a frequent problem. The skin heals well inside the areola proper. Slight asymmetry may occur, requiring an additional touch-up, so patients are usually advised that they may require a touch-up and that there will be an additional fee for performing this procedure. Most of the patients who are well counseled preoperatively do have very satisfactory and happy outcomes as a result of the procedure.

The breast size for augmentation in the transsexual tends to be considerably larger than in the female patient because of the larger pectoral diameter and also frequently because of the greater height of the patient. The author's average size used ranges from 500 ml to 550 ml, but several patients have had 750–800-ml and larger breasts. Breast transsexuals do often request a significantly larger breast, and the author asks them to bring in magazine pictures of breasts they consider to be of adequate size. Patients are shown before-and-after photos of patients to again determine which size they feel would be comfortable for them.

43.4
Conclusions

Breast augmentation in the transsexual is usually a very positive and uplifting experience for patients who were prescreened well (Fig. 43.1).

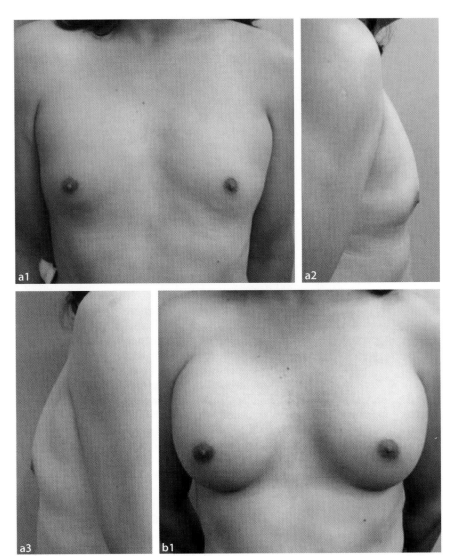

Fig. 43.1 a *1–3* Preoperative.
b *1–3* Postoperative

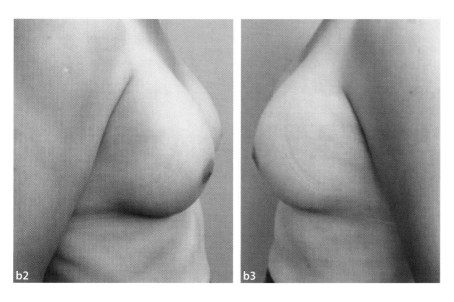

Fig. 43.1 *(continued)*
b *1–3* Postoperative

Chapter 44

Anesthetic Drip System to Reduce Pain in Cosmetic Surgery

44

Melvin A. Shiffman

44.1
Introduction

Controlling postoperative pain is an important aspect of patient care. Patient comfort in the postoperative period varies with the patient's tolerance to pain. Oral nonnarcotic pain medications are most often used, and some patients cannot get relief until narcotics are administered.

A new system has been devised that delivers local anesthetic through small catheters placed in the wound using a drip method. The amount of anesthetic administered is controlled by the system so that only 4 ml/h is delivered (2 ml/h from each catheter in the dual-catheter system or 4 ml/h in the single-catheter system), with 400 ml in the pump. This gives 4 days of administration without refill.

44.2
Technique

44.2.1
Filling and Priming the Pump

All the materials for the On-Q PainBuster (I-Flow, Lake Forest, CA, USA) are supplied in a sterile package. Aseptic technique is used to fill the pump. The clamp on the tubing is closed and the protective cap from the port removed. The syringe filled with anesthetic solution (the type of solution being decided upon by the surgeon) is attached to the port and injected into the pump (Fig. 44.1). This is repeated until the total amount of anesthetic solution is in the pump (Table 44.1). The cap is replaced, and the clamp is opened to prime the catheter.

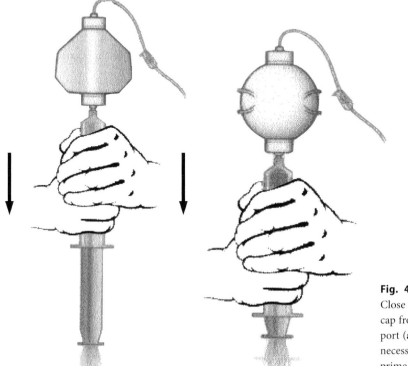

Fig. 44.1 Filling and priming the pump. Close clamp on tubing. Remove protective cap from fill port. Attach filled syringe to fill port (**a**) and inject into pump (**b**). Repeat as necessary. Replace cap and open clamp to prime

Table 44.1 Product information for pain relief system

Delivery days	Description
5	65 ml at 0.5 ml/h
2	100 ml at 2 ml/h
5	270 ml at 2 ml/h
2 ¼	270 ml at 5 ml/h
3	270 ml at 4 ml/h (dual; 2 ml per catheter)
3 ½	400 ml at 5 ml/h
2	400 ml at 10 ml/h
4	400 ml at 4 ml/h (dual; 2 ml per catheter)

44.2.2
Priming the Catheter

To ensure that no air is trapped that can cause air lock, the syringe with the medication should be attached to the catheter connector and the catheter slowly primed (Fig. 44.2). The medication must infuse out of all the holes along the length of the catheter before the catheter is fully primed.

44.2.3
Placing the Catheter

The needle guard is removed, and the introducer needle is inserted through the skin 3–5 cm from the incision site (Fig. 44.3). While the T-handle is held, the needle is withdrawn, leaving the sheath and the catheter inserted through the sheath into the wound. The catheter is advanced into the wound site until the catheter segment is visible (Fig. 44.4). While the catheter tip is held, the T-handle is withdrawn from the puncture site while splitting the sheath and peeling it from the catheter. The surgeon can reposition the catheter in the wound.

44.2.4
Attaching the Pump

The syringe is disconnected from the catheter, and the catheter connector is attached to the pumping tube (Fig. 44.5). The pump clamp is opened to begin infusion.

44.2.5
Securing the Catheter

An occlusive dressing is applied over the insertion site and coiled catheter (Fig. 44.6). This keeps the catheter separate from the wound. The flow restrictor is taped to the skin to ensure accuracy of the flow rate.

44.2.6
Completed Setup

The pump is secured to the patient with an E-clip attached to the pump or placed in a carrying case (Fig. 44.7). Drug infusion occurs between the catheter marking and marked tip (Fig. 44.8).

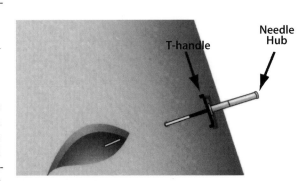

Fig. 44.3 Placement of the catheter. Remove needle guard and insert introducer needle 3–5 cm from the incision site. While holding the T-handle, withdraw the needle and insert the catheter through the sheath into the wound

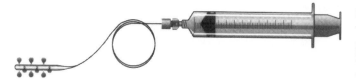

Fig. 44.2 Priming of the catheter. Attach syringe with anesthetic to catheter connector and slowly prime catheter until medication infuses out all the holes along the length of the catheter; trapped air can cause air lock

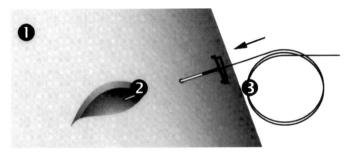

Fig. 44.4 The catheter is advanced into the wound until the catheter tip is visible. While holding the catheter tip (*1*), withdraw the T-handle from the puncture site (*2*). Split the introducer sheath and peel it away from the catheter (*3*)

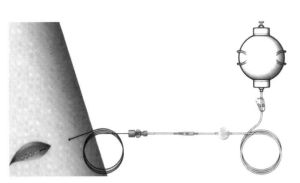

Fig. 44.5 Disconnect syringe and attach catheter to the pump tubing. Open clamp to begin infusion

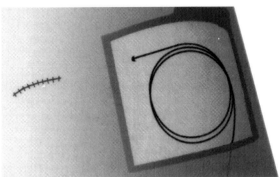

Fig. 44.6 Apply occlusive dressing over insertion site and coiled catheter. This keeps the catheter separate from the wound site. Tape the flow restrictor to the skin to ensure accuracy of flow rate

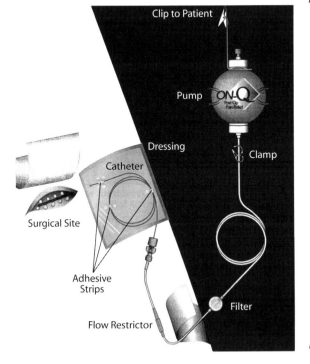

Fig. 44.7 Completed setup. The pump is secured to the patient with an E-clip attached to the top of the pump, or a carrying case can be used

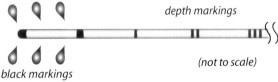

Fig. 44.8 Infusion area. Drug infusion occurs between the catheter *marking* and the *marked tip*

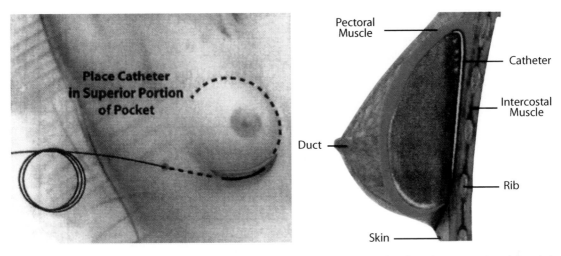

Fig. 44.9 Catheter placement for breast augmentation (Geldner method). **a** Insertion from lateral puncture site and threaded to superior portion of implant. **b** Catheter around the implant

44.2.7
Catheter Wound Placement

The catheter should be placed so that gravity will take the medication to the raw surfaces of the wound. In breast augmentation, the catheter is brought from a lateral or inferior position and is placed at the high segment of the implant (Fig. 44.9).

44.3
Discussion

Placement and securing of the catheter and pump are easily learned, and the instructions in the package are very specific. In abdominoplasty patients, the author advises a 4-0 chromic loosely tied suture near the end of the catheter to hold the catheter in the superior aspect of the wound. The patient can be ambulatory with the pump. The pump is noiseless and will not keep the patient awake because the internal plastic bulb with the anesthetic is filled under pressure and decompresses through a very thin catheter with a flow regulator

Patients can be essentially pain-free 24 h a day while being infused. The pump holds 65–400 ml of anesthetic solution that lasts 2–4 days. If 0.5% lidocaine with epinephrine 1:200,000 is used, the total amount of lidocaine infused with 400 ml in the pump is 40 mg/h or 480 mg/day. Any local anesthetic agent may be used as long as the amount does not exceed a safe limit. Physicians should be extremely careful with Marcaine (bupivicaine), which has a low safe total dosage of 300 mg/24 h. Caution should also be taken with 2% lidocaine because the maximum recommended dosage can easily be exceeded at 10 ml/h.

The drip anesthesia technique can be used in any cosmetic surgical procedure and is beneficial in breast augmentation as well as abdominoplasty, in which pain is a common problem. Another area where there is potential use with a longer needle with peelable sheath for insertion is in liposuction (especially the abdominal wall).

Aseptic technique is essential to prevent infection. The catheter hub should never be left open or exposed. The catheter should be removed promptly after the infusion is completed. The pump should not be refilled because of the risk of contamination. The patient and incision site should be monitored for signs or symptoms of infection.

Pacik et al. [1], who had the patient give intermittent injections of a local anesthetic agent (bupivicaine) through catheters in the wounds, recommended for augmentation mammoplasty patients that the breasts be jiggled for 15 min after each dose.

The use of continuous infusion of local anesthetic for pain management has been reported in abdominoplasty [2]. Continuous infusion of local anesthetic agents has been reported to reduce the rates of infection [3].

The available products of the On-Q PainBuster pain relief system, with the amounts that can be infused, are shown in Table 44.1. Accessories are listed in Table 44.2.

Note: The author has no financial arrangements from On-Q PainBuster pain relief system or with any company that sells the system.

Table 44.2 Accessories

Description
T-Peel needle (3.25-in)
T-Peel needle (6-in)
T-Peel needle (8-in)
Large E-clips for use with 270-ml pumps
Fill extension sets

References

1. Pacik PT, Werner C, Jackson N, Lobsitz C: Pain control in augmentation mammaplasty: the use of indwelling catheters in 200 consecutive patients. Plast Reconstr Surg 2003;111(6):2090–2096

2. Mills DC: Safety of continuous infusion of local anesthesia via elastomeric bolus pump for pain management following abdominoplasty. Presented at the Annual Meeting of the American Society for Aesthetic Plastic Surgery, April 2004

3. Dine AP: Surgical site infection rates reduced with the use of continuous incisional infusion of local anesthetic. Presented at the 50th Annual Meeting of the Association of Perioperative Registered Nurses, 23–27 March 2003

Part V
Position of Implant

Chapter 45

Submammary Versus Subpectoral Implant

Chin-Ho Wong, Bien-Keem Tan, Colin Song

45.1
Introduction

Breast augmentation is one of the most common cosmetic surgery procedures performed today [1]. Pocket selection is one of the main surgical decisions in breast augmentation [2–6]. This important decision determines not only the aesthetic outcome but also the adequacy of long-term soft tissue coverage and the potential for complications [7–8]. Understandably, critical factors in pocket selection revolve around the craft of creating an aesthetically pleasing breast and selecting a plane that minimizes complications and reoperation rates [8–14]. Although this decision is largely driven by personal preference and experience, understanding the scientific basis for specific recommendations serves as a useful guide in breast implant pocket selection [5–8]. Ultimately, personal preferences aside, this decision should be individualized to each patient and based on clearly defined tissue criteria to achieve the surgical goals [7]. The surgeon should be aware that each pocket or plane has specific indications and a unique set of limitations and trade-offs. This chapter aims to outline these indications and define patient tissue characteristics that should be considered in selecting either a submammary or a subpectoral pocket in breast augmentation. Recent technical refinements, such as the subfascial plane and dual-plane techniques, are also discussed.

45.2
Markings

Preoperative markings are made with the patient standing or sitting upright with her arms resting comfortably by her side. Markings must take into consideration the necessary adjustments to address preexisting asymmetry to achieve an optimal balance. The extent of dissection is determined by the existing and targeted breast size and the type of implant used. The limits of the pocket usually extend from the 2nd rib superiorly, the anterior axillary line laterally, and the medial extent of the pectoralis muscle origin. Care should be taken not

to dissect beyond the medial origin of the pectoralis to avoid synmastia. The inferior extent is at the inframammary fold when the crease is positioned normally. When asymmetry of the inframammary fold exists, the lower pole is constricted with a high fold, or when the distance of the lower areola-to-inframammary crease is <5 cm, the inframammary fold may need to be lowered. Also, if a large implant is planned, the fold may be lowered accordingly, with the aim to place the nipple–areola complex over the center of the implant. A generous pocket should be created for smooth implants to facilitate implant massage postoperatively. For a textured implant, however, the pocket should correspond more precisely to the implant dimensions so as to minimize the risk of malposition [5].

45.3
Submammary Pocket

Submammary breast augmentation is defined as implant placement below the breast tissue and above the pectoralis muscle and fascia. This pocket is the most anatomically advantageous location to site an implant to augment the breast. Many surgeons believe that submammary placement gives a more aesthetically pleasing breast that hangs more naturally from the chest wall and moves more subtly with body motion. A full cleavage is also more readily achievable [3] (Fig. 45.1).

The indications for submammary placement include breast hypoplasia in patients with adequate native breast tissue (pinch test >2 cm), mild ptosis that could be addressed concurrently with augmentation, and the presence of pectoralis muscle hypertrophy, which relatively contraindicates subpectoral placement because of the potential for implant distortion [3, 5, 7].

The submammary pocket may be accessed with the usual periareolar, inframammary, or axillary incisions. After the incision is deepened, the submammary plane is identified in the loose areolar layer between the posterior breast capsule above and the musculofascial layer below. Dissection is performed sharply with electrocautery or bluntly with breast dissectors. Careful hemosta-

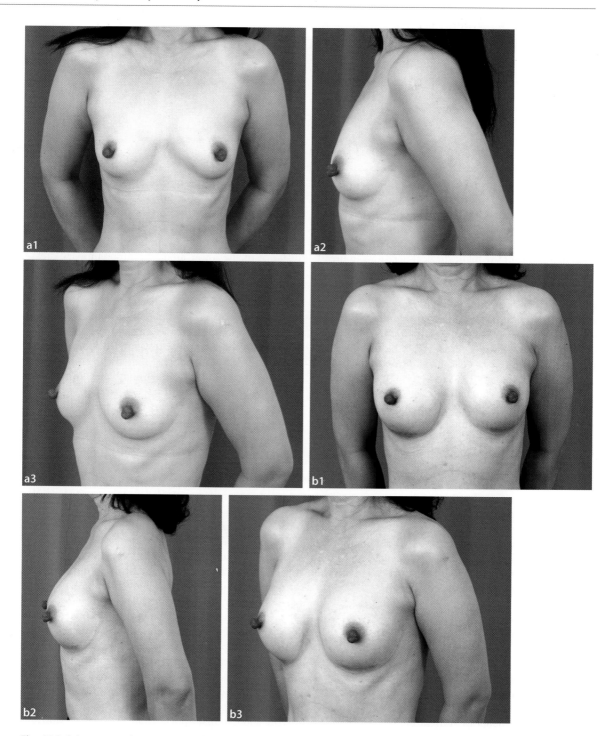

Fig. 45.1 Submammary breast augmentation. **a** *1–3* Preoperative. **b** *1–3* Six months postoperative, with Mentor 175-ml round
cohesive-gel implants inserted in the submammary pocket bilaterally

sis is essential. Lateral dissection should be performed bluntly to avoid injuring the intercostal neurovascular bundle that supplies breast and nipple sensation. These can safely be stretched to create an adequate pocket, but sharp dissection in this area should be avoided.

Disadvantages of submammary implant placement include a greater chance of implant visibility, palpability, and rippling. Capsular contracture, one of the most problematic complications of breast augmentation, is also more common when a submammary pocket is used compared with a subpectoral pocket [15–23]. In this context, it has been demonstrated that use of a textured implant, regardless of whether a saline or silicone implant is used, reduces the incidence of capsular contracture in the submammary pocket [23]. A textured implant is therefore recommended in this pocket. Finally, mammographic visualization to screen for breast cancer is reduced to a greater extent in submammary augmentation.

45.4
Subpectoral Pocket

Subpectoral breast augmentation is defined as implant placement under the pectoralis major muscle. The implant sits on the chest wall and pectoralis minor muscle. This is a partial submuscular pocket because the implant is covered by the pectoralis major muscle superiorly, and a variable portion of the implant is covered by breast tissue inferiorly [2–4]. Subpectoral augmentation has been criticized for creating an unnaturally shaped breast. However, in appropriately selected patients, many authors have shown long-term results of subpectoral augmentations to be indistinguishable from submammary augmentations [3–5] (Fig.45.2).

Subpectoral placement is indicated for patients with severe breast hypoplasia (soft tissue pinch test <2 cm) [7] to provide better coverage for the implant. The subpectoral pocket is also indicated to provide more durable soft tissue coverage for the implant. As mentioned, one of the main benefits of placing an implant in the subpectoral pocket is the lower incidence of capsular contracture [15–23]. By virtue of the thicker soft tissue cover, subpectoral augmentation has a lower incidence of visibility and palpability of the implant and disturbing rippling seen with breast motion [24].

The subpectoral space can be approached from the inferior border of the pectoralis major muscle via the periareolar and inframammary incisions or from the superior lateral aspect of the muscle via an axillary incision. Sharp dissection of the costal origin of the pectoralis muscle down to the chest wall is performed.

Blunt dissection is done to develop the plane between the pectoralis major muscle and the chest wall. Again, lateral dissection should be done bluntly to avoid injury to the intercostal neurovascular bundle. Superiorly, the plane should be developed above the pectoralis minor muscle. The costal (inferior) origin of the pectoralis muscle along the inframammary fold and sternal (medial) origin of the pectoralis major muscle up the superior margin of the areola are divided [9–12]. This allows better aesthetic contouring, giving a better projection to the lower pole of the breast and a more natural inframammary fold. Costal and sternal releases also prevent ridging and lateral and superior displacement of the implant with muscle contractions. The division of the sternal origin of the muscle, however, is somewhat controversial. This maneuver improves medial envelope fill and reduces the intermammary distance to achieve a fuller cleavage, which is a very desirable aesthetic effect [13, 14]. However, some authors have advocated that this should not be performed to preserve the crucial medial coverage of the implant by the muscle [25, 26]. Division may therefore risk deformities such as medial implant edge visibility, traction rippling, and synmastia. The shortcomings of preserving the medial origins, however, are potential lateralization of the implant and the fact that a full cleavage would be more difficult to achieve [25].

The subpectoral pocket has some limitations and potential problems. It is relatively contraindicated for patients with mild breast ptosis because placement here may result in a double-bubble deformity [9–12]. Placement in this pocket may produce superior and lateral displacement of the implant with pectoralis muscle contraction, especially if the costal (inferior) origins of the muscle have not been divided. Patients with hypertrophic muscles, such as bodybuilders, are more prone to this problem. Asymmetry and implant distortion are further potential problems [9–12]. Unless the medial (sternal) insertions of the pectoralis muscle are divided, it is more difficult to achieve the full cleavage that many patients desire [13, 14].

45.5
Discussion

When Cronin and Gerow [27] introduced the first breast implant in 1963, they placed the prosthesis in the subglandular pocket because this was the most logical site to place it to enhance the breast. However, the unacceptably high incidence of capsular contracture noted with these early implants cast severe doubts on their viability as a means augmenting the breast [5]. This led

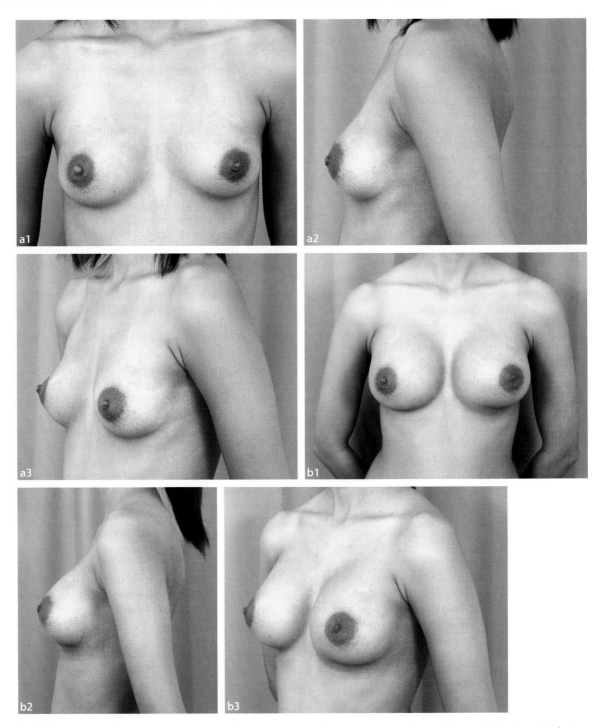

Fig. 45.2 Subpectoral breast augmentation. **a** *1–3* Preoperative. **b** *1–3* One year postoperative, with Mentor 200-ml round cohesive-gel implants inserted in the subpectoral pocket bilaterally

implant manufacturers to improve product design with the development of subsequent generations of breast implants: thicker shells, textured shells, saline-filled implants, double-lumen implants, and form-stable silicone fillers. At the same time, surgeons then began to explore alternative pockets in which to place breast implants in order to reduce complications, particularly that of capsular contracture. The use of the submuscular pocket for this purpose was first suggested by Dempsey and Latham in 1968 [28]. Initially reported as a total submuscular placement beneath the pectoral major and serratus anterior muscles, this technique limits the anterior projection of the implant and fails to produce an aesthetically shaped breast. Subsequently, in 1977 Regnault [29] introduced the technique of partial submuscular placement under the pectoralis major muscle only with the release of its lower medial origins. This dramatically improved the aesthetic results and revived interest in the submuscular pocket. Regnault's technique evolved into the subpectoral pocket used today.

Today, submammary and subpectoral pockets are the most common pockets in which breast implants are sited [2, 3]. Refinements of these techniques, including the subfascial and dual-plane techniques, have been described more recently, with the aim of improving aesthetic results while reducing complication rates. Table 45.1 briefly describes the various pockets currently used in breast augmentation, along with their advantages, disadvantages and indications.

It is generally claimed that the submammary pocket is the most ideal and anatomically sound place to site an implant to augment the natural shape and form of the breast. Many consider submammary augmentation to deliver superior results compared with subpectoral augmentation in the absence of capsular contracture [3, 6]. However, many authors have demonstrated that the subpectoral pocket can deliver equally satisfying aesthetic results with proper redraping of the pectoralis muscle over the implant [4, 5]. The subpectoral pocket has the added advantage of reducing the incidence of capsular contracture, rippling, and implant palpability and visibility [23, 24]. Two main theories explain the etiology of capsular contractures: subclinical infection and hypertrophic scarring of the capsule that forms around the breast [3, 5]. The lower incidence of capsular contracture in the subpectoral pocket therefore has been attributed to two factors. First, the pectoral muscle functions as a well-vascularized tissue barrier that protects the implant from the potentially contaminated breast parenchyma. This reduces subclinical infection rates in subpectoral pockets. Second, placement here allows the pectoralis muscle to continuously massage the implant with muscle contractions, thereby modulating tendencies toward hypertrophic scarring. With greater

patient awareness and expectations, consideration for pocket selection has evolved from merely creating an aesthetically pleasing breast to the concept of optimizing soft tissue coverage of the breast in the interest of providing stable long-term coverage and reducing complications and reoperation rates [9–12]. In this context, using the pectoralis major muscle as an additional soft tissue cover has a definite advantage. Therefore, while the subglandular pocket continues to be favored by many plastic surgeons, more authors have moved from using this pocket to using a subpectoral pocket [2, 3, 7].

To improve the long-term results of the submammary pocket, the subfascial pocket has recently been developed [30–37]. First described by Graf et al. [30], this modification of the submammary pocket places the implant under the deep fascial layer covering the pectoralis major muscle This plane is created by incising the deep fascia covering the pectoralis major and elevating it off the muscle. The pectoralis fascia originates from the clavicle and sternum and extends laterally over the pectoralis major muscle to form the axillary fascia. Inferiorly it continues as the fascia over the external oblique, rectus, and serratus anterior. This fascial layer is thickest superiorly and becomes more attenuated toward the inframammary fold. Proponents of this technique argue that placing the implant under the deep muscle fascia has the advantage of providing additional soft tissue coverage of the implant. This has been claimed to reduce implant edge palpability and visibility [35, 37]. The thickness of the deep fascia has been reported by various authors to range from 0.1 mm to 1.14 mm [34, 38]. It is difficult to imagine that such a thin layer of fascia can provide significant additional soft tissue coverage [38]. No long-term follow-up of breast implants placed in the subfascial plane has been reported to date, and based on the best current knowledge, surgeons should consider subfascial augmentation to be equivalent to submammary augmentation in terms of soft tissue coverage [38]. However, the real appeal of the subfascial pocket is that it potentially may reduce the incidence of one of the biggest problems in submammary breast augmentations, that of capsular contracture.

Subclinical infection is one of the main theories for the etiology of capsular contractures [39, 40]. Placing the implant in the subfascial pocket enables the well-vascularized deep fascia to separate the implant from the breast parenchyma, thus acting as a biological barrier and shielding the implant from a potentially contaminated area. However, it remains to be seen in prospective controlled studies whether this additional fascial layer confers a significant advantage.

To improve aesthetic results of the subpectoral implant, it has been recommended that medial pectoral release of the sternal muscle origin be done up to the superior margin of the areola [9–12]. This is done primarily to prevent distortion and lateral displacement of the implant with contractions of the pectoral muscle and to improve lower-pole projection. This maneuver also improves the medial fill of the breast and decreases the intermammary distance to produce a fuller cleavage. However, some authors have advised against medial pectoral release, arguing that this sacrifices crucial medial coverage of the implant and hence may potentially be complicated by problems that are difficult to correct surgically: medial implant visibility, palpability, traction rippling, and, rarely, synmastia [24–26]. It is acknowledged that preserving the medial pectoral origin may result in a wider intermammary distance (cleavage gap), but this is considered a necessary compromise or trade-off in order to adequately cover the implant medially. By preserving this medial origin, Tebbetts [41] has demonstrated that no reoperations for problems related to inadequate medial coverage, such as visible implant edges, rippling, or synmastia, were necessary in his cohort of 1,414 patients after a follow-up of up to 12 years. He also noted that none of his patients underwent revisional surgery for excessively wide intermammary distance. Lindsey [26] compared patients in whom medial pectoral release was performed versus patients in whom this was not done and noted a significantly higher incidence of medial implant visibility and palpability in the former group. Furthermore, he noted that aesthetic outcomes in terms of the intermammary distance and lateral breast protrusion were not statistically different between the groups.

On balance, however, medial pectoral release, when done judiciously, can deliver excellent, long-lasting aesthetic results, and it is perhaps premature to recommend one technique over the other. What is important is for the surgeon to be aware of the potential problems due to inadequate medial coverage and to assess the need to divide or preserve the sternal (medial) origin of the pectoral muscle based on the specific tissue characteristics of each individual patient.

Although the subpectoral pocket has many advantages, it has several major drawbacks [9–14] (see Table 45.1). To improve on its limitations, Tebbetts [25] introduced the concept of dual-plane breast augmentation. By incorporating dissection in both the submammary space and the subpectoral space, this technique places the implant partially subpectoral and partially submammary. This is a refinement of the subpectoral pocket, which seeks to harmonize soft tissue implant dynamics. The purpose of the dual-plane placement is to optimize soft tissue coverage, minimize forces that displace the implant with muscular contraction, and optimize expansion of the lower pole, especially in patients with breast ptosis and a constricted lower pole.

Types 1, 2, and 3 dual-plane augmentation have been described, with the lower pole of the implant progressively contacting more of the lower breast parenchyma (Fig. 45.3). This is achieved by complete division of the pectoralis major origin along the inframammary fold for type 1 dual-plane. In addition, for type 2 dual-plane, the breast parenchyma is separated from the pectoralis muscle up to the inferior edge of the areola, and for type 3 up to the superior edge of the areola. The selection of type of dual-plane technique is made intraoperatively and is based on the needs to match coverage of the implant of the selected size with individual breast tissue characteristics. In this technique, the sternal origin of the pectoralis muscle is preserved. Tebbetts stresses that the sternal origin should be preserved and attributes his favorable long-term results of up to 12 years to this [41]. Limitations include breast ptosis grades 2 and 3 and patients with a nipple-to-inframammary-fold distance >10 cm.

Total muscular coverage has a limited role in primary aesthetic breast augmentation. This technique was originally developed to reduce implant visibility and palpability and to reduce capsular contracture, but it has considerable disadvantages, including inadequate shape of lower-pole breast projection and inframammary fold definition [28]. Long-term complications such as superior implant migration and pseudoptosis resulting from the breast parenchyma slipping inferiorly over the relatively well-supported submuscular implant are also unique problems with total submuscular placement [3]. With improved implant designs (which have contributed to the reduction of capsular contracture rates both in the subglandular and subpectoral planes) and development of techniques such as subpectoral placement (in which implants are partially covered by muscle) that have been demonstrated to be effective in reducing implant visibility and palpability in patients with minimal breast tissue, the necessity of total submuscular coverage of the implant has been reduced considerably [29]. The use of total submuscular placement today is therefore mostly restricted to cases where maximal soft tissue coverage is necessary; these are usually indicated in breast reconstruction cases rather than primary aesthetic augmentation [3].

Oncologic issues are relevant when considering breast augmentation in general; in particular, the use of submammary versus submuscular implant relates to interference with detection of early breast cancer. Some patients are particularly concerned about this aspect of breast augmentation, so it is important for the plastic surgeon to be familiar with the literature in this area. Despite earlier concerns, recent studies have demonstrated that breast implants do not cause breast cancer [42–45]. Breast augmentation does interfere with

Table 45.1 Pros and cons of different implant pockets and specific recommendations for the use of each. The subglandular and subpectoral pockets are the two most common worldwide. A total submuscular pocket is used for selected indications. Subfascial and dual-plane augmentations are promising techniques described recently; they represent refinements of the subglandular and subpectoral techniques, respectively

	Subglandular	Subpectoral	Subfascial	Total submuscular	Dual-plane
Pocket description	The pocket is created between the breast parenchyma and the deep fascia over the pectoralis major muscle	The pocket is created between the pectoralis major muscle and the chest wall. The inferior (costal) and medial (sternal) origins of the muscle may be divided up to the superior margin of the areola to allow the muscle to retract superiorly to achieve better aesthetic contouring of the breast	The pocket is created by elevating the deep fascia off the pectoralis major muscle	The implant is totally covered by muscle. The pectoralis major covers the superior and medial aspects of the implant, and the serratus anterior muscle the inferior and lateral aspects of the implant	The pocket is subpectoral in the superior aspect and submammary in the inferior aspect, hence the name "dual plane." Types 1, 2, and 3 are described with increasing contact of the inferior portion of the pocket with the breast parenchyma. Sternal origin is left intact to minimize risk of medial implant palpability, visibility, rippling, and synmastia
Advantages	Better control of breast shape Better control of inframammary fold position and shape Faster postoperative recovery Minimal distortion with pectoralis muscle contraction	Less risk of capsular contracture Less risk of palpable or visible implant Better visualization of breast tissue on mammography	All the advantages of the subglandular pocket with potentially less risk of capsular contracture	Better soft tissue coverage of the inferolateral part of the implant	Affords better control of lower breast shape while providing for better coverage of the implant in the upper pole Lower risk of medial implant visibility, palpability, and synmastia

Table 45.1 (*continued*) Pros and cons of different implant pockets and specific recommendations for the use of each. The subglandular and subpectoral pockets are the two most common worldwide. A total submuscular pocket is used for selected indications. Subfascial and dual-plane augmentations are promising techniques described recently; they represent refinements of the subglandular and subpectoral techniques, respectively

	Subglandular	Subpectoral	Subfascial	Total submuscular	Dual-plane
Disadvantages	Increased risk of edge visibility and palpability; Increased incidence of capsular contracture; More bleeding compared with subpectoral pocket; Greater interference with mammography	Less control of the upper and medial breast fill; Risk of lateral displacement of implant over time with widening of the intermammary distance; More postoperative pain and slightly longer recovery; Distortion of breast with pectoralis contraction	Same disadvantages as for subglandular pocket	In addition to the disadvantages of subpectoral plane, total submuscular pocket have the following problems: Greater risk of superior and lateral displacement of implants over time; Less control of inframammary fold position, depth, and shape; Pseudoptosis of the breast with the gland slipping under the well-supported implant	Wider intermammary distance and more difficulty in achieving a full cleavage because of the preservation of the sternal origin of the muscle; Increased risk of palpable or visible implant edges inferiorly; Generally, types 2 and 3 dual-plane breast augmentation cannot be performed through an axillary incision
Patient selection/indications	Adequate breast tissue (soft tissue pinch test >2 cm); Mild glandular ptosis	Severe hypomastia with soft tissue pinch test <2 cm	Same as the subglandular breast augmentation	Patients in whom maximal soft tissue coverage of the implant is necessary to minimize complications and implant exposure. Usually for breast reconstruction cases	Dual-plane techniques can be used for a wide range of breast types. It should not be used in patients with severe breast ptosis or downward-pointing nipples or in patients with a nipple-to-inframammary-fold distance >10 cm
Specific recommendations	Textured implant, either silicone or polyurethane, should be used, as these have been demonstrated to reduce capsular contracture in this pocket	Muscle coverage is recommended if the soft tissue pinch thickness of the upper pole is <2 cm, to minimize implant palpability and visibility	Same as for subglandular breast augmentation	Limited role in primary aesthetic breast augmentation; more for reconstructive cases where the soft tissue coverage is deficient	Can be used for a wide range of breast types

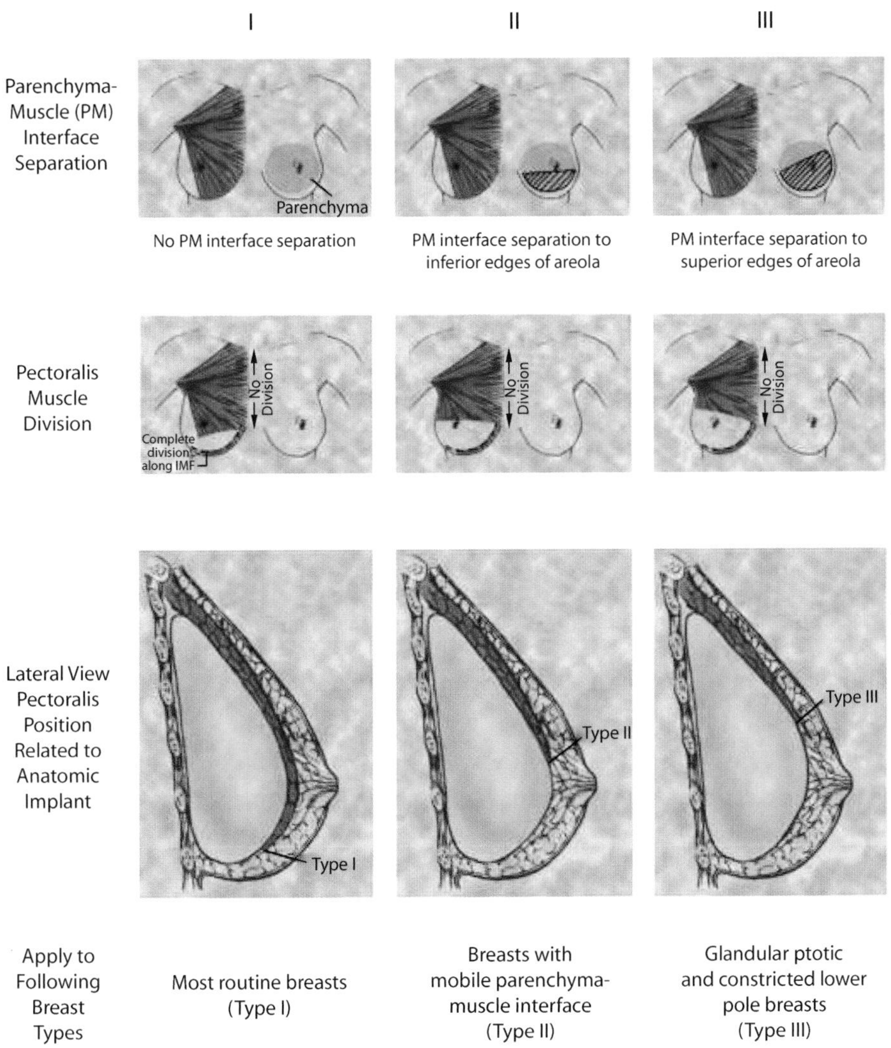

	I	II	III
Parenchyma-Muscle (PM) Interface Separation			

Parenchyma

No PM interface separation

PM interface separation to inferior edges of areola

PM interface separation to superior edges of areola

Fig. 45.3 Dual-plane breast augmentation. (Reproduced with permission from Tebbetts [25])

Pectoralis Muscle Division

No Division

Complete division along IMF

No Division

No Division

Lateral View Pectoralis Position Related to Anatomic Implant

Type I

Type II

Type III

Apply to Following Breast Types

Most routine breasts (Type I)

Breasts with mobile parenchyma-muscle interface (Type II)

Glandular ptotic and constricted lower pole breasts (Type III)

screening mammography, even with the implant-displaced views that are currently used for all patients with breast implants [42, 46–48]. However, implant pockets interfere with mammography to a varying extent, with subpectoral implants reducing the area visualized to a lesser extent than submammary implants [46–48]. Handel et al. [48] studied factors that affect mammographic visualization of the breast after augmentation. They found that the two most important factors compromising mammographic visualization are the presence of capsular contracture and placement of the implant in a submammary plane. Considering that capsular contracture itself is more common in the submammary pocket, subpectoral placement is therefore clearly preferable from an oncologic surveillance point of view.

Women concerned about the potential for breastfeeding after breast augmentation should be informed that there are currently no studies demonstrating that either the submammary or the subpectoral pocket results in a higher incidence of lactation insufficiency [49–52]. However, they must be informed that breast augmentation itself makes it three times more likely for a woman to be unable to fully breastfeed her babies and that the periareolar incision has the most adverse effect on breastfeeding potential, with a five times greater likelihood of lactation insufficiency compared with patients with no prior surgery on the breast.

45.6
Conclusions

As with many procedures in cosmetic surgery, pocket selection should be individualized to each patient's specific needs. Placing the implant either in the submammary pocket or in the subglandular pocket can deliver long-lasting, aesthetically excellent results in appropriately selected patients. The surgeon's preference continues to be a major factor in pocket selection, and it is this variation in preferences that makes breast augmentation both a science and an art to be mastered.

The authors did not receive any funding for this work and declare no conflict of interest in this present work.

References

1. American Society of Plastic Surgeons National Clearinghouse of Plastic Surgery Statistics. Cosmetic surgery trends, 1992–2001, published results. Arlington Heights, IL, American Society of Plastic Surgeons 2002

2. Hidalgo DA: Breast augmentation: choosing an optimal incision, implant, and pocket plane. Plast Reconstr Surg 2000;105(6):2202–2216

3. Spear LS, Bulan EJ, Venturi ML: Breast augmentation. Plast Reconstr Surg 2004;114(5):73E–81E

4. Vazquez B, Given KS, Houston GC: Breast augmentation: a review of subglandular and submuscular implantation. Aesthet Plast Surg 1987;11(2):101–105

5. Maxwell GP, Hartley RW: Breast augmentation. In: Mathes SJ (ed). Plastic Surgery, 2nd edn, vol 6. Philadelphia, Saunders, pp 1–33

6. Lesavoy MA: Breast augmentation techniques. In: Mathes SJ (ed). Plastic Surgery, 2nd edn, vol 6. Philadelphia, Saunders, pp 35–46

7. Tebbetts JB: A system for breast implant selection based on patient tissue characteristics and implant-soft tissue dynamics. Plast Reconstr Surg 2002;109(4):1396–1401

8. Tebbetts JB: The greatest myths in breast augmentation. Plast Reconstr Surg 2001;107(7):1895–1903

9. Tebbetts JB: Dimensional Augmentation Mammoplasty. Santa Barbara, McGhan Medical Publishing 1994

10. Bostwick J: Plastic and Reconstructive Breast Surgery. St. Louis, Quality Medical Publishing 2000, pp 274–308

11. Matarasso A, Hutchinson OHZ: Augmentation mammoplasty: subpectoral augmentation using the periareolar or inframammary approach. Oper Tech Plast Reconstr Surg 2000;7(3):93–99

12. Grubber RP, Friedman GD: Submuscular augmentation mammoplasty. In: Noone RB (ed). Plastic and Reconstructive Surgery of the Breast. St, Louis, Mosby Year Book 1991, pp 142–157

13. Elliot LF: Breast augmentation with round, smooth-saline or gel implants: the pros and cons. Clin Plast Surg 2001;28(3):523–529

14. Codner MA, Cohen AT, Hester RT: Complications in breast augmentation. Clin Plast Surg 2001;28(3):587–595

15. Hakelius L, Ohlsen L: Tendency to capsular contracture around smooth and textured gel-filled silicone mammary implants: a five-year follow-up. Plast Reconstr Surg 1997;100(6):1566–1569

16. Coleman DJ, Sharpe DT, Naylor IL, Chander CL, Cross SE: The role of the contractile fibroblast in the capsules around tissue expanders and implants. Br J Plast Surg 1993;46(7):547–556

17. Malata CM, Feldberg L, Coleman DJ, Foo IT, Sharpe DT: Textured or smooth implants for breast augmentation? Three year follow-up of a prospective randomised controlled trial. Br J Plast Surg 1997;50(2):99–105

18. Collis N, Coleman D, Foo IT, Sharpe DT: Ten-year review of a prospective randomized controlled trial of textured versus smooth subglandular silicone gel breast implants. Plast Reconstr Surg 2000;106(4):786–791

19. Tarpila E, Ghassemifar R, Fagrell D, Berggren A: Capsular contracture with textured versus smooth saline-filled implants for breast augmentation: a prospective clinical study. Plast Reconstr Surg 1997;99(7):1934–1939

20. Fagrell D, Berggren A, Tarpila E: Capsular contracture around saline-filled fine textured and smooth mammary implants: a prospective 7.5-year follow-up. Plast Reconstr Surg 2001;108(7):2108–2112; discussion 2113

21. Burkhardt BR, Demas CP: The effect of Siltex texturing and povidone-iodine irrigation on capsular contracture around saline inflatable breast implants. Plast Reconstr Surg 1994;93(1):123–128

22. Burkhardt BR, Eades E: The effect of Biocell texturing and povidone-iodine irrigation on capsular contracture around saline-inflatable breast implants. Plast Reconstr Surg 1995;96(6):1317–1325

23. Wong CH, Samuel M, Tan BK, Song C: Capsular contracture in subglandular breast augmentation with textured versus smooth breast implants: a systematic review. Plast Reconstr Surg 2006;118(5):1224–1236

24. Tebbetts JB: Patient evaluation, operative planning and surgical technique to increase control and decrease morbidity and reoperations in breast augmentation. Clin Plast Surg 2001;28(3):501–521

25. Tebbetts JB: Dual plane (DP) breast augmentation: optimizing implant-soft-tissue relationships in a wide range of breast types. Plast Reconstr Surg 2001;107(5):1255–1272

26. Lindsey JT: The case against medial pectoral releases. A retrospective review of 315 primary breast augmentation patients. Ann Plast Surg 2004;52(3):253–256

27. Cronin TD, Gerow FJ: Augmentation mammoplasty: a new "natural feel" prosthesis. Transactions of the rd International Congress of Plastic Surgery, 13–18 October 1968, Amsterdam, Excerpta Medica Foundation

28. Dempsey WC, Latham WD: Subpectoral implant in augmentation mammoplasty. Plast Reconstr Surg 1968;42(6):515–521

29. Regnault P: Partial submuscular breast augmentation. Plast Reconstr Surg 1977;59(1):72–76

30. Graf RM, Bernades A, Rippel R, Araujo LR, Damasio RC, Auersvald A: Subfascial breast implant: a new procedure. Plast Reconstr Surg 2003;111(2):904–908

31. Graf RM, Bernades A, Auersvald A, Damasio RC: Subfascial endoscopic transaxillary augmentation mammaplasty. Aesthet Plast Surg 2000;24(3):216–220

32. Benito-Ruiz J: Subfascial breast implant. Plast Recons Surg 2004;113(3):1088–1089

33. Goes JC, Landecker A: Optimizing outcomes in breast augmentation: seven years of experience with the subfascial plane. Aesthet Plast Surg 2003;27(3):178–184

34. Lin J, Song JL, Chen XP, Tan XY, Lou JQ, Men Q, Li B: Anatomy and clinical significance of pectoral fascia. Plast Reconstr Surg 2006;118(7):1557–1560

35. Evangelos K: Personal experience following 350 subfascial breast augmentations. Plast Reconstr Surg 2006;118(5):1276–1277

36. Munhoz AM, Fells K, Arruda E, Montag E, Okada A, Aldrighi C, Aldrighi JM, Gemperli R, Ferreira MC: Subfascial transaxillary breast augmentation without endoscopic assistance: technical aspects and outcome. Aesthet Plast Surg 2006;30(5):503–512

37. Barbato C, Pena M, Triana C, Zambrano MA: Augmentation mammoplasty using the retrofascia approach. Aesthet Plast Surg 2004;28(3):148–152

38. Tebbetts J: Does fascia provide additional meaningful coverage over a breast implant? Plast Reconstr Surg 2004;113(2):777–779

39. Burkhart B, Dempsey P, Schnur P, Tofield J: Capsular contracture: a prospective study of the local antibacterial agents. Plast Reconstr Surg 1986;77(6):919–932

40. Shah Z, Lehman JA Jr, Tan J: Does infection play a role in breast capsular contracture? Plast Reconstr Surg 1981;68(1):34–42

41. Tebbetts JB: Dual plane (DP) breast augmentation: optimizing implant-soft tissue relationships in a wide range of breast types (update discussion). Plast Reconstr Surg 2006;118(7 suppl):81S–98S, discussion 99S–102S

42. McCarthy CM, Pusic AL, Disa JJ, Cordeiro PG, Fey JV, Buchanan C, Sclafani L, Mehrara BJ: Breast cancer in the previously augmented breast. Plast Reconstr Surg 2007;119(1):49–58

43. Deapen DM, Bernstein L, Brody GS: Are breast implants anticarcinogenic? A 14-year follow-up of the Los Angeles Study. Plast Reconstr Surg 1997;99(5):1346–1353

44. Deapen DM, Brody GS: Augmentation mammaplasty and breast cancer: a 5-year update of the Los Angeles study. Plast Reconstr Surg 1992;89(4):660–665

45. Deapen D, Hamilton A, Bernstein L, Brody, GS: Breast cancer stage at diagnosis and survival among patients with prior breast implants. Plast Reconstr Surg 2000;105(2):535–540

46. Silverstein MJ, Handel N, Gamagami P, Waisman E, Gierson ED: Mammographic measurements before and after augmentation mammaplasty. Plast Reconstr Surg 1990;86(6):1126–1130

47. Destouet JM, Monsees BS, Oser RF, Nemecek JR, Young VL, Pilgram TK: Screening mammography in 350 women with breast implants: prevalence and findings of implant complications. AJR Am J Roentgenol 1992;159(5):973–978

48. Handel N, Silverstein MJ, Gamagami P, Jensen JA, Collins A: Factors affecting mammographic visualization of the breast after augmentation mammaplasty. J Amer Med Assoc 1992;268(14):1913–1917

49. National Academy of Sciences Institute of Medicine: Safety of Silicone Breast Implants. National Academy Press, Washington, DC 1999, p 197

50. Neifert M, DeMarzo S, Seacat J, Young D, Leff M, Orleans M: The influence of breast surgery, breast appearance, and pregnancy-induced breast changes on lactation sufficiency as measured by infant weight gain. Birth 1990;17(1):31–38

51. Hurst NM: Lactation after augmentation mammoplasty. Obstet Gynecol 1996;87(1):30–34

52. Strom SS, Baldwin BJ, Sigurdson AJ Schusterman MA: Cosmetic saline breast implants: a survey of satisfaction, breast-feeding experience, cancer screening, and health. Plast Reconstr Surg 1997;100(6):1553–1557

CHAPTER 46

Treatment of the Submammary Fold in Breast Implantation

46

Adrien Aiache

46.1
Introduction

The inframammary fold is the most important anatomical element in breast augmentation. Its elusive symmetry and its location are defining factors in the aesthetic surgical outcome.

46.2
Anatomy

The submammary fold is situated at the junction of the mammary gland and the chest tissues below it. Histologically, it consists of a loose connective tissue reinforcement barely different from the subcutaneous tissues above and below it [1, 2].

Women's breasts are often asymmetrical in size, shape, and location. In approximately 90% of women, the left breast is larger and lower than the right breast (Fig. 46.1). The physician must take these elements into consideration because attempts at symmetry during surgery are often impossible due to these differences that cannot be changed, namely the actual breast location with its attendant vessels, nerves, and connective tissues. Although simple to understand, these factors are often troublesome to women interested in augmentation, especially when they wish to return to "the way they were before their pregnancies." The surgeon has to evaluate how much improvement he or she can get and how much correction of existing discrepancies is possible, and then convey this assessment to an understanding patient.

46.3
Factors Distorting the Inframammary Fold

Aside from improper location of the breast pocket due to a surgeon's inability to develop it at the same level on both sides, other factors can distort the location of the fold. An excess of bleeding and hematoma formation will in turn become excess scarring and secondary

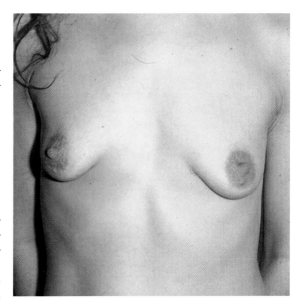

Fig. 46.1 Left breast is larger and lower than the right

capsule contracture, leading to an elevated fold in the breast.

Early postoperative activity of the arms and pectoralis friction are known to increase capsule contracture. Early trauma during the healing period can also result in contracture. Low-grade infection has been questioned as a cause for a long time; to prevent such an occurrence, preoperative and postoperative antibiotics are advised.

The question of subpectoral versus submuscular implantation [3] also adds a new dimension to the occurrence of fold irregularities. The placement of a submuscular implant can often be marred by the actual anatomical dissection of the pocket. Fully submuscular pockets are developed in a plane under the fascia of the rectus muscle medially and the external oblique, internal oblique, and transversus abdominus muscles laterally (Fig. 46.2). In such cases, especially in transumbilical breast augmentation or the axillary approach, the deep planes have a strong tendency to close early, re-

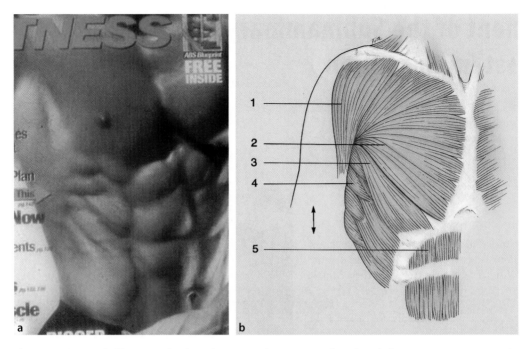

Fig. 46.2 a External oblique muscles (*arrow*) to pectoralis major muscle and medial to serratus anterior muscle. **b** Deltoid muscle (*1*), pectoralis major muscle (*2*), external oblique muscle (*3*), serratus anterior muscle (*4*), rectus muscle (*5*)

sulting in an elevated fold. The actual cause of this problem is the fact that these are flat muscles coming from the same surface on the chest wall, and their tendency to close early pushes the implant superiorly.

46.4
Surgical Maneuvers
To Improve the Submammary Fold

If the fold is higher on one side secondary to capsule contracture, the repair is performed by ensuring a certain excess in lowering the fold to fight the contracture, although the implant may also end up lower than the opposite side if the lowering is too extensive. This is a difficult problem to evaluate at the time of the operation because the behavior of the scar contracture is impossible to foresee.

In subpectoral implants, the technique consists of an attempt to place the fold and the pocket in a more superficial plane to be able to avoid early closure of the fold due to the chest muscles. Less often the fold is too low, creating secondary problems because of the pressure of the implant on the lower chest area. Although simple suturing of the submammary pocket is possible, it is again difficult to foretell whether a secondary contracture will develop after the capsulorrhaphy to correct a pocket that is too large.

If the implant pocket is made too low on the chest, some problems can result. In subglandular implants, a low pocket will be well below the original fold and often leads to patient discomfort from the pressure of the implant on the ribs, which are thinly covered by subcutaneous tissues. The implant that is too high or higher than the fold will tilt the breast, resulting in a drooping, downward-pointing nipple (Fig. 46.3).

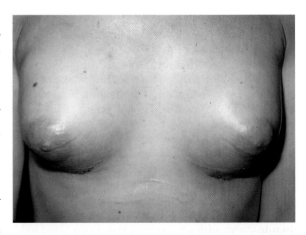

Fig. 46.3 Tight inferior poles and downward tilting of the nipple when the inframammary fold is too high after breast augmentation

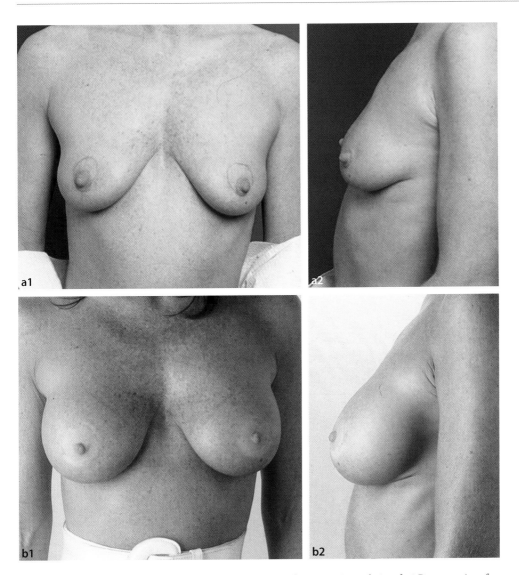

Fig. 46.4 a *1* Preoperative patient with slight asymmetry and ptosis. *2* Lateral view. **b** *1* Postoperative after circumareolar mastopexy and breast implants. *2* Lateral view

If the pocket is lower than the original fold, the nipple will rise about 30° in a normal breast. A slightly larger or drooping breast might not raise the nipple as much, and it is a good idea to raise the low nipple–areola complex with a crescent or circumareolar incision while the pocket is made to the level of the fold or lower than the opposite fold (Fig. 46.4).

46.5 Nipple–Inframammary Fold Relationships

Lowering the inframammary fold followed by breast implantation might result in "stargazing" of the nipple (Fig. 46.5). This phenomenon can be used to improve a drooping nipple only if there is excess upper pole tissue, as this condition would make the technique useless and might result in a "double-bubble" phenomenon. The surgeon has to be careful when using this maneuver.

After the implants are inserted during surgery, the location of the fold is made with the patient in a sitting position, even under general anesthesia. During the maneuver, the patient's shoulders should be level for proper evaluation of the fold. A long ruler is applied under the fold, and every attempt is made to judge the horizontal level of the fold. It is useful to apply a second ruler at the point above the implants to judge whether the superior poles are level.

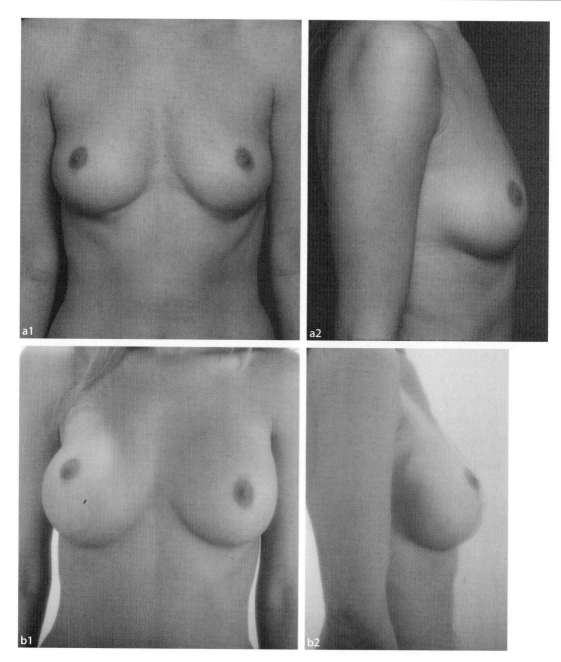

Fig. 46.5 a *1* Preoperative 31-year-old woman with bilateral breast implants and slight asymmetry. *2* Lateral view. **b** Postoperative with low inframammary fold on right side, resulting in "stargazing" of the nipple. *2* Lateral view

To correct a high upper pole secondary to a higher pocket, the inframammary pocket is lowered, and a decision has to be made concerning the shape of the upper pole as opposed to the inframammary fold. In asymmetrical breasts, the question of size differences for the implants can help somewhat to correct the discrepancy. At the time of surgery, scrutiny of the upper poles will help determine whether the breasts and upper poles

are even. The anesthesiologist's position is important in that respect.

An important factor is to measure the actual distance from the clavicle to the nipple, as opposed to the distance from the nipple to the inframammary fold. If the superior distance is shorter, the result can be stargazing nipples, with the nipples becoming too high and difficult to conceal with a regular bra, sometimes even coming out of the top border of the bra. Correction of the problem consists of shortening the distance from the areola to the submammary fold by either a submammary excision of skin or sometimes an inferior periareolar skin excision between the areola and the inferior pole if any of the anatomical conditions allow these techniques. There must be sufficient skin to excise and to use to obtain horizontally oriented nipples.

For instance, if the left breast is larger and lower than the right breast, one can use a smaller implant in the right breast and probably end up with better symmetry but also with a lower upper pole on the right side. Thus, fully symmetrical upper poles are not obtained (Fig. 46.6).

46.6
Implant Size and Submammary Fold Problems

Limiting the size of breast implants is not always conducive to improved surgical results. Smaller implants may fail to fulfill patients' goals regarding cleavage, slightly round upper poles, and good projection without the lateral breast fullness that is often objectionable to patients. Larger implants give better cleavage and better upper pole fullness, but they can stretch the breast tissues and the chest wall, resulting in drooping breasts, an overstretched inframammary fold with pressure on the lower ribs, and an uncomfortable feeling, sometimes with lack of nipple sensitivity and stretching and thinning out of the skin (Fig. 46.7).

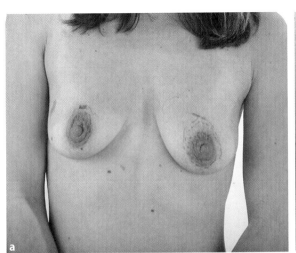
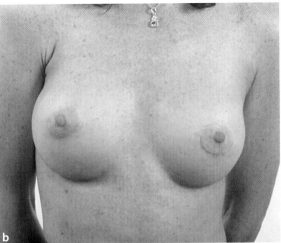

Fig. 46.6 a Preoperative 30-year–old woman with left breast larger and lower than the right. **b** Postoperative

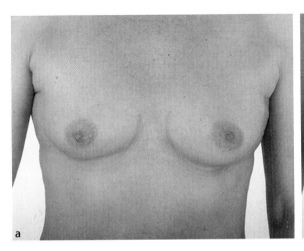
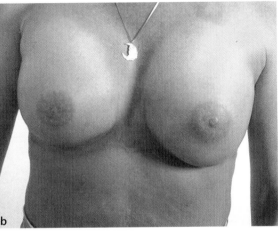

Fig. 46.7 a Preoperative patient with a short lower pole and high inframammary fold. **b** Postoperative with inframammary fold not lowered enough. The volume of the implant contributes to the problem when the right fold is too high and the breast implants too large

The choice of breast implant size is a problem, and each case has to be treated differently to obtain proper results.

46.7
Conclusions

The elusive submammary fold is an important factor in breast implant surgery. Even when the surgeon has excellent knowledge and understanding of the problems, the outcome is not always ideal. Breast implantation can be a simple operation; however, a critical eye from the patient, the surgeon, or an observer can call the surgical results into question in most cases. Striving for perfection is an endless journey.

References

1. Boutros S, Kattash M, Wienfeld A, Yuksel E, Baer S, Shenaq S: The interdermal anatomy of the inframammary fold. Plast Reconstr Surg 1998;102(4):1030–1033
2. Bayati S, Seckel BR: Inframammary crest ligaments. Plast Reconstr Surg 1995;95(3):501–508
3. Puckett CL, Croll GH, Reichel TAA, Concannon MT: A critical look at capsule contracture in subglandular versus subpectoral mammary augmentation. Aesthet Plast Surg 1987;11(1):23–28

CHAPTER 47

Subfascial Prepectoral Implant Using the Inframammary Approach

47

Toma T. Mugea

47.1 Introduction

Since the initial use of implants for breast augmentation, surgeons have been looking for the proper plane for the augmentation. The orthodox implant plane is submuscular or subglandular [1].

The subglandular plane (Fig. 47.1) usually has implant edge visibility, especially in thin women, and causes a high incidence of fibrous capsular contracture. The submuscular plane can lead to implant distortion, a two-peak breast, and a relatively long recovery period [2, 3]. Advocates of the subglandular approach believe that it produces a better breast shape. This implant placement is generally effective in patients with some amount of breast tissue and subcutaneous fat and with first-degree breast ptosis. It works best when there is adequate soft tissue coverage of the implant. In patients with less soft tissue, there is a higher risk of implant visibility, and a sharp transition can often be seen in the upper pole. It is also clear that the subglandular plane is less satisfactory for mammography [4].

Graf et al. [5] first reported that the subfascial plane for breast augmentation (Fig. 47.2) has some advantages over conventional technique, such as good breast shape and rapid recovery, and avoids some shortcomings, such as implant edge visibility, implant distortion, a two-peak breast, and a relatively long recovery period. Furthermore, it can also provide the breast implant with more soft tissue.

Although the pectoral fascia is very thin, it is a dense tissue, and its integrity can be carefully preserved during dissection. Even if it cannot provide more soft tissue for the implant than the subglandular location, subfascial positioning does not disturb the breast architecture as an entity, keeping the deep layer of superficial fascia that covers the base of the breast in continuity and the retromammary space undisturbed. The retromammary space will allow the breast tissue to glide naturally over the implant. The connective tissue that support the structures of the breast (Cooper's ligaments) runs from the deep muscle fascia through the breast parenchyma to the dermis of the overlying skin (Fig. 47.3).

The attachments of these suspensor ligaments between the deep layer of the superficial fascia and the deep muscular fascia are not tight and allow the breast mobility. These attachments can be stretched and attenuated by weight changes, pregnancy, and aging, which can result in excess breast mobility and ptosis.

At the upper breast near the 2nd rib space, the pectoral fascia tightly connects with the superficial fascia of the breast and is difficult to dissect bluntly [6]. This

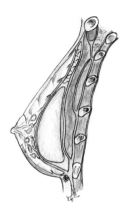

Fig. 47.1 Subglandular pocket location in breast augmentation

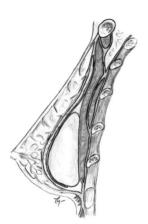

Fig. 47.2 Subfascial breast augmentation

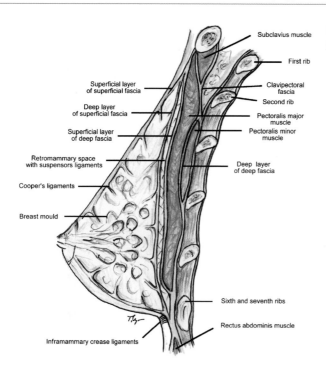

Fig. 47.3 Schematic representation of breast and pectoral fascia

is the meeting point of three fasciae, which hang to the clavicle. The superficial layer of the superficial fascia joins the deep layer of the superficial fascia (including the breast mound between them) and the superficial pectoralis fascia. At the upper and middle pectoral fascia, many thin fibers are found between the pectoral fascia and the deep layer of the superficial fascia of the breast [7]. The breast suspensory ligaments [8] will be in continuity and will support the breast over the implant [9]. The upper pole of the anatomic implant will have an anatomic soft tissue coverage with a natural-looking augmented breast (Fig. 47.4).

47.2
Incision Site

Because of the ever-present patient concerns about scars, various techniques have been devised to minimize or hide the incisions. Current choices include inframammary, periareolar, transaxillary, and periumbilical incisions [10]. Patients present with certain anatomic variables, constraints, and desires that may make one approach more advantageous than another. When a large areola is present, an inferior periareolar incision can be used, or the implants can be inserted in conjunction with a circumareolar mastopexy.

One advantage of the saline-filled implant is that it is equally useful with all incisions. When using silicone gel breast implants, it is more difficult to use the transaxil-

lary incision, and the periumbilical incision would clearly not be appropriate. Silicone implants require a larger incision than saline-filled implants do, and the larger the silicone implant and the more cohesive the gel, the larger the incision needs to be.

The inframammary incision represents the simplest and most straightforward approach to breast augmentation. Direct access to both the subglandular and subpectoral planes can be achieved without violating the breast parenchyma, and visualization of the breast pocket is unsurpassed by the other incision options. For us, using Mentor Contour Profile Gel implants with memory gel in the majority of cases (95%), the inframammary approach is routine.

The patient with an augmented breast will have in her future, sooner or later, other surgical operations to correct the problems that may became visible and to restore the aesthetic appearance. For this situation, the inframammary approach can be the best option.

The scar is frequently inconspicuously hidden in the well-developed inframammary fold and can often be seen only in the recumbent position. In addition, the length of the incision can be of generous size to fit various implants. In patients with significant hypoplasia that causes an ill-defined inframammary fold or with a constricted breast and a breast fold too close to the areola, placement of the incision is less obvious. Therefore, the incision should be at or just above the site of the anticipated new fold, as governed by the vertical diameter of the implant [11].

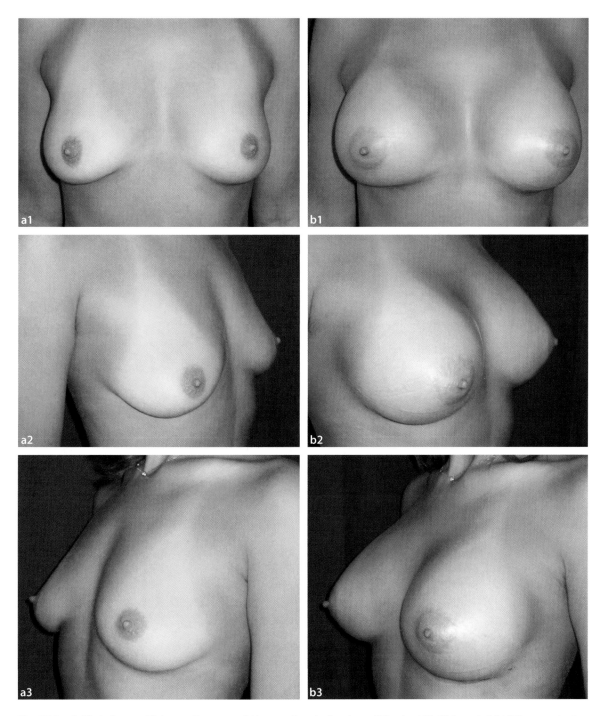

Fig. 47.4 a *1* Clinical case with breast diameters of 11 cm and normal soft tissue elasticity (R:P=2.5) and mild ptosis. *2,3* Lateral views. **b** *1* Subfascial breast augmentation with anatomic breast implant Mentor CPG style 322 (moderate-plus projec-tion), volume 255 ml, width 10.5 cm, height 9.9 cm, projection 4.4 cm. Implant perimeter height is 14.59 cm. *2,3* Lateral views. (Courtesy of Mentor)

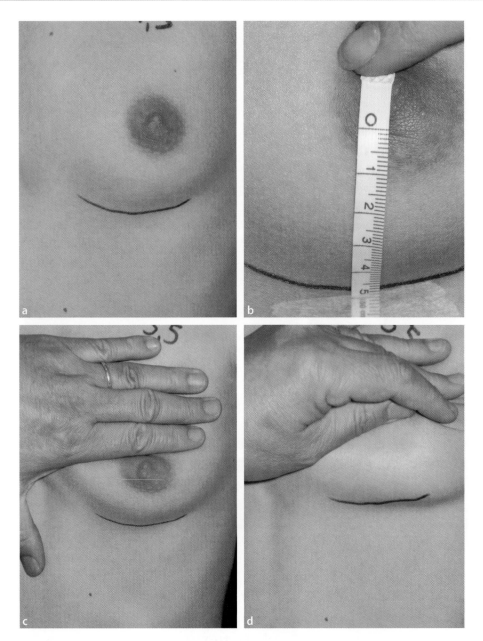

Fig. 47.5 The maneuver for defining the new inframammary fold location and the site of the incision, comparative with the old inframammary fold position. **a** The actual inframammary fold level. **b** Nipple–inframammary measurement of 5 cm. **c** Upper-pole compression of the breast mould. **d** The second maneuver, pulling the nipple and areola upward

To measure the distance from the nipple to the new inframammary line location, the nipple is held between the index finger and thumb and lifted up, and the breast's upper pole is compressed with the palm (Fig. 47.5). With this maneuver, the breast mound will simulate an implant effect, and the skin expansion will show its elasticity and relative excess.

For breast augmentation in thin patients, this maneuver help define the position of the future inframammary fold if an inframammary approach is the option (Fig. 47.6). If the thin patient does not have any glandular tissue, the areola is too small, and the inframammary approach is the option, the distance between the breast upper pole anatomic landmark and the inferior

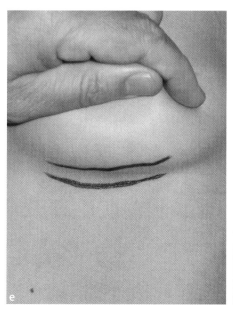
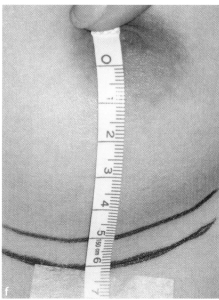

Fig. 47.5 *(continued)* The maneuver for defining the new inframammary fold location and the site of the incision, comparative with the old inframammary fold position. **e** In combination with the upper pole pressure, this maneuver will show the new inframammary fold level where the incision should be done. **f** New nipple–inframammary distance of 6 cm

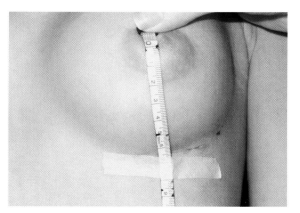

Fig. 47.6 Postoperative, demonstrating the incision position relative to the new inframammary fold location

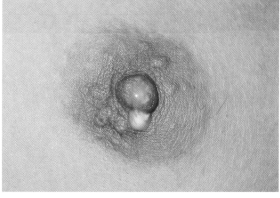

Fig. 47.7 Nipple discharge from a normal breast and possible implant contamination if the periareolar and transglandular approach is the option

margin of the nipple is measured and then divided by two. The result represents the distance from the nipple to the future inframammary fold.

The periareolar incision [12, 13] gives central access to all breast quadrants and is compatible with all of the various breast implants and planes of dissection. It is the most versatile incision when the inframammary fold is being lowered significantly, as well as the logical choice when considering or planning a simultaneous mas-

topexy or when breast parenchyma alteration is needed, as with tuberous breast deformity. Preliminary reports [14] suggest an increased risk of implant contamination with bacteria normally growing in the ducts, as well as changes to nipple sensation and lactation ability with the periareolar approach [15, 16]. Sometimes we face the situation of nipple discharge (Fig. 47.7) without any specific pathology. Implant contamination could be the trigger for the early capsular contraction.

47.3
Pocket Dissection

Patients give informed consent at least 3 days before surgery. Surgery is performed through a 5-cm inframammary fold incision. An incision size less than 5 cm is not recommended because an internal gel fracture can occur on insertion of the implant, even with smaller implant sizes. With the patient under general anesthesia, her arms are abducted to 90° and the dorsum is elevated slightly. The incision is made precisely at the planned location. Cephalexin is administered intravenously at surgery and then orally for 3 days after the procedure.

The midline, the midclavicular line, and the planned lowered inframammary fold were previously marked with the patient in an upright position. The medial edges of the 3rd, 4th, and 5th intercostal spaces are also marked (Fig. 47.8). These represent the exit points of the medial neurovascular pedicles (internal mammary perforators and anteromedial intercostal nerves) and should not be touched by overzealous medial dissection. This will be the landmark of medial dissection (Fig. 47.9). Laterally, the dissection will stop close to the edge of the pectoralis major muscle, where anterolateral intercostal nerves are located.

Pocket dissection is carried out under direct vision us-

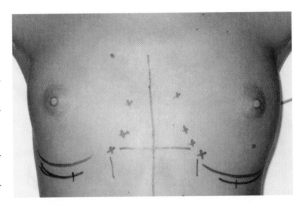

Fig. 47.8 Preoperative marking of the medial edges of the 3rd, 4th, and 5th intercostal spaces

ing the electrocautery unit. Precise pocket dissection is necessary to minimize postoperative implant rotation.

After the incision of the Scarpa fascia, the retroglandular space is opened, and the superficial pectoralis fascia can be seen (Fig. 47.10). The dissection starts at the level of the lateral border of the pectoralis muscle down to the fascia of the pectoralis major muscle, initially in a sagittal direction, up to the areolar level. Dissection of the fascia in the lower portion of the pectoralis major

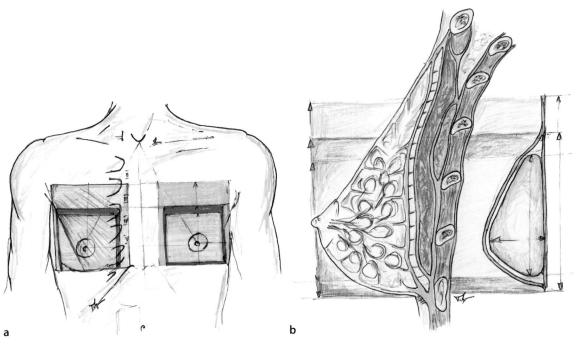

a   b

Fig. 47.9 a Breast rectangles: *yellow rectangle* for anatomic landmarks and pocket dissection, *red rectangle* for breast mould limits, and *blue rectangle* for implant dimension. **b** Lateral view

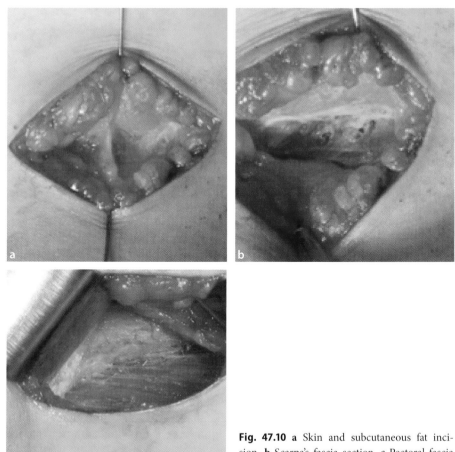

Fig. 47.10 a Skin and subcutaneous fat incision. **b** Scarpa's fascia section. **c** Pectoral fascia elevated

muscle is sometimes associated with increased bleeding [17, 18].

The ease of dissection has to do mostly with the quality of the breast tissue. In some cases, breast tissue that presents with a very loose connection with the underlying tissue can be dissected quite easily and quickly, with no blood loss. In other cases, though, numerous small vessels can be found at this dissection level, which require continuous and careful coagulation and can result in a longer and more demanding dissection. In a few cases in which the breast tissue is attached very firmly to the underlying tissue, dissection to create the subfascial pocket becomes very difficult.

Along the level of the 4th intercostal space, the horizontal septum originating from the pectoral fascia connects with the nipple, as Würinger and Tschabitscher [19] have reported. Here, a strong vascular pedicle for the nipple–areola complex (Fig. 47.11) has to be carefully sectioned after bipolar coagulation.

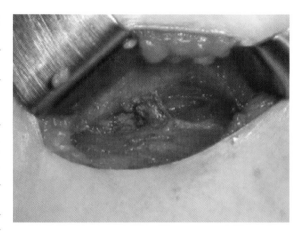

Fig. 47.11 Vascular pedicle for the nipple–areola complex emerging through the pectoralis muscle at the 4th intercostal space level

After this central point is reached, the dissection is carried out with the needle-pointed electrocautery unit through the medial and then lateral edge of the pocket. Superior dissection is carried up to the 2nd intercostal space level.

This upper pole dissection allows adequate redraping of the breast and soft tissues following implant insertion, moving together and hanging to the clavicle. Inferiorly, dissection should be carried exactly to the level of the inframammary fold, if there is no indication to alter this.

When the entire subfascial space is created, meticulous hemostasis is reviewed and finally established. The pocket height is measured, with no tension on the overlying tissues. After that, the dissected fascia is grasped with forceps at its inferior pole and tension is applied, pulling in a sagittal direction. This maneuver will give the dimension of the implant's perimeter height to be selected (Fig. 47.12), taking into account the soft tissue's ability to move and stretch over the implant, especially in breast ptosis cases (Fig. 47.4).

After insertion, anatomic positioning of the implant is assessed by palpating the orientation tabs on both the anterior and posterior surfaces of the implant. There should be perfect hemostasis to prevent any fluid accumulation around the implant. Drains are used for 12 h. The pocket is closed with interrupted sutures using Vicryl 2-0.

A postoperative sports bra is then put on the patient, and she is advised to wear it permanently for the first 6 weeks and after that during sports and fitness activities. This helps promote implant stability during the initial healing period, which is particularly important when using an anatomically shaped device.

47.4
Discussion

The subfascial placement of breast implants has many of the advantages of the submuscular position without lifting the muscle attachments from the ribs [20–22]. The subfascial placement is definitely less injurious to the patient than the submuscular procedure [23]. During subglandular placement, there is an increased risk of injury to the 4th intercostal nerve [24]. Subpectoral placement usually results in temporary numbness because the nerve is stretched with the approach. Subfascial breast augmentation also has less morbidity [25], and the patient is more comfortable. It prevents muscle movement. The subfascial implant location does not prevent the stuck-on teacup appearance caused by interruption of the clavicle-to-nipple line, as does the submuscular. It is somewhat less efficient in this because it is not as thick as the muscle. The subfascial position minimizes rippling above the areola, just as the subglandular position does.

One additional advantage of subfascial positioning is a tighter implant pocket. This may be particularly desirable as shaped gel implants become more widely used. The biggest negative of shaped implants is the potential for device rotation. It may be that subfascial positioning will be helpful in terms of both camouflaging the margins of the implant as well as providing a slightly tighter space around the implant to discourage rotation as well as capsular formation [26–28]. This observation of a lower capsular contracture rate due to additional fascial tissue as a biological barrier between the soft tissue and the implant has recently been supported by an animal study [29].

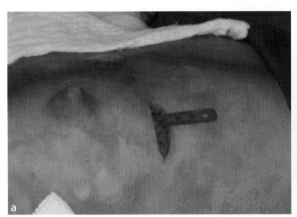
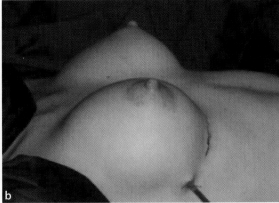

Fig. 47.12 a Intraoperative pocket length measurement shows 13 cm. This corresponds to an implant cover with normal soft tissue elasticity with a similar dimension (13 cm) and to an implant with a 13-cm perimeter height. **b** The selected implant for this case was a 322 CPG implant, 195 ml, medium profile, height 9.4 cm, width 10.0 cm, projection 4.2 cm. Implant perimeter height is 13.26 cm. (Courtesy of Mentor)

Implant dislocation is also reduced because the upper pole is placed between the muscle and the fascia, which leads to a stronger supporting system than the breast parenchyma alone. The creation of this stronger supporting system for the implant's superior pole is one of the main advantages of subfascial augmentation.

The subfascial implants gives the breast shape and contour a more natural look (Figs. 47.13, 47.14).

Subfascial placement has become the preferred position in our practice for placing breast implants. Compared with the subpectorally located implant, the subfascially positioned implant gives the breast a nicer contour and a more natural look. Subfascial breast augmentation can be highly recommended. However, we have not recommended that augmentation mammaplasty using the subfascial plane substitute for either subglandular or subpectoral augmentation; this augmentation mammaplasty is an alternative technique, depending on patient characteristics and tissue conditions as well as the patient's requests and the surgeon's preferences.

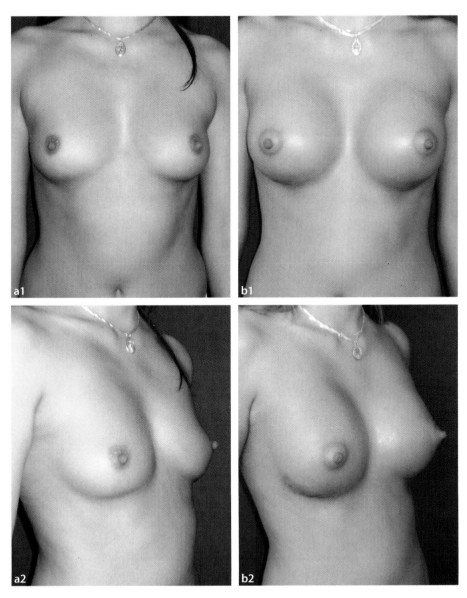

Fig. 47.13 a *1* Clinical case with breast diameters of 11 cm and tight soft tissues (R:P=1.5). *2,3* Lateral views. **b** *1* Subfascial breast augmentation with anatomic breast implant Mentor CPG style 321 (moderate projection), volume 180 ml, width 10.5 cm, height 9.9 cm, projection 3.8 cm. Implant perimeter height is 13.74 cm. *2,3* Lateral views. (Courtesy of Mentor)

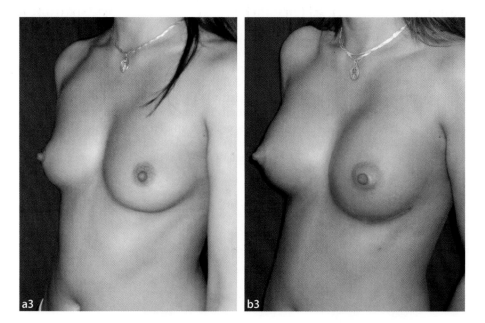

Fig. 47.13 *(continued)* **a** *2,3* Lateral views. **b** *2,3* Lateral views. (Courtesy of Mentor)

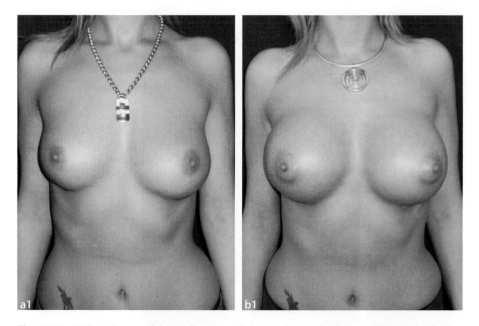

Fig. 47.14 **a** *1* Clinical case with breast diameters of 12 cm and normal soft tissues (R:P=2). **b** *1* Subfascial breast augmentation with anatomic breast implant Mentor CPG style 322 (moderate-plus projection), volume 225 ml, width 10.5 cm, height 9.9 cm, and projection 4.4 cm. Implant perimeter height is 13.93.

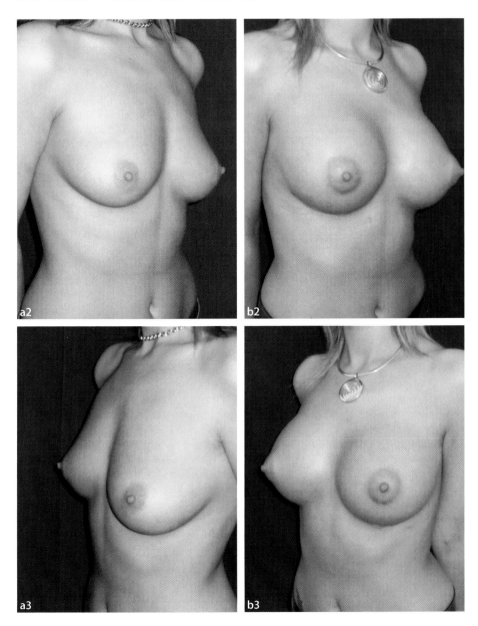

Fig. 47.14 *(continued)* **a** *2,3* Lateral views. **b** *2,3* Lateral views. (Courtesy of Mentor)

References

1. Biggs TM, Yarish RS: Augmentation mammaplasty: a comparative analysis. Plast Reconstr Surg 1990;85(3):368–372
2. Silverman BG, Bright RA, Kaczmarek RG, Arrowsmith-Lowe JB, Kressler DA: Reported complications of silicone gel breast implants. An epidemiologic review. Ann Intern Med 1996;124(8):744–756
3. Gabriel SE, Woods JE, O'Fallon WM, Beard CM, Kurland LT, Melton LJ III: Complications leading to surgery after breast implantation. N Engl J Med 1997;336(10):677–682
4. Silverstein MJ, Handel N, Gamagami P: The effect of silicone gel-filled implants on mammography. Cancer 1991;68(5 suppl):1159–1163

5. Graf RM, Bernardes A, Rippel R, Araujo LR, Damasio RC, Auersvald A: Subfascial breast implant: a new procedure. Plast Reconstr Surg 2003;111(2):904–908

6. Graf RM, Bernardes A, Auerswald A, Damasio RCC: Subfascial endoscopic transaxillary augmentation mammaplasty. Aesthetic Plast Surg 2000;24(3):216–220

7. Jinde L, Jianliang S, Xiaoping C, Xiaoyan T, Jiaging L, Qun M, Bo L: Anatomy and clinical significance of pectoral fascia. Plast Reconstr Surg 2006;118(7):1557–1560

8. Würinger E, Mader N, Posch E, Holle J: Nerve and vessel supplying ligamentous suspension of the mammary gland. Plast Reconstr Surg 1998;101(6):1486–1493

9. Mugea TT: Subfascial breast augmentation. XIIas Jornadas Mediterraneas de confrontations terapeuticas en cirurgia cosmetica, 30 April–2 May 2004, Barcelona

10. Hidalgo DA: Breast augmentation: choosing the optimal incision, implant, and pocket plane. Plast Reconstr Surg 2000;105(6):2202–2216

11. Spear SL, Beckenstein M: The inframammary approach to augmentation mammaplasty. In: Spear SL (ed). Surgery of the Breast: Principles and Art. Philadelphia, Lippincott-Raven 1998

12. Jones FR, Tauruas AP: A periareolar incision for augmentation mammaplasty. Plast Reconstr Surg 1973;51(6):641–644

13. Stoff-Khalili MA, Scholze R, Morgan WR, Metcalf JD: Subfascial periareolar augmentation mammaplasty. Plast Reconstr Surg 2004;114(5):1289–1291

14. Mugea TT: Aesthetic complications in breast aesthetic surgery—can we avoid it? Limberg Meeting of Plastic, Reconstructive and Aesthetic Surgery, 22–24 September 2005, St. Petersburg

15. Neifert M, DeMarzo S, Seacat J, Young D, Leff M, Orleans M: The influence of breast surgery, breast appearance, and pregnancy-induced breast changes on lactation sufficiency as measured by infant weight gain. Birth 1990;17(1)31–38

16. Hurst NM: Lactation after augmentation mammaplasty. Obstet Gynecol 1996;87(1):30–34

17. Tebbetts JB: Does fascia provide additional, meaningful coverage over the breast implant? Plast Reconstr Surg 2004;113(2):777–779

18. Tebbetts JB: Subfascial periareolar augmentation mammaplasty (discussion). Plast Reconstr Surg 2004;114:1289

19. Würinger E, Tschabitscher M: New aspects of the topographical anatomy of the mammary gland regarding its neurovascular supply along a regular ligamentous suspension. Eur J Morphol 2002;40(3):181–189

20. Goes JC, Landecker A: Optimizing outcomes in breast augmentation: seven years of experience with the subfascial plane. Aesthetic Plast Surg 2003;27(3):178–184

21. Benito-Ruiz J: Subfascial breast implant. Plast Reconstr Surg 2004;113(3):1088–1089

22. Barbato C, Pena M, Triana C, Zambrano MA: Augmentation mammaplasty using the retrofascia approach. Aesthetic Plast Surg 2004;28(3):148–152

23. Papillon J: Pros and cons of subpectoral implantation. Clin Plast Surg 1976;3(3):321–337

24. Schlenz I, Kuzbari R, Gruber H, Holle J: The sensitivity of the nipple–areola complex: an anatomic study. Plast Reconstr Surg 2000;105(3):905–909

25. Stoff-Khalili MA, Scholze R, Morgan W, Metcalf JD: Subfascial periareolar augmentation mammaplasty. Plast Reconstr Surg 2004;114(5):1280–1288

26. Duman A, Dincler M, Findik H, Uzunismail A: Further advantages of using the subfascial implant in terms of capsular formation. Plast Reconstr Surg 2005;115(3):950–952

27. Rohrich RJ, Kenkel JM, Adams WP: Preventing capsular contracture in breast augmentation: in search of the Holy Grail. Plast Reconstr Surg 1999;103(6):1759:1760

28. Burkhardt BR: Prevention of capsular contracture. Plast Reconstr Surg 1999;103(6):1769

29. Riefkohl R: Augmentation mammaplasty. In: McCarthy JG (ed). Plastic Surgery, vol. 6. Philadelphia, Harcourt Brace 1990, pp 3879–3884

CHAPTER 48

Subfascial Transaxillary Breast Augmentation   48

Ruth Graf, Daniele Pace

48.1
Introduction

Breast augmentation is a very common procedure nowadays in plastic surgery, but women are concerned about breast size and breast contour when requesting this surgery. Therefore, different techniques have been developed to offer better results with regard to scar position and natural contour of the breast.

The subfascial plane is well recognized and widely used among plastic surgeons to improve the results in breast augmentation. The authors first described the technique in 1999 and published it in 2000 and 2003 [1–3]. The subfascial position gives a good shape and a natural result. There is additional soft tissue between the implant and skin, also improving mammary glandular tissue resistance in the upper pole and leading to a less noticeable implant edge [4, 5].

The major advantage of transaxillary breast augmentation is to not place a scar in the breast unit. Through the transaxillary access, the implant pocket can be undermined by direct visualization, and the final result can be obtained with a scar at a natural axillary crease [6–8].

Transaxillary subfascial breast augmentation is indicated for patients with hypomastia or micromastia with good skin quality or mild breast ptosis and a normal position of the nipple–areola complex. It is contraindicated for patients with severe breast ptosis and poor skin quality who will need mastopexy. Asians and Afro-American patients are good candidates for the transaxillary approach because they have a greater tendency to develop hypertrophic scarring or keloids mainly at the sternal and breast areas. Patients who present with keloids from previous surgeries can be included in this group.

During the first consultation, it is important to discuss with the patient the size and shape of the implant and the position of the scar. All of these aspects depend on the patient's desires and the appearance of the breast, e.g., if she has only hypomastia or associated ptosis (after pregnancy or massive weight loss).

48.2
Technique

The markings are done a day before or just before the surgery. With the patient in the supine position, a midline marking is drawn, and the inframammary crease is marked. The neosulcus line is drawn 2 cm below the crease if the distance between the areola and the inframammary fold needs to be increased. The lateral border of the pectoralis major muscle is drawn with the patient placing her hands on her waist and contracting the pectoralis muscle. The design of the pocket for the implant is delineated 1 or 2 cm from the midsternum line and extended cephalically to the level of the upper pole of the breast and laterally to the anterior axillary line (Fig. 48.1). The axillary incisions are placed in a natural crease in an "S" shape, 1 cm posterior to the pectoralis major muscle border and 4 cm in length (Fig. 48.2).

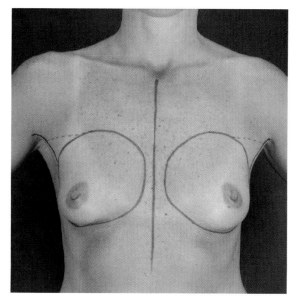

Fig. 48.1 Breast markings

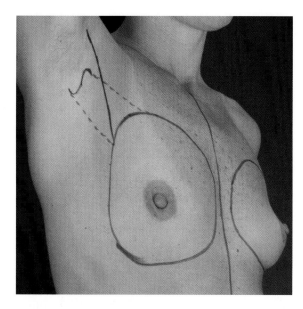

Fig. 48.2 Axillary markings

To perform an endoscopic transaxillary breast augmentation, specific instruments are necessary:

1. 10-mm 30° breast endoscope
2. Endoscopic camera with compatible ring connector
3. Tebbetts breast "L" retractor with 90° angle
4. Fiber optic cable connected to the endoscope
5. Suction tube connected to the retractor
6. Insulated cautery dissector – one set in three different sizes: 3, 10, and 30 cm
7. Endoscopic cart containing camera-video output and monitor with DVD recorder
8. Biggs retractor for implant input

The patient is placed in the prone position on the operating room table, her arms are placed at 90°, and the dorsum is slightly elevated. After the patient is prepped and draped, the position is checked. The areas are infiltrated with epinephrine 1:300,000, starting at the axillary incision and going to the periphery of the drawn circle, using an average of 50 ml in each side. The axillary incision is in the natural crease in an "S" shape, 1 cm posterior to the pectoralis major muscle border and 4 cm in length. A tattoo point at the middle of the incision is made to facilitate skin closure, and a retaining suture is placed at the anterior part of the incision to avoid accidental laceration of the skin during retraction. A skin incision is made using a #15 blade.

The lower side of the incision is retracted at the skin, and the subcutaneous tissue flap is created and dis-

sected until the pectoralis major muscle is identified (Fig. 48.3). Careful dissection with electrocautery exposes the lateral border of the pectoralis muscle, where the fascia is incised along the muscle fibers and the subfascial plane created.

The plane between the pectoralis muscle and the superficial pectoralis fascia is undermined to the areolar level with a light-handle retractor, and then using video endoscopy or continuing by direct view, the subfascial pocket is created at exactly the premarked position. After the introduction of video endoscopy, it is possible to see the fascia and the muscle (Fig. 48.4). In the cephalic portion, the fascia is more defined and resistant. Its inferior portion is thinner and more friable. This undermining should be done very carefully to avoid fascia rupture, trying to keep fascia in the roof and muscle below. If there is doubt about the plane, some muscle fibers may be left attached to the fascia. Once the dissection is completed, a careful evaluation for bleeding is carried out.

The surgeon changes gloves and washes his or her hands to remove the talc. As previously discussed with the patient, an implant of the appropriate size, shape, and texture is placed. The patient is placed in a sitting position on the operating table to check the placement and symmetry of the implants. If an anatomical implant is used, it is necessary to be sure that it is in the correct position (Fig. 48.5)

The skin is closed with a running suture of 4-0 Monocryl (Fig. 48.6). No drain is used, and a band is placed at the upper pole of the breast to compress the axillary dissected area. After that, a soft bra is placed on the patient.

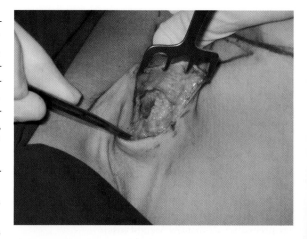

Fig. 48.3 Subcutaneous tissue flap and pectoralis major muscle

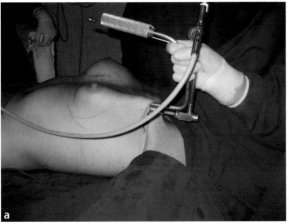 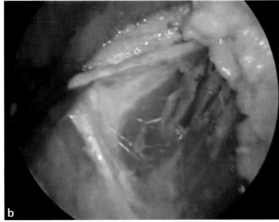

Fig. 48.4 **a** Introduction of video endoscopy. **b** Direct vision of the pectoralis fascia and pectoralis major muscle

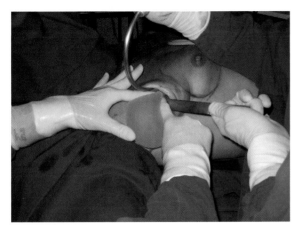

Fig. 48.5 Introduction of the implant

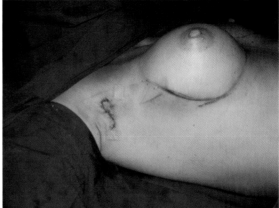

Fig. 48.6 Skin closure

48.3
Postoperative Care

The patient is recommended to wear a soft bra for 1 month and a band on the upper pole for 1 week. She should avoid rough movements with her arms for 1–2 weeks. Analgesics starting 12 h before surgery and anti-inflammatory drugs (cyclo-oxygenase-2 inhibitors) starting 1 h before surgery are used for 1 week to help achieve adequate pain control. (These drugs must be avoided in patients allergic to these medications.) The use of leukotriene inhibitors such Accolate and vitamin E is advisable to prevent capsular contracture, beginning 1 week postoperatively and continuing for 3 months. Monthly liver function tests are recommended while the patient is taking these medications. If the patient presents with any side effects, their use must be discontinued.

Lymphatic drainage twice a week for 1 month is advisable to reduce the duration of edema and pain, starting on postoperative day 5. Physical activities are allowed 1–2 weeks after the procedure, but the patient should avoid high-impact activities for 2 months.

48.4
Results

Patient satisfaction is higher with this procedure, mainly because of the natural breast shape, the lack of scar on the breast, and the lack of implant edge visibility (Figs. 48.7–48.9).

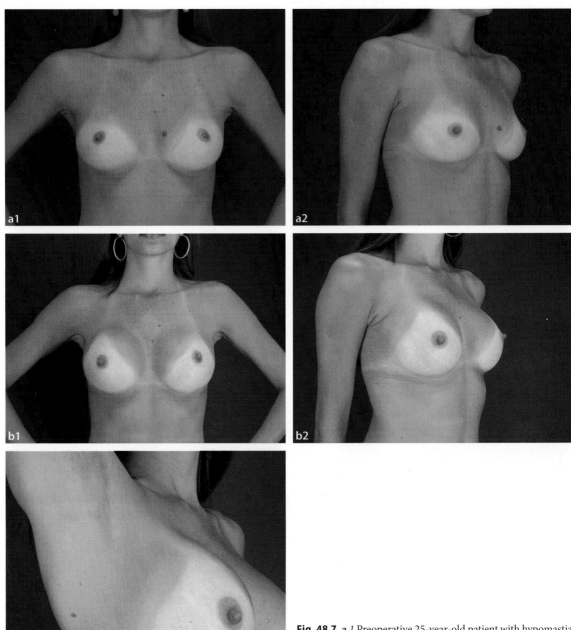

Fig. 48.7 a *1* Preoperative 25-year-old patient with hypomastia. *2* Lateral view. **b** *1* Two years postoperative following transaxillary breast augmentation with 275-ml textured round implant in subfascial plane. *2* Lateral view. **c** Axillary scar after 2 years

48.5
Discussion

The position of an implant in the subglandular space has significant disadvantages if the soft tissue cover is inadequate. In addition to implant palpability and visibility, the rates of fibrous capsular contracture, rippling, and nipple sensation alteration, such as numbness, are higher. To correct these problems encountered with subglandular placement, use of the retropectoral space has become commonplace [9].

The disadvantages of submuscular placement include a more invasive procedure, increased postoperative discomfort, and visible flattening or distortion of the breast

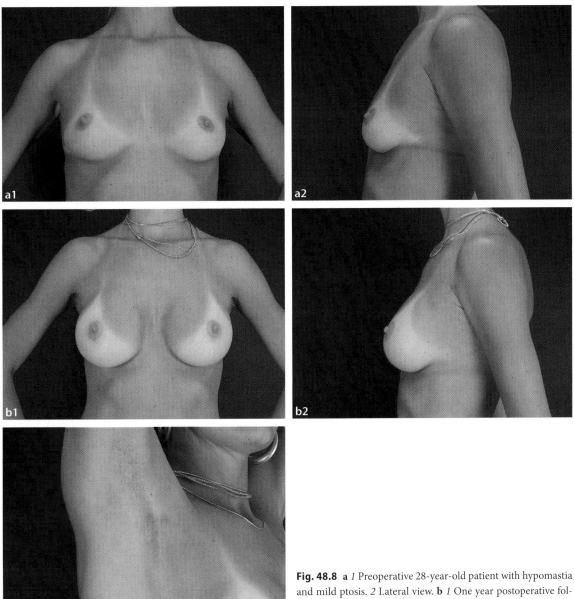

Fig. 48.8 a *1* Preoperative 28-year-old patient with hypomastia and mild ptosis. *2* Lateral view. **b** *1* One year postoperative following transaxillary breast augmentation with 375-ml textured high-profile anatomic implant in subfascial plane. *2* Lateral view. **c** Axillary scar after 1 year

when the pectoral muscle is contracted. If the muscle is released inadequately medially, the implant may ride too high, or if the muscle is released excessively, the implant may be displaced inferiorly and laterally [10, 11].

A reasonable solution to the problem of acquiring adequate soft tissue coverage without distorting the implant through muscle contracture has been to use the subfascial plane. Because the pectoralis muscle fascia is a well-defined structure and very consistent in the upper thorax, it can be used to minimize the appear-ance of the edges of the implant on the skin, making the implant less noticeable. The integrity of the muscle is preserved, and the implant is totally covered. Additionally, the strong attachment between fascia and muscle provides muscle elevation when the implant is placed, giving an extra cover at the limits of the implant pocket and providing a pleasing and natural aesthetic result. In the subfascial plane, there will be no alteration to the breast shape by muscular contraction or displacement due to muscular movement.

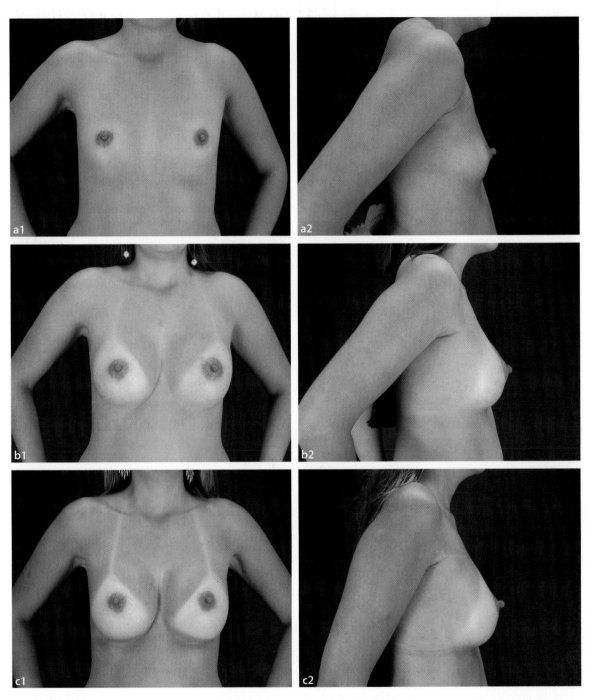

Fig. 48.9 a *1* Preoperative 26-year-old patient with hypomastia and asymmetry, with right breast smaller than the left breast. *2* Lateral view. **b** *1* Six months postoperative following transaxillary breast augmentation with textured high-profile anatomic implants—315 ml in the right breast and 290 ml in the left breast—in subfascial plane. Note the rippling in the medial aspect of the right breast; the patient was also dissatisfied with the size. *2* Lateral view. **c** *1* Two years following transaxillary breast augmentation to change the implant to 375 ml in the right breast and 310 ml in the left breast (textured high-profile anatomic implant in subfascial plane). They were maintained with the same approach. *2* Lateral view

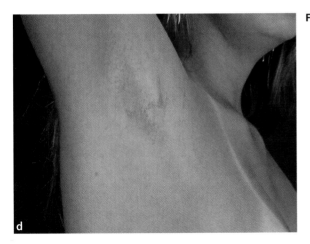

Fig. 48.9 *(continued)* **d** Axillary scar after 2 years

It is very important during the physical examination to take measurements such as the breast base or breast width, the distance between the inframammary fold and the inferior areola, and the distance between the xyphoid process and the superior areola, and to determine the position of the upper pole of the breast tissue by pressing the breast superiorly. The pinch test with a special instrument is used to measure the subcutaneous fat thickness.

Taking the breast base measurements and the pinch test measurements, we can choose the base of the implants and, consequently, the implant size. If the measurement of the inframammary fold to the areola is too short—less than 4 cm—an anatomically shaped implant is the best choice to spread and increase this distance and to move up the nipple–areola complex. If the patient has almost no breast tissue and so we need to give shape to the breast, an anatomical implant also is the best choice. If the patient has nicely shaped breasts and wants only augmentation and better upper-pole fullness, a round implant will be better.

Regarding breast projection, the majority of patients want good projection. Therefore, a high-profile implant is the best choice for them. If the patient has enough breast tissue, an implant with moderate profile can be chosen.

The implant size can be defined in conjunction with the patient at the first consultation. For example, if the breast base or breast width is 12 cm and the pinch test is 1.0 cm, the base of the implant can be 11–12 cm, depending on the patient's desire . After that, the surgeon can look at the tables that the implant companies provide and automatically choose the size of the implant. At the same time, it is possible to choose the implant's projection and shape.

Smooth-surface devices are acceptable for the submuscular position because they are safer compared with textured devices, despite the probability of double the incidence of capsular contracture and seroma with muscular movement. The textured device is better for the subfascial and subglandular positions because it provides better adherence to the tissue and a lower capsular contracture rate.

The complications that can occur with this technique are hematoma in the early postoperative period, late seroma, malposition, and implant rotation. In any reoperation, the axillary incision is maintained. Late seroma is seen mainly in textured implants when the patient makes rough movements that undermine the capsular adherence, detaching and provoking bleeding between the capsular tissue and the implant shell and resulting in an intracapsular hematoma. In some cases, treatment with ultrasound-guided aspiration can resolve the problem; otherwise, it is necessary to reoperate to perform rigorous hemostasis and change the implant. One year after surgery, it is possible to perform mammography studies (Fig. 48.10).

48.6 Conclusions

Transaxillary breast augmentation is indicated in patients with good position of the nipple–areola complex. Patients with severe breast ptosis are not good candidates. The goal of transaxillary breast augmentation is to not place a scar in the breast unit, and the goal of the subfascial position is to promote good shape and a natural result.

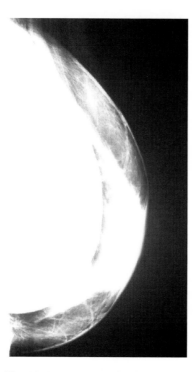

Fig. 48.10 Mammography in a patient with breast implant in subfascial plane. Note the pectoralis fascia covering the implant in the upper pole of the breast

References

1. Graf RM: Mamaplastia de aumento transaxilar videoendoscópica subfascial. Rev Bras Cir Plást 1999;14(2):45–54
2. Graf RM, Bernardes A, Auersvald A, Damasio RCC: Subfascial endoscopic transaxillary augmentation mammaplasty. Aesthet Plast Surg 2000;24(3):216–220
3. Graf RM, Bernardes A, Rippel R, Araujo LR,Damasio RCC, Auersvald A: Subfascial breast implant: a new procedure. Plast Reconstr Surg 2003;111(2):904–908
4. Goes JC, Landecker A: Optimizing outcomes in breast augmentation: seven years of experience with the subfascial plane. Aesth Plast Surg 2003;27(3):178–184
5. Barbato C, Pena M, Triana C, Zambrano MA: Augmentation mammoplasty using the retrofascia approach. Aesth Plast Surg 2004;28(3):148–152
6. Barnett A: Transaxillary subpectoral augmentation in the ptotic breast: augmentation by disruption of the extended pectoral fascia and parenchymal sweep. Plast Reconstr Surg 1990;86(1):76–83
7. Howard PS, Oslin BD, Moore JR: Endoscopic transaxillary submuscular augmentation mammaplasty with textured saline breast implants. Ann Plast Surg 1996;37(1):12–17
8. Tebbetts JB: Transaxillary subpectoral augmentation mammaplasty: long-term follow-up and refinements. Plast Reconstr Surg 1984;74(5):636–649
9. Papillion J: Pros and cons of subpectoral implantation. Clin Plast Surg 1976;3(2):321–337
10. Regnault P: Partially submuscular breast augmentation. Plast Reconstr Surg 1977;59(1):72–76
11. Biggs TM, Yarish RS: Augmentation mammaplasty: a comparative analysis. Plast Reconstr Surg 1990;85(3):368–372

CHAPTER 49

Modified Subfascial Breast Augmentation

Richard A. Baxter

49.1
Introduction

Techniques for breast augmentation have undergone continuous evolution since breast implants were first introduced in the early 1960s. In addition to improvements in the procedure itself, preoperative planning relative to assessment of the adequacy of the soft tissue envelope has been emphasized [1]. This can then be applied to an algorithm to determine whether the implant should be placed in the submuscular or the subglandular plane. Because the subfascial plane is not generally believed to contribute to the thickness of the soft tissue coverage, it has received less emphasis.

Each plane has advantages and disadvantages. For subglandular placement, trade-offs include a potentially less supportive envelope, visible rippling, and a less natural upper-pole contour compared with the submuscular plane. These considerations are balanced against ease of dissection and quick recovery. The subpectoral or "dual-plane" approach improves coverage and contours for many patients, but some patients will develop a dynamic deformity that occurs with muscle flexion. This is related to the requisite detachment of the costal portion of the muscle origin, so that the free edge of the muscle fuses with the anterior capsule. Additionally, muscle activity over time may contribute to implant malposition, in particular a wide intermammary space.

Although the subfascial plane does not contribute to padding, it does add support [2–4]. The author has found it especially useful in athletic women who present a particular challenge: With low body fat, a subglandular implant will appear unnatural, while a subpectoral implant is often subject to considerable and unacceptable distortion with activity. This problem is especially acute in bodybuilders. In some of these cases, the author uses a variation of the subfascial technique in which the pectoral muscle is split so as to preserve the attachments, while using the upper portion for implant coverage [5]. The lower portion of the pocket is in the subfascial plane. It may be helpful to think of the subfascial plane as a continuum with the subpectoral plane, providing a range of options.

The subfascial plane has been employed primarily by surgeons outside the United States, and the form-stable implant (cohesive gel, Inamed style 410) is the most popular choice. This may be due to the fact that these are shaped implants, so the potential for upper-pole step-off deformity and visible rippling is mitigated. These benefits come at the expense of a firmer implant, which some may find unappealing, and lack of natural-appearing motion as with a round implant. The split subpectoral/subfascial plane is an adaptation to the round implant, harmonizing a variety of competing factors. Upper-pole coverage is optimized with muscle; muscle flexion deformity is minimized by leaving the costal origin of the muscle intact behind the implant; and the round implant has compliance and motion characteristics more similar to a natural breast.

49.2
Technique

There are four useful variations on the subfascial technique: "standard" subfascial, split subpectoral/subfascial, and conversion of subpectoral or subglandular to subfascial.

Total subfascial placement is straightforward. Regardless of the incisional access, the dissection must be done under direct vision. Electrocautery is quite helpful as there are several vascular perforators. I most often use the periareolar incision, and then dissect in the deep subcutaneous plane toward the inframammary fold. Most often, the chest wall is encountered above the fold and over the attachments of the rectus abdominis muscle. This muscle has a thick fascia that is elevated down to the desired level for the inframammary fold. This provides good lower-pole support. The fascia is then elevated from the pectoral muscle, and it gets noticeably thicker in its superior portion. A precise match of pocket dimensions to the base diameter of the implant is the goal.

The first stage of the split-muscle approach is similar to the total subfascial approach. However, the fascia is elevated only up to the level of the muscle where it is to be divided. Most commonly, this is on a line from the junction of the costal to the sternal heads of the muscle toward the axilla. It is a muscle-splitting technique, as opposed to a muscle-cutting technique as with the dual-plane approach. For some athletic individuals, only the uppermost portion of the muscle is elevated. It is occasionally helpful to suture the edge of the upper portion of the muscle to the fascia with 2-0 or 3-0 polyglactin sutures to avoid having it pop behind the implant with activity before the capsular scar secures it.

Conversion from dual-plane to split submuscular/subfascial is indicated for muscle flexion deformity. Most often, when the patient flexes the pectoral muscle, the implant moves superiorly and laterally, and a transverse groove or depression is visible on the lower pole where the muscle has fused with the capsule (Fig. 49.1). This area is marked preoperatively. After implant removal, the anterior capsule is dissected off of the subglandular portion of the breast until the edge of the muscle is encountered (Fig. 49.2). The muscle is then dissected down, leaving the fascia on the deep aspect of the breast tissue. The muscle is split along the line extending from the junction of the sternal and costal portions. The costal segment is then sutured to the posterior capsule at the level of its original attachment, using 2-0 polyglactin horizontal mattress sutures. The split edge of the upper muscle is secured to the fascia as well.

For conversion of subglandular to split subpectoral, the muscle is easily exposed within the posterior capsule. It is divided with cautery, and the upper portion is then mobilized as with a standard subpectoral approach. The edge is sutured to the anterior capsule, and the lower and lateral portions of the capsule remain unaltered.

49.3 Results

The author has used the split subpectoral/subfascial technique as a "default" method in more than 300 cases. Round implants are used exclusively, providing a reasonable balance between form, feel, and motion. Distortion with active pectoral muscle flexion is minimal, and it is helpful to include a flexion pose in the postoperative set of photographs (Fig. 49.3).

The technique is especially useful for correcting the flexion deformity related to dual-plane implant placement. In these cases, splitting the muscle and reattaching the lateral portion to the chest wall while preserving the sternal origin reliably minimizes the deformity while maintaining upper-pole coverage and contour (Fig. 49.4).

49.4 Complications

Control of bleeding can be problematic if the muscle is split too high toward the axilla. This resulted in two hematomas early in the series. Capsular contracture has been seen in approximately 2% of cases, with none more than Baker grade 3.

49.5 Discussion

The subfascial plane has been used for a number of years but has had limited popularity in North America, where

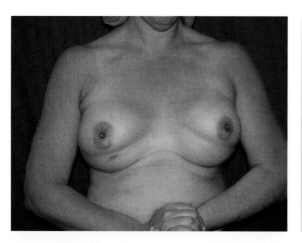

Fig. 49.1 When the patient flexes the pectoral muscle, the implant moves superiorly and laterally, and a transverse groove or depression is visible on the lower pole where the muscle has fused with the capsule

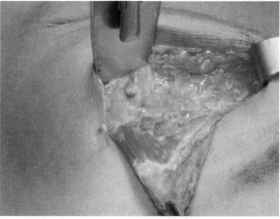

Fig. 49.2 After implant removal, the anterior capsule is dissected off the subglandular portion of the breast until the edge of the muscle is encountered

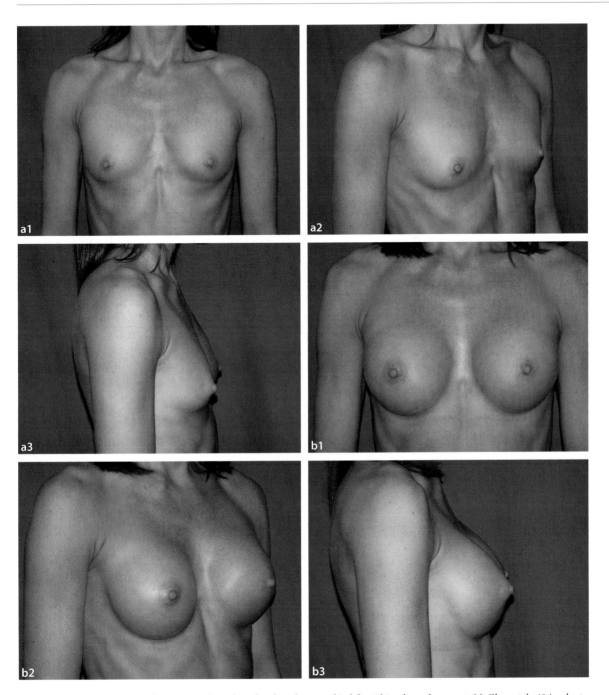

Fig. 49.3 a *1–3* Preoperative. **b** *1–3* Typical result with split subpectoral/subfascial implant placement, McGhan style 40 implants, 300 ml

shaped implants have declined in use for a variety of reasons. Round implants have a number of advantages, but enhanced soft tissue coverage is frequently required for optimal results; for this reason, the subpectoral plane is most frequently employed. Breast deformity with muscle contraction may result from this, although the incidence has not been determined, and no grading scale has been put forth. Nevertheless, it must occur by definition to some degree with every case of dual-plane subpectoral augmentation because of the detachment of the muscle origin and fusion to the anterior capsule at some point above the inframammary fold.

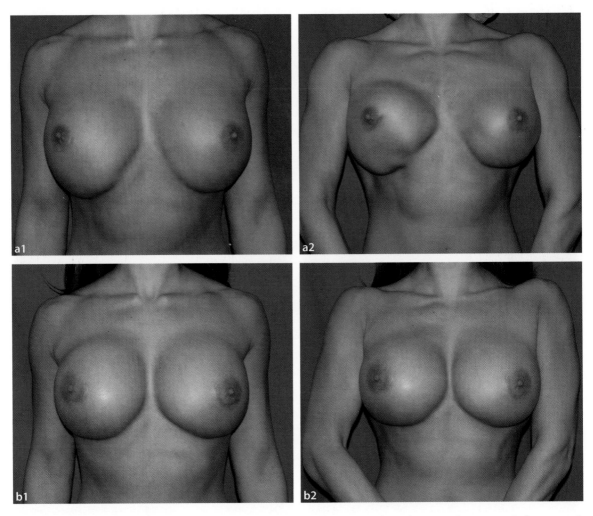

Fig. 49.4 a Precorrection. *1* Fitness model with 600-ml round gel implants. *2* Muscle flexion distortion. **b** *1* This was corrected by reattaching the muscle to the chest wall behind the implant, leaving a strip of muscle across the upper pole for a smooth transition. *2* Flexion shows minimal distortion

Total subfascial augmentation is most successful with either cohesive (form-stable) gel implants or round implants with at least a 1–2-cm subcutaneous fat layer for contour camouflage. The most useful variation is the split subpectoral/subfascial approach with round implants. This allows for upper-pole muscle coverage, natural implant contours, natural implant motion, no risk of implant rotation deformity, a low risk of flexion deformity, and adequate implant support.

Authors debate whether the pectoral fascia contributes to support. Jinde et al. [6] measured the thickness of the fascia in a series of cadaver dissections and found that it ranged from 0.2 mm to 1.14 mm. The fascia is continuous with the rectus fascia and the serratus anterior fascia [7], so total subfascial coverage is possible.

These findings support the notion that the fascia provides meaningful implant support. However, variations including muscle coverage address this shortcoming.

49.6
Conclusions

The subfascial plane is a versatile option for breast augmentation. It can be used with round implants by employing the split subpectoral/subfascial pocket. Competing factors can be balanced in order to optimize implant coverage and aesthetics while minimizing the risk of implant malposition and distortion with muscle flexion.

References

1. Tebbetts JB: Dual plane breast augmentation: optimizing implant-soft-tissue relationships in a wide range of breast types. Plast Reconstr Surg 2006;18(7 suppl):81S–98S

2. Góes JCS, Landecker A: Optimizing outcomes in breast augmentation: seven years of experience with the subfascial plane. Aesthetic Plast Surg 2003;27(3):178–184

3. Graf RM, Bernardes A, Auersvald A, Damasio RC: Subfascial endoscopic transaxillary augmentation mammaplasty. Aesthetic Plast Surg 2000;24(3):216–220

4. Graf RM, Bernardes A, Rippel R, Araujo LR, Damasio RC, Auersvald A: Subfascial breast implant: a new procedure. Plast Reconstr Surg 2003;111(2):904–908

5. Baxter R: Subfascial breast augmentation: theme and variations. Aesthetic Surg J 2005;25(5):514–520

6. Jinde L, Jianliang S, Xiaoping C, Xiaoyan T, Jiaging L, Qun M, Bo L: Anatomy and clinical significance of pectoral fascia. Plast Reconstr Surg 2006;118(7):1557–1560

7. Hwang K, Kim DJ: Anatomy of pectoral fascia in relation to subfascial mammary augmentation. Ann Plast Surg 2005;55(6):576–579

Submuscular Fascial Dual-Plane Breast Augmentation

50

Toma T. Mugea

50.1
Introduction

The optimal technique for breast augmentation has always been debated, and numerous variables fit the needs of the variously shaped patients. A subpectoral pocket is favored because this implant location provides for more soft tissue cover in the upper pole of the breast and less difficulty when performing screening mammography [1]. A subglandular position is selected only if there is adequate tissue cover, especially in the superior pole. Adequate tissue cover is defined as a minimum of 2 cm of tissue when pinching the breast in the middle segment of the upper pole. When glandular ptosis exists in the presence of minimal upper pole tissue, a dual-plane pocket is selected. This approach maintains adequate soft tissue cover in the upper pole and results in improved breast shape by allowing the lower portion of the implant to sit in a subglandular position [2].

Total muscle coverage (Fig. 50.1) was developed as an option to reduce implant visibility and palpability and, ideally, to decrease the incidence of capsular con-

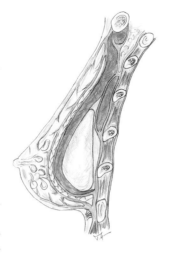

Fig. 50.1 Breast augmentation with total muscle coverage

tracture. This was at the expense of adequate lower-pole shape and inframammary fold definition. Late superior migration of the implants or pseudoptosis of the breast (Figs. 50.2, 50.3) was seen in a significant number of

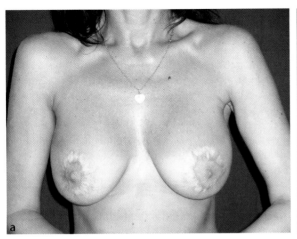
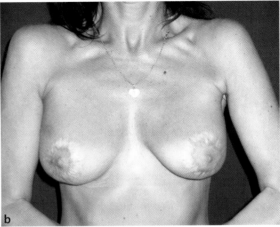

Fig. 50.2 a This 32-year-old woman was first seen after periareolar mastopexy and submuscular breast augmentation. No details about implant size, shape, or filler were available. **b** She had a poor scar, breast mould ptosis, and implant migration with pectoralis muscle contraction

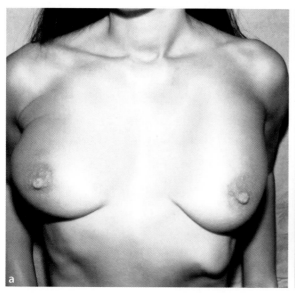
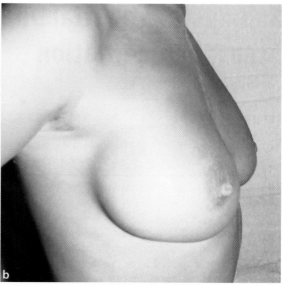

Fig. 50.3 This 35-year-old woman had a total submuscular breast augmentation. No details about implant size, shape, or filler were given. **a** Note breast mould ptosis (hanging breast), breast asymmetry, and lateral implant migration at the pectoralis muscle contraction. **b** Lateral view

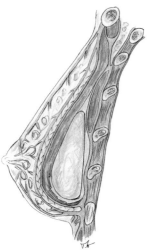

Fig. 50.4 Breast augmentation with subpectoral placement

women. In such cases, bad surgery also augments the problems. This was a result of the gravitational effects on the breast against an implant still supported by the lower muscle panel. The development of newer devices has seemed to reduce the risk of capsular contracture, so there became less need for total muscle coverage [3].

Subpectoral placement (Fig. 50.4) generally refers to partial muscle coverage of the implant in its upper pole by the pectoralis major, with the lower portion of the implant being subglandular. This plane seems to achieve about as low a rate of capsular contracture as total submuscular positioning while also facilitating mammography. The pectoral muscle is divided close to the origin (1-cm inferior margin left), and will retract by itself, leaving a thin muscular layer attached to the superficial pectoral fascia. Usually, the muscle retracts upward to the nipple–areola complex level.

There is improved upper-pole breast contour because the muscle blunts the transition between the upper breast and the implant superiorly. The pocket dissection is easier overall in the subpectoral loose areolar plane, and the breast parenchyma is less devascularized, which is optimal for any planned breast shaping or mastopexy.

Subpectoral implantation should be used with caution in patients with significant postpartum atrophy, glandular ptosis, or significant native tissue volume, because the lower pole of the breast cannot be properly filled, and the breast will hang in front of the augmented pectoral region (Fig. 50.5). Also, these clinical situations are at higher risk for developing a double-bubble deformity (Fig. 50. 6) [4].

50.2
Retromuscular Glandular Dual-Plane Breast Augmentation

When glandular ptosis exists in the presence of minimal upper-pole tissue, a dual-plane pocket is selected.

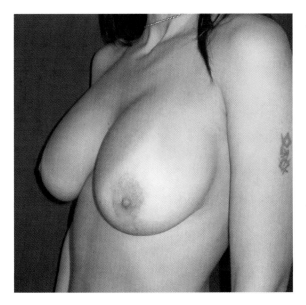

Fig. 50.5 Subpectoral breast augmentation with "hanging breast" appearance. The implant volume does not fill the breast

This approach maintains adequate soft tissue cover in the upper pole and results in improved breast shape by allowing the lower portion of the implant to sit in a subglandular position (Fig. 50.7).

The dual-plane augmentation has developed as a variation of subpectoral plane augmentation to minimize the risk of a double-breast-contour deformity. This variation, described by Tebbetts [5], helps create a desirable breast shape by using the subpectoral plane in conjunction with the subglandular plane, which is ad-

justable for the less ptotic nulliparous breast to the more ptotic or loose breast.

The key difference between dual-plane and subpectoral implant sites is the use of a subglandular dissection that may extend superiorly above the level of the inferior border of the pectoralis major.

After complete division of the pectoralis origins across the inframammary fold, stopping at the medial aspect of the inframammary fold, three variations of the parenchyma–muscle interface dissection are used by Tebbetts [5, 6]:

Type I dual-plane: *No dissection in the retromammary plane to free the parenchyma–muscle interface. This corresponds to the retromuscular implant position.* According to Tebbetts, a type I dual-plane technique is selected for most *routine breasts,* with all of the breast parenchyma located above the inframammary fold and tight attachments at the parenchyma–muscle interface. The drawback of this last situation could be a downward-looking nipple and a straight lower pole of the breast (Fig. 50.8).

Type II dual-plane: *Dissection in the retromammary plane to approximately the inferior border of the areola.* According to Tebbetts, a type II dual-plane technique is selected for breasts with *highly mobile parenchyma*: "The goal in this type of breast augmentation was to perform more dissection at the parenchyma–muscle interface to allow the muscle to retract more superiorly, reducing the risks of highly mobile parenchyma sliding off the anterior surface of the pectoralis postoperatively."

Type III dual-plane: *Dissection in the retromammary plane to approximately the superior border of the areola.* According to Tebbetts, a type III dual-plane technique is selected for *glandular ptotic* and *constricted lower pole breasts*: "The goal in both glandular ptotic and con-

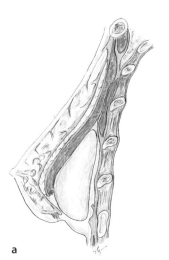

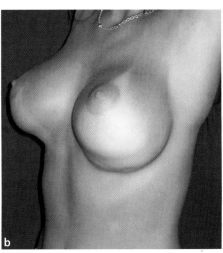

Fig. 50.6 a Double-bubble deformity in subpectoral implantation. Because of the inferior insertions of the superficial fascia to the pectoral fascia, the breast mound and fascial system, including the inframammary crease ligaments, are pulled upward, leaving the hanging implant to protrude. **b** Double bubble in patient

a   b

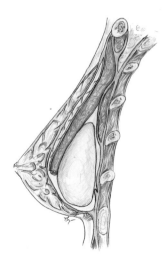

Fig. 50.7 The dual-plane (retromuscular-glandular) breast augmentation maintains adequate soft tissue cover in the upper pole and results in improved breast shape by allowing the lower portion of the implant to sit in a subglandular position

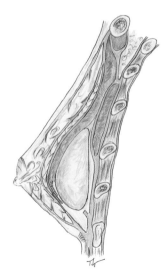

Fig. 50.8 Downward-looking nipple deformity in type I dual-plane subpectoral implantation. Because of the tight attachments at the parenchyma–muscle interface (musculofascial connections), the breast mound and fascial system are pulled upward. The implant cannot fill the lower pole of the breast

stricted lower pole breasts was to maximally free the pectorals inferiorly and to incrementally free the parenchyma from the pectoralis major at the parenchyma–muscle interface to allow the inferior edge of the pectoralis to move superiorly. In both constricted lower pole and glandular ptotic breasts, the implant must maximally contact parenchyma and project interiorly without muscle restriction to optimally correct the deformities. In constricted lower pole breasts, the implant must contact large areas of parenchyma to achieve parenchymal redistribution after scoring and to optimally expand the inferior envelope" [5, 6].

50.3
Retromuscular Fascial Dual-Plane Breast Augmentation

Soon after Graf and colleagues [7, 8] published their experiences with subfascial breast augmentation, the author started using this procedure in selected cases (cases that were supposed to have the "classical" retroglandular implant position) [9]. With more extensive experience, the retroglandular plane is no longer used. The retrofascial approach is very friendly, and this is the first choice (without pushing the limits) in breast augmentation, keeping the retropectoral pocket as the "B plan" for revision surgery in the same cases.

In the retromuscular plane technique for breast augmentation, when the soft tissue is not thinner than 2 cm, the dissection is started 1–2 cm in the retrofascial plan above the inframammary fold level. This small techni-

cal modification provides good visibility with better control of pectoralis muscle division and hemostasis. Also, the pectoralis muscle can retract upward, without tension on the lower pole of the breast (Fig. 50.9).

With the fascial dual-plane approach, the aesthetic outcome is improved. The superficial pectoralis fascia is lifted as in subfascial breast augmentation, keeping the dissection at the nipple level (the areola has a wide variety of diameters, so it is not appropriate to use it as a landmark).

The main features and surgical steps of this technique are as follows:
1. Dissection in the retrofascial plan
2. Retropectoral dissection
3. Pectoralis muscle division

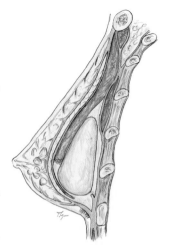

Fig. 50.9 The pectoralis muscle can retract upward, without tension on the lower pole of the breast

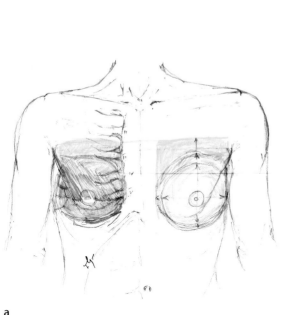

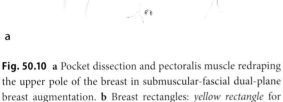

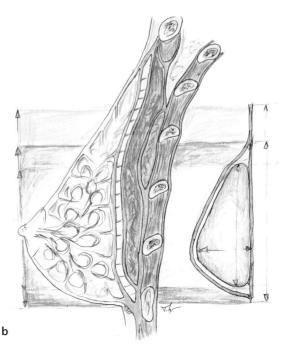

a

b

Fig. 50.10 a Pocket dissection and pectoralis muscle redraping the upper pole of the breast in submuscular-fascial dual-plane breast augmentation. **b** Breast rectangles: *yellow rectangle* for anatomic landmarks and pocket dissection, *red rectangle* for breast mould limits, and *blue rectangle* for implant dimension

50.4
Technique

All patients undergoing breast augmentation surgery are informed that this type of procedure is not a once-in-a-lifetime operation. The patient is told to expect that secondary surgery may be necessary at certain times in her life to either change or reposition an implant or to perform surgery on the overlying breast tissue. The most common reasons for reoperation include capsular contracture and correction of changes in breast tissue caused by aging, pregnancy, or effects from the underlying implant. On the basis of the preceding discussion, it is reasonable to suggest that the inframammary incision is the simplest and most straightforward approach to breast augmentation. Direct access to both the subfascial and subpectoral dual planes can be achieved without violating the breast parenchyma, and visualization of the breast pocket is unsurpassed by the other incision options. The length of the incision can be of generous size to fit various implants.

Usually, surgery is performed through a 5-cm inframammary fold incision. An incision less than 5 cm is not recommended because internal gel fracture can oc-

cur when the implant is inserted, even with smaller implant sizes.

Pocket dissection is carried out under direct vision using the electrocautery unit. Precise pocket dissection is necessary to minimize postoperative implant rotation (Fig. 50.10).

The retrofascial dissection will stop cranially at the level of the nipple–areola complex, medially at the exit points of the medial neurovascular breast pedicles, and laterally close to the edge of the pectoralis major muscle where anterolateral intercostal nerves are located.

The retropectoral dissection starts laterally, close to the inframammary fold, where the space is easiest to enter because there are no attachments to the pectoralis minor or serratus anterior muscles. It is carried out superiorly up to the nipple–areola complex and then medially. The pectoralis muscle is free with two dissected spaces anterior and posterior to its belly. With the pectoralis fibers held with an anatomical forceps, the surgeon begins muscle origin division, going from lateral to medial (Fig. 50.11) parallel to the inframammary fold and 1 cm above it.

The pectoralis muscle division stops at the medial edge of the inframammary fold, joining the retrofascial

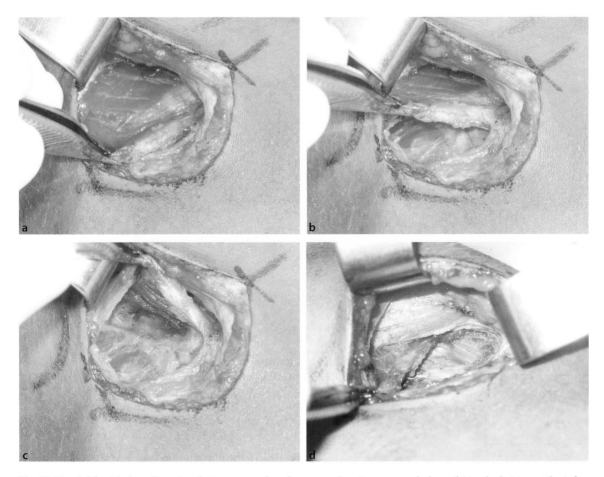

Fig. 50.11 a Subfascial plane dissection. **b** Retropectoral pocket approach. **c** Retropectoral plane. **d** Muscle division at the infra-mammary fold level

dissection level. The retropectoral dissection continues according to the anatomic landmarks. The surgeon should stop dissection at the lateral border of the pectoralis minor to avoid overdissecting the lateral pocket and then dissect superiorly, opening the superior subpectoral pocket until the thoracoacromial pedicle is visible, dissecting from lateral to medial, and then opening the medial pocket from superior to inferior along the sternum. Excessive medial or superior release of this muscle risks creating synmastia, "window-shading," or unnatural medial breast fullness.

Partial division of the main body of the pectoralis origins along the sternum, although often mentioned, is difficult to define, and partial division can inadvertently become complete division, sacrificing coverage and increasing risks of the previously mentioned deformities.

The implants are handled as little as necessary to minimize possible contamination. All patients receive perioperative antibiotics; most receive a first-generation cephalosporin.

Postoperative tape and a sports bra are then applied and left for 5 days. This helps promote implant stability during the initial healing period, which is particularly important when using an anatomically shaped device.

50.5
Clinical Cases

For all of the retromuscular-fascial dual-plane breast augmentations, the author uses the TTM computer program for Mentor implant selection and the inframammary approach.

Three clinical cases are presented here, each having the same breast horizontal and vertical diameters (11 cm) but different quality of the soft tissue: tight (Fig. 50.12), normal (Fig. 50.13), and loose (Fig. 50.14). Fig. 50.15 shows a clinical case with normal soft tissue elasticity [pinch (P) and relax (R) tests: R:P=2.5] but a low breast vertical diameter (10 cm) and prominence of

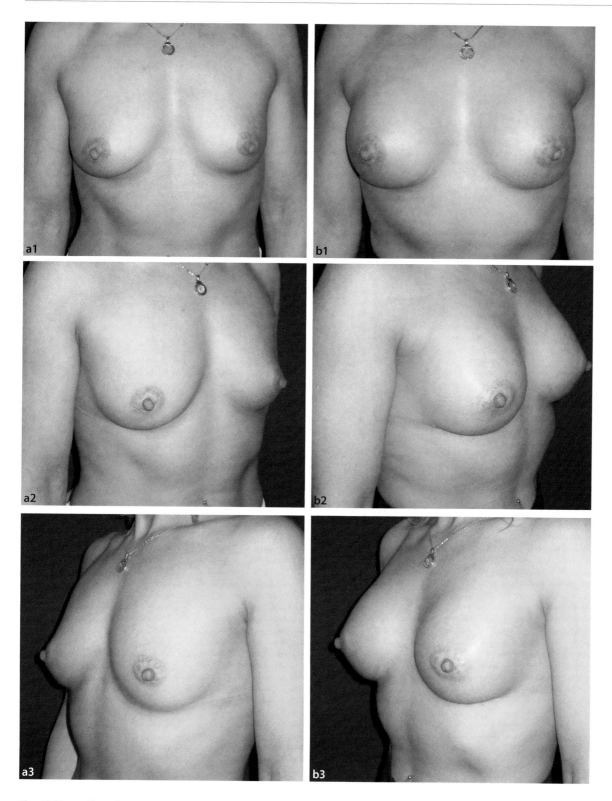

Fig. 50.12 a *1* Clinical case with breast diameters of 11 cm and tight soft tissue (R:P=1.5). *2,3* Lateral views. **b** *1* Submuscular-fascial dual-plane breast augmentation with anatomic breast implant Mentor CPG style 321 (moderate projection), volume 180 ml, width 10.5 cm, height 9.9 cm, projection 3.8 cm, implant perimeter height 13.74. *2,3* Lateral views. (Courtesy of Mentor)

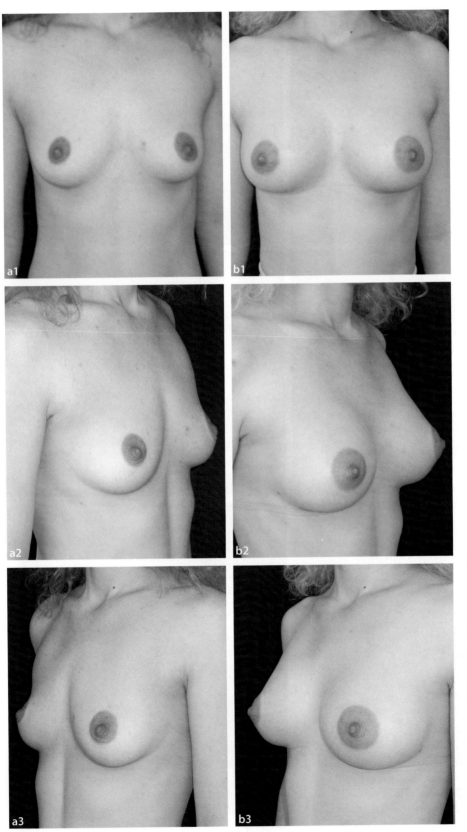

Fig. 50.13 **a** *1* Clinical case with breast diameters of 11 cm and normal soft tissue elasticity (R:P=2.5). *2,3* Lateral views. **b** *1* Submuscular-fascial breast augmentation with anatomic breast implant Mentor CPG style 322 (moderate-plus projection), volume 255 ml, width 10.5 cm, height 9.9 cm, projection 4.4 cm, implant perimeter height 14.59 cm. *2,3* Lateral views. (Courtesy of Mentor)

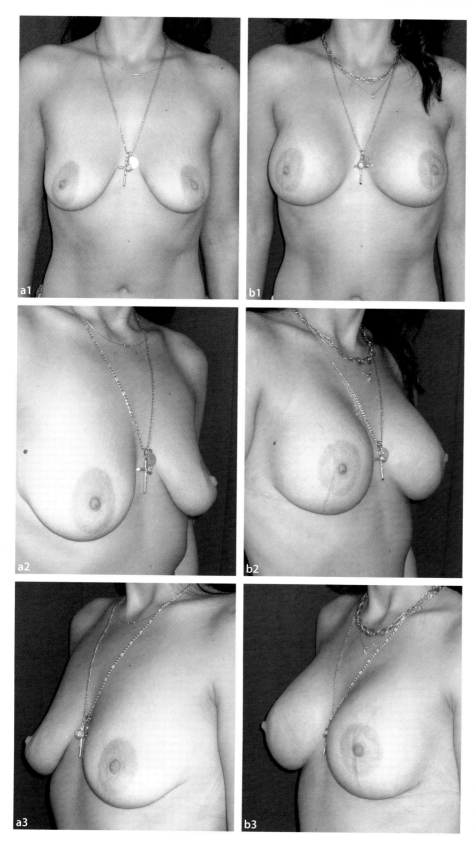

Fig. 50.14 a *1* Clinical case with breast ptosis, breast diameters of 11 cm, and loose soft tissue (R:P=3.5). *2,3* Lateral views. **b** *1* Dual-plane retromuscular-fascial breast augmentation with anatomic breast implant Mentor CPG style 323 (high projection), volume 260 ml, width 10.5 cm, height 9.9 cm, projection, 5.3 cm, implant perimeter height 15.23 cm. *2,3* Lateral views. (Courtesy of Mentor)

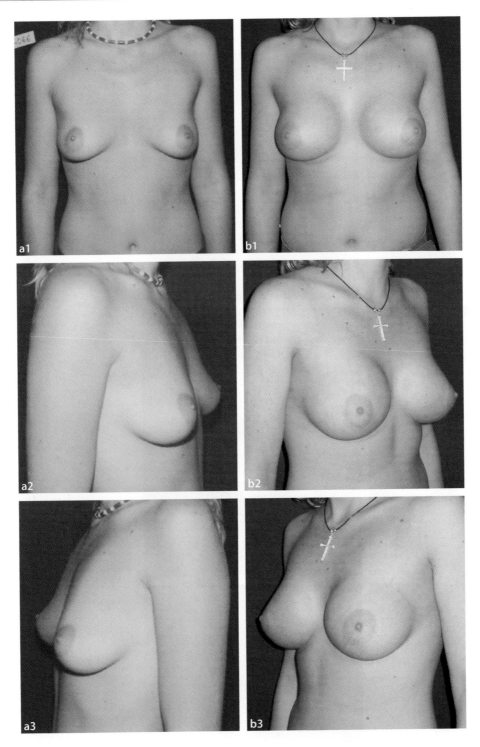

Fig. 50.15 a *1* Clinical case with normal soft tissue elasticity (R:P=2.5) but low breast vertical diameter (10 cm) and prominence of the 3rd rib in the medioclavicular line. Horizontal diameter is 11 cm. *2,3* Lateral views. **b** *1* Submuscular-fascial dual-plane breast augmentation with anatomic breast implant Mentor CPG style 312 (moderate profile, low height), volume 195 ml, width 10.5 cm, height 9.3 cm, projection 4.4 cm, implant perimeter height 13.62 cm. *2,3* Lateral views. (Courtesy of Mentor)

the 3rd ribs on the medioclavicular line . A thin patient with normal soft tissue elasticity (R:P=2.5) and small breast diameter (10 cm) is presented in Fig. 50.16. For a patient with a long chest and pectus carinatum (pigeon chest), the program selects a moderate-profile tall height (Fig. 50.17).

Compared with other techniques of dual-plane dissection, this technique has several advantages:

1. The implant benefits from the advantages of both retropectoral and retrofascial techniques; the additional coverage is provided by connective tissue of greater tension than the mammary gland, with a lower compressive effect than the muscle (leading to less deformity of the implant and maintaining the superior pole with a very natural projection).
2. It keeps the breast and pectoral fascia in their normal anatomic relation, in the lower pole of the breast.
3. It allows good redraping of the soft tissues over the lower pole of the anatomic implants.
4. The pectoral muscle sectioning at the inframammary fold level is done under direct vision.
5. The pectoral division is done with minimal bleeding, allowing good hemostasis as the muscle is held free with the forceps.
6. Even deep subcutaneous fascia overlying the pectoralis at the inframammary fold does not provide meaningful additional coverage. It can provide fold

accuracy, especially when the soft tissue thickness is thinner, and prevent implant palpation.
7. It allows a good secondary revision in certain cases with complete retropectoral position.

50.6 Conclusions

The following conclusions can be made:

1. Breast aesthetic surgery requires accurate evaluation of the patient's chest and breast.
2. All of the clinical data should be included in the patient's chart.
3. The chart and computer program give aesthetic dimensions of the breast suited to the patient's chest dimensions, weight, and height. All of the anomalies are very well documented and can be discussed with the patient, emphasizing the possible outcome of surgery.
4. The quality of the soft tissue of the breast can be assessed by the pinch (P) and relaxed (R) tests in the upper pole.
5. The selected implant must fit the pocket dimensions.
6. The new implant dimension of perimeter height should correspond to the soft tissue cover length.

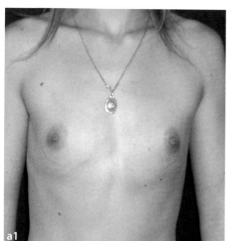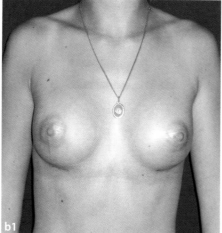

Fig. 50.16 **a** *1* Clinical case with normal soft tissue elasticity (R:P=2.5) and breast diameters of 10 cm. **b** *1* Submusculo-fascial dual-plane breast augmentation with anatomic breast implant Mentor CPG style 322 (moderate profile), volume 165 ml, width 9.5 cm, height 8.9 cm, projection 4.0 cm, implant perimeter height 12.60 cm

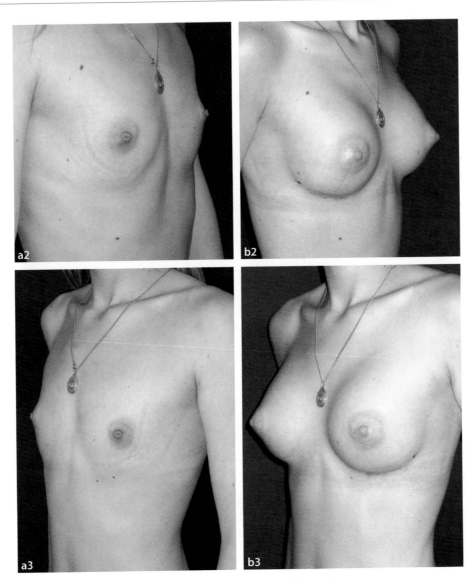

Fig. 50.16 **a** *2,3* Lateral views. **b** *2,3* Lateral views. (Courtesy of Mentor)

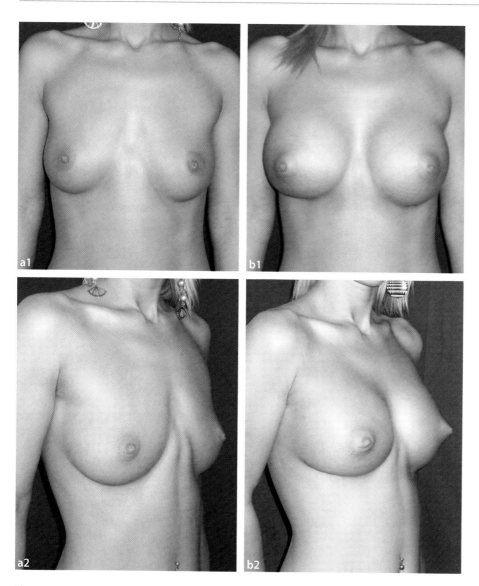

Fig. 50.17 *(continued)* **a** *1* Clinical case with pectus carinatum. Normal soft tissue elasticity (R:P=2.5) but high breast vertical diameter (12 cm) and prominence of the 3rd ribs on the medioclavicular line. Horizontal diameter is 11 cm. *2,3* Lateral views. **b** *1* Dual-plane submuscular-fascial breast augmentation with anatomical breast implant Mentor CPG style 332 (moderate profile, tall height), volume 235 ml, width 10.5 cm, height 10.9 cm, projection 44 cm, implant perimeteral height 14.97 cm. 2,3 Lateral views. (Courtesy of Mentor)

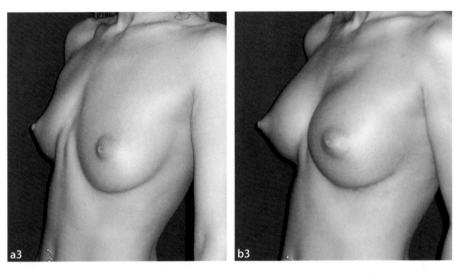

Fig. 50.17 *(continued)* **a** *2,3* Lateral views. **b** *2,3* Lateral views. (Courtesy of Mentor)

References

1. Eklund GW, Busby RC, Miller SH, Job JS: Improved imaging of the augmented breast. AJR Am J Roentgenol 1988;151(3):469–473
2. Tebbetts JB: Dual plane breast augmentation: optimizing implant-soft tissue relationships in a wide range of breast types. Plast Reconstr Surg 2001;107(5):1255–1272
3. Spear SL, Bulan EJ, Venturi ML: Breast augmentation. Plast Reconstr Surg 2004;114(5): 73E–81E
4. Hidalgo DA: Breast augmentation: choosing the optimal incision, implant, and pocket plane. Plast Reconstr Surg 2000;105(6):2202–2216
5. Tebbetts JB: A system for breast implant selection based on patient tissue characteristics and implant-soft-tissue dynamics. Plast Reconstr Surg 2002;109(4):1396–1409
6. Tebbetts JB: Achieving a predictable 24 hour return to normal activities after breast augmentation: part II. Patient preparation, refined surgical techniques and instrumentation. Plast Reconstr Surg 2002;109(1):293–305
7. Graf RM, Bernades A, Auerswald A, Damasio RCC: Subfascial endoscopic transaxillary augmentation mammaplasty. Aesthetic Plast Surg 2000;24(3):216–220
8. Graf RM, Bernardes A, Rippel R, Araujo LR, Damasio RC, Auersvald A: Subfascial breast implant: a new procedure. Plast Reconstr Surg 2003;111(2):904–908
9. Mugea TT: Subfascial breast augmentation. XIIas Jornadas Mediterraneas de Confrontations Terapeuticas en Cirurgia Cosmetica, 30 April–2 May 2004, Barcelona

Chapter 51

"Reverse" Dual-Plane Mammaplasty

51

Gianpiero Gravante, Gaetano Esposito

51.1
Introduction

Augmentation mammaplasty is nowadays the most common operation in aesthetic surgery; however, two important issues still remain unsolved. The first relates to the choice of prosthesis positioning. After long years of debate, still no definitive conclusions have been reached, so the approach should be selected according to each patient's own physical characteristics and expectations [1–3]. The second is related to prosthesis shape. Initially, manufacturers warned against the retropectoral use of teardrop prostheses because of the increased risk of displacement and shape modifications due to muscular contractions. Round prostheses reduced that risk, while retropectoral placement avoided the superior-pole fullness present with the subglandular approach. But even in this case, no definitive conclusions could be reached [4, 5]. To combine the benefits of both retroglandular and retropectoral positions, the subfascial and the dual-plane techniques were introduced [6–9]. The former is used to blunt the implant edge visibility that has been described with retroglandular implants and to avoid the shape distortion by muscular contraction that has been described for retropectoral implants. The latter consists of subglandular positioning in the inferior portion of the breast to give a more aesthetic appearance and retropectoral positioning in the superior portion to avoid superior-pole fullness. Initial results seemed encouraging [6–9].

In January 2000 the authors developed a different type of dual-plane mammaplasty with a subglandular approach and teardrop prosthesis. It is called "reverse" for the subglandular positioning in the superior part of the breast and retrofascial in the inferior part, in contrast to the standard dual-plane approach (Fig. 51.1). The technique can be used for patients with sufficient adequate breast tissue to disguise the implant, those affected by asymmetric hypoplasia, and those who do intense workout activities that could alter prosthesis shape.

51.2
Technique

51.2.1
Preoperative

The superior, inferior, medial, and lateral margins of the future pockets are measured preoperatively. Briefly, lateral sternal and anterior axillary lines are drawn and their distance measured. Normally, the authors select prostheses with a horizontal diameter 1 cm less than this distance; patients looking for greater volumes receive those that correspond perfectly. Subsequently, a horizontal line passing through both nipples is drawn with the patients' arms placed in a crossed position. Selected prostheses are placed over the breast with their vertical diameters halfway over this line. Margins of the future pocket are marked. Necessary modifications of the horizontal line and of the pocket's inferior margin are made for patients affected by asymmetric bilateral hypoplasia in order to obtain final symmetry. If the patient is taking oral anticoagulants, they are discontinued 7 days before surgery.

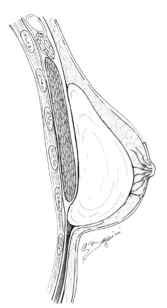

Fig. 51.1 Reverse augmentation mammaplasty: subglandular positioning in the superior part of the breast and retrofascial-precostal positioning in the inferior part

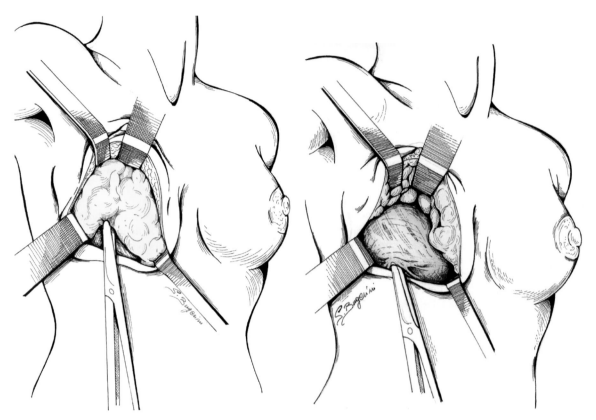

Fig. 51.2 Dissection proceeds throughout the breast tissue until the pectoral muscle sheath is reached. A pocket is then created with scissors and finger dissection, spreading devices, or a sponge on a stick

Fig. 51.3 The point at which a small incision is performed, where the inferior fibers of the major pectoral muscle gradually evolve into a thin connective tissue

51.2.2
Procedure

Pocket creation (superior, lateral, and medial borders): An inferior semicircular incision is made 2–3 mm within the external rim of the areola. Dissection proceeds throughout the breast tissue until the pectoral muscle sheath is reached. A pocket is then created with scissors and finger dissection, spreading devices, or a sponge on a stick (Fig. 51.2). Superiorly, according to preoperative markings, it reaches approximately the 3rd–4th rib. Medial dissection of the pocket is taken down until the preoperative markings, approximately corresponding to the lateral sternal border, are reached. The lateral dissection is taken approximately to the anterior axillary line according to the preoperative markings. Once the superior, medial, and lateral parts of the pocket are ready, dissection is extended to the lower border of the pectoral muscle.

Tunnel creation (inferior border of the pocket): A small incision (3 cm wide) is performed on the mid-

clavicular line where the inferior fibers of the major pectoral muscle gradually evolve into a thin connective tissue (Fig. 51.3). Through this incision, finger dissection reaches the precostal sheath (Fig. 51.4) and, without opening it, continues caudally on this plane until the inferior preoperative markings are reached (Fig. 51.5). This maneuver creates a tunnel that extends over the precostal sheath for approximately 3–4 cm beyond the inferior border of the major pectoral muscle. At this point, most of the pocket located over the pectoral muscle and the tunnel deep over the precostal sheath have been dissected. Both join together medially and laterally. The tunnel's medial border consists superiorly of the pectoral muscle insertion fibers and inferiorly of the dense connective tissue covering the precostal sheath (Fig. 51.6). Some of the muscular insertion fibers are sectioned about 2 cm for better lodging of the prosthesis (Fig. 51.7). The tunnel's lateral border consists of the dense connective tissue over the precostal sheath.

Meticulous hemostasis using electrocautery is done. Usually, dissection is performed on one side, a few

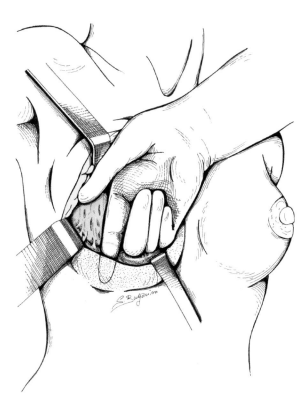

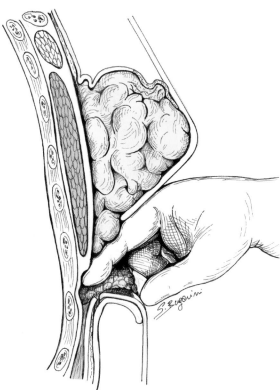

Fig. 51.4 Through this incision, finger dissection reaches the precostal sheath

Fig. 51.5 Dissection of the "tunnel" over the precostal sheath to create the lower part of the pocket

sponges are placed in the pocket, and then the other side is dissected. When returning to the first side, small bleeders are occasionally apparent and cauterized. Teardrop-shaped prostheses (McGhan style 410, Soft Touch "L" series) are then inserted. Finger dissection further extends the pocket's margin only if necessary to improve the final appearance of the breast. Usually no drains are left in place.

Incision is closed in layers (superficial fascia and subcutaneous with interrupted absorbable sutures; skin with continuous nonabsorbable subcuticular suture; Fig. 51.8). A compressive dressing is maintained for 24 h.

51.3
Postoperative Care

The authors usually prescribe postoperative antibiotics for the first 3 days after surgery and pain medications (usually ketorolac) as required by the patient. The patient is told to avoid aspirin and ibuprofen for the first 2 weeks. An elastic bra forcing the prostheses downward

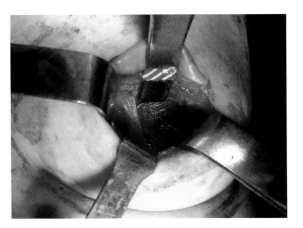

Fig. 51.6 Tunnel's medial border, consisting superiorly of the pectoral muscle insertion fibers and inferiorly of the dense connective tissue covering the precostal sheath

is required for 9 days after surgery. Although the patient could return to work in approximately 3 days, physical exercise (especially workouts) needs to be avoided for

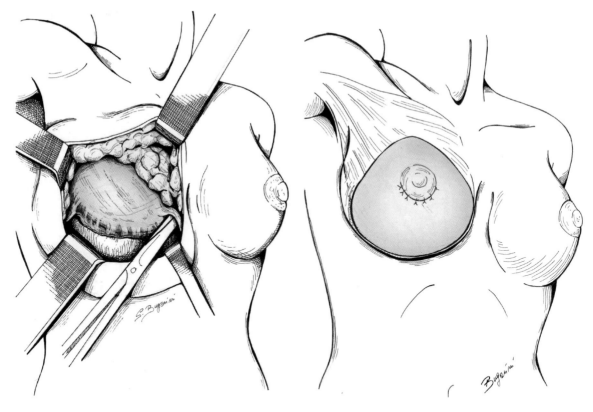

Fig. 51.7 Sectioning of a few muscular insertion fibers

Fig. 51.8 Incision is closed in layers

the first 3 weeks. Follow-up consists of outpatients visits 2 and 10 days after the operation and at 1, 3, and 12 months. The continuous subcuticular sutures are removed after 10 days.

51.4
Results

The authors have operated on 119 patients since January 2002. The primary diagnoses were moderate hypotrophy in 63 patients, hypotrophy following breastfeeding in 20 patients, tuberous breast in five patients, and different degrees of breast asymmetry in 31 patients. Mean age was 31 years (range 20–68). Mean operating time was 100 min (range 60–160). In 93% of cases, good final shapes were obtained, according to the patients' and surgeons' judgement (Figs. 51.9, 51.10). Even in cases of breast asymmetry, the technique gave good aesthetic results. No postoperative bleeding, hematoma, or seroma was recorded, nor was any displacement, asymmetry, or rupture after 1 year of follow-up. Six patients (5.2%) showed unilateral capsular contractures (Baker type III), which were resolved with capsulotomy and prosthesis removal.

51.5
Discussion

Although many approaches to prostheses placement are used worldwide, no definitive agreement exists about the perfect technique. Despite the numerous possibilities of implant positioning, there is still no single best answer that is appropriate for every patient, and each person's own physical characteristics determine the choice. For this reason, each approach must still be balanced according to the patient's characteristics and requirements.

Searching for the perfect augmentation mammaplasty technique, the authors developed the "reverse dual-plane" technique. The main characteristics of this technique are a more anatomic appearance of the final breast with no risk of prosthetic displacement. The anatomic appearance derives from three factors. First, the implant is subglandular in the superior portion behind only the tissue to be augmented. This likely yields the most natural-looking result and avoids the circular-shaped breasts that are frequently seen with retropectoral operations. Second, prostheses are of the teardrop type, more resembling breasts of Caucasian women for the horizontal, medial, and lateral development. Third,

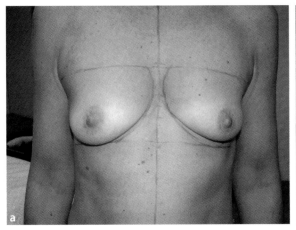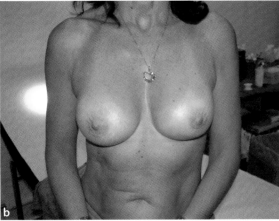

Fig. 51.9 A 35-year-old woman affected by severe hypotrophy. **a** Preoperative. **b** One year postoperative

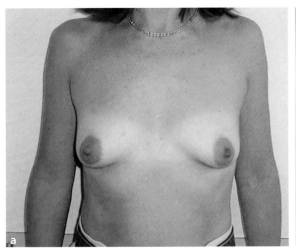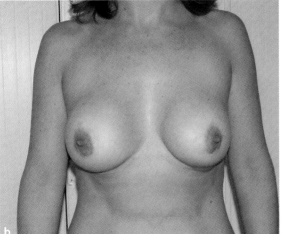

Fig. 51.10 A 28-year-old woman affected by severe hypotrophy. **a** Preoperative. **b** One year postoperative

the inferior part of the pocket (tunnel), which is specific to this technique, is subfascial and lessens tension on the overlying skin.

The absence of postoperative displacement derives from three factors. First, the tunnel (the pocket's inferior border) adds stability to the prosthesis because it creates a stable floor for implants. Second, the overlying fibers of the pectoralis muscle (medial border, partially sectioned fibers) give additional firmness, creating a sort of "natural bra" for implants. Third, teardrop prostheses, with their larger inferior horizontal cores, are less unstable than the round types.

51.6
Conclusions

Reverse dual-plane mammaplasty is a new technique of aesthetic breast augmentation and a valid alternative to classic approaches. The low risk of complications renders it a feasible and safe option for the aesthetic surgeon. In the future, such a technique also deserves experimentation for reconstructive surgery (cancer patients), in which cases the high rates of capsular contracture seen with the classic techniques often endanger the final results.

References

1. Sarwer DB, Nordmann JE, Herbert JD: Cosmetic breast augmentation surgery: a critical overview. J Womens Health Gend Based Med 2000;9(8):843–856

2. Biggs TM, Yarish RS: Augmentation mammaplasty: retropectoral versus retromammary implantation. Clin Plast Surg 1988;15(4):549–555

3. Vazquez B, Given KS, Houston GC: Breast augmentation: a review of subglandular and submuscular implantation. Aesthetic Plast Surg 1987;11(2):101–105

4. Reynaud JP, Tassin X: Past, present and... future of breast implants. Ann Chir Plast Esthet 2003;48(5):389–398

5. Young VL, Watson ME: Breast implant research: where we have been, where we are, where we need to go. Clin Plast Surg 2001;28(3):451–483

6. Graf RM, Bernardes A, Rippel R, Araujo LR, Damasio RC, Auersvald A: Subfascial breast implant: a new procedure. Plast Reconstr Surg 2003;111(2):904–908

7. Graf RM, Bernardes A, Auersvald A, Damasio RC: Subfascial endoscopic transaxillary augmentation mammaplasty. Aesthetic Plast Surg 2000;24(3):216–220

8. Tebbetts JB: Dual plane breast augmentation: optimizing implant-soft-tissue relationships in a wide range of breast types. Plast Reconstr Surg 2001;107(5):1255–1272

9. Spear SL, Carter ME, Ganz JC: The correction of capsular contracture by conversion to "dual-plane" positioning: technique and outcomes. Plast Reconstr Surg 2003;112(2):456–466

Part VI
Breast Augmentation with Autologous Tissue

CHAPTER 52

History of Breast Augmentation with Autologous Fat

Melvin A. Shiffman

52.1
Introduction

There has been some controversy about the use of autologous aspirated fat for mammary augmentation. The complaint has been that small calcifications can occur in the breast that are indistinguishable from cancer and thus may prevent the diagnosis of cancer.

52.2
Historical Contributions

Czerny (1895) [1] reported the first use of autogenous fat (a lipoma) in breast reconstruction. Lexer (1931) [2] described removal of the glandular breast in a patient with chronic cystic mastitis and reconstruction with fat rotated from the axilla. May (1941) [3] reported on a patient with bilateral breast reconstruction using a free fat autograft on one side and a free fascia-fat autograft on the opposite side.

Bames (1953) [4] used fat from the buttocks denuded of epidermis in the breast and found a 40% loss of volume because of fat liquefaction. B placing the graft with its dermal side in contact with the breast tissue and the fascial side in contact with the pectoral fascia, there was about 90% graft survival. Reversal of the placement resulted in 60% survival.

Peer (1956) [5] stated that dermal-fat grafts provide a readily available transplantation material for establishing normal contour in small breasts instead of using foreign implants.

Schorcher (1957) [6] reported autogenous free-fat transplantation to treat hypomastia. He noted that the connective tissue elements remained intact, with fat shrinkage to 25% of the original size by 6–9 months. He believed that if the graft were in several pieces, it would receive better nourishment for the recipient site.

52.3
Recent History with Liposuctioned Fat

Bircoll (1984) [7] was the first to inject autologous fat from liposuction to augment the breast. This helped avoid the complications of breast prostheses [8]. He used small droplets of fat (1 cc for each deposit), with a maximum of approximately 130 cc [9].

Bircoll and Novack (1987) [10] described the use of insulin to pretreat the fat in order to increase the survival percentage. Their report concerned one patient who had autologous fat injection into one breast to allow better symmetry with the opposite reconstructed breast (which had been removed for cancer and reconstructed with a transverse abdominal rectus flap).

Asken (1987) [11] reported the use of autologous fat obtained by liposuction to augment the hypoplastic breast. He advised the fat injection to be done on withdrawal to avoid a large amount of fat in one location. Johnson (1987) [12] reported more than 50 augmentation mammoplasties performed by macroinjection from liposuctioned fat. Krulig (1987) [13] reinjected fat into the breast area and noted more than 50% resorption.

In a panel discussion at a meeting of the American Society for Aesthetic & Plastic Surgery, Bircoll [14] reported calcifications in three patients following breast augmentation with fat. All were biopsied and showed normal fat. Ousterhout [15] felt that the audience did not agree with the procedure in light of the calcifications and stated that "to create calcifications in the breast by fat injections could cause considerable dilemma in mammogram diagnosis and possibly a missed malignancy diagnosis if each area of calcification was not biopsied."

There followed a flurry of letters in the journal *Plastic and Reconstructive Surgery*. Linder [16] stated that fat necrosis may require removing some of the breast. Calcifications may occur in areas of fat necrosis, an inflammatory reaction may produce a tumor-like mass, and "…extreme reservation should be exercised in performing this procedure in the breast." Ettelson's [17] impression was that the "preoperative and postoperative results both in the anterior and lateral views are virtually interchangeable as far as I am concerned. I am frankly shocked that the *Journal* would publish an article with such an unimpressive result." Hartrampf and Bennett [18] had the impression that the fate of nonvascularized fat in the breast is fat necrosis and that this causes thickening and hardening, which are clinically indistinguishable from carcinoma. Also, calcifications can occur in areas of fat necrosis. They stated that "injection of any material into the breast, including autogenous fat, should be condemned." Baibak [19] complained about Bircoll's report [14], saying that there was no documentation of any change in the patient's overall appearance.

Bircoll [20] responded by stating that no patient had developed hard, lumpy breasts. Calcifications in two patients had occurred within 3 months of fat transplantation, and the calcifications were in the fatty tissues surrounding the breast, which are distinguished by comparison with preoperative mammograms. Calcifications that remain stable can be observed rather than removed, and the calcifications in areas of micronecrosis are distinguishable from carcinoma.

Microcalcifications occur following breast augmentation with implants, open and closed capsulotomy, and breast reduction. As with any new technique, the problem of microcalcifications in fat augmentation of the breast should be fully evaluated and understood before the procedure is discarded. Bircoll [21, 22] reported an estimate of 1.4% microcalcifications following fat augmentation of the breast; these were periparenchymal and were not multidensity, rodlike, punctuate, or branching spicules.

Miller et al. [23] noted calcifications on mammogram in three (12.5%) of 24 patients who had undergone reduction mammoplasty. These postsurgical calcifications all had a benign appearance. Brown et al. [24] reported finding asymmetric densities on mammograms in approximately 50% of patients who underwent reduction mammoplasty. Out of 42 patients, a few developed calcifications on mammogram during the first year, and over 50% had calcifications after 2 years. The calcifications were coarse and usually occurred in the periareolar and inferior portions of the breast. Only one patient with calcifications required biopsy. These authors concluded that "knowledge of the expected mammographic alterations and their time course may help to distinguish between postoperative change and carcinoma and thus eliminate the need for biopsy in some cases."

Mitnick et al. [25] used mammography to study 152 patients who had reduction mammoplasty. The incidence of calcifications was 24.3%. The calcifications were mainly rounded and well formed with occasional lucent centers. Gradinger [26] declared that, "The use of the autologous fat injection for breast augmentation as advocated by Bircoll [in 1987] is deplored because some patients can develop calcifications and esthetic results are marginal." Grazer [27] continued to denounce the procedure when he stated that "autologous fat grafting should never be used as a breast augmentation procedure.... Calcifications have been found to be a problem in some patients, masking malignant and premalignant changes. Biopsies must be performed in patients with nodules, pain, or calcification ... the aesthetic results are marginal if large-volume augmentation is required." Pitman [28] opined that the "presence of calcifications in the breasts of injected patients makes the technique unacceptable."

The Society of Plastic and Reconstructive Surgeons (ASPRS) produced a position statement on October 1, 1992, which stated that the society "strongly condemns the use of fat injections for breast enlargement," warning that the procedure "may hamper the detection of early breast cancer or result in a false-positive cancer screening. ... Furthermore, women who seek the procedure for breast enlargement are sometimes not informed that much of the injected fat will die, causing scar tissue and calcifications ... In a worst-case scenario, a patient may face painful exploratory surgery or even mastectomy because of an uncertain mammography result."

It is this author's opinion that medicolegally it would be a breach of the standard of care to do a "mastectomy" because of an uncertain mammography result. Stereotactic needle biopsy is simple, accurate, and almost painless. "Exploratory surgery" would be virtually unnecessary in the hands of a capable and knowledgeable mammographer and surgeon.

An article appeared in *Cosmetic Surgery Times* in 1998 [29] quoting Robert W. Alexander, MD, DMD, who described satisfactory results and 60–70% fat retention from autologous fat injection for breast augmentation. There was a 3–4% incidence of small fat cysts, or spherical calcifications, that were easily differentiated mammographically from malignancy. What followed were letters objecting to the article and procedures. Lynch (president of the American Society of Plastic and Reconstructive Surgery) and Penn (president of the American Society for Aesthetic Plastic Surgery) [30] reiterated the 1992 ASPRS position statement. Gorney [31] (executive vice president of marketing services for The Doctors Company, a medical malpractice insurer) stated that "the installation of fat grafts in the breast is an extremely poor idea which will lead to highly undesirable consequences ... As any sensible surgeon knows, fat grafts to the breast are notoriously unreliable because the vast majority of the material reabsorbs within a matter of weeks to months, and what remains behind is merely the stroma of the cell, which very quickly calcifies and closely initiates the appearance of early cancer." He stated that four claims (presumably regarding breast fat injection) had been defended by The Doctors Company. One was lost, one was tried and won, and two were settled. The Doctors' Company specifically excludes fat injection to the breast from coverage. Stone [32] stated that he would not incorporate the procedure into his practice because "injecting autologous fat into the breast" will cause "at some future date mammogram abnormalities" that will "lead to unneeded biopsies," and "… my malpractice carrier specifically will not cover the procedure."

The letters regarding the article in *Cosmetic Surgery Times* were responded to by Schaeffer (editor-in-chief) [33]. She stated that the political scientist John Stuart Mills wrote, "If all mankind minus one, were of one opinion, and only one person were of the contrary opinion, mankind would be no more justified in silencing that one person, than he, if he had the power, would be justified in silencing mankind … If the opinion is right, they are deprived of the opportunity of exchanging error for truth: if wrong, they lose what is almost as great a benefit, the clearer perception and livelier impression of truth, produced by its collusion with error."

Breast augmentation with fat has been reported by a number of authors [34–45]. Da Silveira [39] reported on 31 patients with hypomastia, asymmetry, postgestational involution, and finishing touches to postmammaplasty who had breast augmentation with fat. Edema usually resolved after 3–4 weeks, and resorption of fat ended around the 3rd or 4th month. Complications included resorption, steatonecrosis, one case of calcification in a cyst wall, and one patient with microcalcifications characteristic of benign disease. Adequate donor areas are needed, and the patient may need more than one lipograft.

Fischer [40], Fournier [41, 42], Hin [43], and Fulton [44, 45] have reported success with fat transfer to augment the breast.

52.4 Discussion

Those same surgeons who denounce fat augmentation of the breast because of calcifications have performed breast augmentation with silicone gel implants, which have up to a 70% capsule contracture rate requiring surgical correction. The silicone-covered saline implants presently used have an approximately 10% incidence of contracture (smooth implants) and a 9% incidence of rippling (textured implants), most cases of which

will require surgical intervention. The fibrous capsule around the implant does develop calcifications, which are readily distinguishable from malignant calcification both by position and character. Breast reduction surgery is still performed with a small but significant incidence of stippled calcifications from fat necrosis "within the breast parenchyma." Despite their appearance some months after surgery, these may need to have stereotactic biopsy because they are within the breast. However, this does not contraindicate breast reduction by any surgeon's standard.

Patients who desire fullness of the breasts, not large breasts, are satisfied with the procedure. To some physician observers, this may appear to be "unimpressive," but they fail to realize that it is the patient who determines whether the surgery is adequate. Many patients fear the problems of implants, such as scars, asymmetry, postoperative pain, deflation, capsule contracture, rippling, decreased mammography sensitivity, the possible need for repeat surgery, and "possible" autoimmune disease.

Fat injection into the breast results in very little discomfort. Lumps that appear are the result of oil cysts from too much fat injected into one area. Calcifications, which may occur months after the injections, can be sampled, if the physician and patient desire, by the simple expedient of stereotactic core needle biopsy. Open biopsy is unnecessary if the core shows benign tissue. These calcifications can then be followed by yearly mammograms, just as is done with other surgeries causing microcalcifications. Properly trained and experienced mammographers should be able to distinguish benign from malignant calcifications in the breast.

The most important fact is that since 1989, most surgeons performing augmentation of the breast with fat are placing the fat outside the breast parenchyma. Up to 300 cc of fat, equally divided, is placed into three areas: the subpectoral space, intrapectoral muscle, and the submammary space. The arguments concerning alteration of the breast parenchyma are now moot except for accidental placement of fat into the breast itself.

It has been reported [46] that use of the nonsurgical Brava breast suction system (see Chap. 56) can increase space and vascularization in order to increase the survival of fat transferred to the breast for augmentation.

In reference to the article by Spear et al. [47] regarding fat injection to correct contour deformities in the reconstructed breast, it is refreshing to see a positive account of fat transfer to the breast area without the controversy that has given fat augmentation of the breast an undeserved bad name. More recently, Coleman and Saboeiro [48] retrospectively studied their patients who had fat transfer to the breast area and found no problems in diagnosing breast cancer.

References

1. Czerny A: Plastischer Ersatz der Brustdrüse durch ein Lipoma. Chir Kongr Verhandl 1895; 2:216

2. Lexer E: Die Gesamte Wiederherstellungs-Chirurgie. Leipzig, Barth 1931

3. May H: Transplantation and regeneration of tissue. Pennsylvania Med J 1941; 45:130

4. Bames HO: Augmentation mammoplasty by lipo-transplant. Plast Reconstr Surg 1953;11:404–412

5. Peer LA: The neglected free fat graft. Plast Reconstr Surg 1956;18(4):233–250

6. Schorcher F: Fettgewebsverpflanzung bei zu kleiner Brust. München Med Wochenschr 1957;99(14):489

7. Bircoll MJ: New frontiers in suction lipoectomy. Second Asian Congress of Plastic Surgery 1984;80(4):647

8. Bircoll M: Autologous fat tissue augmentation. Amer J Cosmet Surg 1987;4(2):141–149

9. Bircoll M: Cosmetic breast augmentation utilizing autologous fat and liposuction techniques. Plast Reconstr Surg 1987;79(2);267–271

10. Bircoll M, Novack BH: Autologous fat transplantation employing liposuction techniques. Ann Plast Surg 1987;18(4);327–329

11. Asken S: Autologous fat transplantation: Micro and macro techniques. Amer J Cosmet Surg 1987;4(2):111–120

12. Johnson GW: Body contouring by macroinjection of autogenous fat. Amer J Cosmet Surg 1987;4(2):103–109

13. Krulig E: Lipo-injection. Amer J Cosmet Surg 1987; 4(2): 123–129

14. Bircoll M: Panel on fat injection. American Society for Aesthetic Plastic Surgery, Los Angeles, 26 March 1987

15. Ousterhout DK: Breast augmentation by autologous fat injection (letter). Plast Reconstr Surg 1987;80(6):868

16. Linder RM: Fat autografting (letter). Plast Reconstr Surg 1987;80(4):646–647

17. Ettelson CD: Fat autografting (letter). Plast Reconstr Surg 1987;80(4):646

18. Hartrampf CR, Jr, Bennett GK: Autologous fat from liposuction for breast augmentation (letter). Plast Reconstr Surg 1987;80(4):646

19. Baibak GJ: Liposuction. Plast Reconstr Surg 1987;80:647

20. Bircoll M: Reply (letter). Plast Reconstr Surg 1987;80(4):647

21. Bircoll M: Autologous fat transplantation to the breast (letter). Plast Reconstr Surg 1988;82:361–362

22. Bircoll M: Autologous fat transplantation: an evaluation of microcalcification and fat cell survivability following (AFT) cosmetic breast augmentation. Amer J Cosmet Surg 1988;5(4):283–288

23. Miller CL, Ferg SA, Fox JW IV: Mammographic changes after reduction mammoplasty. Amer J Roentgenol 1987;149:35–38

24. Brown FE, Sargent SK, Cohen SR, Morain WD: Mammographic changes following reduction mammoplasty. Plast Recontr Surg 1987;80:691–698

25. Mitnick JS, Roses DF, Harris MN, Colen SR: Calcification of the breast after reduction mammoplasty. Surg Gynecol Obstet 1990;171:409–412

26. Gradinger GP: Breast augmentation by autologous fat injection (letter). Plast Reconstr Surg 1987;80(6):868–869

27. Grazer FM: Special reconstruction and therapeutic procedures. In: Grazer FM (ed). Atlas of Suction Assisted Lipectomy in Body Contouring. New York, Churchill Livingstone 1992, pp 319–329

28. Pitman GH: Odds and ends: lipomas, flap debulking, lymphedema, fat reinjection, and additional complications. In: Pitman GH (ed). Liposuction & Aesthetic Surgery. St. Louis, Quality Medical Publishing 1993

29. Moyer P: Breast augmentation—results are "satisfying" using autologous fat as filler. Cosmetic Surgery Times 1998;2(4):4

30. Lynch DJ, Penn JG: Fat injection to breast compromises safety. ASPRS and ASAPS do not recommend procedure. Cosmetic Surgery Times 1998;2(6):3

31. Gorney M: Fat injection to breast compromises safety. Commenting on calcifications. Cosmetic Surgery Times 1998:2(6):3

32. Stone A: Fat injection to breast compromises safety. Questioning the procedure. Cosmetic Surg Times 1998;2(6):3

33. Schaeffer I: Fat injection to breast compromises safety. Editorial response. Cosmetic Surg Times 1998;2(6):3

34. Illouz Y-G: Fat injection: a four year clinical trial. In: Hetter GP (ed). Lipoplasty: The Theory and Practice of Blunt Suction Lipectomy, 2nd edn. Boston, Little, Brown 1990, pp 239–246

35. Skouge J: Autologous fat transplantation in facial surgery. In: Coleman WP III, Hanke CW, Alt TH, Asken S (eds). Cosmetic Surgery of the Skin: Principles and Techniques. Philadelphia, BC Decker 1991, pp 239–249

36. Yoho RA, Brandy-Yoho J: Fat transplantation. In: Yoho RA, Brandy-Yoho J (eds). A New Body in One Day: A Guide to Local Anesthetic Cosmetic Surgery Procedures. Studio City, CA, First House Press 1999, pp 79–87

37. Fulton JE: Breast contouring by autologous fat transfer. Am J Cosmet Surg 1992;9(3):273–279

38. da Silveira JW: Autologous lipograft for augmentation mammoplasty. A new treatment of breast hypoplasia. Rev da Soc Beras Plast Est Reconstr 1993;8(1, 2, 3):12–19

39. da Silveira JW: Breast augmentation with autologous lipograft. Am J Cosmet Surg 1998;15(2):109–115

40. Fischer G: Autologous fat implantation for breast augmentation. Workshop on liposuction and autologous fat reimplant. Isola d'Elba, September 1986

41. Fournier PF: Breast augmentation with fat transfer. In: Fournier P (ed). Body Sculpting. Solana Beach, CA, Samuel Rolf International 1987, pp 65–70

42. Fournier PF: The breast fill. In: Fournier PF (ed). Liposculpture: The Syringe Technique. Paris, Arnette 1991, pp 357–367

43. Hin LC: Syringe liposuction with immediate lipotransplantation. Am J Cosmet Surg 1988;5(4):243–248

44. Fulton JE: Stabilization of fat transfer to the breast with autologous platelet gel. Int J Cosmet Surg 1999;7(1):60–65

45. Fulton JE: Stabilization of fat transfer to the breast with autologous platelet gel. In: Shiffman MA (ed). Autologous Fat Transplantation. New York, Marcel Dekker 2001, pp 207–218

46. Schwanke J: New reasons to consider breast augmentation using autologous fat. Cosmet Surg Times 2006;9(6):29–29

47. Spear SL, Wilson HB, Lockwood MD: Fat injection to correct contour deformities in the reconstructed breast. Plast Reconstr Surg 2005;116(5):1300–1305

48. Coleman SR, Saboeiro AP: Fat grafting to the breast revisited: safety and efficacy. Plast Reconstr Surg 2007;119(3):775–785

CHAPTER 53

Breast Augmentation with Autologous Fat

53

Tetsuo Shu

53.1
Introduction

Liposuction was introduction in 1975 by Fisher [1]. The fat retrieved from liposuction ultimately began to be used to augment tissues. Since the introduction of tumescent liposuction by Klein in 1987 [2], there has been less blood loss in liposuction, and more fat can be retrieved.

The author has been performing breast augmentation with autologous fat for over 20 years. In 1989 the author stopped injecting the fat into the breast but rather into the surrounding tissues, with great success.

53.2
Technique

Intravenous sedation or general anesthesia is used in all patients.

The fat retrieved by liposuction should be washed with normal saline and squeezed in cheesecloth to wash out the blood and broken fat cells (Fig. 53.1). Fat should be injected as pure fat without contaminants (Fig. 53.2). The amount of fat injected into each breast depends on the original size of the breast. If the breast is large and ptotic, up to 300 ml of fat is injected into each breast.

The fat is injected while withdrawing the 3-mm cannula in linear fashion to prevent pooling of the fat, which may result in cyst formation and necrosis with calcifications. The fat is injected in one plane through radiating tunnels. The layers of injection are the submuscular, muscular, subglandular, and subcutaneous planes. The fat areas are then massaged to help distribute the fat evenly; massage prevents cyst formation.

53.3
Case Reports

Case 1 (Fig. 53.3): This patient had hypoplastic breasts. Multiple fat transfers to augment the breasts were performed over a period of 4 years. Fat was taken from multiple sites in the body and transferred to both breasts in four sessions (Tables 53.1, 53.2). The breasts were enlarged slowly over a period of time until the patient was satisfied.

Case 2 (Fig. 53.4): This patient had right breast lumpectomy for cancer. Fat was retrieved from multiple areas, and there were four sessions of fat transfer to the right breast performed over a 4.5-year period (Table 53.3). The fat filled the breast so that the breasts were almost equal.

Case 3 (Fig. 53.5): This patient had breast implant removal from prior augmentation. After three sessions over 3 years, fat was taken from multiple areas and transferred to both breasts (Table 53.4). The result was very full, normal-appearing breasts.

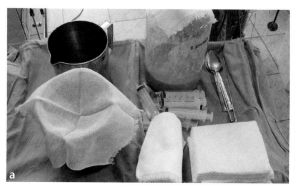
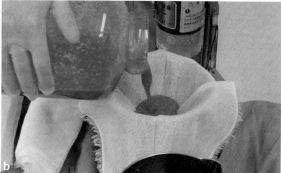

Fig. 53.1 Preparation of aspirated fat. **a** Equipment for fat transfer to augment the breasts. **b** Aspirated fat poured into cheesecloth

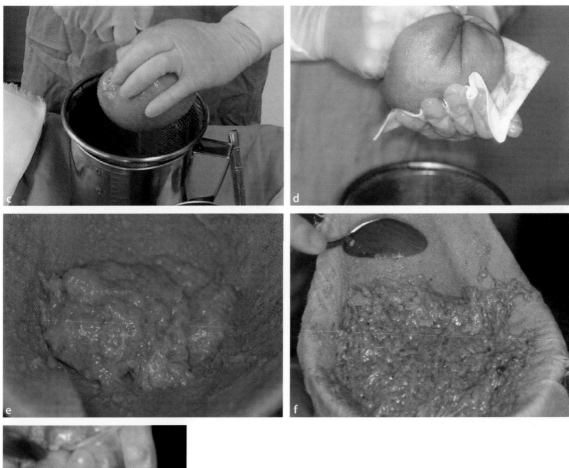

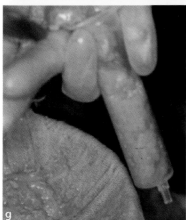

Fig. 53.1 *(continued)* Preparation of aspirated fat. **c** Cheesecloth wrapped around fat and squeezed to remove excess liquid. **d** Excess fluid cleaned from around cheesecloth. **e** Fat is now very thick. **f** Fat removed with a spoon. **g** Fat inserted into syringe

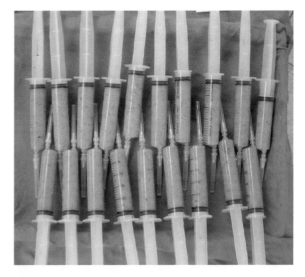

Fig. 53.2 Clean fat in syringes ready for insertion

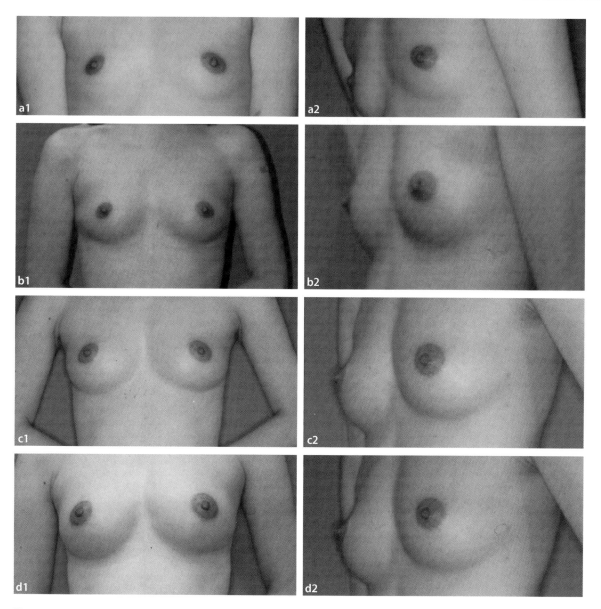

Fig. 53.3 a *1,2* Preoperative. **b** *1,2* One year postoperative after first fat transfer and before second fat transfer. **c** *1,2* Three years postoperative after second fat transfer and before the third fat transfer. **d** *1,2* Four years postoperative after third fat transfer and before fourth fat transfer

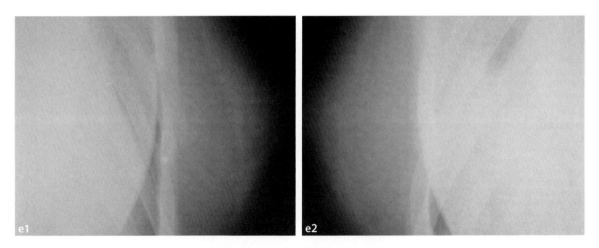

Fig. 53.3 *(continued)* **e** *1,2* Postoperative mammograms showing darkened areas of fat transfer posterior to the breast gland, with no calcifications

Table 53.1 Case 1: Breast augmentation with fat. Sites of fat retrieval and amounts injected into breasts in four sessions

		Right	Left	Liposuction
1st injection	17 Mar. 1992	140 ml	100 ml	Abdomen: 450, hip: 800
2nd injection	29 Mar. 1994	180 ml	120 ml	Thighs: 1,400
3rd injection	14 Sept. 1995	50 ml	50 ml	Back, waist: 500
4th injection	1 Mar. 1996	54 ml	54 ml	Legs: 330

Table 53.2 Case 1 measurements before fat transfer and after each fat transfer

	Height (cm)	Weight (kg)	Breast, top (cm)	Breast, under (cm)	Abdomen (cm)	Abdomen, waist (cm)	Hips (cm)
Before	160	46.5	75.0	67.0	76.1	67.5	88.5
Before 2nd surg.	160	47.0	81.4	67.5	73.0	67.0	83.0
Before 3rd surg.	160	47.0	79.3	68.0			
Before 4th surg.	160	47.5	79.2	66.6			

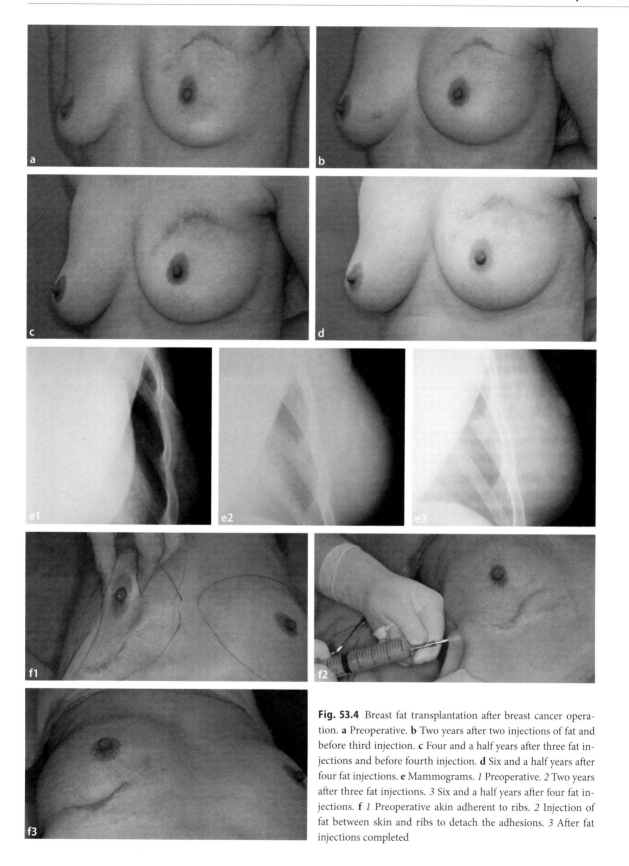

Fig. 53.4 Breast fat transplantation after breast cancer operation. **a** Preoperative. **b** Two years after two injections of fat and before third injection. **c** Four and a half years after three fat injections and before fourth injection. **d** Six and a half years after four fat injections. **e** Mammograms. *1* Preoperative. *2* Two years after three fat injections. *3* Six and a half years after four fat injections. **f** *1* Preoperative akin adherent to ribs. *2* Injection of fat between skin and ribs to detach the adhesions. *3* After fat injections completed

Table 53.3 Case 2: Right breast augmentation with fat following left breast lumpectomy for cancer. Sites of fat retrieval and amounts injected into breasts in four sessions

		Right	Left	Liposuction
1st injection	8 Oct. 1997	122 ml	187 ml	Hips, waist
2nd injection	16 Jan. 1998	175 ml	233 ml	Thighs
3rd injection	17 May 1999	75 ml	200 ml	Abdomen
4th injection	19 Mar. 2002	50 ml	75 ml	Arms, back

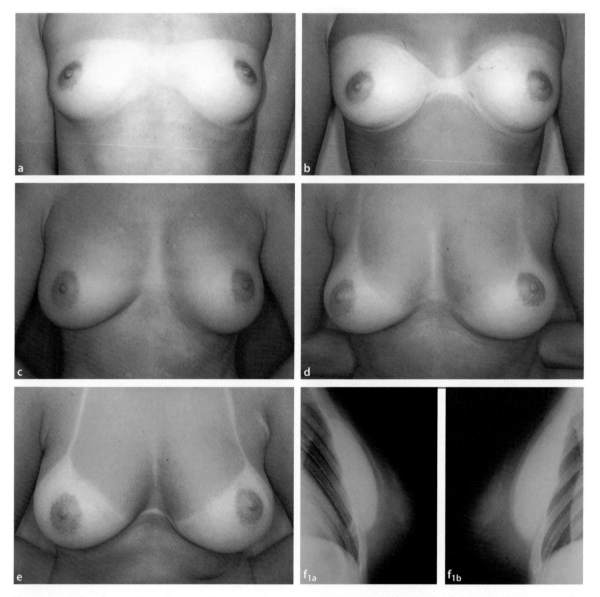

Fig. 53.5 a Before fat transfer with 115-ml breast prostheses. **b** One month postoperative. **c** Six years after three fat injections. **d** Removal of breast prostheses 5 years after fat transfers had begun. **e** Ten and a half years after fat transfers. **f** Mammography. *1a,b* Five years after three fat transfers. *2a,b* Nine years after fat transfers and removal of breast prostheses

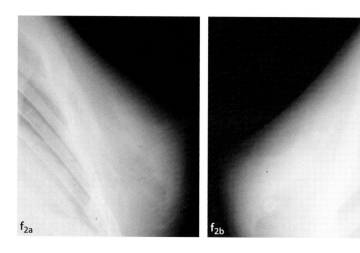

f_{2a}   f_{2b}

Fig. 53.5 *(continued)* **f** Mammography. *1a,b* Five years after three fat transfers. *2a,b* Nine years after fat transfers and removal of breast prostheses

Table 53.4 Case 3: Breast augmentation with fat transfer and then removal of breast augmentation prostheses. Sites of fat retrieval and amounts injected into breasts in three sessions over 3 years

		Right	Left	Liposuction
1st injection	5 Apr. 1991	55 ml	55 ml	Abdomen, silicone bag 150 ml
2nd injection	29 Apr. 1993	180 ml	160 ml	Thighs, legs
3rd injection	2 Aug. 1994	145 ml	112 ml	Abdomen, hips, waist
	3 Apr. 1996			Removal of silicone bag

53.4 Discussion

Fat transfer to the breast is relatively easy. Before transfer, the fat should be washed thoroughly to remove blood products. Injection of fat should be through tunnels at various levels outside the breast gland. Care should be taken that the fat is not injected into pools, and the fat should be massaged after injection so that it will not necrose and calcify.

The results of fat augmentation of the breast have been excellent, with minimal complications.

References

1. Fischer G: Surgical treatment of cellulitis. Third International Congress of International Academy of Cosmetic Surgery, Rome, 31 May 1975
2. Klein JA: The tumescent technique for liposuction surgery. Am J Cosm Surg 1987;4:263–267

CHAPTER 54

Fat Transfer with Platelet-Rich Plasma for Breast Augmentation

54

Robert W. Alexander

54.1
Introduction

It is generally acknowledged that tissue augmentation with autologous elements is considered the ideal choice for transplantation and volume augmentation surgery. As is well recognized, the ideal graft tissue should offer the standard features of ready availability, low antigenicity, minimal donor site morbidity, predictable and reproducible retention, and avoidance of disease transmission.

Autologous fat grafting meets all of these fundamental criteria, and therefore represents a very appealing resource for soft tissue volume augmentation. It is well established that autologous tissue grafts survive the harvest and transfer procedures to a healthy recipient site by the principles of induction and conduction [1–7]. Autologous fat grafting has rapidly become a very important treatment modality over the past 15 years. Fat tissue survival, although well documented, has often been reported as somewhat unpredictable in its effectiveness or longevity. It was not until the early 1990s that many surgeons recognized the actual mechanism of liposuction surgery and harvest. Since the advent of low-pressure, closed-syringe-system harvest and super-smooth harvest and transfer cannulas, fat grafting (large and small volumes) has become one of the most frequently used therapies in face and body contouring procedures [8–13].

Gradual standardization of consistent harvesting, manipulation, and transfer protocols is improving the ability to accurately predict volume enhancements and appreciate the long-term survival of the grafted tissues [14]. Many opinions expressed in the surgical community regarding the efficacy of autologous fat grafting seem in conflict with our experiences with regard to the amount of graft retained and long-term success [1, 4, 5, 8, 15, 16]. Most of the claims of high-resorption rates (40–60%) do not account for the fluid volumes needed to transport the harvest and transfer tissues. For example, if the harvested and transferred graft materials are comprised of 30% fluid and 60% cellular elements, the observed reduction in mass volume seen in the first few weeks most likely represents the gradual extraction of the carrier fluids, not failure of survival of the graft's cellular element. In-vitro studies demonstrate very high survival rates in tissue culture. It appears that survival following low-pressure suction harvest is in the high 90th percentile for intact cells observed [4, 5, 11, 13, 17, 18].

Many factors appear to exert substantial influence on the success of autologous fat transplantation. Some of these include the patient's systemic health, genetic predisposition for cellular fat storage from the preferred donor sites (so-called primary fat deposit locations), pre-graft and postgraft nutrition, basal metabolic rate, use of minimally traumatic harvest and handling techniques, proper preparation of the recipient bed, and relatively early graft immobilization in the recipient sites during the initial graft acceptance and healing cascade [9].

The value of additives to autologous fat grafts is becoming much better documented and understood. With the ability to favorably influence the body's wound-healing efforts through the use of such additives, recognition of the value, safety, and predictability in autologous fat grafts has greatly increased [1, 10].

In addition, perhaps one of the most important advances in the use of adult lipocytes and stimulating mesenchymal stem cell component as fillers has been the use of platelet-derived factors added to the harvested graft materials [1].

Platelets are living but terminal cytoplasmic portions of marrow megakaryocytes. They have no nucleus for replication and typically last for 5–9 days in vivo. For many years their role was considered only to contribute to the hemostatic process, in which they become tacky and adhere together to form a plug. They are now understood to extrude important initiators of the coagulation cascade. In more recent research, it is now known that they also actively extrude multiple growth factors that are very important to early wound-healing processes.

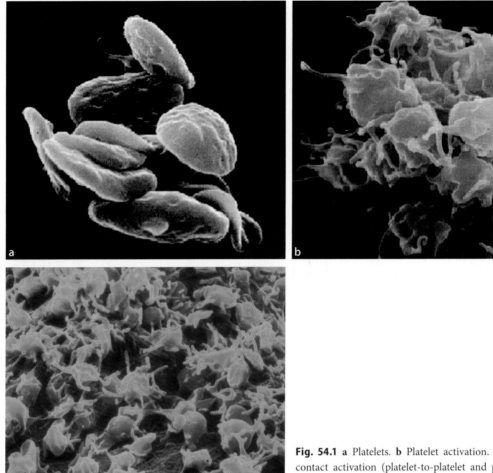

Fig. 54.1 a Platelets. **b** Platelet activation. Receptor site and contact activation (platelet-to-platelet and platelet-to-fibrous-matrix) to initiate growth factor release and healing-cascade mechanisms. **c** Activated platelets

In response to platelet-to-platelet or platelet-to-connective-tissue contact, the platelet cell membrane is "activated" (Fig. 54.1) to release these products from the alpha granules via active extrusion. When these extruded growth factors are released, histones and carbohydrate chains are added to receptor sites, thereby creating their unique chemistries and making the "active" growth factors. It is important to have this basic appreciation of the contribution that platelet-derived products make in wound healing and to extrapolate this to autologous fat graft acceptance.

Since the advent of a very convenient harvest and preparation system (Harvest Technology) to isolate platelet-rich plasma (PRP), the ability to use PRP (also known as autologous platelet concentrate, or APC) has become a reality in the outpatient surgical and hospital settings [10].

As is scientifically clearly appreciated, wound healing is initiated in a relatively complex environment, typically started and maintained from elements specifically derived from platelets. Besides initiating coagulation processes, platelets undergo a degranulation process that releases a complex group of growth factors and cytokines (peptides) essential for wound-healing mechanisms. The platelet-derived growth factors (PDGF) are characterized as regulatory peptides that have specific tissue site receptors [19–22]. These serve to regulate and deregulate cellular activity, enzymes, angiogenic factors, antiangiogenic factors, induction agents for gene expression, and much more [21, 23–25]. Initial studies demonstrating the powerful expression of PDGF have been reported for bone healing (also from a mesenchymally derived stem cell set) [3]. It is now considered that use of the platelet-derived factors in autologous fat transplantation and wound healing are equally important.

It is beyond the scope of this chapter to provide a complete explanation of the biology of wound healing, but it is important to express the potential enhancement of known pathways to improve and enhance the survivability of grafted cells for long-term volume success. It is also important to have a basic understanding of the scientific relevance of the use of PRP in autologous fat-grafting techniques [26–29]. The potential of enhanced viability and clinical success in using transplanted fat in both small-volume and large-volume applications explains the importance of such a combination to promote natural wound-healing mechanisms. Introducing such concentrated growth factors during the preparation and transfer phases may greatly potentiate wound healing through normal physiologic mechanisms that control cellular recruitment, migration, and differentiation within the recipient sites. In addition, such additives contribute to the induction and conduction aspects of both the donor's and recipient's undifferentiated mesenchymal stem cell population and, thereby, may significantly contribute to the overall graft success. The author's experience suggests that the use of PRP and calcium chloride with or without thrombin increases the long-term retention of the transplanted fat cells and increases the rate of revascularization and survival of the transplanted cells [10]. This enhancement of the healing rate and graft acceptance is thought to decrease the potential for liponecrosis, lipid cyst formation, and incidence of spherical microcalcifications within the breast tissues [1].

54.2
General Biology of Wound and Graft Healing with PRP

The clinical value of PRP as a promoter of wound healing is very well documented [22, 25–30]. PRP is rich in both PDGF and transforming growth factor beta 1 (TGF-B1), which are derived directly from degranulating platelets and which contain the highest concentrations of those elements. These growth factors are recognized as key elements in initiation and subsequent progression of the wound-healing cascade. The addition of PDGF has been shown to stimulate actual repair of the damaged cytoplasmic membrane, to permit a return to metabolic activity in the in-vitro cultured lipocytes, and to synergistically promote the healing of wounds by the ability of PDGF to restore plasma function [22, 25; M. Lyles, personal communication, 2006]. It is also well established that the key cytokines derived from the platelet degranulation processes are intrinsically involved in maintaining the actual healing process. The cytokines most implicated in this wound-healing process are listed in Table 54.1.

Both PDGF and TGF-B1 are concentrated in the alpha granule of the platelet and are released with platelet cellular activation and degranulation. Each has shown a marked beneficial effect on wound healing [10, 31]. Initial extrusion of such factors leads to complete growth factors via the process of extrusion of the growth factors, which meet with histones and carbohydrate side chains in a wound site to result in "active" growth factors. As an example of activation, PDGF has a direct mitogenic influence on the target cells by binding to specific cell surface receptors and indirectly enhancing the proliferative response even in cells lacking detectable PDGF receptors [22, 27]. Platelets are the richest known source of PDGF, although PDGF have also been identified within macrophages, fibroblasts, and some endothelial cells [30]. Likewise, TGF-B1 concentrates are primarily released from the alpha granule but have also been isolated in macrophages. TGF-B1 is also chemotactic

Table 54.1 Some of the most common platelet-derived cytokines implicated in wound healing

Cytokine	Abbreviation
Platelet-derived growth factor -AA, -BB, -AB	PDGF
Transforming growth factor -B1, -B2	TGF-B1, TGF-B2
Platelet-derived epidermal growth factor	PDEGF
Platelet-derived angiogenesis factor	PDAF
Platelet factor 4	PF-4
P-selectin	GMP-140
Interleukin 1	IL-1
Fibroblast growth factor	FGF
Interferons: alpha, gamma	I-A, I,G
Insulin-like growth factor	IGF

for recruitment of macrophages and fibroblasts and is a potent stimulator of granulation tissue formation. Working synergistically, PDGF initially acts as an attractant for monocytes, macrophages, or both, and then becomes an activator to begin production and secretion of additional PDGF into the wound area. This is known as an autocrine amplification system and is important in sustaining the wound-healing processes [1, 22].

In autologous fat cell transfer, placement of harvested cells into a created potential space (pretunneling) permits recipient-site cellular contact with graft cells. This tunneling and placement also produces some degree of platelet-containing blood to be released in the field from native sources. The addition of highly concentrated PRP then enhances the activity of these processes and offers important acceleration of the early inflammatory activities. This complements the native (recipient) site processes that began with mild injury.

In graft situations, the initial wound oxygen concentration is decreased, resulting in relatively hypoxic conditions (partial pressure of oxygen 5–10 mmHg) and acidosis (pH 4–6) within the graft itself. This area is surrounded by recipient tissues that are normal (partial pressure of oxygen 45–55 mmHg) and have a physiologic pH (7.42). With placement of PRP with the graft materials, the lipocyte activity, mesenchymal stem cell element (in both donor and recipient tissues), interstitial collagen, and fibroblasts are more rapidly activated to respond. The recipient site provides the needed circulation and the cellular element access for structural cells, healing-capable cells, and intact capillaries. It is in this junctional area that small capillaries develop terminal clots and offer exposed endothelial cells for revascularization. It has been suggested that this may explain why small aliquots of graft placed in prepared tunnels to provide surrounding native fat cells and stroma contribute to enhanced graft survival and success.

The establishment of oxygen tension potential between the graft and the surrounding recipient bed tissues is capable of inducing macrophage recruitment and promoting angiogenesis by secreting macrophage-derived angiogenesis factor and macrophage-derived growth factor [32–34]. The angiogenic effect of macrophages is selectively induced by mild hypoxia and may be potentiated by hyperbaric oxygen therapy. In the presence of normal oxygen tension, the number of fibroblasts, the amount of collagen deposit, and the number of capillaries can be increased by increasing the number of macrophages present. Therefore, it can be concluded that the healing potential of a wound is influenced not only by the presence or absence of chemotactic agents but also by the number of competent cells. Working synergistically, the recipient site conditions

plus the concentrated factors derived from PRP serve to enhance the healing environment.

This very complex environment, simplified for the sake of this discussion, represents the basic model of wound healing in any tissue injury. The endogenous system of repair starts, maintains, and promotes repair related to the needs of the injury and offers an opportunity for surgeons to encourage enhanced tissue regeneration and graft tissue acceptance.

The use of concentrated platelet gels, "activated" in PRP by the addition of calcium chloride and thrombin, appears to offer a unique biologic sealant and graft carrier (gel) to the recipient sites. This combination has been used extensively in a variety of disciplines, with remarkable clinical success [1, 5–7, 16, 21, 26, 27, 35]. In the activated PRP (PRP+) graft, the gel matrix may provide some helpful early graft immobilization, known to be contributory to a variety of autologous grafts.

54.3
Autologous Fat Graft Healing Model

Some early investigators suggested that some or all transplanted mature adipocytes might de-differentiate into a precursor phenotype, or might maintain characteristics of donor-site adipose tissue. Work by Jones et al. clearly demonstrated in vitro that low-pressure, syringe-harvested fat did not regress but did become metabolically active to begin to store lipid within the cells [31].

In addition, considering the fact that autologous fat grafts do best where existing adipose tissues exist, it is considered very likely that additional induction stimuli within the recipient and/or donor cell populations do exist. This promotes differentiation of precursor elements into new adipocytes, making additional graft cellular tissues within the recipient bed [36–39].

Later studies that involved placing PRP into the cell culture further demonstrated actual repair of damaged cytoplasmic membranes to an intact, metabolically active state. In addition, it appeared that some induction of pluripotential cells into mature adipocytes was stimulated and that liponeogenesis was initiated in a three-dimensional tissue culture matrix [M. Lyles, personal communication, 2006].

In the autologous fat graft, it is convenient to characterize three stages of graft acceptance. During the first stage, cellular differentiation and activation of preadipocytes begin with release of PDGF and TGF-B1 during degranulation of platelets. PDGF is believed to stimulate both mitogenesis and differentiation of the preadipocyte. Simultaneously, angiogenesis is stimulated, resulting in capillary budding and ingrowth via induction of endothelial cell mitosis. This initial stage of graft healing is measured in hours and days, with high activity persisting for up to 1 week. The second stage, typified by fibroblast activation, usually lasts for up to 2 weeks. It is suggested that the TGF-B1 is responsible for initial fibroblastic activation, resulting in increased numbers of fibroblasts, and stimulates additional differentiation of precursor adipocyte cells. The prolonged presence of TGF-B1 further acts to stimulate adipocyte lipogenesis, while fibroblasts begin to synthesize procollagen type 1 in preparation for deposit of the collagen matrix to support the capillary ingrowth activities. The activated fibroblasts begin synthesis of fibronectin and hyaluronic acid, which are known essential elements of the new extracellular matrix. The third stage represents the beginning of wound maturation and typically remains active for up to 1 year. During this time, the TGF-B1 continues to be active, encouraging additional fibroblast activity. PDGF activates the secretion of certain enzymes (e.g., collagenase) to assist in collagen remodeling and wound maturation. The action of these growth factors is clearly synergistic in promotion of acceptance of autologous fat grafts [22]. PDGF participates in development of the autocrine amplification system. This feedback system both initiates and maintains healing and integration of the newly transplanted and differentiated cells by capillary ingrowth and collagen remodeling within the recipient bed.

54.4
Technique

54.4.1
Isolation of Platelet-Rich Plasma

Early experiences with isolation techniques for PRP were difficult due to the equipment size, cost, and need for a perfusionist, making its use inconvenient and expensive and requiring a substantially larger blood-volume draw than the current system [1].

Since the development of simple, precise equipment in a complete kit format, the costs of isolation and ease of use have greatly improved [10]. It is now practical to have the isolation capability within an ambulatory surgical center, hospital setting, or a practice's surgical suite without the need of additional personnel, requiring only an 18–48-cc patient blood draw. In addition, the cost is dramatically less. We currently use an automated, dual-spin process (SmartPReP®2, Harvest Technologies, Plymouth, MA, USA; Fig. 54.2). The patient is phlebotomized to obtain a whole blood sample, the volume

of which depends on the amount of autologous platelet concentrate needed for a given protocol. For large-volume grafting, as in breast or buttock augmentation, we use 10–20 ml PRP following the simple protocol. The kits contain everything needed to properly isolate the platelet concentrate. The drawn specimen is placed in the provided sterile container, which contains citrate phosphate dextrose as an anticoagulant. This container is then placed in the SmartPReP dual-spin centrifuge for an automated cycle, resulting in separation into its three primary components: red blood cells, PRP, and platelet-poor plasma (PPP). Because of the differing densities of the above components, each isolates in its own respective layer following timed centrifugation. The cell separator allows removal of the least dense top layer of PPP (which offers the ability to form a fibrin glue when mixed with thrombin, which is useful in many open surgical and graft procedures). Following removal of the PPP layer, the remaining specimen is centrifuged at 2,400 rpm, allowing accurate separation of the PRP layer from the denser blood-cell layer. The isolated PRP is then introduced into the sterile field for use directly in surgical wound sites or is mixed with graft materials in preparation for tissue transfer. In large-volume transfers, PRP is added as a ratio ranging from 10 cc per 500 cc of harvested graft materials to 20 cc per 500 cc of graft (0.5–1% concentration). Additional studies are underway to try to identify the minimal PRP concentration to graft volume to maximize effects [10].

Grafts may be transplanted in either a fibrin gel form (i.e., "activated" after the addition of the proper proportions of thrombin and calcium chloride) or in the isolated graft-plus-PRP form with no additional additives [40–43]. Based on current clinical observations, in fat grafting there seems to be no distinct difference between the two techniques, unlike in bone and cartilage graft applications, which are improved by placing grafts in a gel matrix.

The remaining blood cells are discarded rather than returned to the patient. Because the volumes now extracted are typically less than 50 cc (some 10 times less than for previous isolation cell-separator devices, which required a 500–600-cc draw), there is no significant concern to the patient about volume loss.

54.4.2
Harvest of Autologous Fat by Closed Syringe

Most experienced fat-transfer surgeons have adopted the use of low-pressure syringe harvesting of autologous fat graft materials. Selecting the donor site for harvest is considered an important issue. It appears that

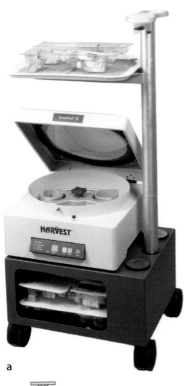

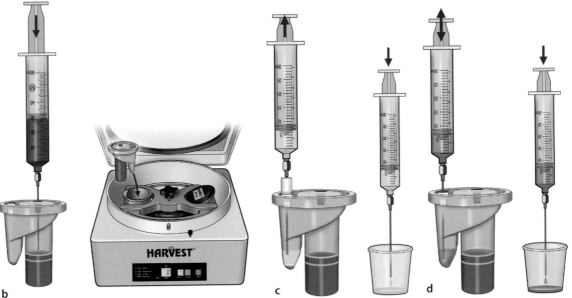

Fig. 54.2 a Stage 1: Transfer total syringe into blood chamber. **b** Stage 2: Load SmartPReP®2. **c** Stage 3: After processing, use syringe with spacer and withdraw platelet-poor plasma (*yellow*). **d** Stage 4: After second spin, the platelet-rich plasma is isolated (*red*)

autologous fat grafts display donor-site memory (that is, they may retain the metabolic and storage characteristics of the adipocytes common to the sites selected for harvest). This suggests that genetic influence varying with the hereditary distribution commonly reported in related individuals may be of great significance [1, 9, 10, 44]. This has significant clinical importance for deter-

mining the ideal donor sites, making such selection not on the basis of the surgeon's convenience or preference but on the basis of demonstrated fat-storage preference and fat metabolic activity levels in each individual patient. These so-called problem areas are recognized as metabolically resistant locations (i.e., to exercise and diet programs) and are commonly referred to as pri-

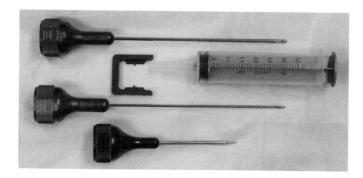

Fig. 54.3 Tulip BioMed closed-syringe system for minimally traumatic harvesting of autologous fat and matrix. Coated external cannulas with internal polish via an extrusion process maximize smoothness and minimize trauma

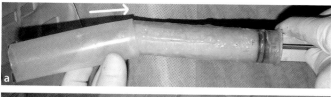

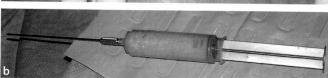

Fig. 54.4 a Tissu-Trans system (Shippert Medical) for large-volume harvesting, rinsing, and platelet-rich plasma insertion of autologous fat. **b** Filled syringe

mary deposit sites. The areas that are influenced with diet and exercise are known as secondary deposit sites.

Harvest is carried out using tumescent fluid infiltration of the selected donor sites, composed of sterile saline with 0.05% Xylocaine with 1:1,000,000 epinephrine. It is common to infiltrate in a ratio of 1:1 up to 2:1 (infiltrate:extraction volumes) via a multiport infiltrator to evenly distribute the fluid throughout the donor site tissues; this provides the liquid vehicle to gently remove the graft tissues. Currently, the use of superpolished cannulas (internal via extrusion techniques, external by coating techniques; Tulip BioMed Cell Friendly™ system) is favored (Fig. 54.3). For large-volume transfers, we attempt to minimize graft harvest trauma by using 2.1–3.7-mm external diameter cannulas, and we displace air from the system by filling the cannula with saline or Ringer's lactate solution before applying negative pressure. During the actual graft harvest, low pressure is applied by limiting the plunger movement to one-half or less of the syringe being used. In large-volume cases, we favor use of the Tulip Cell-Friendly System, which was patented for use with 60-ml Toomey syringes, and the superpolished, coated titanium cannula and the bi-beveled cobra tip [9, 10]. Recent advances in harvesting large volumes are seen in the use of the Tissu-Trans™ system (Fig. 54.4) to harvest, rinse, and permit the addition of PRP in 60-ml Toomey syringes [14].

The actual ideal diameter of a cannula for harvest is

not certain. There is an evolving belief that transfer of some stromal matrix (which actually contains the majority of undifferentiated precursor cells) may, in fact, contribute to long-term graft success. Use of larger harvesting cannulas may be more effective in large-volume scenarios from a minimal pressure extraction. Regardless, larger harvest cannulas are considered to potentially be more efficient in harvest speed, substantially reducing the time for harvesting viable cellular and stromal (containing adult stem cell) materials, with average operating times of 1–2 h maximum.

After the harvested graft material is rinsed to effectively reduce the intracellular lidocaine concentration [45] and permit removal of extracellular lipid materials and debris, the PRP is added to the autologous graft materials in an approximate ratio of 0.5–1% of the total graft prepared for large-volume transplantation. Very-low-speed centrifugation has been used to further concentrate the graft materials from infranatant fluids. In the event that the thrombin–calcium chloride additive is introduced into the graft materials, the condensation of the graft is found to be equally effective to concentrate it without using any additional centrifugation. Following gentle agitation to thoroughly mix the graft and PRP, it is left for 5–10 min to permit release of platelet concentrate component elements. Following this interval to biologically "activate" the graft, it is ready to be placed in the recipient sites [1].

54.4.3
Autologous Fat-Graft Breast Augmentation with PRP

To prepare for transfer augmentation of the breasts, the patient is marked in an upright position in a fashion similar to that for alloplastic augmentation, but the breasts are also marked in quadrants centered on the nipple–areola complex (Fig. 54.5). The line intersecting the inframammary crease and the vertical quadrant line represents the primary 3-mm access point for pretunneling and graft placement in layers (Fig. 54.6).

With the glandular breast tissues elevated, pretunneling is carried out using a 3-mm bi-beveled cobra-style cannula along the deeper aspects of native fat on the fascia surface of the pectoralis major muscle, then layering more superficially toward the breast glandular elements in preparation for subsequent grafting. There has been some suggestion that intramuscular or submuscular grafting may be advantageous, but this has not been well documented [40].

Pretunneling is considered very important to provide loosened tunnels of "native" fat tissues, to initiate recipient site-healing efforts, and to provide a resident cellular and precursor cell matrix to receive the graft materials. Stacking layers of graft is recommended to provide the desired increase in volume in an evenly distributed and effective manner. As in small-volume experiences with autologous fat, it is clear that grafted fat does best in areas where existing fat is found and where

the graft can be surrounded by these native elements [10, 46]. TenderCups™ are used to immobilize autologous fat grafts (Fig. 54.7).

In the clinical trial period of 1992–1996, graft volumes were electively limited to 150 ml (±10%) evenly distributed within the four quadrants of breast. Since that time, volumes of up to 300 ml per breast have been transferred effectively, with placement of more volume within the upper hemispheres where significant volume losses are commonly found [47]. It is very important to understand that the amount of graft volume that can be placed correlates directly with the existing native fat volumes. That is, in patients with greater amounts of native breast fat, larger volumes may be transplanted and well vascularized during the healing process [10]. Very thin patients or patients with essentially no palpable retroglandular fat deposits may not be ideal candidates for fat-graft augmentation of the breasts. In those with very limited recipient-site fat tissues, it is common to transfer lower volumes (such as 150 ml or less to each side) and to plan on a secondary transfer in 4–6 months. With the initial stage increasing the volume of adipose tissue, the breasts may effectively accommodate larger graft volume placement in the subsequent treatment. In our experience, out of approximately 240 fat-graft augmentations since the clinical trial experience, 28% of patients opted to have a second transfer for this reason, or simply to further augment their breasts. The average clinical volume increase at 1 year is estimated to be one

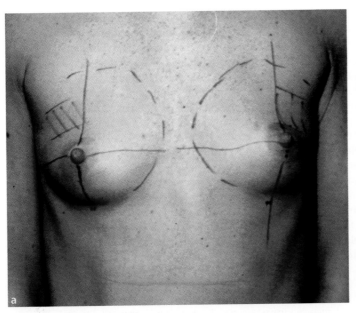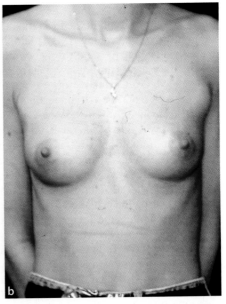

Fig. 54.5 Marking of patient. **a** A 38-year-old woman marked in upright position. **b** One year postoperatively after fat grafting with platelet-rich plasma (150 ml bilateral)

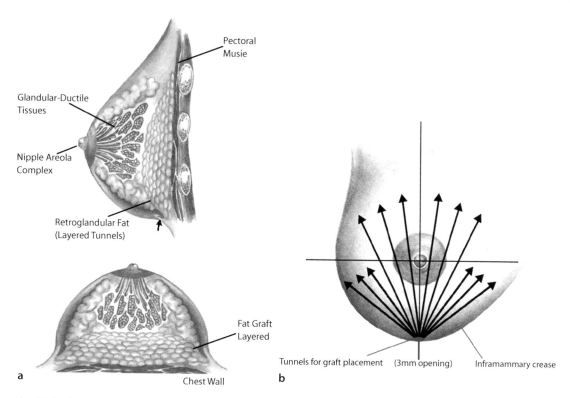

Fig. 54.6 a Separation into quadrants for breast augmentation with autologous fat. A single access point is located within the inframammary crease intersection with vertical marking centered through nipple–areola complex. **b** Placement of fat in autologous fat graft augmentation

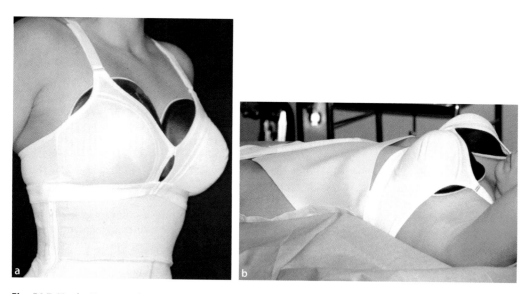

Fig. 54.7 TenderCups™ used to immobilize autologous fat grafts. **a** Tenderfoam™ on abdomen postharvest, TenderCups™ posttransfer. *Black* area is dense, closed-cell foam cup lined with *pink* TenderFoam™ layer next to skin surface

cup size, with some patients achieving larger enhancements. Placement options to accurately deal with small asymmetries, depressions, and alloplastic implant rippling and to help restore the upper hemisphere fullness that many augmentation patients need is available via this technique [47, 48].

Retention of grafted tissues taken from the hereditary (genetic) sites is considered to be very high. Observations coupled with in-vitro studies confirm that cell viability may be well within the 90th percentile. Research on the ability to provide a quantitative analysis based on biochemical characteristic differential is underway at this time. Furthermore, the longevity of such volume increases that have been followed over the past 15 years confirms that volume retention is a long-term effect, taking into account the anticipated loss of subdermal fat deposits in the face and breast areas associated with normal aging processes [1, 10]. It is very important to understand that many reports regarding the "take" rate are often misinterpreted because authors do not account for the fact that at least 30–40% of the transferred volumes do not represent cellular tissues but rather the carrier fluids introduced with the graft cell placement at the time of transfer. It should not be surprising to see initial volume reductions following graft surgery resulting from the gradual removal of these carrier fluids during the healing and graft acceptance process. Experience in breast augmentation via autologous fat grafting suggests that volumes achieved at 4–6 weeks represent the graft placed, with most of the edema and transfer fluids moving away from the graft sites [1, 47–49].

The timing of secondary transfers is typically 4–6 months to permit wound healing and inflammatory stabilization. It is suggested that early regraft intervention while active inflammatory processes are in progress is detrimental to the graft's success. This is consistent with the suggestions to rinse harvested graft materials to remove the red blood cell components (which stimulate inflammatory processes) [45]. In addition, this concept is consistent with the findings reported by Clark and Clark [50] in studies of fat retention in granulation tissue beds. Those studies concluded that lipocytes did not flourish in the acidic environment of active inflammatory activities in granulating tissues until neovascularization and extravasation of red blood cells were complete.

54.5
Results and Complications

Fifteen years of experience confirms that breast augmentation using autologous fat grafting can be safe, predictable, and effectively accomplished. The use of additives, such as PRP, appears to further enhance the success and rate of graft acceptance in both small-volume and large-volume applications. PRP has proven to provide such improvements, and it can be inexpensively isolated and applied to multiple surgical applications, including breast augmentation by fat grafting (Fig. 54.8).

There appears to be minimal morbidity associated with transplantation of autologous fat in the retroglandular breast, and those effects described appear to be similar or less severe than those associated with alloplastic choices.

The limited size of the access points (<3 mm), the gentle blunt tunneling in the recipient bed, and the autologous nature of grafts appear favorable for breast augmentation by this modality.

It is noted that most of the encountered limitations and complications with this group of procedures relate to the harvesting, preparation, and delivery of the autologous grafts to the prepared recipient bed. One of the ongoing difficulties in interpreting many reports relates directly to limited or no standardization of technique for each step in the process. This being the case, accurate comparisons or the ability to duplicate results of the studies is essentially impossible, making it difficult to draw valid scientific conclusions. Recently, the American Society of Liposuction Surgery prepared a preliminary standardization of protocols that will, it is hoped, improve the ability of surgeons to interpret and compare reports in scientific sessions and publications. There is no single "correct" way to perform the harvest, preparation, or transfer, but the ability to observe consistency of results and long-term efficacy may be improved by better understanding the nuances that enhance the patient results [14].

The basic risks associated with conventional liposuction harvest techniques, even though relatively infrequent, are encountered even less, based on the limited volumes typically extracted for fat transfer. The morbidity of this procedure seems to be directly proportional to the instrumentation, technique, and aggressiveness of the harvesting procedure. As a secondary benefit, donor areas often achieve a desired benefit—reduction of unwanted, exercise- and diet-resistant deposit and improved contouring [10, 50].

Autologous fat grafting has advantages and limitations compared with alloplastic augmentation. Advantages include the lack of implant-related difficulties such as neurological nipple–areola injury, deflation, leakage, rippling, visible implant margins, limited expected longevity of the capsule, or capsular contraction [10, 48–50].

Limitations observed in fat-graft augmentation of the breast area make patient selection extremely important. Because there is no limiting capsule filled with

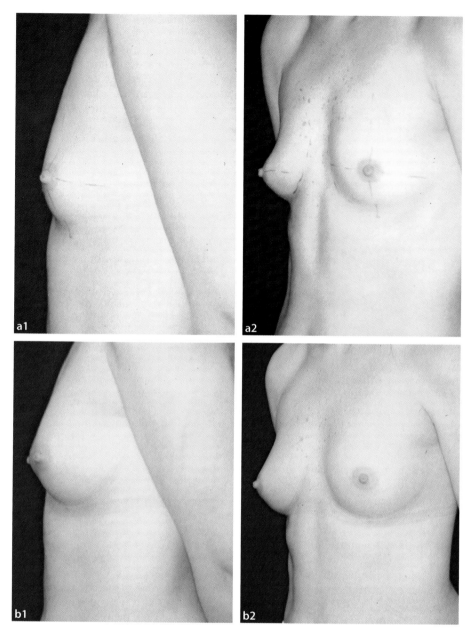

Fig. 54.8 a *1, 2* Preoperative views of 30-year-old patient. **b** *1, 2* Three years after single-stage grafting of 160-ml bilateral grafts without platelet-rich plasma

volume material, the resultant volume increases that are realized may be somewhat limited. In other words, for patients whose primary concern is increased size, it is often better to recommend implants to achieve their goals. With structural augmentation via fat grafting, the tissues are more diffusely infiltrated in stacked tunnels that are feathered along the margins. This permits the opportunity to provide specific area support and volumes in the areas of the inframammary crease, sternum (cleavage), and upper hemispheres, where many patients demonstrate loss of fullness such as follow-

ing pregnancy and aging. The candidates selecting the fat-graft alternative tend to be moderately older, in the 26–55-year age group. In this mature population, restoration of fullness and support often exceeds the desire for large volume increases. There may be a modest difference in the realized graft enlargement based on vascular patterns altered because of pregnancy or hormonal cycle changes. This variable is the subject of additional study, including a retrospective analysis of volume increases and patient satisfaction analysis [49]. Reports of additional unanticipated disproportional enlargement has been reported up to 10 years after grafting in patients having substantial weight gains in that period. This is interpreted as consistent with the genetic predisposition of grafted cells to store lipid.

Structural grafting may also permit better implant margin masking, and can be used in select postlumpectomy or minor asymmetric areas. In the very thin patient with minimal retroglandular native volumes, the addition of such volume via grafting is often completed before actual alloplastic implant placement, knowing that implant margins may be difficult to hide.

It is believed that recipient site characteristics (such as thickness, density, and vascularization of the recipient bed) may contribute to limitations of graft volumes that are readily accepted in the site. As mentioned, it has been well documented that autologous fat grafts do better in sites rich in existing "native" fat cellular and stromal elements. Whether this is involved in cellular survival, is a function of induction effects on undifferentiated stem cells (preadipocytes and mesenchymal types), or is simply related to the presence of favorable infrastructure and environment remains unclear at this time. Early tissue culture evidence suggests that stimulated harvested cells experience a more rapid return to an active metabolic state when directly enhanced with the addition of autologous platelet concentrates (APC, PRP). This has been demonstrated in examples of cytoplasmic closure and repair following suction harvest, with return to fat metabolic activity in vitro [M. Lyles, personal communication, 2006].

Recipient site morbidities are similar to those cited for small-volume transfers. The development of palpable cystic or nodular accumulations in the recipient site following transplantation is possible [33, 34]. This is postulated to represent small areas of extracellular lipid accumulation or steatonecrosis with failure of cellular acceptance [50–59]. It is important to note that the clinical frequency of such changes has substantially decreased since the advent of the use of platelet concentrates. It is believed that the presence of palpable nodules or cystic accumulations may be a direct function of delayed healing or poor circulation within the grafted recipient site [10].

Cytosteatonecrosis, resulting in a low-grade inflammatory response, may encourage formation of microcysts and spherical calcifications, as has been documented as morbidities associated with traditional autologous fat grafting. Such findings, an early expressed concern of many breast surgeons, are relatively easily differentiated via mammography and ultrasound studies. Current studies using review with magnetic resonance imaging to gain greater detail of any suspicious areas—much like the current recommendations for silicone implant evaluations—are ongoing.

Patients are recommended to have preoperative mammography to serve as a baseline prior to breast augmentation by either alloplastic or autologous means. Following autologous fat graft augmentation, we recommend a follow-up study to reset the baseline. After several hundred experiences, it appears that any changes are typically visible within 6–18 months. On four occasions, the findings did not appear for more than 24 months. Imaging specialists report comfort in differentiating the spherical-type cysts and/or microcalcifications from those potentially harmful to the patient [56]. In the clinical trial, the radiologists were blinded to any procedure, and in many instances their only findings were reported as "greater retroglandular fat matrix of unknown origin" as the only changes noted [49].

The occurrence of the above described morbidity can be related to graft trauma at the time of placement, delayed revascularization, or increased inflammatory response within the recipient bed. It has been postulated that the addition of PRP may enhance the healing cascade rates and specifically stimulate greater revascularization processes [10, 47, 49]. Recent approval from the U.S. Food and Drug Administration for the use of PRP with bone marrow aspirate confirms the efficacy and safety associated with PRP and mesenchymal stem cell tissues. As a source of mesenchymal stem cells, fat tissue has been well documented to provide higher numbers of such cells than are present in bone tissues [36]. The importance of stem cell induction and differentiation in both bone and fat grafting is a current subject of extensive investigations.

54.6
Discussion

The scientific literature contains numerous studies to date that have sought to elucidate a biochemical additive or agent that can improve or speed the acceptance and outcome of autologous fat grafts. Numerous additives such as heparin, calcium, thyroid hormone, bezafibrate, vitamin E, albumin, and insulin have been studied, with little or no evidence supporting greater graft acceptance [1, 10, 60–71]. Suggestions that use of osmotic gradients (e.g., albumin) may stabilize adipocyte cellular membranes need to be further explored. It is possible that a portion of the effects of PRP additives may also relate to the osmotic characteristic in addition to the wound-healing factors.

Growth factors are the biologically active signal peptides released from local tissue or blood products (particularly the platelet fraction) that play a critical role in influencing the initiation and progression of the normal wound-healing process. Such factors coordinate the processes of epithelialization, angiogenesis, and collagen-matrix formation—the key steps in the wound-healing sequence. Growth factors function in paracrine, endocrine, and autocrine manners to guide the dynamic stages of wound healing. No single growth factor appears to maintain a total physiologic task, but instead these peptides work in a coordinated fashion to orchestrate the normal wound-healing processes. A substantial volume of basic research has displayed the efficacy of these bioactive peptides with regard to healing in both soft and osseous tissues. Steed et al. [72], in a randomized, prospective, double-blind, placebo-controlled study of 118 patients with chronic, full-thickness lower-extremity diabetic neurotrophic ulcers of at least 8 weeks in duration, displayed a statistically significant difference in both numbers of patients healed and healing rates after daily application of topical recombinant growth factors. Forty-eight percent of patients randomized to the growth factor application group achieved complete wound healing, compared with only 25% wound closure in the control group. Knighton et al. [73] displayed a 93% reepithelialization rate in 41 patients displaying a total of 71 chronic wounds, after receiving daily treatments with autologous platelet concentrate (PRP). In a second study by Knighton et al. [74], they confirmed the first study, with complete wound resolution in 17 of 21 chronic lower-extremity ulcerations treated with an 8-week course of twice-daily PRP/APC application. Of those patients in the placebo group, only two of 13 displayed the same results. Upon crossover treatment of the control group with APC (PRP), all previously unresponsive wounds displayed reepithelialization. Extensive reports in other mesenchyme-derived tissues have documented enhanced healing in bone and cartilage models in vivo. Powell et al. [75] reported trends suggesting enhanced recovery with decreases in postoperative edema and ecchymoses in a pilot randomized, prospective, controlled clinical trial involving patients undergoing standard deep-place facelifting. The effect of growth factors on enhancement of neovascularization was reported by Khouri et al. [76]. This study demonstrated that after basic fibroblast growth factor was applied to ischemic flaps in a rat model, greater flap survival rates were seen, as well as a greater increase in the number of new blood vessels upon histologic examination.

PRP, as a clinical enhancement to native wound-healing capabilities, contains supraphysiologic concentrations of growth factors. Reports extrapolating the basic wound-healing model with respect to transplantation of autologous fat show improved efficacy of such small-volume and large-volume grafts in the clinical setting. In those, it is postulated that the effects of PRP with regard to enhancement of the normal wound-healing processes mean that it can be safely and effectively used as an additive in autologous fat grafting. The addition of PRP to grafts appears to actively promote increased graft-volume retention and a return to metabolic activity. Based on those clinical observations, it is reported that the addition of PRP (and the attendant addition of high concentrations of growth factors and cytokines) increased retention of the transplanted fat cells, increased the rate of revascularization of the grafts, and aided differentiation of preadipocyte precursor cells into mature adipocytes to further enhance the retained graft volumes [1, 10, 17, 39]. The use of mesenchymal stem cells derived from fat tissue is the current subject of study, as they appear to be able to undergo induction and differentiation into a variety of tissues of similar origin and are more prevalent and easier to obtain than bone marrow cells [36–39].

In the case of autologous fat transplantation, the recipient bed represents a basic model of soft tissue injury. There appears to be clinical enhancement of wound repair within that site following introduction of grafts with the PRP additive, favoring maintenance of graft volumes and acceptance. Autologous fat cells are injected into a created potential space that is subjected to mild tissue injury as a result of pretunneling in the recipient locations. Following grafting, these created spaces consist of transplanted cellular elements, clotted blood containing platelets, exposed endothelial cells, interstitial collagen, fibroblasts, and undifferentiated stem cell elements.

The use of activated PRP gel or plain PRP-added grafts appears to actively initiate the hemostatic phase of wound healing, which is expected to last for the first few minutes following injury. With the initial tissue injury, the damaged recipient bed cells (native) release their own growth factors (notably PDGF and TGF). Concurrently, activation of the clotting cascade results in the transformation of fibrinogen to fibrin, a potent stimulus for the further release of growth factors from the alpha granules within the aggregated platelets. These factors then activate their target cells (polymorphonuclear leukocytes, macrophages, lymphocytes, fibroblasts, endothelial cells, epithelial cells, and so on) to proliferate and migrate to the wound site and carry out important functions regarding graft acceptance and site healing.

Knowledge of the inflammatory stage of wound healing (3–5 days after the initial injury) is important. It is during this time that success or failure of free grafting may be determined. In this stage, activation of inflammatory cells, such as macrophages secreting growth factors; induction of fibroblast proliferation; early collagen synthesis; endothelial cell replication and mobilization; and epidermal cell mobility and proliferation must be appreciated.

Next, the proliferative phase (days 3–12 following injury) of the process continues the graft acceptance processes. During this phase, fibroblasts are activated to lay down a new extracellular matrix. Angiogenic growth factors are simultaneously released by injured cells, platelets, macrophages, and extracellular matrix aimed at inducing early vascularization.

The remodeling phase (approximately 2 weeks after injury) is a gradual process, lasting for up to 1 year, and is considered to be less critical to the success of individual grafts. During this time, a balance is achieved between synthesis of new matrix and degradation by proteases, and a permanent infrastructure is provided for long-term graft volume maintenance. Type III collagen is gradually replaced by type I collagen. The final result of the remodeling phase is formation of the supportive fibrous matrix.

Thus, the conclusion drawn regarding the addition of concentrated platelet-derived factors to a wound bed is that it will markedly augment and improve the healing process. This enhancement of healing rate and graft survival may result in more favorable and reliable results with regard to the success of transplantation of autologous fat in small-volume and large-volume applications.

The importance of growth factors in initiating the differentiation of adipose precursor cells into mature adipocytes is currently under extensive study. In-vitro studies have shown that such factors do, in fact, stimulate the proliferation and differentiation of precursor adipose cell cultures [31, 36–39].

This bioactivation phenomenon has been studied successfully in a number of clinical trials. Yuksel et al. [60] demonstrated quantitative increases in weight maintenance and adipocyte area percentage means in the rat model following the addition of insulin-like growth factor 1 and basic fibroblast growth factor delivered by PLGA/PEG microspheres in conjunction with autologous fat grafts. Small-volume fat graft survival after growth factor application in the facial region has been studied by Eppley et al. [30]. Ninety days after grafting, those treated with dextran beads soaked with basic fibroblast growth factor exhibited greater graft weight maintenance. In addition, the grafts in the experimental group histologically displayed greater numbers of intact cells compared with those in the control group. Eppley et al. [71], in a later study, observed near-complete graft weight maintenance, larger adipocyte volume, increased numbers of intact cells, and the presence of numerous smaller adipocyte-like cells 1 year after grafting, compared with the controls. These small adipocytes may represent a group of newly differentiated cells slowly beginning to return to the metabolic activity of a mature adipocyte. In some autologous fat-grafting cases, delayed volume increases have been observed, particularly in cases of large-volume transfer. This may suggest a differentiation of precursor cells to adipocyte form, and the delay may represent restoration of the metabolic activities of cytoplasmic lipid storage.

Suggestions that growth factors enhance graft volumes as well as increase the actual number of adipocytes with grafted tissues are very significant. With these observations, it is possible that those mature adipocytes lost in the harvest and transplantation process may be replaced by newly inducted and differentiated cells, allowing the overall graft volume to be retained.

54.7
Conclusions

The conclusions drawn from scientific and experiential pathways is that autologous fat grafting offers a viable and safe alternative means of breast augmentation in selected patients [49, 77]. Long-lasting natural contouring and volume increases are attainable.

Since the advent of the closed-syringe system for lipocontouring and harvesting for grafts, the predictability and safety are gaining recognition. Many of the early contributions to the literature have made the use of autologous fat grafting a feasible and useful modality in volume augmentations to the breasts [78].

The use of additives to bioactivate the grafts and recipient bed appears to substantially improve the augmentation achieved and to reduce the incidence of lipid cysts, cellular loss, and microcalcifications. The exact incidence of microcalcifications is not established, but based on the author's personal experience, the incidence was found to be 12% in the non-PRP-treated grafts versus 8% in the PRP-treated grafts (Fig. 54.9). This trend suggests improvement in the acceptance of low-pressure, syringe-harvested free-fat grafts. The literature is now beginning to provide more reporting of such findings, and the actual incidence of lipid cysts and characteristic microcalcifications in a large sample should be forthcoming.

Fat-graft augmentation may be of value as a simple aesthetic enlargement or to correct some asymmetries and breast deformities in a reconstructive application. Patient satisfaction is very high, especially in those in the older median age group and those with major aversion to the use of artificial implants of any kind [10].

Patient selection and communication remain the most important determinants in successful augmentation with grafts. Establishing the patient's expectations remains the crucial point for selecting grafting techniques. The use of additives such as PRP appears

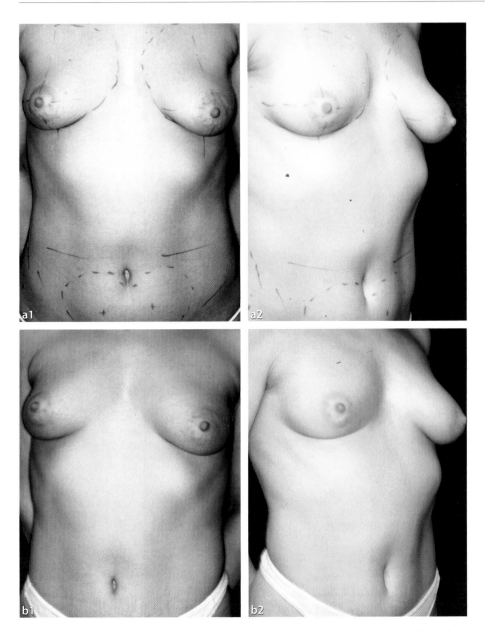

Fig. 54.9 **a** *1, 2* Preoperative views of patient. **b** *1, 2* Postoperative views following fat transfer without platelet-rich plasma (PRP)

to have improved the efficacy, speed of recovery, and safety of the graft alternative.

As mainstream practitioners begin to report their findings of these techniques, much-needed reproducibility of results and qualitative/quantitative analysis of the augmentation volume will be available. Standardization of techniques is needed to permit practitioners to more effectively appreciate the results of and satisfac-

tion with structural fat grafting in both small-volume and large-volume applications.

The importance of autologous fat grafting may be further enhanced with increased understanding of the stem cell implications associated with the tissue. Additional research relative to the induction and differentiation of transplanted cellular elements is underway at this time. Such information may provide much greater

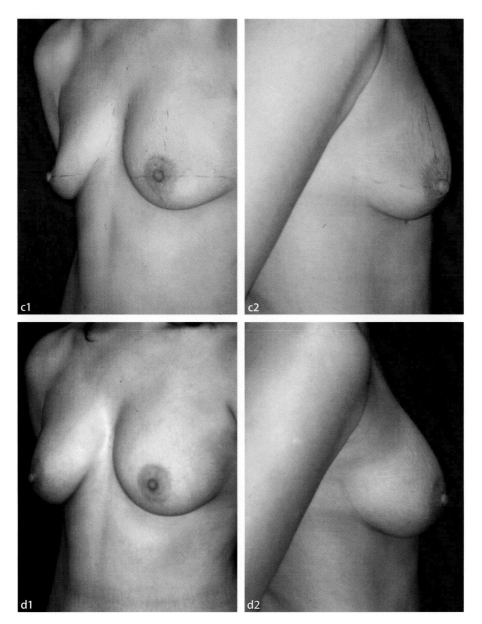

Fig. 54.9 *(continued)* **c** *1, 2* Preoperative views of patient. **d** *1, 2* Postoperatively following fat transfer with PRP

understanding of our clinical experience and explanation of the success for long-term maintenance of results. With the rush to explore the possibilities of precursor cells, there may be many more clinical applications for the use of mesenchymally derived adult stem cell tissues in medicine and surgery.

The author has no financial interest in Harvest Technology, Tulip Medical, or Shippert Medical companies.

References

1. Alexander RW, Abuzeni PZ: Enhancement of autologous fat transplantation with platelet rich plasma. Am J Cosmet Surg 2001;18:59–70
2. Whitman DH: Platelet gel: an autologous alternative to fibrin glue with applications in oral and maxillofacial surgery. J Oral Maxillofacial Surg 1997;55(11):1294–1299

3. Marx RE: Platelet-rich plasma: growth factor enhancement for bone grafts. Oral Surg Oral Med Oral Path Oral Radiol Endod 1998;85(6):638–646

4. Fagrell D, Sverker E, Kniola B: Fat cylinder transplantation: an experimental comparative study of three different kinds of transplants. Plast Reconstr Surg 1996;98(1):90–96

5. Niechajev I, Sevcuk O: Long-term results of fat transplantation: clinical and histologic studies. Plast Reconstr Surg 1994;94(3):496–506

6. Billings E, May JW Jr: Historical review and present status of free fat graft autotransplantation in plastic and reconstructive surgery. Plast Reconstr Surg 1989;83(2):368–381

7. Nguyen A, Pasyk KA, Bouvier TN: Comparative study of survival of autologous tissue taken and transplanted by different techniques. Plast Recon Surg 1990;85(3):378–386

8. Fulton JE, Suarez M, Silverton K, Barnes T: Small volume fat transfer. Dermatol Surg 1998;24(8):857–865

9. Alexander RW: Liposculpture in the superficial plane: closed syringe system for improvement in fat removal and free fat transfer. Am J Cosmet Surg 1994;11:127–134

10. Alexander RW, Sadati K, Corrado A: Platelet-rich plasma (PRP) utilized to promote greater graft volume retention in autologous fat grafting. Am J Cosmet Surg 2006;23(4):203–221

11. Obaji S: Selecting for fat transfer success. Cosmet Surg Times 2006;9(4):26

12. Bircoll M: A nine-year experience with autologous fat transplantation. Am J Cosmet Surg 1992;9(1):55–61

13. Coleman SR: Structural Fat Grafting. St. Louis, Quality Medical Publishing 2004, pp 30–175

14. Shippert R: Autologous fat transfer: eliminating the centrifuge, decreasing lipocyte trauma, and establishing standardization for scientific study. Am J Cosmet Surg 2006;23(1):21–27

15. Ersek RA: Transplantation of purified autologous fat; a three year follow-up is disappointing. Plast Recon Surg 1991;87(2):219–227

16. Pinski KS, Roenigk HH : Autologous fat transplantation long-term followup. J Dermatol Surg Oncol 1992;18(3)179–184

17. Lyles MB: Adipocytes hearty: certain storage conditions favor pre-adipocyte survival. Cosmet Surg Times 2003;6:10–11

18. Coleman SR: Structural fat grafting: more than a permanent filler. Plast Reconstr Surg 2006;118(3 suppl):108S–120S

19. Forgue-Lafitte ME, Van RL, De Gasquet P, Rosselin G: The presence of epidermal growth factor receptors in cultured human adipocyte precursors. Scand J Clin Lab Invest 1982;42(8):627–631

20. Lau D, Roncari D, Yip D, Kindler S, Nilsern S: Purification of a pituitary polypeptide that stimulates the replication of adipocyte precursors in culture. FEBS Lett 1983;153:395–398

21. Zapf J, Schoenle E, Froesch R: Insulin-like growth factor I and II: some biological actions and receptor binding characteristics of two purified constituents of nonsuppressible insulin-like activity of human serum. Eur J Biochem 1978;87(5):285–296

22. Reeder GD, Hood A, Hill A: Perioperative autologous sequestration I: physiology, phenomena, and art. Proceedings of the American Academy of Cardiovascular Perfusion. San Antonio, 1993

23. Haystead T, Hardie DG: Both insulin and epidermal growth factor stimulate lipogenesis and acetyl-CoA carboxylase activity in isolated adipocytes. Inportance of homogenization procedure in avoiding artifacts in acetyl-CoA carboxylase assay. Biochem J 1986;234(2):279–284

24. Ng TB, Wong CM: Epidermal and nerve growth factors manifest antilipolytic and lipogenic activities in isolated rat adipocytes. Comp Biochem Physiol B 1985;81(3):687–689

25. Chai Y, Salvkin HC: Biology of bone induction and its clinical applications. Oral Maxillofacial Surg Clin 1994;7:739–753

26. Cromak DT: Current concepts in wound healing: growth factor and macrophage interaction. J Trauma 1990;30:130–132

27. Pierce GF: Platelet-derived growth factor-BB and transforming growth factor beta 1 selectively modulate glycosaminoglycans, collagen, and myofibroblasts in excisional wounds. Am J Pathol 1991;138(3):629–646

28. Ross R: The biology of platelet-derived growth factor. Cell 1986;46(2):155–169

29. Pierce GF: Role of platelet-derived growth factor in wound healing. J Cell Biochem 1991;45(4):319–326

30. Eppley BL, Snyders RV, Winkelmann T, Delfino JJ: Autologous facial fat transplantation: improved graft maintenance by microbead bioactivation. J Oral Maxillofacial Surg 1992;50(5):477–482

31. Jones JK, Lyles M: The viability of human adipocytes after closed-syringe liposuction harvest. Am J Cosmet Surg 1997;14:275–279

32. Marx RE, Carlson E: Growth factor enhancement for bone grafts. J Oral Maxillofacial Surg 1993;51:1181–1193

33. Knighton DR, Hunt TK, Scheuenstuhl H, Halliday BJ, Werb Z, Banda MJ: Oxygen tension regulates the expression of angiogenesis factor by macrophages. Science 1983;221(4617):1283–1285

34. Marx RE, Ehler WJ., Tayapongsak P, Pierce LW: Relationship of oxygen dose to angiogenesis induction in irradiated tissue. Am J Surg 1990;160(5):519–524

35. Carpaneda CA, Ribiero MT: Study of histologic alterations and viability of the adipose graft in humans. Aesth Plast Surg 1993;17(1):43–47

36. Zuk PA, Zhu M, Mizuno H, Huang J, Futrell JW, Katz AJ, Benhaim P, Lorenz HP, Hedrick MH: Multilineage cells from human adipose tissue: implications for cell-based therapies. 2001;7(2):211–228

37. Aust L, Devlin B, Foster SJ, Halvorsen YD, Hicok K, du Laney T, Sen A, Willingmyre GD, Gimble JM: Yield of human adipocyte-derived adult stem cells from liposuction aspirates. Cytotherapy 2004;6(1):7–14

38. Strem BM, Hicok K, Zhu M, Wulur I, Alfonso Z, Schreiber RE, FraserJK, Hedrick MJ: Multipotential differentiation of adipose tissue-derived stem cells. Keio J Med 2005;54(3):132–141

39. Gimble J, Guilak F: Adipose-derived adult stem cells: isolation, characterization, and differentiation potential. Cytotherapy 2003;5(5):362–369

40. Fulton JE: Breast contouring with "gelled" autologous fat: 10 year update. Int J Cosmet Surg Aesthet Dermatol 2003;5:155–161

41. Santrach PJ, Hoffman M: Laboratory validation of autologous platelet gel. Transfusion 2004, 44 (12 supp):68A–69A

42. Sacchi MC, Maresca P, Tartuferi L, Bellanda M, Micheletti P, Riva S, Borzini P, Levis A, Rosti G: Platelet gel as a new routine method to improve wound healing and regeneration. Transfus Med 2000;10:325–329

43. Man D, Plosker H, Winland-Brown J.E: The use of autologous platelet-rich plasma (platelet gel) and autologous platelet-poor plasma (fibrin glue) in cosmetic surgery. Plast Reconstr Surg 2001;107(1):229–237

44. Fulton JE: Breast contouring by autologous fat transfer. Am J Cosmet Surg 1992;9:273–279

45. Alexander RW, Maring T, Aghabo T: Autologous fat grafting: a study of residual intracellular adipocyte lidocaine concentrations after serial rinsing with normal saline. Am J Cosmet Surg 1999;16:123–126

46. Ersek RA, Chang P, Salisbury M: A lipo layering of autologous fat: an improved technique with promising results. Plast Reconstr Surg 1998;101(3):820–826

47. Alexander RW: Breast augmentation by injection of autologous fat. Proceedings of the American Society of Cosmetic Breast Surgery, Newport Beach, CA, 1996

48. Alexander RW: Use of fat transfer for facial and breast augmentation. Proceedings of World Congress on Liposuction Surgery, San Francisco 1996

49. Alexander RW: Use of fat grafts for augmentation mammoplasty. Summary of clinical information with radiographic documentation. Proceedings of the American Society of Cosmetic Breast Surgery, Newport Beach, CA, 1998

50. Clark ER, Clark EL: Microscopic studies of new formation of fat in living adult rabbits. Am J Anat 1940;67:255–281

51. Coleman SR: Fat grafting to the breast revisited: safety and efficacy. Plast Reconstr Surg 2007;119(3):775–787

52. Bircoll M: Cosmetic breast augmentation utilizing autologous fat and liposuction techniques. Plast Reconstr Surg 1987;79(2):267–271

53. Bircoll M: Autologous fat transplantation: an evaluation of microcalcification and fat cell survivability following (AFT) cosmetic breast augmentation. Am J Cosmet Surg 1998;5:283–288

54. Hogge JP, Robinson RE, Magnant CM, Zuurbier RA: The mammographic spectrum of fat necrosis of the breast. Radiographics 1995;15(6):1347–1356

55. Johnson GW: Benign breast calcifications. Am J Cosmet Surg 1988;5:177–180

56. Pulagam SR, Poulton T, Mamounas EP: Long-term clinical and radiologic results with autologous fat transplantation for breast augmentation. Breast J 2006;6(1):63–67

57. Fine RE, Staren ED: Updates in breast ultrasound. Surg Clin North Am 2004;84(4):1001–1006

58. Chala LF, de Barros N, de Camargo Moraes, P, Endo E, Kim SJ, Pinceraato KM, Carvalho FM, Cerri GG: Fat necrosis of the breast: mammographic, sonographic, computed tomography, and magnetic resonance imaging findings. Curr Probl Diagn Radiol 2004;33(3):106–126

59. Kneeshaw PJ, Lowry M, Manton D, Hubbard A, Drew PJ, Turnbull LW: Differentiation of benign from malignant breast disease associated with screening detected microcalcifications using dynamic contract enhanced magnetic resonance imaging. Breast 2006;15(1):29–38

60. Yuksel E, Weinfeld AB, Cleek R, Wamsley S, Jensen J, Boutros S, Waugh JM, Shenaq SM, Spira M: Increased free fat-graft survival with the long-term local delivery of insulin, insulin-like growth factor-1, and basic fibroblast growth factor by PLGA/PEG microspheres. Plast Reconstr Surg 2000;105(5):1712–1720

61. Wabitsch M, Hauner H, Heinze E, Teller WM: The role of growth hormone/insulin-like growth factors in adipocyte differentiation. Metabolism 1995;44(10 suppl 4):45–49

62. Boney CM, Moats-Staats BM, Stiles AD, D'Ercole AJ: Expression of insulin-like growth factor-1 (IGF-1) and IGF-binding proteins during adipogenesis. Endocrinology 1994;135(5):1863–1868

63. Alexander RW: Platelet rich plasma offers vast fat graft benefits. Cosmet Surg Times 2004;7(3):18–20

64. Menschik Z: Vitamin E and adipose tissue. Edinburgh Med J 1944;51:486–489

65. Sidman RL: The direct effect of insulin on organ cultures of brown fat. Anat Rec 1956;124(4):723–739

66. Reynold AE, Marble A, Fawcett DW: Action of insulin on deposition of glycogen and storage of fat in adipose tissue. Endocrinology 1950;46:55–66

67. Krawisz BR, Scott RE: Coupling of proadipocyte growth arrest and differentiation. I. Induction by heparinized medium containing human plasma. J Cell Biol 1982;94(2):394–399

68. Flores-Delgado G., Marsch-Moreno M, Kuri-Harcuch W: Thyroid hormone stimulates adipocyte differentiation of 3T3 cells. Molec Cell Biochem 1987;76(1):35–43

69. Brandes R, Hertz R, Arad R, Nashtat S, Weil S, Bar-Tana J: Adipocyte conversion of cultured 3T3-L1 pre-adipocytes by benzafibrate. Life Sci 1987;40(10):935–941

70. Ullmann Y, Hyanms M, Ramon Y, Beach D, Peled IJ, Lindenbaum ES: Enhancing survival of aspirated human fat injected into nude mice. Plast Reconstr Surg 1998;101(7):1940–1944

71. Eppley BL, Sidner RA, Platis JM, Sadove MA: Bioactivation of free-fat transfer: a potentially new approach to improving fat survival. Plast Reconstr Surg 1992;90(6):1022–1030

72. Steed DL: Clinical evaluation of recombinant human platelet-derived growth factor for the treatment of lower extremity diabetic ulcers. J Vasc Surg 1995;21(1):79–81

73. Knighton DR, Ciresi K, Fiegel V, Schumerth S, Butler E, Cerra F: The use of topically applied platelet growth factors in chronic non-healing wounds. Wounds 1998;1:71–78

74. Knighton DR, Ciresi K, Fiegel VD, Schumerth S, Butler E, Cerra F: Stimulation of repair in chronic, non-healing cutaneous ulcers using platelet-derived wound healing formula. Surg Gynecol Obstet 1990;170(1):56–60

75. Powell DM, Chang E, Farrior EH: Recovery from deep-plane rhytidectomy following unilateral wound treatment with autologous platelet gel. Arch Plast Surg 2001;3(4):245–250

76. Khouri RK, Brown DM, Leal-Khouri SM, Tark KC, Shaw WW: The effect of basic fibroblast growth factor on the neovascularization process: skin flap survival and staged flap transfers. Br J Plast Surg 1991;44(8):585–588

77. Alexander RW: Results are satisfying using autologous fat: breast augmentation with autologous fat transfer. Cosmet Surg Times 1998;2(4):4

78. Fournier PF: The breast fill. In: Fournier PF (ed). Liposculpture: The Syringe Technique. Paris, Arnette-Blackwell 1991, pp 357–367

CHAPTER 55

Fat Transfer and Implant Breast Augmentation   55

Katsuya Takasu, Shizu Takasu

55.1
Introduction

Since the controversy over the safety of silicone-gel-filled breast implants, inflatable saline-filled implants have been popular materials for augmentation mammoplasty in Japan. Saline solution is short of viscosity; therefore, saline-filled implants provide a somewhat firmer and less elastic touch to the overlying breasts compared with silicone gel implants. This shortcoming has caused patients dissatisfaction, especially when the saline-filled implants are used for very small breasts. Many of the Japanese patients seen in our office are thin, and their breasts are extremely hypoplastic. The authors have found that saline-filled implants are palpable through these patients' thin chest skin even though they are placed under the pectoral muscles.

Fat injection has been used for breast augmentation [1, 2]. Although some of the reported results have been encouraging, this technique is not free of complications. Clinical trials have shown problems related to unpredictable postoperative resorption, fat necrosis, calcification, and cyst formation [3–5]. Researchers have discussed the rationale of transplanting a limited amount of fat in an area in contact with well-vascularized tissue [6–8]. The major problem lies in injecting enough fat to obtain the desired volume. This is particularly the problem when fat transplantation alone is used for patients with small breasts.

The authors have considered that the combination of the above two procedures might eliminate the problems associated with either approach alone.

55.2
Technique

The procedure is performed under general anesthesia. Fat is harvested from convenient sites, such as the abdomen, buttock, and thighs, using a suction machine. Tumescent technique is used to fill out the donor areas [9]. The aspirate is rinsed repeatedly with saline solution to remove the blood component. The collected fat is packed into multiple 20-cc syringes for injection.

Through a small stab wound along the inframammary fold, the fat is then injected into the breast using a fine blunt-tip cannula (2.0 mm in diameter). It is important to inject a small amount of fat at each location in order to secure sufficient nutrition for the cells [1, 2, 6–8]. The fat is thereby grafted into multiple areas of the entire breast, including the subcutaneous tissue, pectoral fascia, and pectoral muscle. At the completion of the injection, the breast is massaged manually to evenly spread out the injected material.

A transverse incision is made in the axilla, and the dissection is performed under the pectoral muscle. At the beginning of the operation, Klein's solution is infiltrated into the subpectoral space to minimize bleeding during the dissection. An inflatable silicone bag implant is then inserted into the submuscular pocket, and the implant is filled with saline.

55.3
Clinical Case

A 23-year-old Japanese woman presented with mammary hypoplasia (Fig. 55.1). She desired considerable enlargement of the breast. Saline-bag implantation was definitely indicated, and the size of implant required should be more than 300 ml to achieve the desired volume. However, her small mammary gland and thin subcutaneous tissue did not seem thick enough to conceal the firm touch of saline-filled implants. It was, therefore, suggested that the combined use of fat injection as an adjacent procedure with the inflatable implant might be of benefit to provide a natural look and palpation to her augmented breast.

Four hundred milliliters of fat was collected by means of liposuction from the woman's abdomen, buttock, and bilateral thighs. Two hundred milliliters of aspirate was injected into each breast area. Using the standard transaxillary approach, 250-ml saline-filled implants were inserted under the pectoral muscle.

The patient's postoperative course was uneventful. Immediately after the surgery, her breast enlargement was somewhat overwhelming (Fig. 55.2). The 1-week postoperative computed tomography (CT) scan showed

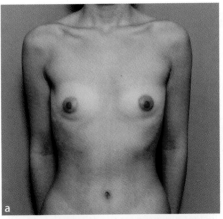

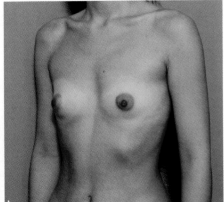

Fig. 55.1 a–c Preoperative views of 23-year-old Japanese female with mammary hypoplasia. Her abdomen is also thin

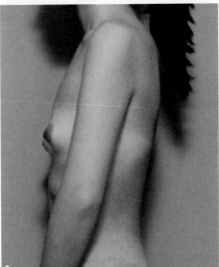

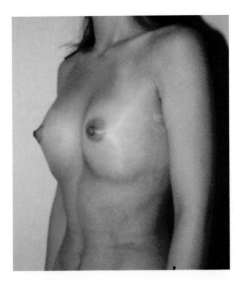

Fig. 55.2 One week postoperatively. Note significant fullness of the breasts

significant thickening of the breast tissue overlying the prosthesis, which was located under the pectoralis major muscle (Fig. 55.3). Over the course of the following 3 weeks, there was observable regression in the fullness of the breast. The breast had lost more than half of the injected volume by that time. Thereafter, the resorption seemed to slow down. The 2-month postoperative CT scan showed no cyst formation in the breast (Fig. 55.3). The breast tissue lost significant volume, about two-thirds of the transplanted fat, compared with that seen 1 week postoperatively. This volume loss was obvious on clinical observation (Fig. 55.4). Only a small amount of the injected fat was retained in the subcutaneous tissue and breast tissue. Nonetheless, the remaining fat helped camouflage the saline-filled implants. The patient was satisfied with her breasts and also pleased with the body contour as a result of liposuction. Both clinical observation and CT scanning demonstrated that this benefit lasted for at least 2 years (Figs. 55.3, 55.5).

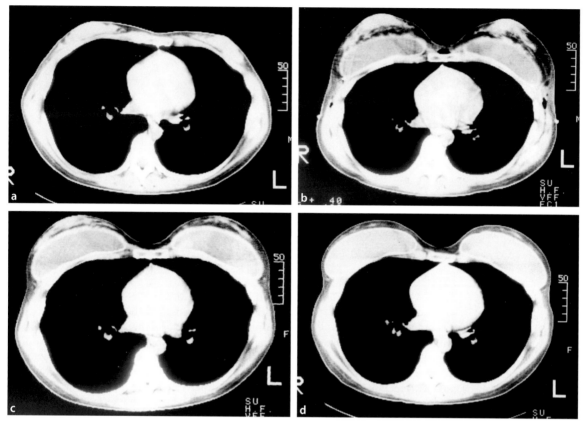

Fig. 55.3 a Preoperative computed tomography (CT) scan. **b** The 1-week postoperative CT scan shows thickening of the breast tissue due to fat injection and inflammatory reaction. Note the saline-filled implant under the pectoral muscle. **c** Two-month postoperative CT scan. Note significant volume reduction (about two-thirds) of breast tissue compared with the 1-week postoperative CT scan. **d** Two-year postoperative CT scan. Note slight thinning of the breast tissue compared with 2-month postoperative CT scan

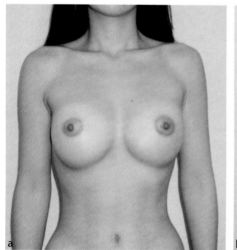

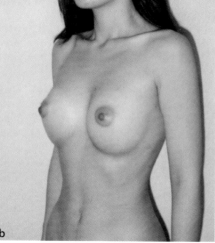

Fig. 55.4 Two months postoperatively. **a** Note significant volume reduction of the breasts compared with 1 week postoperatively(Fig.55.b). **b** Lateral view

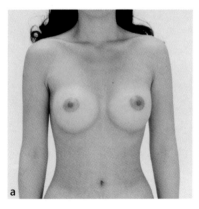 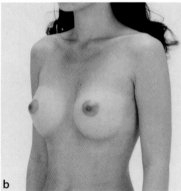 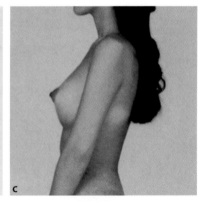

Fig. 55.5 Two years postoperatively. **a** A further volume decrease, although small, is noted compared with that 2 months postoperatively (Fig. 55.4). **b, c** Note improvement of the lower body contour as well as breast augmentation

55.4 Discussion

The technique of transplanting autologous fat obtained via liposuction has been generally accepted for soft tissue augmentation. Many reports have shown that much, if not all, of the transplanted fat is retained when small quantities are placed in adequately vascularized areas [4, 6–8]. Accordingly, when this method is used for breast augmentation, the injected amount needs to be limited to avoid remarkable resorption related to liquidization, necrosis, and cyst formation. However, there has been no definitive answer to the volume limit of how much can be successfully transplanted. Bircoll [1] described that this volume limitation appeared to be about 130 ml, whereas Fulton [2] mentioned that his limit was 300–350 ml. Although the illustrations in the latter report show attractive improvement in the breast appearance, the x-ray study showed the development of eggshell calcification around the lipid droplets. This suggests that the amount of fat injected was too much, resulting in liquefaction and/or necrosis of injected fat.

In the present case, the authors transplanted 200 ml of fat, which lost more than two-thirds of the volume during the follow-up period. This resorption was much more than was expected. The amount of injection, 200 ml, was considered too large for the small breast of our patient. The breast size is an important issue when determining the injection volume. The smaller the breasts are, the smaller the amount of fat injection should be.

Although the volume retention of the transplanted fat was low in our case, the remaining fat provided sufficient thickness to the breasts and prevented the firm feel resulting from saline-filled implants. This method of using fat injection together with saline-filled breast prostheses was found very useful for producing a natural look and soft touch of the breast.

Unfortunately, this procedure cannot be used for every patient. The search for donor sites can be a problem because many of the patients seeking augmentation mammoplasty seen in our clinic are very thin. The combined method described here is useful for those individuals who would benefit from fat injection for breast augmentation as described by Fulton [2]. The candidates should have a sufficient amount of disharmonious obesity. It has been described that the fat transplantation alone is indicated for a woman who will be satisfied with a small to modest size increase, such as increase by a single bra size or less [1, 2]. In contrast, a modest to even large augmentation of a small breast can be obtained with the presented technique.

References

1. Bircoll M: Cosmetic breast augmentation utilizing autologous fat and liposuction techniques. Plast Reconstr Surg 1987;79(3):267–271
2. Fulton JE: Breast contouring by autologous fat transfer. Am J Cosmet Surg 1992;9(3):273–279
3. Ersek RA: Transplantation of purified autologous fat: a 3-year follow-up is disappointing. Plast Reconstr Surg 1991;87(2):219–227
4. Horl HW, Feller AM, Biemer E: Technique for liposuction fat reimplantation and long-term volume evaluation by magnetic resonance imaging. Ann Plast Surg 1991;26(3):248–258
5. Har-Shai Y, Lindenbaum E, Ben-Itzhak O, Hirshowitz B: Large liponecrotic pseudocyst formation following cheek augmentation by fat injection. Aesth Plast Surg 1996;20(5): 417–419

6. Bircoll MA: Nine-year experience with autologous fat transplantation. Am J Cosmet Surg 1992;9:55–59

7. Niechajev I, Sevcuk O: Long-term results of fat transplantation: clinical and histologic studies. Plast Reconstr Surg 1994;94(3):496–506

8. Fournier PF: Facial recontouring with fat grafting. Dermatol Clin 1990;8(3):523–537

9. Klein J: Tumescent technique for regional anesthesia permits lidocaine doses of 35 mg/kg for liposuction. J Dermatol Surg Oncol 1990;16(3):248–262v

CHAPTER 56

Breast Augmentation with the Brava® External Tissue Expander

56

Ingrid Schlenz

56.1
Introduction

Millions of women all over the world are dissatisfied with the size of their breasts and are interested in breast enlargement [1, 2]. However, less than 1% of these per year have a surgical augmentation [3]. The majority of women are still reluctant to undergo surgery for cosmetic reasons; they fear possible complications of surgery and implants or are deterred by the costs [2].

56.2
History

In 1999 an external breast tissue expander (Brava® External Tissue Expander, Brava LLC, Miami, FL, USA, www.brava.com) was introduced as a nonsurgical alternative to breast augmentation. This device is based on the principle that any tissue (skin, bone, nerves, vessels, muscles) can grow if subjected to sustained gentle distraction. The Ilizarov procedure for lengthening extremities, the use of tissue expanders, and the new devices that have been developed to correct hypoplastic facial bones are all based on this principle [4–8]. In contrast to all of these other current approaches that require surgical intervention to introduce the force-transducing device into the body, Brava® can be applied from the outside. The device consists of two semi-rigid polyurethane domes with a silicone rim that are placed around the breasts and that interface the skin with gel-filled donut bladders. These bladder rims serve to maintain an airtight seal and to dissipate pressure and shear forces. A small battery-operated and microchip-controlled mini-pump maintains a 20-mmHg negative pressure inside the domes. This vacuum effectively exerts an isotropic distractive force to the breast. The entire system is contained within fabric and worn like a bra (Fig. 56.1).

Since 1999, several reports have confirmed that the distractive force exerted on the breast by the device can stimulate tissue growth and thereby effectively enlarge the breasts [9–13]. The first study was conducted with 17 participants who were advised to wear Brava® 10 h/day

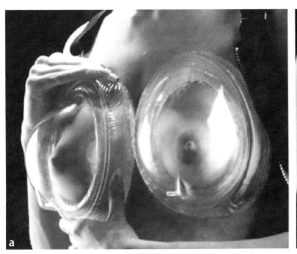 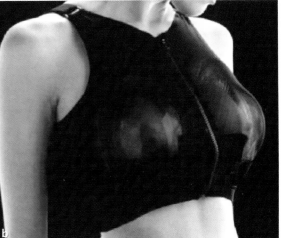

Fig. 56.1 a Woman wearing the Brava® system. **b** System is worn like a bra. (Reproduced with permission of Brava LLC, Miami, FL, USA)

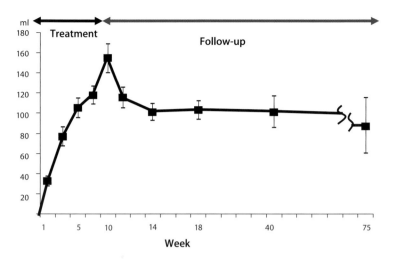

Fig. 56.2 Breast volume increase over the course of 10 weeks of treatment and an additional 30 weeks of follow-up. Measurements obtained by the bead displacement method. (Reproduced with permission of *Plastic and Reconstructive Surgery*)

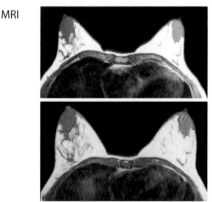

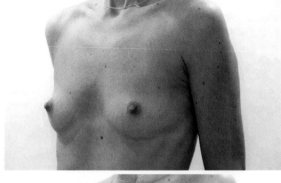

No edema

Even growth of glandular and fatty tissue

Normal architecture

Fig. 56.3 T1-weighted coronal magnetic resonance images of a participant at baseline (*above*) and after treatment (*below*) show an increase in size with a proportionate increase in fatty tissue (*white*) and fibroglandular tissue (*grey*). Note that there is no change in the distribution or appearance of the fatty or fibroglandular components. (Reproduced with permission of *Plastic and Reconstructive Surgery*)

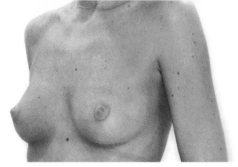

Fig. 56.4 a Pretreatment 42-year-old patient, one child, from the first study. **b** Thirty weeks after treatment. (Reproduced with permission of *Plastic and Reconstructive Surgery*)

for 10 weeks [9]. They were monitored closely for breast growth and compliance. Every 2 weeks, photographs were taken, and the breast volume was measured using three different methods. Twelve women completed the study, and five had to be excluded because of noncompliance to the wear protocol. At the end of the treatment period, the women's breast volume had doubled, and after 4 weeks the average increase was 100 ml (Fig. 56.2). All women had breast magnetic resonance imaging (MRI) before the study began and 4–6 weeks after the study ended, on days 6–12 day of their menstrual cycle. The MRI revealed an overall increase of breast size with preservation of the original breast architecture

(Fig. 56.3). All women were satisfied with the treatment (Fig. 56.4). Psychological testing revealed positive changes with regard to self-esteem and body image.

Because 10 weeks were considered too short after the first study, women were allowed to use Brava® as long as they wanted to in the second study, which was performed as a multicenter study throughout the United

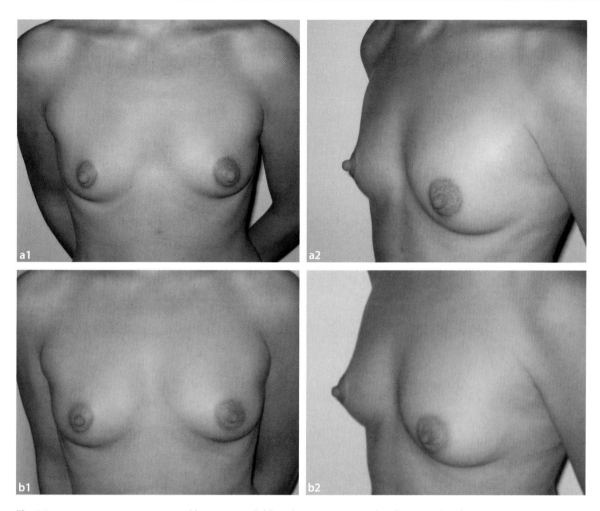

Fig. 56.5 a *1, 2* Pretreatment 27-year-old patient, no children. **b** *1, 2* Sixteen months after 22 weeks of treatment

States in 1999 [13]. In this study, 125 women were enrolled, and 95 finished. Noncompliance was again the major reason for dropping out (24 women). Skin problems and excessive weight changes (>5% body weight) were minor reasons. The results were similar to those of the first study—the women used Brava® for an average of 13.5 weeks (range 10–25 weeks), and the average increase was 108 ml (range 30–250 ml; see Fig. 56.5). This study provided a better understanding of how tissue growth takes place. Breast enlargement can already be seen after 2–3 days of use of the external breast expander.

In the beginning, the enlargement is due only to tissue edema. Real tissue growth takes place very slowly and only after prolonged use (Fig. 56.6). Therefore, longer and intensive wear results in better growth. At the end of treatment, the dissolution of the edema is responsible for the volume loss, while the real tissue

growth remains and seems to be long-lasting. So far, the longest follow-up has been 18 months (Fig. 56.7).

The second study also made clear that women respond differently to the Brava® treatment. Women who have children and have breastfed before experience visible tissue growth much more quickly because their breast skin has been stretched before. On the other hand, young women with a more masculine breast take much longer because their tight skin envelope is more resistant to stretching. This made clear that patience and motivation are prerequisites for successful treatment.

After the second study, Brava® became commercially available, and thousands of women all over the world used it, aiming at the one-cup enlargement promised in the media. However, in clinical experience, not all patients achieved the promised one-cup enlargement, and satisfaction with the results was variable among physicians and patients [9–13].

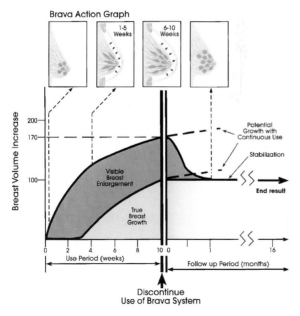

Fig. 56.6 Brava growth graph. (Reproduced with permission of Brava LLC, Miami, FL, USA)

A third study was undertaken to identify factors associated with a successful outcome [14]. Fifty women seeking breast enlargement without surgery were followed for up to 2 years. They purchased Brava® from Brava LLC, Miami, FL, USA. All women were informed about the need for consistent wear and that the minimum wear time was 10 h/day for a minimum of 10 weeks. Standardized photographs and volume measurements were made as proven successful by the other studies. At the final visit, the women completed a questionnaire to judge their results, any side effects, and their satisfaction with the treatment.

Data were analyzed statistically to evaluate the potential influences of body mass index (BMI), childbearing, initial breast volume, and intensity of wear (total use of the breast tissue expander, measured in hours) on the measurable breast volume increase. Of the 50 women enrolled, 40 (ages 17–53) could be evaluated. They used Brava® an average of 11 h/day for a median of 18.5 weeks (14–52 weeks). Posttreatment follow-up averaged 10 months (range 7–20 months). The median volume increase measured with the GRD was 155 ml (range 95–300 ml). Chest circumference at the height of the nipple increased by a median of 4.4 cm (1–11 cm). Measurements taken 4 weeks after the end of treatment remained constant until the latest follow-up.

All women stated that the treatment was painless. Side effects included sweating, itching, and skin irritation. Skin rashes were the most common problem; they occurred either within the first week when women with sensitive skin used the expander more than 10 h or after 6–8 weeks when the silicone rim was worn out or colonized with bacteria due to improper cleaning. Ten women developed rashes when they used the roll-on that was part of the first-generation skincare by Brava LLC. With the second-generation skincare and the development of a special dome cleanser, the skin rash problem was essentially resolved.

Thirty women (75%) were satisfied or very satisfied with the results. They felt that their breasts were fuller, firmer, and filled up or even outgrew their bras (Fig. 56.8). Five women (12.5%) acknowledged enlargement of their breasts but considered the treatment too bothersome for the result. Five women (12.5%) were disappointed because of little growth.

Factors associated with poor growth included lesser intensity of wear and low BMI (<18). Although most women stated that Brava® was not comfortable to wear and that their social life was quite restricted during the treatment period, 85.5% would recommend it to a friend.

56.3 Discussion

The principle of tissue expansion is well established in plastic and orthopedic surgery and is the only proven method of permanent tissue generation in the adult [4–8, 14]. The mechanisms by which sustained gentle mechanical tension induces tissue growth have recently been reviewed [15–18]. The external soft tissue expander Brava® for nonsurgical breast enlargement is the latest development based on this principle. Several controlled studies have proven that it is effective [9–13]. It is a good alternative for women looking for natural enlargement of their breasts if they fear the risks of surgery and implants. However, several factors make it difficult for the patient and physician to achieve the desired results [14].

As an external tissue expander, Brava® is compliance dependent and works well only for women willing to put up with the rigorous wearing schedule. Ten hours per day is the minimum required, and patients who are able to wear it longer show statistically significant better growth. While this does not seem to be a problem for some women who work or study while wearing the device, the majority of women have to restrict their social lives and spend their evenings at home in order to manage 10 h of wear per day. Because they have to do that for several months, it becomes understandable that some lose interest or do not manage to wear the device long enough. Therefore, it is of utmost importance to

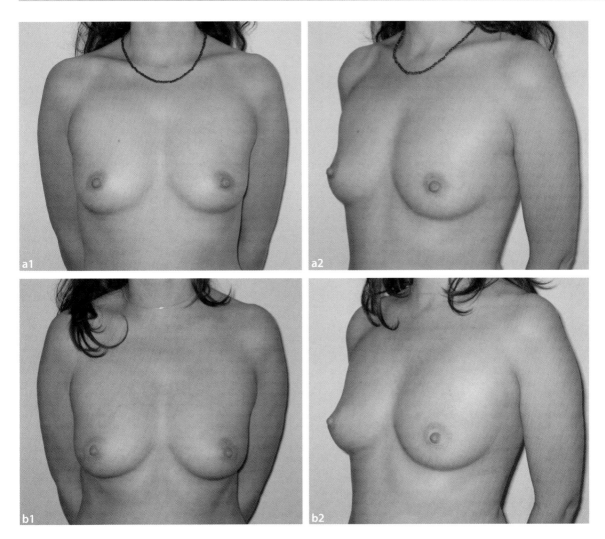

Fig. 56.7 **a** Pretreatment 41-year-old patient, one child. **b** Eighteen months after 24 weeks of treatment

inform women about the strict wearing protocol. They must consider whether they can comply before they decide to buy Brava®.

Second, it is difficult to keep women motivated if they perceive that their breasts are not growing. All of the studied women kept comparing their deflated breasts in the evening to the swollen, edematous breasts in the morning after taking off the domes, and they would forget how small their breasts were originally. Tissue growth takes place very slowly at about 1–1.5 ml per day of sustained use [1, 15] and is not comparable with the amount of swelling observed during the first weeks. Even after 10 weeks, 50% of the volume increase is due to swelling [9, 13]. Therefore, it is important to keep the women motivated by measuring their breasts and taking pictures to show them their progress.

Third, it is difficult to satisfy a woman with only 160 ml of growth, for example, after she has seen and prefers what her breasts look like with a 300-ml increase due to the swelling. Although all women were informed, before starting, that breast enlargement with Brava® is not comparable to that of an implant, and even though they had all stated that they would be happy with just a little more volume, they always wanted more once they had seen what their breasts could look like. Therefore, the physician has to critically evaluate the woman's breast size, BMI, and desired growth. It is unrealistic to fill a B cup if one starts with an AA and grows only 100–150 ml. However, more growth is unlikely if the BMI is <18 due to the small amount of body fat and a metabolic balance that is not permissive.

Another problem that led to complaints is that

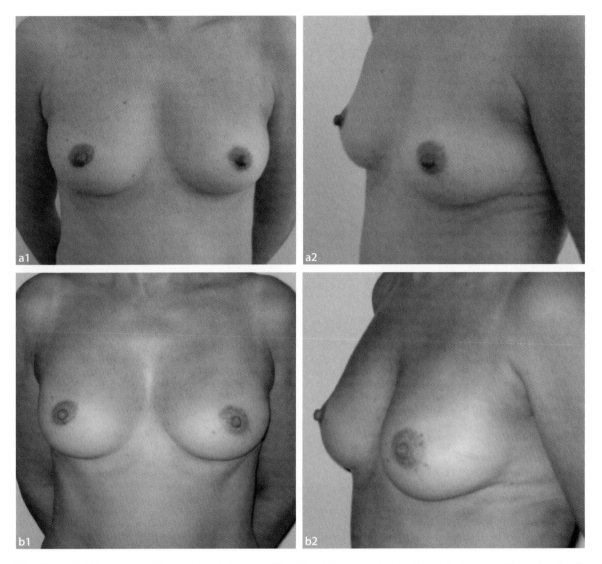

Fig. 56.8 a *1, 2* Pretreatment 39-year-old patient, two children. **b** *1, 2* Nine months after 16 weeks treatment (Reproduced with permission of *Plastic and Reconstructive Surgery*)

women were made to believe by advertisements that they could grow one cup within 10 weeks. It takes 16–20 weeks to grow that much. Women with small breasts tend to wear bras that are too big for them to make their breasts look bigger under clothes. After the treatment, they complained that they still wore the same bras, not considering that they now fit them. If before-and-after picture are taken with the same bra, this can easily be demonstrated (Fig. 56.9).

Most women use the Brava® system while they sleep. They have to be informed that it will take about 1 week to get used to it. Only six out of 120 women treated

since 1998 stated that they could not sleep with the device. Four of these stopped wearing it, and two stated that they would not have bought it if they had known how bothersome it was.

These difficulties and complaints must not make one overlook the fact that in the end, 75% of the women were satisfied or very satisfied with the results, and 85% would recommend it to a friend. In comparison to patients looking for breast implants [19], women interested in Brava® tend to have reached higher levels of education (72% had finished high school or acquired a university degree) and are very health-conscious as indicated by

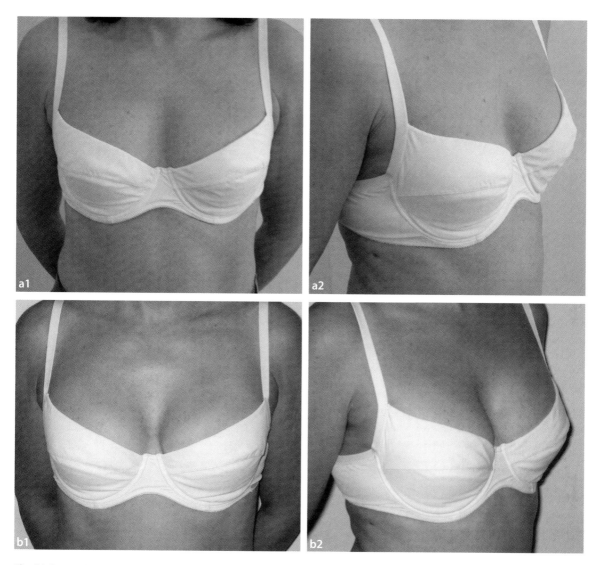

Fig. 56.9 a *1, 2* Pretreatment 39 year-old patient, with two children. **b** *1, 2* Nine months after 16 weeks of treatment (Reproduced with permission of Plastic and Reconstructive Surgery)

their diet and regular sport activities. The majority have been unhappy with the size of their breasts for many years but would never consider implants because they know of and fear their possible side effects. All women with children had lost volume after breastfeeding and stated that they just wanted to regain the size they had before pregnancy. The others also initially stated that they would rather have less growth than implants in their healthy breasts. The women were followed up to 2 years after the end of treatment, and they had kept the volume growth measured 1 month after discontinuing use. Figure 56.2 shows that after the initial volume loss

within the first 3 weeks after the end of the treatment, the volume remains constant. This confirms what has been found in the other studies: The remaining volume is real tissue growth and is long-lasting [13, 14].

56.4
Conclusions

The Brava® system is an alternative method of breast enlargement. It is aimed at a completely different group of women than breast implants and it works best for women who look for a one-cup enlargement and are happy with the shape of their breasts. Because the Brava® system can naturally enlarge breasts with virtually no side effects, every woman looking for a breast enlargement should be informed about it. However, to avoid disappointments and dropouts, patients have to be closely screened with respect to their motivation and expectations, as well as be informed about the rigorous wearing schedule and the time realistically necessary to achieve a one-cup enlargement. They should also be made aware that their social life will be restricted during the treatment period. Women with a BMI <18 and very small breasts should not be considered as Brava®candidates. Brava® will not replace implants but will bring women to the physician's office who otherwise would not have considered visiting a plastic surgeon.

References

1. National Clearinghouse of Plastic Surgery Statistics. Cosmetic surgery telephone survey, 1998
2. Hase/Shannen quantitative market research, 1999
3. American Society of Plastic and Reconstructive Surgeons. Plastic Surgery News, June 1999
4. Ilizarov GA: Clinical application of a tension-stress effect for limb lengthening. Clin Orthop 1990;250:8–26
5. Ilizarov GA: The tension-stress effect of the genesis and growth of tissues. Part I. The influence of stability of fixation and soft-tissue preservation. Clin Orthop 1989;238:249–281
6. Yasui N, Kojimoto H, Shimizu H, Shimomura Y: The effect of distraction on bone, muscle and periosteum. Orthop Clin North Am 1991;22(4):563–567
7. McCarthy JG, Schreiber J, Karp N, Thorne CH, Grayson BH: Lengthening the human mandible by gradual distraction. Plast Reconstr Surg 1992;89(1):1–8
8. Polley JW, Figueroa AA: Management of severe maxillary deficiency in childhood and adolescence through distraction osteogenesis with an external, adjustable, rigid distraction device. J Craniofac Surg 1997;8(3):181–185
9. Khouri RK, Schlenz I, Murphy B, Baker TJ: Nonsurgical breast enlargement using an external soft-tissue expansion system. Plast Reconstr Surg 2000;105(7):2500–2512
10. Greco RJ: Nonsurgical breast enhancement—fact or fiction? Plast Reconstr Surg 2002;110(1):337–339
11. Khouri RK, Rohrich RJ, Baker TJ: Multicenter evaluation of an external tissue expander system (Brava®) for breast enlargement. Proceedings of the Plastic Surgical Forum, ASPS Annual Scientific Meeting, 2–6 November 2002, p 168
12. Smith CJ: Initial experience with the Brava nonsurgical system of breast enhancement. Plast Reconstr Surg 2002;110(6):1593–1595
13. Baker TJ, Schlenz I, Khouri RK: A new device for nonsurgical breast enlargement: fifteen months follow-up. Proceedings of the Plastic Surgical Forum, ASPS Annual Scientific Meeting, October 2000, pp 113–114
14. Schlenz I, Kaider A: The Brava® external tissue expander: is breast enlargement without surgery a reality? Plast Reconstr Surg 2007;120(6):1680–1689
15. Neumann CA: The expansion of skin by a progressive distension of a subcutaneous balloon. Plast Reconstr Surg 1957;19(2):124-130
16. Ingber DE: Tensegrity: the architectural basis of cellular mechanotransduction. Annu Rev Physiol 1997;59:575–599
17. Sachs F: Biophysics of mechanotransduction. Memb Biochem 1986;6(2):173–195
18. De Filippo RE, Atala A: Stretch and growth: the molecular and physiologic influences of tissue expansion. Plast Reconstr Surg 2002;109(7):2450–2462
19. Brinton LA, Brown SL, Colton T, Burich MC, Lubin J: Characteristics of a population of women with breast implants compared with women seeking other types of plastic surgery. Plast Reconstr Surg 2000;105(3):919–927

Autogenous Augmentation Mammaplasty with Microsurgical Tissue Transfer

57

Mary E. Lester, Robert J. Allen

57.1
Introduction

Even though aesthetic surgery underwent an overall decline in 2006, the number of breast augmentation procedures increased 5% in the United States to over 380,000 [1]. Implant technology has improved since the first breast augmentations in the early 1960s; however, there are multiple sequelae from implant use, including capsular contracture, displacement, and rupture. Silicone implants can have a rupture rate of 26% [2]. Early complication rates have been estimated to be 9% and long-term complications as much as 23% [3].

The Mentor study found reoperation rates of breast augmentation procedures of 25% at 7 years [4]. For patients undergoing implant breast reconstruction, reoperative rates and capsular contracture rates at 7 years are 50% and 49%, respectively [4]. The dissatisfaction with implant breast cancer reconstruction has led to the use of autologous tissue. Similarly, implant complications have initiated alternative approaches to breast augmentation.

The benefits of autogenous tissue that have been learned from breast reconstruction can also be applied to breast augmentation. Autologous tissue has a decreased rate of infection, and treatment consists primarily of antibiotics. Avoiding the use of implants eliminates capsular contracture. The breast consists of skin, fibrofatty tissue, and glandular tissue. Autogenous flaps allow replacement of the breast with skin and fibrofatty tissue, thereby replacing like with like. Flaps will gain and lose weight with patients and also age appropriately. The ability of autologous tissue to mimic ptosis improves the natural appearance of the breast. Microsurgical flaps have additional benefits by providing adequate tissue from multiple sites while minimizing donor site morbidity. The most common flaps used are the superficial inferior epigastric artery flap (SIEA) and perforator flaps including the deep inferior epigastric artery flap (DIEP), superior gluteal artery flap (SGAP), and inferior gluteal artery flap (IGAP).

57.2
History

Partial breast reconstruction has been described with autologous tissues including flaps from the chest wall [5, 6]. The first reported autologous augmentation was with a deepithelialized latissimus dorsi myocutaneous flap by Hollos [7]. This procedure involves harvesting the skin and fat with a small strip of latissimus while preserving the thoracodorsal nerve and the majority of the latissimus muscle. Intercostal artery perforator (ICAP) and thoracodorsal artery perforator (TAP) flaps have been used in breast augmentation and take advantage of excess tissue in the lateral axillary fold [8]. TAP and ICAP flaps have primarily been used in partial breast reconstructions or symmetry procedures [6, 8].

However, in the patient with massive weight loss, the ICAP flap can be of sufficient volume for augmentation. Patients with massive weight loss may have complications with prosthetic augmentation because of poor soft tissue coverage. Their body habitus offers large volumes of tissue in the thoracodorsal artery and intercostal artery distribution for augmentation [9].

Other options for autologous augmentation include abdominal flaps and fat grafting. Transverse rectus abdominis myocutaneous (TRAM) flaps have been used to reconstruct the implant failure patient [10] and for primary augmentation [11]. Lai et al. [11] described difficulties in prosthetic augmentation in Asian women secondary to small body habitus. A small amount of breast tissue and a thin chest wall predispose to wrinkling and palpability of the implant. To circumvent this problem, they performed bilateral deepithelialized pedicled TRAM flaps in 14 patients. Mizuno et al. [12] described free-TRAM augmentation after excision of injected silicone. Fat grafting has also been performed for breast augmentation with large volumes injected in small aliquots [13].

SIEA, gluteal artery perforator (GAP), and DIEP flaps have been used for breast reconstruction since the early 1990s and have multiple advantages over the other autologous reconstructive techniques [14, 15]. They offer more volume than the axillary and latissimus donor sites. Compared with the TRAM flaps, they have less donor site functional impairment, less donor site hernia, less postoperative pain, and a shortened recovery time [16].

57.3
Technique

The abdominal tissue is the preferred donor site for the DIEP and SIEA flaps. The superficial vessels are always explored during abdominal flap harvest. The superficial inferior epigastric artery is present in 65% [17] to 72% [16] of patients. It involves harvest of the abdominal tissue without opening the anterior rectus sheath. The superficial inferior epigastric vein is also explored because it is frequently used to alleviate venous congestions. The DIEP flaps are based on one, two, or three perforators and involve no muscle sacrifice. Occasionally, the abdominal tissue is unavailable because of previous abdominal surgery, liposuction, or abdominoplasty. Patients may also be thin or nulliparous, or desire buttock flaps [18]. The SGAP and IGAP are based on one or two perforators.

The breast incision is most frequently inframammary, which allows adequate exposure of the internal mammary vessels. The incision length varies according to preoperative breast size and skin laxity. This incision can be extended along the lateral margin of the breast (Fig. 57.1). If the thoracodorsal vessels are used for recipient vessels, then an axillary incision can be used. Problems with the use of the thoracodorsal vessels and an axillary incision include a laterally displaced flap and fullness in the axilla.

A submammary pocket is created, which places the flap in a natural position, allowing for ptosis and decreased pain from lack of pectoral muscle stretching. A tissue expander can be placed within the pocket during flap harvest to stretch the skin envelope. The internal mammary vessels are the most frequently used recipient vessels. The 4th rib cartilage is removed for access to the internal mammary vessels during microsurgical anastomoses. The 5th rib can also be removed, but typically the internal mammary vein is small at this level. The Synovis Microvascular Anastomotic Coupler System (Synovis, Minneapolis, MN, USA) is often used for venous anastomosis in both the internal mammary and thoracodorsal recipient veins. Postoperative monitoring is performed via skin paddle assessment of color, temperature, capillary refill, and turgor. A small skin island is left in the inframammary fold (Fig. 57.2) [19]. If an

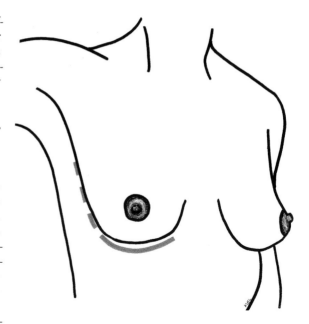

Fig. 57.1 The inframammary incision is most commonly used and can be extended along the lateral aspect of the breast. This incision is used with internal mammary recipient vessels. If the thoracodorsal vessels are the planned recipient vessels, then the incision is made along the anterior axillary line and extended to the inframammary area if needed

axillary incision is used, a skin island can be left in place also. However, if leaving a lateral skin paddle results in axillary fullness, then the Cook implantable Doppler probe (Vandergrift, PA, USA) is placed for monitoring. The implantable Doppler probes are usually a second choice compared with skin paddles for monitoring.

57.4
Results and Complications

From 1993 to 2002, 16 patients underwent autogenous augmentation. The age range was 16–62 years, with an average age of 35 years. Indications for augmentation included failed cosmetic implant augmentation, congenital deformity, symmetry in breast reconstruction, breast hypoplasia, and pectus excavatum (Table 57.1). These patients' photographs were evaluated by independent observers using the Netscher five-point grading system (Figs. 57.2–57.5) [20]. The observers were presented randomized photographs and were also blinded to preoperative or postoperative status.

The independent observers noticed a 65% improvement in Netscher points (Table 57.2). Patients also eval-

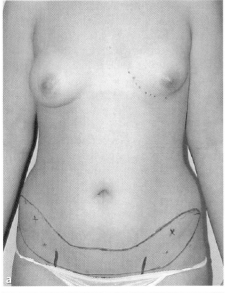
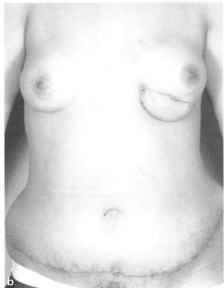
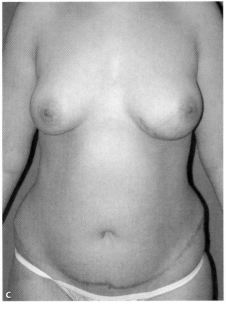

Fig. 57.2 a Preoperative 16-year-old with Poland's syndrome. **b** Early postoperative after superficial inferior epigastric artery flap. Note the skin island in place. **c** Postoperative photograph. Note that the skin island has been excised

uated their own postoperative results using Netscher points. Symmetry was rated at 3.8 on the right and 4.3 on the left, upper pole projection 3.8 on the right and 4.7 on the left, aesthetic proportions 4.3 on the right and 4.7 on the left, and ptosis 4.3 bilaterally [18].

Complications were associated with recipient and donor sites. Recipient complications included flap venous insufficiency, wound dehiscence, hematoma, seroma, and partial or total flap loss. Donor site complications included contour irregularities and seromas (Table 57.3). Donor site revisions primarily involved simple excision of dog ears with occasional liposuction or scar excision.

57.5
Discussion

Prosthetic breast augmentation has experienced increasing popularity without a significant decrease in the complications associated with implants. These complications have prompted numerous techniques for

Table 57.1 Indications for augmentation

	No. of flaps	No. of patients
Failed implant augmentation	6	3
Breast hypoplasia	3	3
Contralateral augmentation for symmetry in breast reconstruction	4	4
Poland's syndrome	3	3
Breast aplasia	3	2
Pectus excavatum	1	1
Total	20	16

From Allen and Heitland [19]

autogenous augmentation. Microsurgical and perforator flap augmentation has multiple benefits. Autologous tissue has a natural feel and appearance. Autologous tissue offers a lifetime reconstruction with the ability to adjust to the patient during weight change and aging. The additional benefits of SIEA, GAP, and DIEP flaps are decreased donor site morbidity and pain [21]. They remove excess tissue in areas that patients desire while providing adequate volume for breast augmentation. Implant complications such as reoperation, loss of nipple sensation, capsular contracture, asymmetry, implant removal, wrinkling, breast pain, infection, deflation, and so on are avoided [4].

Although microsurgical augmentation costs more than implant augmentation, it involves a decreased hospital stay, cost, and operating time compared with TRAM flaps [22]. We do not advocate using microsur-

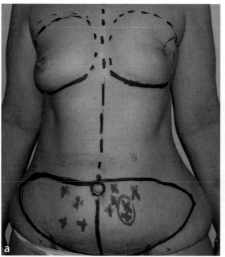
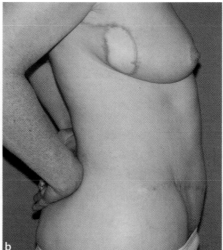
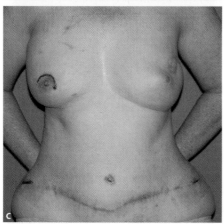

Fig. 57.3 a Preoperative 52-year-old woman who underwent lumpectomy and radiation for a left breast cancer. She desired left partial breast reconstruction and right augmentation for symmetry. **b** Early postoperative following left partial reconstruction and right augmentation using bilateral deep inferior epigastric artery flaps. Thoracodorsal vessels were used, and the incision was based on the anterior axillary line. The skin island is in place. **c** Postoperative after second-stage excision of the skin island, crescent mastopexy, and revision of dog ears

Table 57.2 Aesthetic outcome as judged by three independent examiners (SD standard deviation)

	Superior		Aesthetic		Summed
	pole	Ptosis	proportions	Symmetry	score
Preoperative score	2.2	3.0	1.9	2.6	9.7
SD	±1.2	±1.5	±1.2	±1.7	±4.1
Postoperative score	3.9	4.2	3.8	4.0	16.0
SD	±0.9	±0.8	±1.0	±1.0	±4.0
Difference	1.7	1.2	2.0	1.4	6.3
Percent change	77%	41%	104%	53%	65%

Adapted from Allen and Heitland [19]

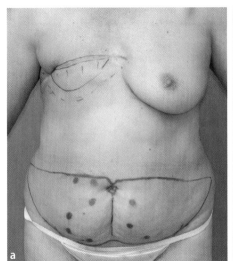
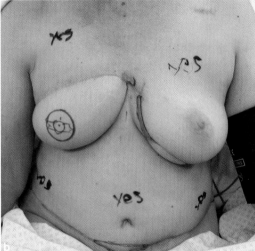

Fig. 57.4 a A 51-year-old patient with right breast cancer, status postmastectomy, chemotherapy, and radiation, who desired right breast reconstruction and left breast augmentation. **b** Postoperative right breast reconstruction and left breast augmentation with bilateral deep inferior epigastric artery flaps prior to a second-stage procedure in which she underwent right nipple reconstruction, excision of left breast skin island, and donor site revision

gical autogenous augmentation in every implant failure or for any other absolute indication. However, many patients desire a more natural and long-lasting augmentation. The ideal patient is one who desires augmentation and has excess abdominal or buttock tissue. Patients desiring symmetry for congenital or breast cancer reconstructions are also good candidates. Furthermore, implant failure patients are often unwilling to undergo another procedure involving a prosthesis and therefore desire autogenous reconstruction.

57.6
Conclusions

Microsurgical techniques provide a large volume of tissue with decreased donor morbidity and are therefore an excellent choice for augmentation. They provide a safe and reliable alternative for augmentation over prosthetic augmentation. Patients must be well informed of the advantages and disadvantages of microsurgical autogenous augmentation.

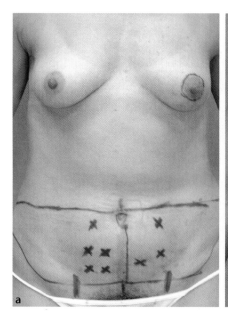
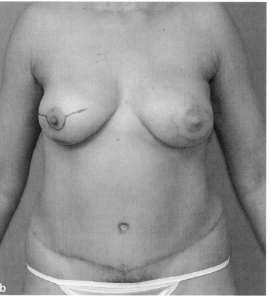

Fig. 57.5 a A 40-year-old patient with left breast cancer who desired immediate left breast reconstruction with right breast augmentation. **b** Postoperative left breast reconstruction with a superficial inferior epigastric artery flap and right augmentation with a deep inferior epigastric artery flap

Table 57.3 Complications at the recipient site and donor site

Complication	No.
Recipient site	
Wound dehiscence	5
Postoperative pain	3
Partial flap loss	2
Hematoma	2
Contour deformity	1
Seroma	1
Hypertrophied scars	0
Total flap loss	0
Total	14
Donor site second-stage procedures	
Skin island removal	10
Revision of abdominal contour deformity	5
Revision of buttock contour deformity	2
Mastopexy	3

Adapted from Allen and Heitland [19]

References

1. American Society for Aesthetic Plastic Surgery: 2006 Cosmetic Surgery National Data Bank Statistics
2. Holmich L, Kjoller K, Vejborg I, Conrad C, Sletting S, McLaughlin JK, Fryzek J, Breiting V, Jorgensen A, Olsen JH: Prevalence of silicone breast implant rupture among Danish women. Plast Reconstr Surg 2001;108(4):848–858
3. Clough K, O'Donoghue J, Fitoussi A, Nos C, Falcou M: Prospective evaluation of late cosmetic results following breast reconstruction: I. Implant reconstruction. Plast Reconstr Surg 2001:107(7):1702–1709
4. Mentor Corporation: Saline-filled breast implant surgery: making an informed decision. January 2004
5. Schneider W, Hill H, Brown R: Latissimus dorsi myocutaneous flap for breast reconstruction. Br J Plast Surg 1977;30(4):277–281
6. Levine J, Souied N, Allen R: Algorithm for autologous breast reconstruction for partial mastectomy defects. Plast Reconstr Surg 2005;116(3):762–767
7. Hollos P: Breast augmentation with autologous tissue: an alternative to implants. Plast Reconstr Surg 1995;96(2):381–384
8. Van Landuyt K, Hamdi M, Blondeel P, Monstrey S: Autologous breast augmentation by pedicled perforator flaps. Ann Plast Surg 2004;53(4):322–327

9. Kwei S, Borud L, Lee B: Mastopexy with autologous augmentation after massive weight loss: the intercostal artery perforator (ICAP) flap. Ann Plast Surg 2006;57(4):361–365

10. Spiro SA, Marshall D: Bilateral TRAM flaps for the reconstruction of the post implantectomy/capsulectomy breast deformity. Aesthetic Plast Surg 1996;20(4):315–318

11. Lai YL, Yu YL, Centeno R, Weng CJ: Breast augmentation with bilateral deepithelialized TRAM flaps: An alternative approach to breast augmentation with autologous tissue. Plast Reconstr Surg 2003;112(1):302–308

12. Mizuno H, Hyakusoku H, Fujimoto M, Kawahara S, Aoki R: Simultaneous bilateral breast reconstruction with autologous tissue transfer after the removal of injectable artificial materials: a 12-year experience. Plast Reconstr Surg 2005:116(2):450–458

13. Coleman S, Saboeiro A: Fat grafting to the breast revisited: safety and efficacy. Plast Reconstr Surg 2007:119(3):775–785

14. Allen RJ, Treece P: Deep inferior epigastric perforator-flap for breast reconstruction. Ann Plast Surg 1994;32(1):32–38

15. Allen RJ, Tucker C: Superior gluteal artery perforator free flap for breast reconstruction. Plast Reconstr Surg 1995;95(7):1207–1212

16. Allen R, Heitland A: The superficial inferior epigastric artery flap for breast reconstruction. Sem Plast Surg 2002;16(1):35–43

17. Taylor G, Daniel R: The anatomy of several free flap donor sites. Plast Reconstr Surg 1975;56(3):243–253

18. Guerra A, Metzinger S, Bidros R, Gill P, Dupin C, Allen R: Breast reconstruction with gluteal artery perforator (GAP) flaps. Ann Plast Surg 2004;52(2):118–125

19. Allen R, Heitland A: Autogenous augmentation mammaplasty with microsurgical tissue transfer. Plast Reconstr Surg 2003;112(1):91–100

20. Netscher D, Sharma S, Thornby J, Peltier M, Lyos A, Fater M, Mosharrafa A: Aesthetic outcome of breast implant removal in 85 consecutive patients. Plast Reconstr Surg 1997100(1): 206–219

21. Kroll S, Sharma S, Koutz C, Langstein HN, Evans GRD, Robb GL, Chang DW, Reece GP: Postoperative morphine requirements of free TRAM and DIEP flaps. Plast Reconstr Surg 2001;107:338

22. Kaplan JL Allen RJ: Cost-based comparison between perforator flaps and TRAM flaps for breast reconstruction. Plast Reconstr Surg 2000;105:943

Part VII
Complications

CHAPTER 58

Complications of Breast Augmentation

58

Anthony Erian, Amal Dass

58.1
Introduction

Breast augmentation is today considered a reliable operation with well-defined parameters and predictable outcomes. As with any other surgery, success of this operation depends on proper patient assessment, surgical planning, familiarity with the procedure, and good postoperative care.

Although the overall incidence of complications from breast augmentation is low, some of the complications are more frequently encountered in cosmetic surgery because of the sheer number of procedures performed. Detailed knowledge of the complications and their etiology is essential and must be considered from the time of initial consultation to postoperative care.

58.2
Capsular Contracture

Capsular contracture is the most common complication of breast augmentation surgery. There are three main themes that need to be considered with regard to capsular contracture:
1. The management of capsular contracture
2. The evolution of implants in response to it
3. Possible etiologies of capsular contracture and their influence on breast augmentation surgery

58.2.1
Management of Capsular Contracture

Capsular contracture is essentially an exaggerated scar around the breast implant. Any foreign material incites an immune response that results in some degree of scar formation, which in the case of breast implants surrounds them. With capsular contracture, however, there is exaggerated scar formation, which, if progressive, contracts around the implant, causing deformity and discomfort. This is in many ways similar to hypertrophic scarring, which can be described as overzealous healing.

The reported incidence of capsular contracture varies from 0.5% to 30% [1]. Capsular contractures are usually detected by palpation, though various other modalities such as applanation tonometry [2], measure of mammary compliance, ultrasonography, and magnetic resonance imaging [3] (Figs. 58.1, 58.2) have been employed, particularly in the context of clinical studies.

The Baker classification [4] remains the prevalent system for grading capsular contracture (Table 58.1). Grades III and IV capsules generally require intervention to correct distortions or alleviate discomfort.

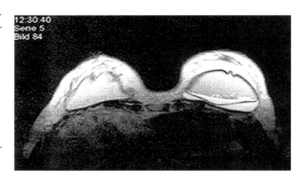

Fig. 58.1 Magnetic resonance image showing capsular contracture of the left breast

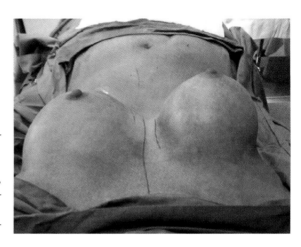

Fig. 58.2 Grade IV capsule of the right breast

Table 58.1 Baker's classification of capsular contracture

Grade I	No palpable capsule	Natural feel and appearance
Grade II	Minimal firmness	Feels harder but natural appearance
Grade III	Moderate firmness	Feels harder, some distortion, implant easily palpable
Grade IV	Severe contracture	Feels harder, tender, marked distortion with pain

Closed capsulotomy used to be a popular method of addressing significant capsular contractures, in which the capsule was torn by manually squeezing the breast until a tear was heard or palpated [5]. However, implant ruptures were common, as were hematomas, dumbbell deformity, silicone bleed, and incomplete capsular rupture [6, 7]. These complications have made this procedure obsolete. However, some surgeons still believe this maneuver may benefit those with early capsules in the immediate months following surgery.

Established capsules are dealt with in two primary ways:

1. Open capsulotomy
2. Open partial or total capsulectomy

Both of these procedures may involve implant removal, exchange, or reinsertion of the implant in a new pocket.

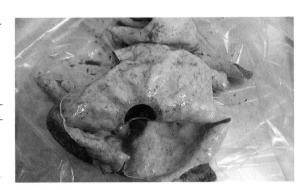

Fig. 58.3 Excised capsule after a total capsulectomy

58.2.1.1
Open Capsulotomy

The implant pocket is opened and reexplored. The capsule is then scored to achieve a release of the contracture caused by the capsule. The scoring may consist of circumferential or cross-hatched incisions of the capsule. Open capsulotomy is effective in early capsules, correction of asymmetries, and in patients with thin tissue cover in whom capsulectomy may result in skin penetration or devitalization of tissue.

58.2.1.2
Open Partial or Total Capsulectomy

Partial or total capsulectomy is indicated in thick fibrous capsules, capsules with significant calcification, and those with silicone granulomas that may need partial or total resection. Total capsulectomy (Fig. 58.3) virtually creates a new pocket for placing a new implant and is usually accompanied by inserting a new implant.

Changing the implant's placement is also a common way of dealing with capsule formation. The implant may be placed subpectorally if previously in a subglandular position and vice versa, providing adequate soft tissue cover [8]. Less commonly, a new pocket is created just in front of or behind the capsule.

58.2.2
Evolution of Implants in Response to Capsular Contracture

The very first implants made by Dow Corning were smooth, teardrop-shaped silicone implants with a Dacron fixation patch on the posterior surface [9]. These were plagued with an unacceptably high capsular contracture rate of up to 40% [10–12].

The Dacron patch was then removed because it was thought to be the cause of capsular contracture. However, the contracture rates still remained unsatisfactory. Thinner shells and less viscous gels were then used in a direct attempt to reduce capsular contracture. They resulted in a far greater incidence of implant leaking or rupture without significantly addressing the intended purpose [7].

Thus, by the 1970s most surgeons had few alternatives to the smooth silicone implant. Emphasis shifted to placing the implant from the subglandular to the subpectoral plane. Earlier trials involving subglandular placement with displacement exercises and implant massage led to improvements in the capsular contracture rate. This led to placement of the implant subpectorally, where massage by pectoral muscle contraction was expected to limit capsule formation around the implant. This was confirmed by a significant decrease in capsule contracture rates [13, 14]. Thus it was believed that the key to limiting capsular contracture was to maintain implant mobility within the pocket [1]. In fact, implant massage and displacement exercises are still recommended after implantation of smooth-walled prostheses. This serves to make the implant capsule more pliable and the implant mobile, with a lower likelihood that the capsule will contract.

The polyurethane-covered silicone implant was first introduced in the late 1960s. The polyurethane was found to shed from the surface of the implant, affecting the collagen orientation in the developing capsule and allowing the implant to remain soft without contracture of the capsule. Thus, it was now possible for implants to remain soft while immobile in a fixed pocket. The dramatic decrease in capsular contracture rates to fewer than 3% [15, 16] made these implants very popular in the 1980s until concern over the breakdown products of polyurethane led the manufacturer to withdraw them from the market in 1991 [8].

Then came advances in surface texturing of silicone implants. Texturing was thought to result in greater adherence of the implant surface to the developing capsule, resulting in thinner, more pliable capsules less likely to contract around them. This surface texturing, along with development of stronger cohesive silicone gels and a double-lumen protective barrier, created an implant less prone to bleeding or rupture that had a very low incidence of capsular contracture when placed subglandularly [17–20].

In a further twist, saline implants came back into vogue after the U.S. Food and Drug Administration (FDA) ruling on silicone implants in 1992. Although the capsular contracture rates were significantly decreased with saline implants, limitations such as rippling, folding, and palpability forced many surgeons to place these implants submuscularly [21].

Thus, the choice and placement of breast implants has been historically influenced by capsular contracture. This remains so today. Most of the data that show a lower rate of capsular contracture with saline implants compare them to the older-generation silicone implants, which were either nontextured or did not have a cohesive gel, leading to a higher bleed rate. Current evidence points to the newer generation of silicone implants as having low rates of capsular contracture in the subglandular position.

58.2.3
Etiology of Capsular Contracture

The cause of capsular contracture is thought to be multifactorial in origin but remains unconfirmed. There are, however, two main theories that attempt to explain it.

These relate to hypertrophic scarring and subclinical infection.

58.2.3.1
Hypertrophic Scarring

Hypertrophic scarring is thought to be triggered by an irritation such as hematoma, seroma, silicone bleed, or the silicone within the capsule itself, stimulating the formation of myofibroblasts within the capsule [22]. These myofibroblasts cause enhanced scar formation and subsequently contract, resulting in capsular contracture. The link between silicone in the implant shell and subsequent capsular contracture, or the link between hematomas and subsequent capsular contracture, has not been confirmed.

Corticosteroids, which are used for treating hypertrophic scarring of the skin, have been shown to decrease capsular contracture rates when used via intracapsular injections within the dissected pocket or when incorporated into the implant's double lumen [23]. However, steroid-related complications such as delayed wound healing, implant herniation, and thinning of tissues have prevented their use [24]. However, low-dose steroid irrigation may see a rise in popularity in the future following the approval of silicone implants for general use [1].

58.2.3.2
Subclinical Infection

Staphylococcus epidermidis is thought to cause an early subclinical infectious process that triggers more vigorous capsule formation [25]. One study suggested a possible link between capsular contracture with a biofilm covering the implant surface, which harbored *Staphylococcus epidermidis*. *Staphylococcus epidermidis* requires special identification techniques, which may explain why swab cultures are routinely negative.

Moreover, capsule formation was shown to be reduced with the use of local antibacterial agents, a finding that is further suggestive of a link. Subclinical infection would logically make total capsulectomy, site drainage, and insertion of a new breast implant the treatment of choice for capsular contracture [26].

The initial response to this link to bacterial infection was irrigation of the implant with Betadine (5% povidone-iodine), antibiotics, and a "no-touch" technique.

Betadine serves to disinfect the implant surface and has been shown to decrease the risk of capsular contracture. However, it was thought to weaken the implant surface, leading the FDA to issue a caution regarding its use. This has since not been substantiated [1].

Many surgeons now use antibiotic irrigation of the implant and the pocket prior to insertion. Commonly used is a combination of 50,000 units of bacitracin, 1 g cefazolin, and 80 mg gentamicin in 500 ml normal saline. This practice has been supported by favorable results from clinical studies that have shown a decreased capsular contracture rate with the use of antibiotic irrigation [27, 28].

The no-touch technique [29] involves handling the implant with fresh gloves with insertion through a sterile plastic sleeve or into a pocket treated with antibiotic irrigation in an attempt to reduce bacterial seeding of the implant. Many surgeons now routinely use both antibiotic irrigation and the no-touch technique with breast augmentation.

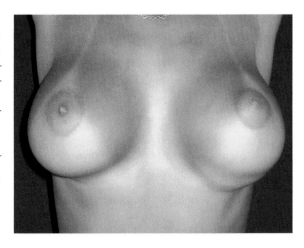

Fig. 58.4 Double bubble on the patient's left breast

58.2.3.3
Leukotriene Receptor Antagonists

Zafirlukast (Accolate) and montelukast (Singulair) are leukotriene receptor antagonists used in the treatment of asthma. Their use has been implicated in the reversal of capsular contracture via an abatement of inflammatory processes [30]. This has led some surgeons to prophylactically prescribe these medications. However, the medications can have side effects (including reversible drug-induced hepatitis), albeit uncommonly, and their use has not been validated by any significant clinical trials to date. Further research into the mechanism of action of these drugs may provide insights into preventing capsular contracture at a cellular level.

58.3
Implant Displacement

After capsular contracture, implant displacement is the second most common source of distress to the patient. It is usually caused by inappropriate dissection, erroneous incisions, capsular contracture, or malposition of initial placement. Displacement is usually inferior and is more commonly seen with the inframammary approach [31], with inferior migration of the implant probably due to disruption of the inframammary fold. Displacement may be associated with the double-bubble phenomenon (Fig. 58.4).

Superior displacement (Fig. 58.5) can also occur, particularly in submuscular augmentations in which repeated contraction of the pectoralis muscle drives the implant upward (although it can cause inferior migration of the implant as well).

If detected early, taping in the desired position for a few weeks may suffice. If this is unsuccessful, surgical correction is often necessary. Surgical correction may

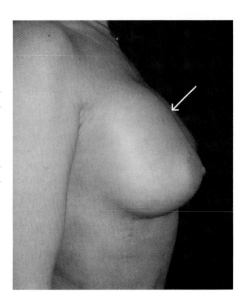

Fig. 58.5 Superior displacement (*arrow*) on the right side

involve dissecting the subcutaneous flap free and reapproximating the fascia of the chest wall with a nonabsorbable suture [31]. Any irregularities of the pockets are also corrected.

Improper or excessive pocket dissection can also result in synmastia and asymmetry.

58.4
Implant Rotation

The placement of anatomic implants requires creating an exact pocket into which the implant fits. Failure to

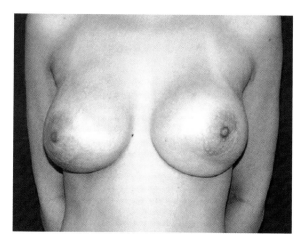

Fig. 58.6 Rotation of anatomic implant on the patient's left breast

accomplish this can result in rotation of the implants, which can be disfiguring (Fig. 58.6).

58.5
Implant Rippling

Rippling is either caused by traction of deficient tissue cover or an underfilled saline implant (Fig. 58.7) [1]. An underfilled saline implant especially has a tendency to knuckle, particularly in the lower poles where the shell actually folds in on itself. This is less commonly seen in silicone gel implants. With saline implants, it is customary to slightly overfill them and place them submuscularly to prevent this deformity. Implants can be palpable or visible (Fig. 58.8).

With traction deformities, the weight of the implant placed subglandularly tugs on the upper poles of the breast, causing traction wrinkles or rippling. This can be avoided by placing the implant submuscularly in women with deficient soft tissue cover.

58.6
Implant Deflation or Rupture

Implant deflation is usually seen with saline implants and can be caused by trauma or can be spontaneous. Underfilling of the implant, intraluminal antibiotics, and steroids are thought to be potential risk factors. Deflation rates of 5.5% have been reported with saline implants [23]. The only treatment is to replace the implant.

The incidence of silicone implant rupture has steadily decreased with successive generations of implants. Rates of less than 1% after 6 years have been reported with 4th-generation silicone implants. Rupture rates vary greatly with the type of implant used. Risk factors

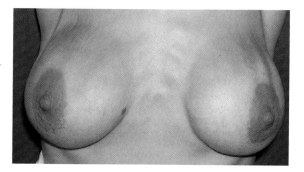

Fig. 58.7 Rippling

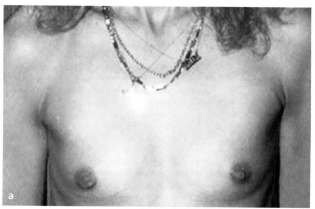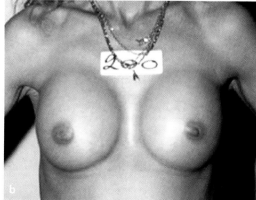

Fig. 58.8 Visible implant edges. **a** Preoperative. **b** Postoperative

are the type of implant [10], implant age [32], degree of capsular contracture, history of trauma (including mammography), and symptoms present [1].

Diagnosis and monitoring are achieved by palpation, mammography, ultrasound, or MRI. Intracapsular gel rupture can be treated by simple implant exchange, whereas extracapsular extravasation requires debulking, washout, and implant replacement.

58.7
Hematoma

The risk of developing a hematoma after breast augmentation is reported to be in the region of 3–4% (Fig. 58.9). Prevention of hematoma is important to minimize blood loss, relieve postoperative discomfort, and limit the incidence of capsular contracture. Before surgery, it should be ensured that the patient has not been on medications that promote bleeding.

Intraoperative hemostasis should be meticulous, with electrocautery of tissues to avoid blunt tissue dissection as far as possible. The dissection pocket should be irrigated with saline and drains inserted where necessary to prevent postoperative collections.

Hematomas usually present as either an expanding hematoma or as a delayed collection some 1–2 weeks after surgery. An expanding hematoma must always be surgically explored. An actively bleeding vessel is usually found; meticulous hemostasis is performed, and the pocket is irrigated and cleared of any excess blood before reinserting the implant. Small delayed collections can be left alone, bearing in mind the higher risk of capsular contracture. All other large or expanding collections are routinely explored.

58.8
Seroma

A seroma is a collection of serous fluid that collects when plasma seeps out of ruptured small blood vessels, with a contribution from inflammatory fluid. Seromas are usually small, nonexpanding collections. However, they can increase the incidence of capsular contracture because they provoke the inflammatory response forming the capsule. Persistent collections can be drained via ultrasonic guidance or by placing drainage catheters.

58.9
Infection

Infections can range from superficial wound infections to deep purulent infections of the implant pocket (Fig. 58.10). *Staphylococcus epidermidis* is the most frequently identified pathogen, making it an opportunistic infection. The risk of infection ranges from 2.0% to 2.5% in most studies.

Surgical technique and the patient's underlying condition are thought to be the most important determinants of infection. Many causes have been suggested but have been hard to pin down. These include a contaminated implant, contaminated saline, the surgery itself or the surgical environment, the patient's skin or mammary ducts, or, as suggested by many reports, seeding of the implant from remote infection sites. Late infection usually results from secondary bacteremia or an invasive procedure at a location other than the breasts.

Any delay in wound healing, unresolving wound erythema, or discharge must be promptly swabbed for culture along with initiation of antibiotics. An oral

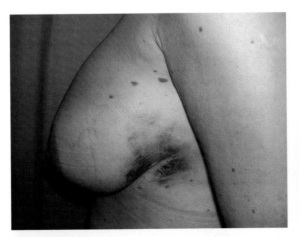

Fig. 58.9 Hematoma on left breast

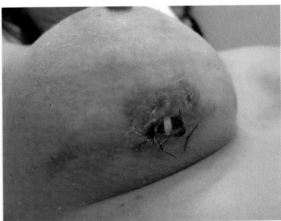

Fig. 58.10 Infection of right inframammary wound with improper scar position

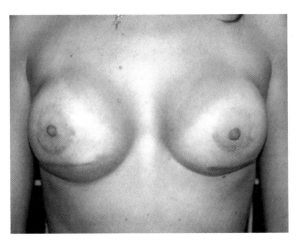

Fig. 58.11 Improper scar placement

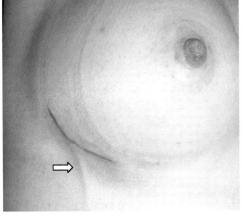

Fig. 58.12 Mondor's disease

2nd-generation cephalosporin is commonly used. Most wound infections are superficial and resolve with oral antibiotics with healing of the wound and tissues by secondary intention.

However, if unresponsive to antibiotics or with worsening symptoms such as pain, tenderness, distension, or cellulitis, reexploration is mandatory. The pocket is reopened and the implant removed, with thorough irrigation and debridement of the pocket. Reimplantation is delayed for at least 3 months. Broad-spectrum intravenous antibiotics are commenced, which can be converted to oral dosing once culture and sensitivity results from the wound swab are available.

As with any surgery, prevention is the key to limiting infections. Intraoperative aseptic technique should be meticulous. Intraoperative antibiotics such as intravenous cephalosporin, with continuation of oral antibiotics for 3–7 days postoperatively, are the norm. Antibiotic irrigation of both the implant and the pocket is usual, as is using the no-touch technique when handling the implant. If ever in doubt, always opt for implant removal with reimplantation after resolution.

58.10
Hypertrophic Scarring

Keloid and hypertrophic scars result from excessive collagen deposition, the cause of which remains elusive. Hypertrophic scarring can occur in 2–5% of patients, whereas true keloidal scars are uncommon.

Incision planning is important. Inframammary scars should be placed more laterally to avoid the sternal area, which is prone to aggressive scarring. Incisions should be planned and placed to maximally camouflage the scars (Fig. 58.11).

The periareolar incision is associated with a slightly lower incidence of hypertrophic scarring. However, if reexploration of the breast via the periareolar incision is required, scarring of the nipple–areolar complex can cause marked distortion or indentation of the nipple–areolar complex. Wound closure should be meticulous and in layers to approximate the epidermis under as little tension as possible.

Prevention remains the best strategy regarding keloid and hypertrophic scarring. Patients with a predisposition to develop excessive scar formation should avoid nonessential surgery. Hypertrophic scars and keloids have been shown to respond to radiation; pressure therapy; cryotherapy; intralesional injections of corticosteroid, interferon, and fluorouracil; topical silicone or other dressings; and pulsed-dye laser treatment. Simple surgical excision is usually followed by recurrence unless adjunctive therapies are employed. No one treatment has been shown to be superior to another, with most treatments only offering some improvement while falling far short of cure [33]. Intralesional steroids are a commonly used treatment modality that suffers from the pitfalls of skin atrophy, striae, and pigmentary changes and thus should be used judiciously.

58.11
Sensory Changes to Nipple–Areolar Complex

Changes in sensation of the nipple–areolar complex are usually due to stretching or irritation of the 4th lateral intercostal nerve, which supplies most of the nipple.

Care should be taken to preserve it during dissection, where it can be found at the 4 o'clock and 8 o'clock positions in the left and right breasts, respectively.

The periareolar approach is thought to have a slightly higher incidence of changes in nipple sensation, although recent evidence suggests otherwise [34]. Reports vary widely in reported incidences. However, it is generally agreed that patients be told that the risk of permanent alteration to nipple sensation is in the region of 3–5%.

58.12
Mondor's Disease

Mondor's disease is a superficial thrombophlebitis that occurs in 1–2% of patients, usually after an inframammary augmentation (Fig. 58.12). It is a self-limiting problem of unknown etiology that resolves several weeks after surgery. Any discomfort should be treated with anti-inflammatory drugs and/or warm compresses. The patient should be reassured.

58.13
Steroids and Other Complications

Steroids have been used intraluminally or via injections and irrigation to prevent capsular contracture. However, complications such as marked atrophy of breast tissues, delayed healing of wounds, and implant herniation due to localized atrophy of tissues quickly brought it into disfavor [24]. However, low-dose steroid irrigation may return in favor with the return of silicone gel implants to the American market.

58.14
Pneumothorax

Pneumothorax is a fortunately uncommon iatrogenic complication and is caused when administering an intercostal block or local anesthetic infiltration of the submammary space. Care should be taken to maintain the needle perpendicular to the ribs to avoid intercostal penetration when infiltrating local anesthetic. A wide-bore needle (18–20-gauge) should be used to administer an intercostal block so that the needle will not deflect or be bent into the intercostal space if a rib is accidentally encountered [31].

References

1. Maxwell PG, Hartley WR: Breast augmentation. In: Mathes SJ (ed). Plastic Surgery, 2nd edn. Philadelphia, Elsevier Saunders 2006, pp 1–33
2. Wong CH, Samuel M, Tan BK, Song C: Capsular contracture in subglandular breast augmentation with textured versus smooth breast implants: a systematic review. Plast Reconstr Surg 2006;118(5):1224–1236
3. Zahavi A, Sklair ML, Ad-El DD: Capsular contracture of the breast: working towards a better classification using clinical and radiologic assessment. Ann Plast Surg 2006;57(3):248–251
4. Baker JL Jr: Breast augmentation and capsular contractures. In: Barrett BM Jr (ed). Manual for Patient Care in Plastic Surgery. Boston, Little, Brown 1982
5. Baker JL Jr, Bartels RJ, Douglas WM: Closed compression technique for rupturing a contracted capsule around a breast implant. Plast Reconstr Surg 1976;58(2):137–141
6. Zide BM: Complications of closed capsulotomy after augmentation. Plast Reconstr Surg 1981;67(5):697
7. Feng LJ, Amini SB: Analysis of risk factors associated with rupture of silicone gel breast implants. Plast Reconstr Surg 1999;104(4):955–963
8. Hester TR Jr, Tebbetts JB, Maxwell GP: The polyurethane-covered mammary prosthesis: facts and fiction (II): a look back and a "peek" ahead. Clin Plast Surg 2001;28(3):579–586
9. Cronin T, Gerow F: Augmentation mammaplasty; a new natural feel prosthesis. Transactions of the 3rd International Congress of Plastic Surgery. Amsterdam, Excerpta Medica Foundation 1964:41
10. Biggs TM, Yarish RS: Augmentation mammaplasty: retropectoral versus retromammary implantation. Clin Plast Surg 1988;15(4):549–555
11. Burkhardt BR: Capsular contracture: hard breasts, soft data. Clin Plast Surg 1988;15(4):521–532
12. Hidalgo DA: Breast augmentation: choosing the optimal incision, implant, and pocket plane. Plast Reconstr Surg 2000;105(6):2217–2218
13. Puckett CL, Croll GH, Reichel CA, Concannon MJ: A critical look at capsule contracture in subglandular versus subpectoral mammary augmentation. Aesthet Plast Surg 1987;11(1):23–28
14. Woods JE, Irons GB Jr, Arnold PG: The case for submuscular implantation of prostheses in reconstructive breast surgery. Ann Plast Surg 1980;5(2):115–122
15. Gasperoni C, Salgarello M, Gargani G: Polyurethane-covered mammary implants: a 12-year experience. Ann Plast Surg 1992;29(4):303–308
16. Pennisi VR: Long-term use of polyurethane breast prostheses: a 14-year experience. Plast Reconstr Surg 1990;86(2):368–371

17. Embrey M, Adams EE, Cunningham B, Peters W, Young VL, Carlo G: A review of the literature on the etiology of capsular contracture and a pilot study to determine the outcome of capsular contracture interventions. Aesthetic Plast Surg 1999;23(3):197–206

18. Coleman DJ, Foo IT, Sharpe DT: Textured or smooth implants for breast augmentation? A prospective controlled trial. Br J Plast Surg. 1991;44(6):444–448

19. Hakelius L, Ohlsen L: Tendency to capsular contracture around smooth and textured gel-filled silicone mammary implants: a five-year follow-up. Plast Reconstr Surg 1997;100(6):1566–1569

20. Gylbert L, Asplund O, Jurell G: Capsular contracture after breast reconstruction with silicone-gel and saline-filled implants: a 6-year follow-up. Plast Reconstr Surg 1990;85(3):373–377

21. Hudson DA: Submuscle saline breast augmentation: are we making sense in the new millennium? Aesthetic Plast Surg 2002;26(4):287–290

22. Baker JL Jr, Chandler ML, LeVier RR: Occurrence and activity of myofibroblasts in human capsular tissue surrounding mammary implants. Plast Reconstr Surg. 1981;68(6):905–912

23. Gutowski KA, Mesna GT, Cunningham BL: Saline-filled breast implants: a Plastic Surgery Educational Foundation multicenter outcomes study. Plast Reconstr Surg 1997;100(4):1019–1027

24. Carrico TJ, Cohen IK: Capsular contracture and steroid-related complications after augmentation mammaplasty. A preliminary study. Plast Reconstr Surg. 1979;64(3):377–380

25. Virden CP, Dobke MK, Stein P, Parsons CL, Frank DH: Subclinical infection of the silicone breast implant surface as a possible cause of capsular contracture. Aesthet Plast Surg. 1992;16(2):173–179

26. Pajkos A, Deva AK, Vickery K, Cope C, Chang L, Cossart YE: Detection of subclinical infection in significant breast implant capsules. Plast Reconstr Surg 2003;111(5):1605–1611

27. Burkhardt BR, Dempsey PD, Schnur PL, Tofield JJ: Capsular contracture: a prospective study of the effect of local antibacterial agents. Plast Reconstr Surg 1986;77(6):919–932

28. Adams WP Jr, Rios JL, Smith SJ: Enhancing patient outcomes in aesthetic and reconstructive breast surgery using triple antibiotic breast irrigation: six-year prospective clinical study. Plast Reconstr Surg 2006;118(7 suppl):46S–52S

29. Mladick RA: "No-touch" submuscular saline breast augmentation technique. Aesthet Plast Surg. 1993;17(3):183–192

30. Scuderi N, Mazzocchi M, Fioramonti P, Bistoni G: The effects of zafirlukast on capsular contracture: preliminary report. Aesthet Plast Surg 2006;30(5):513–520

31. Baker JL Jr: Augmentation mammaplasty. In: Peck GC (ed). Complications and Problems in Aesthetic Plastic Surgery. Hampshire, UK, Gower 1992

32. Rohrich RJ, Adams WP Jr, Beran SJ, Rathakrishnan R, Griffin J, Robinson JB Jr, Kenkel JM: An analysis of silicone gel-filled breast implants: diagnosis and failure rates. Plast Reconstr Surg 1998;102(7):2304–2308; discussion 2309

33. Leventhal D, Furr M, Reiter D: Treatment of keloids and hypertrophic scars: a meta-analysis and review of the literature. Arch Facial Plast Surg 2006;8(6):362–368

34. Mofid MM, Klatsky SA, Singh NK, Nahabedian MY: Nipple–areola complex sensitivity after primary breast augmentation: a comparison of periareolar and inframammary incision approaches. Plast Reconstr Surg 2006;117(6):1694–1698

CHAPTER 59

Less Common Complications of Breast Augmentation

Melvin A. Shiffman

59.1
Introduction

There are a number of complications from breast augmentation that are not common. The surgeon performing breast augmentation should be aware of these complications and understand the possible cause and the treatment.

59.2
Areolar Retraction

Areolar retraction occurs from fibrotic bands extending from the areola to the underlying fascia (Fig. 59.1). Treatment consists of changing the implant from the submuscular position to the submammary position. Transecting or resecting the fibrous band alone will almost always result in recurrence of the indentation.

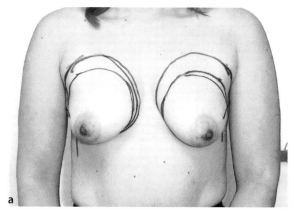

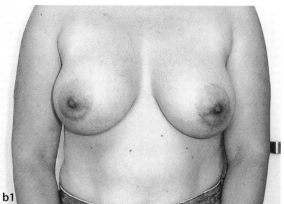

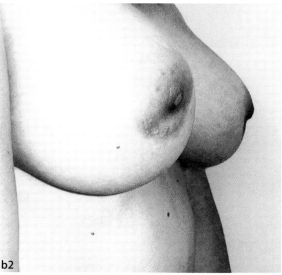

Fig. 59.1 Areolar retraction. **a** Preoperative. **b** *1, 2* Postoperative with areolar retraction

59.3
Axillary Banding

There have been reports of transient axillary banding in patients following the transaxillary approach to breast augmentation [1–4]. Maximovich [1] reported that microscopic examination (done by Ellenbogen) showed the band to be "lymphatic" in origin.

The band is more likely a phlebitis of a superficial vein of the axilla and medial upper arm (branch of basilic vein) [5, 6] that is another form of Mondor's disease. A superficial lymphatic vessel has never been reported to form a thick subcutaneous band and superficially would not be large enough to form a fibrous band that would be palpable and visible.

Mondor's disease (superficial breast phlebitis, sclerosing breast phlebitis) is an obliterative phlebitis of the thoracoepigastric vein, frequently with a history of trauma. The phlebitis normally crosses the anterior chest region and breast from the epigastrium or hypochondriac region to the axilla. The symptoms are usually a red linear cord attached to the skin, not to the deep fascia, with slight to no discomfort. Manifestations usually disappear in 3–6 weeks without treatment. For discomfort, minor analgesics and the application of heat will help. Injection of steroids is not usually necessary, and surgical transection is unnecessary.

A recent suggestion by Rassel, Borsand, and Jonov for symptomatic Mondor's disease is to stabilize the proximal portion of the vessel with the operator's thumb. Very firm pressure is placed along the direction of the vessel with the operator's opposite thumb, as if "milking" the vessel (Fig. 59.2). While the operator's upper hand is stabilizing the vessel, the inferior hand applies a firm downward stroke. This disrupts the cord and resolves the problem, including the pain (Fig. 59.3).

59.4
Autoinflation, Spontaneous

There have been reports of spontaneous autoinflation of implants [7–11].

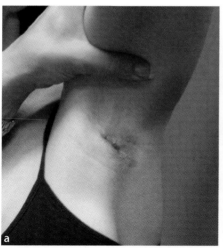
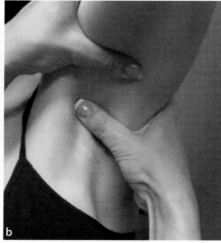

Fig. 59.2 Mondor's disease (axilla). **a** Thumb firmly on proximal portion of the cord. **b** Opposite thumb on distal portion of the cord for firm stretch of cord

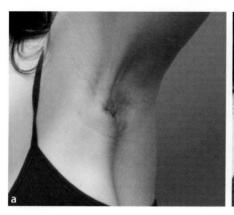
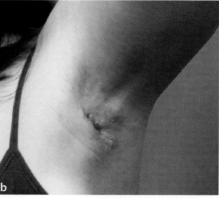

Fig. 59.3 Mondor's disease (axilla). **a** Prior to stretch type of manipulation. **b** After manipulation

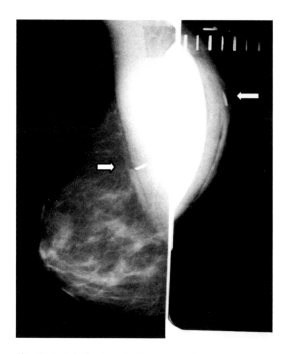

Fig. 59.4 Calcifications in fibrous capsule

59.5
Calcifications

Any long-standing fibrous capsule can develop calcifications (Fig. 59.4). These are usually asymptomatic. The calcifications appear benign on mammography. When the fibrous capsule is thick and calcifications occur, capsule contracture may be present as well. Calcifications may be associated with the presence of the implant stabilization patch [12].

If the calcifications are extensive and associated with symptomatic capsule contracture, capsulectomy should be performed rather than capsulotomy. Otherwise, the remaining calcified fibrous capsule may be palpable.

59.6
Chronic Pain

Chronic pain can occur following breast augmentation from capsule contraction, nerve entrapment (Fig. 59.5), neuromas, or submuscular placement of the prosthesis. With 4th intercostal nerve entrapment, the pain may be sharp or burning in character, starting in the lateral breast, over the nerve, and radiating to the nipple–areola complex. Regional block of the 4th intercostal nerve may help, but surgical neurolysis is usually necessary.

Delayed onset (years) of breast and subscapular pain was reported in eight out of 146 patients who had sub-

muscular placement of prostheses (under the pectoralis major and serratus anterior muscles) [13].

59.7
Capsule Contracture

Instead of surgical treatment of capsule contracture, there have been proposals that Accolate (zafirlukast; AstraZeneca Pharmaceuticals, Wilmington, DE, USA) be used. There has been some success with softening of the capsule with the drug. The dose is 20 mg twice daily.

59.8
Double Bubble

The cause of the appearance of a double bubble is usually that the implant was placed under the pectoralis major muscle and the inframammary fold lowered. The attachment of the skin to the underlying fascia from the original inframammary fold, if it was not adequately broken up during surgery, gives the appearance of a double bubble (Fig. 59.6). During surgery the ligament between the muscle fascia and the skin should be transected, and it may be necessary to make multiple incisions into the fibrous tissue before expanding the crease with the finger and/or a dissection paddle. This can be resolved postoperatively by postoperative compressions to push the fold outward (Fig. 59.6).

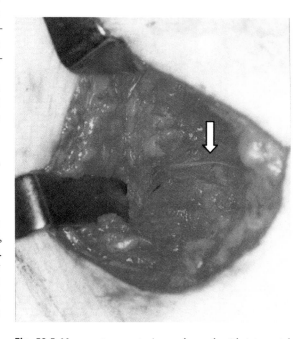

Fig. 59.5 Nerve entrapment. *Arrow* shows the 4th intercostal nerve on the fibrous capsule of the implant

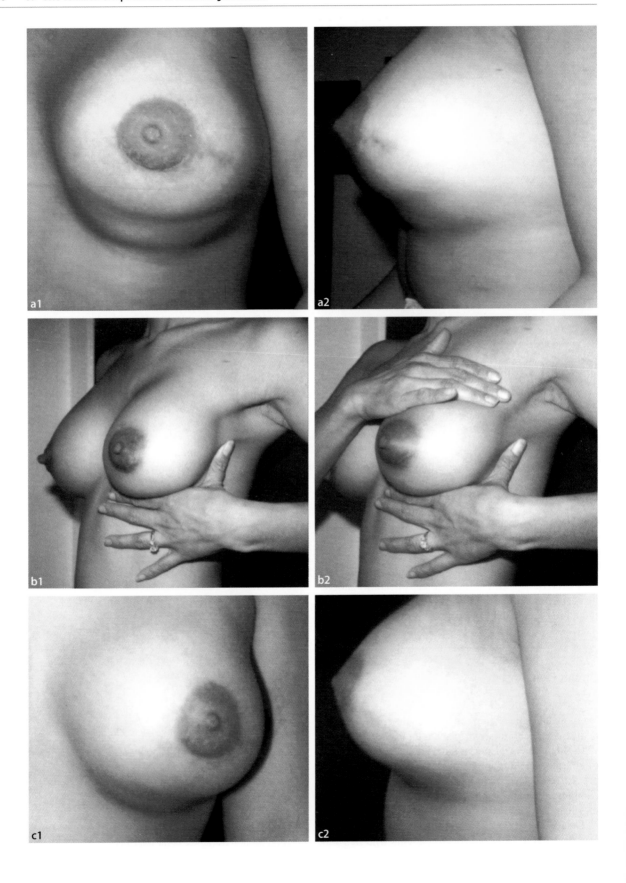

◄ **Fig. 59.6** **a** *1, 2* Immediate postoperative double bubble with submuscular implant. **b** Treatment consists of compressing the inframammary fold with the ipsilateral hand (*1*) and then compressing the upper breast and implant with the contralateral hand (*2*), using firm pressure several times, at least four times daily, to stretch the attachment. **c** One month after treatment (*1*). Only minimal attachment remains (*2*), which resolved completely after 3 months

The treatment would be to take the implant out of the subfascial space and replace it in the submammary space. The use of Gore-Tex or autologous fat to fill the defect is unnecessary.

59.9
Elevated Platinum Levels

There has been one report, by Lykissa and Maharaj [14], on the platinum levels in a variety of tissues of patients who had silicone and saline implants for augmentation. There was an increase in the platinum levels in implant patients that was higher than in the normal population. However, no symptoms or disorders have been attributed to these elevated levels.

59.10
Fibrotic Retraction

Fibrosis at the inferior margin of the implant is rare (Fig. 59.7). It is probably caused by excessive scarring in the area, such as with capsule contracture.

59.11
Galactorrhea

Rothkopf and Rosen [15] reported on a patient with galactorrhea following breast augmentation. The patient's

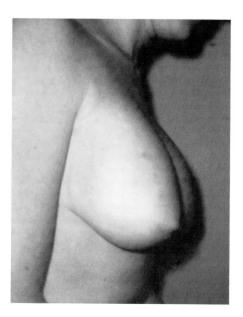

Fig. 59.8 Implant placed too high

prolactin levels were elevated. It was presumed that the lactation was secondary to prolactin elevation due to stimulation of the thoracic nerve endings, which produced impulses that traveled via the dorsal nerve roots to the hypothalamus and pituitary, causing a rise in prolactin secretion.

There have been other reports of lactation following breast augmentation [16, 17]. Oral bromocriptine 1.25 mg daily will usually resolve the problem.

59.12
Idiosyncratic Allergic Reaction

There is one report of an idiosyncratic reaction to textured Becker expander saline implants [18] (see Chap. 70). The patient developed erythematous papules and pustules that showed a perivascular lymphohistiocytic infiltrate, a condition that resolved with removal of the implants. The textured shell patch was placed on the skin, and itching, hives, and urticarial plaques developed under the patch.

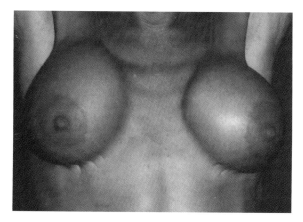

Fig. 59.7 Fibrotic retraction

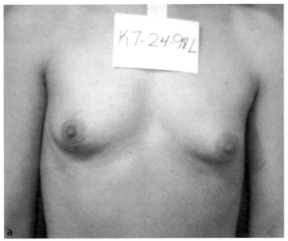
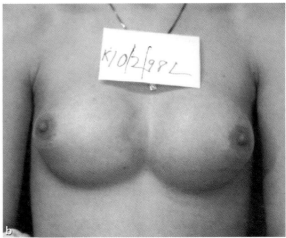

Fig. 59.9 a Preoperative. **b** Implant placed too medially to give the patient more cleavage

59.13
Improper Implant Placement

Implants may be placed too high because of inadequate dissection of the pocket at the inframammary fold (Fig. 59.8). This is most common during the learning phase of the umbilical approach. More often the implant shifts upward when the patient is at home and remains in that position too long. Postoperatively compressing the superior portion of the breasts with an Ace bandage will usually prevent the upward shift of the prosthesis. In the umbilical approach for breast augmentation, there is a learning curve to produce an adequate pocket and compression to keep the implant in position. Many times in the umbilical approach, the implant will slowly settle into the proper position.

When a patient requests a large cleavage fold, there is only so much the surgeon can do, depending on the nipple position and what will occur with the implant placement centered under the nipple. Placing the implant too medially just to create cleavage is a serious error: This is a cosmetic procedure, and nipples shifted outward are aesthetically poor (Fig. 59.9).

59.14
Lactation Problems

There have been reports of inability to produce enough breast milk to breastfeed an infant following breast augmentation [19–22].

The causes of unsuccessful lactation include inadequate glandular development [22], the periareolar approach [19], severed milk ducts [19], altered nipple sensation [19], and lack of or few breast changes during pregnancy, with little or no postpartum engorgement [19].

59.15
Late Bleeding After Breast Augmentation

There are multiple reports of late bleeding into the pocket after breast augmentation [23–28]. Some of the causes have been attributed to chronic inflammatory reaction to a polyurethane-coated implant, granulating tissue with new capillary ingrowth, and the use of corticosteroids in saline prostheses. Another cause that should be ruled out is blood dyscrasia.

59.16
Malposition of the Inframammary Scar

Breast augmentation scars should be as inconspicuous as possible. Scars can be hidden in the transumbilical approach as well as the axillary approach. Axillary scars can become thickened. The position of an inframammary scar should be close to the inframammary crease, within a centimeter, but not in the crease itself because this can result in irritation of the scar by the brassiere's elastic band or wire rubbing the scar.

If the incision is placed too far above the inframammary fold, it will cause a problem when a surgeon is performing a repeat augmentation and inserting a larger prosthesis. This can result in an inframammary scar appearing even higher on the breast and away from the inframammary fold (Fig. 59.10).

59.17
Methicillin-Resistant *Staphylococcus aureus* Infection

Methicillin-resistant *Staphylococcus aureus* (MRSA) is now the most common contaminant of surgical infections. (Previously it was *Staphylococcus aureus* and *Pseudomonas*.)

In one legal case that involved the author, the plastic surgeon delayed taking a culture and sensitivity of an infected wound following insertion of expanders in a patient with breast carcinoma treated with bilateral mastectomies [29]. Culture and sensitivity after the implants were removed showed MRSA sensitive to vancomycin, tetracycline, rifampin, and trimethoprim-sulfamethoxazole. For 5 months the patient was treated with antibiotics that were not sensitive to MRSA despite the sensitivities on the culture and sensitivity having been received, patient temperatures ranging from 102° to 104.4°, and even the need for debridement of the chest wound, with infection invading the rib. The patient developed extensive osteomyelitis involving the sternum and ribs that required resection of ribs and sternum.

59.18
Community-Acquired Methicillin-Resistant *Staphylococcus aureus* (CA-MRSA)

Community-acquired methicillin-resistant *Staphylococcus aureus* (CA-MRSA) is becoming an increasingly important, major pathogen [30–32]. Particular strains of MRSA have recently arisen in community-acquired cases that have been identified by pulsed-field gel electrophoresis typing as USA300; these strains have genetic differences from the typical strain that has been circulating [33].

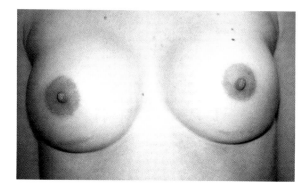

Fig. 59.10 Scar malposition with inframammary incision sites too high on the breast

The USA300 and USA400 strains are quite different from the typical hospital-acquired MRSA (HA-MRSA) [34, 35]. The USA300 strain occurs in diverse regions of the United States [36], while the USA400 strain has been found in several outbreaks and "endemic" CA-MRSA infections in the U.S. Midwest [37].

CA-MRSA accounts for 59% of skin infections (ranging from 15% to 74% in different cities). The drug-resistant strain can cause painful skin lesions that resemble infected spider bites, necrotizing pneumonia, or toxic shock syndrome. CA-MRSA is resistant to erythromycin, cephalexin (Keflex), and dicloxacillin (Diclocil), and is more or less susceptible to clindamycin, fluoroquinolones, tetracycline, rifampin, and trimethoprim-sulfamethoxazole [34, 35, 38].

Moran et al. [38] studied skin and soft tissue infections seen in emergency departments in Los Angeles with cultures and clinical information. Staphylococcus aureus isolates were characterized by antimicrobial susceptibility testing, pulsed-field gel electrophoresis, and detection of toxin genes. On MRSA isolates, typing of the staphylococcal cassette chromosome mec (SCCmec), the genetic element that carries the mecA gene encoding methicillin resistance, was performed. The presence of MRSA was 57% overall (ranging from 15% to 74%). Pulsed-field type USA300 isolates accounted for 97% of MRSA isolates; 74% of these were a single strain (USA300-0114). SCCmec type IV and the Panton–Valentine leukocidin (PVL) toxin gene were detected in 98% of MRSA. Among the MRSA isolates, 100% were susceptible to rifampin and trimethoprim-sulfamethoxazole, 95% to clindamycin, 92% to tetracycline, and 60% to fluoroquinolones. When antimicrobial therapy is indicated to treat skin and soft tissue infections, clinicians should consider obtaining cultures and modifying empiric therapy to provide MRSA coverage.

59.18.1
Virulence

Virulence factors may allow pathogens to adhere to surfaces and invade or avoid the immune system while causing toxic effects to the host [39]. Exotoxins related to the infection may be produced [40]. Superantigens that have been identified include toxic shock syndrome toxin-1 (TSST-1), staphylococcal enterotoxin serotype B (SEB), and staphylococcal enterotoxin serotype C (SEC). Along with PVL, these toxins are associated with toxic shock syndrome, purpura fulminans, and hemorrhagic necrotizing MRSA pneumonia [40–42]. The superantigens induce massive cytokine release from T cells and macrophages. The ensuing hypotension and shock are believed to be the result of activity mediated by tumor necrosis factor-α (TNF-α) and tumor necrosis factor-β (TNF-β) [40]. There is a 70% mortality rate from community-acquired pneumonia caused by PVL-positive CA-MRSA [42].

PVL has a possible role in virulence, either directly or as a marker for closely associated pathogenic factors. PVL is a two-component staphylococcal pore-forming membrane cytotoxin that operates by targeting mononuclear and polymorphonuclear cells, producing severe inflammatory lesions, capillary dilation, chemotaxis, polymorphonuclear karyorrhexis, and tissue necrosis [34, 39].

59.18.2
Reservoirs and Transmission

Humans serve as a reservoir for Staphylococcus aureus through asymptomatic colonization [34]. Higher carriage rates of Staphylococcus aureus compared with the general population are associated with intravenous drug users, insulin-dependent diabetics, patients with dermatologic conditions, patients with indwelling catheters, and healthcare workers [34, 43].

59.18.3
Prevention and Management

To prevent the spread of MRSA in hospitals, it is recommended that those at higher risk for MRSA carriage be screened at admission and isolated if found to be colonized [44]. Surfaces in examination rooms should be cleaned with commercial disinfectants or diluted bleach (1 tablespoon to 1 quart of water), and wound dressings and other materials that come into contact with pus, nasal discharge, blood, or urine should be disposed of carefully [31]. Healthcare providers need to wash their hands between contact with patients [25] and should use barrier precautions and don fresh gowns and gloves for contact with each patient [45, 46].

Guidelines have been developed by the Centers for Disease Control (CDC) for preventing infection among members of competitive sports teams and others in close contact: Individuals should avoid sharing equipment and towels, common surfaces should be cleaned on a regular basis, wounds should be covered, individuals with potentially infectious skin lesions should be excluded from practice and competition until the lesions have healed or are covered, and frequent showering and the use of soap and hot water should be encouraged [32].

A rapid, easy-to-use identification of MRSA in nasal carriers has been developed that consists of real-time polymerase chain reaction assay.

59.18.4
Clinical Management

The CDC has recommended guidelines for CA-MRSA (Table 59.1) [47].

Once an infection has been established, wound cultures should be obtained, ideally from pus or grossly infected tissue. Cultures from ulcers are of dubious value because any bacteria isolated may be due to colonizing strains rather than pathogens [48]. Antibiotics may not be needed in skin and soft tissue infections when adequate surgical drainage can be achieved [48–50]. When antibiotics are not prescribed, patients should have follow-up care and be instructed to seek medical care if symptoms worsen or do not resolve. When antibiotics are used, local patterns of antibiotic susceptibil-

Table 59.1 Centers for Disease Control recommendations for clinical management of community-acquired methicillin-resistant Staphylococcus aureus (MRSA) skin and soft tissue infections (SSTIs) [40]

1. Consider MRSA in diagnosis of SSTIs.
2. "Spider bites" may be MRSA.
3. Consider MRSA in the event of syndromes such as a) Sepsis b) Osteomyelitis c) Septic arthritis d) Severe pneumonia e) Pneumonia following flu-like illness
4. Culture and test susceptibility of abscesses/purulent SSTIs
5. Incise and drain furuncles, abscesses, septic joints
6. Initiate empiric antibiotic therapy if infection is a) Severe b) Progressive
7. Initiate empiric antibiotic therapy in the presence of a) Cellulitis b) Systemic illness c) Immune suppression d) Serious comorbidities e) Very young and elderly patients f) Lack of response to incision/drainage

ity for CA-MRSA should be used to help direct empiric therapy against this pathogen.

59.18.5
Antibiotics

Antimicrobial therapy is critical [51]. Vancomycin has been a mainstay of treatment for serious infections that are resistant to beta-lactams [52]. However, in the treatment of methicillin-sensitive Staphylococcus aureus (MSSA), vancomycin has been associated with a slower clinical response and longer duration of bacteremia compared with the beta-lactams [35]. There has been a recent emergence of vancomycin-resistant Staphylococcus aureus (VRSA) and vancomycin-intermediate-susceptible Staphylococcus aureus (VISA) [35].

Fluoroquinolones have variable activity against CA-MRSA strains, and in some locales there has been over 40–50% fluoroquinolone resistance among MRSA strains [53–55]. Susceptibility to ciprofloxacin indicates that low-level or partial fluoroquinolone resistance is probably not present. Little clinical data are available on the use of moxifloxacin and gemifloxacin to treat CA-MRSA.

Clindamycin has been useful to treat CA-MRSA disease [47, 56, 57], but resistance greater than 10–15% has been encountered [34, 53, 54]. In a Taiwan study, the resistance was 93% [58]. Some strains that are clindamycin-susceptible and erythromycin-resistant can develop resistance when exposed to clindamycin (lincosamide), erythromycin (macrolide), and quinupristin/dalfopristin (streptogramin B). This inducible resistance can be detected by the D-test, which, if positive, is considered diagnostic for inducible resistance [59]. It is believed that clindamycin should not be used to treat D-test-positive strains, especially in a serious syndrome [59].

For multidrug-resistant infections caused by MRSA that require parenteral therapy, vancomycin, linezolid, daptomycin, and quinupristin/dalfopristin are the only agents that are reliably active against many HA-MRSA infections [57]. Trimethoprim-sulfamethoxazole, tetracyclines, clindamycin, and fluoroquinolones may be alternatives if susceptibility to these agents is documented.

59.18.6
Guidelines

The CDC developed, with internationally recognized experts, guidelines to control MRSA through hospitals and healthcare facilities [60]. These include the following:

1. Ensure that prevention programs are funded and adequately staffed.
2. Carefully track infection rates and related data to monitor the impact of prevention efforts.
3. Ensure that staff use standard infection control practices and follow guidelines regarding the correct use of antibiotics.
4. Promote the best practices with health education campaigns to increase adherence to established recommendations.
5. Design robust prevention programs customized to specific settings and local needs.

59.18.7
Discussion

A postoperative infection with MRSA in the pocket of a breast implant patient must be treated promptly and properly. This is a hospital-acquired MRSA. The correct antibiotic must be used, from cultures and sensitivities, for at least 1 week, and then the wound should be recultured. The antibiotic is continued as long as the wound cultures MRSA on a weekly basis. The implant must be removed and not replaced for at least 3 months from the time the infected wound has completely healed (not from the time when the culture was negative).

59.19
Migration of Implant

There is one report of a left breast implant migrating into the thoracic cavity [61]. An axillary approach had been used, and the patient developed sudden dyspnea during the operation on the left side, but this was alleviated by the administration of oxygen. The basis for the migration was believed to be from a large defect of the chest wall, breast massage after surgery, and the difference in pressure between the outside and the inside of the chest wall. However, it is this author's opinion that perforation into the thoracic cavity during surgery caused the sudden dyspnea during the procedure, and this evolved into the large defect in the chest wall with subsequent migration of the implant.

59.20
Myospasm of Pectoralis Major Muscle

Myospasm with spontaneous myoclonic jerks of the left pectoralis muscle was reported following subpectoral breast augmentation [62]. This disorder did not respond to Klonopin, excision of a segment of the lateral

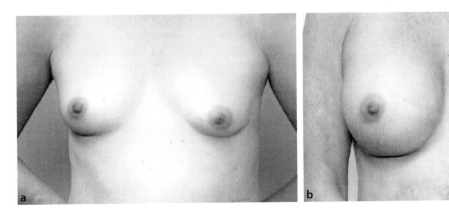

Fig. 59.11 a Preoperative. **b** Residual scarring of left breast following breast augmentation in a smoker

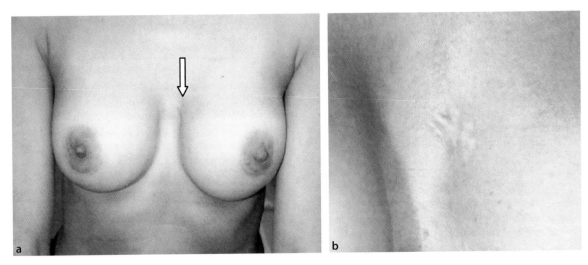

Fig. 59.12 a Skin necrosis with residual scar (*arrow*) from electrocoagulation too close to the skin. **b** Scar

pectoral nerve, or open capsulotomy and transection of the pectoralis major muscle head to the humerus. Explantation relieved the spasms. The presumptive cause was myospasm from mechanical irritation of the nerve from the implant.

59.21
Necrosis

Causes of necrosis include prior radiation therapy for breast cancer, uncontrolled diabetes followed by infection, late diagnosis of hematoma, smoking (Fig. 59.11), infection, electrocoagulation too close to the skin (Fig. 59.12), or a combination of these factors (Figs. 59.13, 59.14). Radiation reduces the vascularity of the exposed area, which makes the breast more sus-

ceptible to complications such as infection and necrosis. In combination with other factors such as uncontrolled diabetes, smoking, or hematoma, the risk of problems increases.

59.22
Neurologic Injury

The axillary approach to cosmetic breast surgery is an excellent alternative to the inframammary, periareolar, areolar, and umbilical incisions. The scar is rarely visible except with the arms raised but does occasionally become hypertrophic. The risks associated with this approach include all the usual risks of any breast implant surgery plus the possibility of neurologic damage, both motor and sensory.

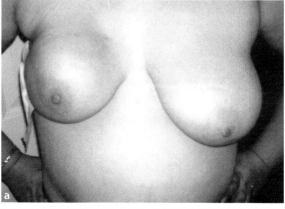

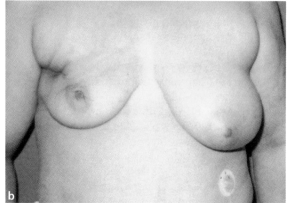

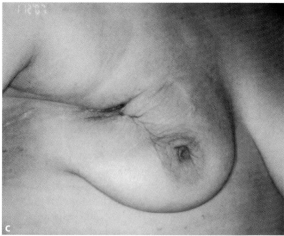

Fig. 59.13 a A diabetic patient, postlumpectomy and radiation therapy for cancer of the right breast, had bilateral augmentation mammoplasty. Capsule contracture occurred on the right side, lifting the breast; there was uncorrected left breast ptosis; and an infection developed in the wound and implant pocket, followed by necrosis. b Skin retraction following removal of the right implant. c Skin retraction

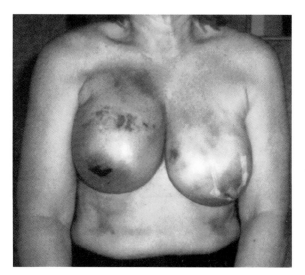

Fig. 59.14 After right lumpectomy and radiation therapy for breast cancer, patient had breast augmentation. Hematoma was diagnosed 1 week postoperatively, and because of the late diagnosis, necrosis of the right nipple areola–complex occurred

The surgeon must be aware of the risks of the axillary approach and convey those risks to the patient to allow a knowledgeable and informed consent to the procedure. The surgery must be performed with cautious attention to the nerves in the area and with methods to avoid injuring those nerves.

A chronic pain syndrome can occur not only from injury to the 4th intercostal nerve but to other sensory nerves higher on the chest wall.

59.22.1
Brachial Plexus

Injury to the brachial plexus is most often caused at the time of surgery by positioning the arm in an abducted position more than 90° from the side of the body. Those patients susceptible to this type of injury usually have some form of actual or potential thoracic outlet syndrome. If the patient's head is turned in the opposite direction during surgery, there is even more likelihood for brachial plexus nerve or vascular compression. There is rarely a need to keep the arm abducted more than 85° except, perhaps, when making the initial skin incision at the high point of the axilla in the axillary approach to breast augmentation.

Although the brachial plexus may be at risk with the axillary approach to cosmetic breast surgery, the plexus is superior to the axillary vessels and is most likely to be injured when bleeding occurs from vessel disruption and a hemostat or clip is placed to control the bleeding without clearly visualizing the surrounding structures. This type of injury can occur following a long period of compression to control the bleeding, without direct injury from a hemostat or clip. There can be permanent injury to the inferior cord of the brachial plexus (ulnar nerve distribution).

The brachial plexus has three cords from which the infraclavicular branches are derived (Table 59.2). The **long thoracic nerve (nerve of Bell)** is located along the side of the chest wall on the outer surface of the serratus anterior, supplying filaments to each of its digitations. This nerve is not normally at risk during breast augmentation from any approach, but it is theoretically possible to injure the nerve when doing a very wide pocket dissection during a capsulectomy or in making a megapocket in a patient with an extremely large implant (over 800 ml). The one medical-legal case [63] encountered by the author concerned a permanent long

Table 59.2 Infraclavicular branches of the brachial plexus

Cord	Nerve	Spinal Origin
Lateral	Musculocutaneous	5, 6, 7 C
	Lateral anterior thoracic	5, 6, 7 C
	Lateral head of median	6, 7 C
Medial	Medial anterior thoracic	8 C, 1 T
	Medial antebrachial cutaneous	8 C, 1 T
	Medial brachial cutaneous	8 C, 1 T
	Ulnar	8 C, 1 T
	Medial head of median	8 C, 1 T
Posterior	Upper subscapular	5, 6 C
	Lower subscapular	5, 6 C
	Thoracodorsal	5, 6, 7 C
	Axillary	5, 6 C
	Radial	5, 6, 7, 8 C, 1 T

thoracic nerve injury causing a winged scapula in a patient who had simple capsulotomies for breast implants and not utilizing an axillary incision. The neurosurgeon expert witness testified that the long thoracic nerve was injured by brachial plexus compression; however, he did not remember that the nerve has three roots (5, 6, and 7 cervical) that do not pass through the thoracic outlet but descend behind the brachial plexus and form the long thoracic nerve inferior to the outlet. The most likely cause of injury in this case was excessively tight dressings that compressed the long thoracic nerve against the chest wall below the axilla, or an unrecorded fall with injury to the lateral chest wall.

The **lateral anterior thoracic nerve** crosses the axillary artery and vein, piercing the coracoclavicular fascia, and enters the deep surface of the pectoralis major muscle. It sends a filament to join the medial anterior thoracic nerve in front of the axillary artery. The nerve supplies the clavicular, manubrial, and sternal portions of the pectoralis major muscle. This nerve can be injured by dissecting too superiorly when forming a submuscular pocket. Injury to the lateral anterior thoracic nerve may affect the strength of the pectoralis major muscle, which flexes, adducts, and rotates the arm medially.

The **medial anterior thoracic nerve** enters and innervates the pectoralis minor muscle, and two or three branches end in the pectoralis major muscle. The nerve supplies the lower sternocostal and abdominal portions of the pectoralis major muscle as well as the pectoralis minor muscle. This nerve is lateral to the lateral anterior thoracic nerve. The medial anterior thoracic nerve may be injured when dissecting a retropectoral pocket using the axillary approach when the lateral edge of the pectoralis major muscle is not identified before dissecting under the muscle and by approaching the muscle from too superior a position. Injury to the medial anterior thoracic nerve leaves no clinical muscle deficit because the nerve sends only a few fibers to the pectoralis major muscle and mainly supplies the pectoralis minor muscle, which helps to adduct the arm by rotating the scapula downward and forward.

59.22.2
Intercostal Nerves

The **sensory nerves** (which are unrelated to the brachial plexus) that are likely to be injured during the axillary approach include the intercostobrachial nerves and the lateral branches of the 3rd and 4th intercostal nerves. When a subpectoral pocket is being formed, injury to the nerves is more likely if the dissection is not started anteriorly against the fascia of the pectoralis major muscle prior to dissecting along the lateral edge and then under the muscle.

One cause of injury to the 4th intercostal nerve is placing a large implant (over 400 cc) in a subpectoral pocket without making sure the nerve is carefully dissected free from the intercostal muscles if the implant impinges on the nerve. The nerve may not be transected, but if folded posteriorly with implant compression, there can be anesthesia of the nipple–areola complex and/or a chronic pain syndrome with associated scarring around the nerve.

59.22.3
Nerve Injury

The most common mistake after making the axillary skin incision at the highest point of the axilla is approaching the lateral edge of the pectoralis major muscle from a superior–lateral direction rather than from an anteromedial–inferior position. The proper method is to make the skin incision and then pull the skin anteromedially over the lateral edge of the muscle and slightly inferiorly, followed by dissecting downward onto the muscle and exposing the lateral edge [64]. By carefully staying on the muscle fascia and dissecting around the muscle edge and under the muscle, the submuscular pocket can be formed without approaching any of the axillary nerves.

Elective intraoperative division of the medial thoracic (pectoral) nerve denervates the lower third of the pectoralis minor muscle, making it more flaccid, and has been used clinically to allow more anterior breast projection and to minimize postoperative flexion-induced breast deformity in the patient with retromuscular breast implants [65, 66]. No clinical problem with transection of the nerve has been described.

Arm position during surgery with abduction to 90° or greater may result in brachial plexus or vascular compression, which can cause temporary or permanent nerve damage. The surgeon should always be aware of arm positioning at the beginning of surgery so that excessive abduction does not occur. The elbow should be padded to prevent ulnar nerve paresis.

59.23
Periareolar Scar Indentation

There have been some instances of depression of the periareolar scar following breast augmentation (S.J. Mirrafati, personal communication, 27 August 2007; Fig. 59.15). The cause has been attributed to the technique, after the skin incision, of extending the dissection under the skin in an oblique method, pointing inferiorly to avoid damage to the breast ducts or to dissect around the inferior portion of the breast gland to

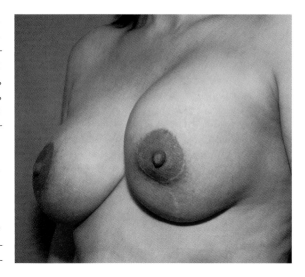

Fig. 59.15 Periareolar scar indentation

avoid cutting through the breast tissue. This creates a potential space after closure of the skin incision because the subcutaneous fat may not line up properly to fill the space under the skin. The usual method is to dissect straight down through the breast tissue to form the underlying pocket in the submammary or subpectoral space. Cutting through the breast tissue does not destroy any major ducts but does cut smaller ductules. No infections have been directly attributed to transecting the small ductules.

59.24
Pneumothorax

Care must be taken when performing breast augmentation under local anesthesia. Any sharp needle inserted into the tissues around the breast has the potential to perforate into the pleural space and cause a pneumothorax or tension pneumothorax.

When an implant pocket is made in the retropectoral area, there is the possibility of pneumothorax when a bleeder is electrocoagulated in the intercostal space. This can leave a hole in the pleura. If this is noted at the time of surgery, the surgeon should insert a Robinson catheter in the pleural space, complete the procedure, and insert the implant. The anesthesiologist should expand the lungs, or if the anesthesia is local, the surgeon can instruct the patient to take a deep breath, and then withdraw the catheter. The implant will plug the small opening until it is fully healed.

General anesthesia can cause a pneumothorax [67] when too much pressure is used in bagging the patient, especially if the patient has lung blebs. It is possible for a spontaneous pneumothorax to occur when a lung bleb ruptures without general anesthesia.

If a pneumothorax is suspected, a chest x-ray should be taken. A pneumothorax that is less than 15% can be observed with repeat chest x-ray. If the air is increasing or if the air is over 15%, then a tube should be inserted into the chest, usually at the anterior 2nd intercostal space, and connected to an underwater seal.

An unusual cause of pneumothorax in breast augmentation was described by Fayman et al. [68]. Four patients developed bilateral pneumothorax and one developed unilateral pneumothorax after the transaxillary approach for submuscular placement of implants. Two patients were symptomatic. The assumption was that air was trapped in the subpectoral pocket, which was sealed by the implant and wound closure. The air was forced into the pleural cavity as a result of the high pressure created in the subpectoral pocket by the advancing implant. The problem was resolved by placing a large-bore suction catheter into the subpectoral pocket before the implant was inserted.

59.25
Rippling

With the use of saline implants, the problem of rippling (skin waviness) has appeared more often. This usually occurs with the use of textured saline implants (Fig. 59.16) and can be resolved by converting to a smooth implant.

59.26
Serous Fluid Drainage

Seroma is a tumor-like collection of serum in the tissues. This postoperative collection of seroma fluid can occur in breast augmentation surgery [69] and can result in increased morbidity and chronic serous drainage.

In a histopathologic study, it was noted that seromas may incite an inflammatory reaction that subsequently becomes a contributing factor in persistent seroma formation [70].

The author has seen one case of persistent serous drainage that was caused by a large amount of granulation tissue in the pocket. When the granulation tissue was cleaned off and the implant replaced, there was no further problem.

Movement of the textured implant in the pocket may cause chronic tissue irritation and inflammation with subsequent seroma formation. Removing and exchanging a textured implant for a smooth one will usually resolve the problem. If a smooth implant is in place, then consider exuberant granulation tissue as a possible cause. Exploration of the wound and curetting all the granulations will allow resolution.

59.27
Synmastia

The meeting of implants in the midline is called synmastia or symmastia. This can result from dissection of the pockets to the midline of the sternum, thus weakening the medial tissues and allowing the implant to migrate medially (Fig. 59.17), or from thin and weak tissues near the sternum that, postoperatively, are pushed medially by the implants. Treatment consists of capsulotomy laterally and closure of the midline tissues with the fibrous capsule sutured to the deep tissues. Postoperatively, compression of the midline is essential for at least 1 week.

59.28
Thromboembolism

Patients who undergo surgery are at risk for venous thromboembolic complications. This is especially crit-

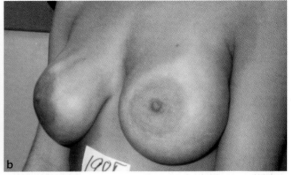

Fig. 59.16 a Rippling in a patient with textured saline implants. **b** Lateral view

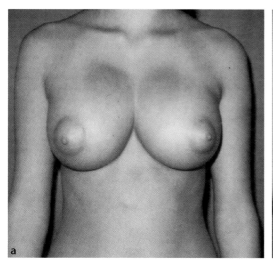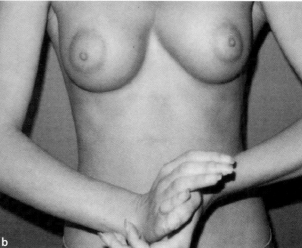

Fig. 59.17 **a** Synmastia secondary to dissection of the pockets to the midline of the sternum. **b** Same patient

ical in the cosmetic surgery patient who, having an elective procedure, would not expect the morbidity or mortality associated with thromboembolic disease. The cosmetic surgeon must be aware of the possibility of thromboembolism in every patient and should take a careful history to disclose predisposing risk factors. The surgeon should also be aware of the clinical manifestations of pulmonary embolus in order to make a timely diagnosis.

59.28.1
Risk Factors

Minor surgery lasting <30 min in patients over 40 years of age without additional risk factors and uncomplicated surgery in patients under 40 years of age without additional risk factors are in the low-risk category. General surgery in patients over 40 years of age lasting >30 min and patients under 40 years who take oral contraceptives are in the moderate-risk category [71]. The high-risk category consists of major surgery in patients over 40 years of age with recent history of deep vein thrombosis or pulmonary embolism, extensive pelvic or abdominal surgery for malignancy, and major orthopedic surgery of the lower extremities.

Predisposing risk factors include age over 50 years, malignancy, obesity, prior history of thromboembolism, varicose veins, recent operative procedures, and thrombophilia. These risks are further modified by the duration and type of anesthesia, preoperative and postoperative immobilization, level of hydration, and the presence of sepsis [72]. Medical problems associated with increased risk include acute myocardial infarction,

stroke, and immobilization [73]. Estrogen therapy and pregnancy are common risk factors, while uncommon factors include lupus anticoagulant, nephrotic syndrome, inflammatory bowel disease, polycythemia vera, persistent thrombocytosis, paroxysmal nocturnal hemoglobinuria, and inherited factors such as antithrombin III deficiency, protein C deficiency, protein S deficiency, plasminogen activator deficiency, elevated plasminogen activator inhibitor, and homocystinuria [74].

Superficial calf vein thrombosis, proximal deep vein thrombosis, and fatal pulmonary embolus increase in incidence as the risk category increases from low to high (Table 59.3).

59.28.2
Clinical Manifestations

Superficial thrombophlebitis (inflamed vein) appears as a red, tender cord. Deep-vein thrombosis may be associ-

Table 59.3 Risk categories and associated thromboembolism

Risk	Calf vein thrombosis	Proximal vein thrombosis	Fatal pulmonary embolism
Low	<10%	<1%	<0.01%
Moderate	10–40%	2–10%	0.1–0.7%
High	40–80%	10–30%	1–5%

ated with pain at rest or only during exercise, with edema distal to the obstructed vein. The first manifestation can be pulmonary embolism. There may be tenderness in the extremity, and the temperature of the skin may be increased. Increased resistance or pain on voluntary dorsiflexion of the foot (Homan's sign) and/or tenderness of the calf on palpation are useful diagnostic criteria.

Pulmonary embolism is usually manifested by one of three clinical patterns: onset of sudden dyspnea with tachypnea and no other symptoms, 2) sudden pleuritic chest pain and dyspnea associated with findings of pleural effusion or lung consolidation, or 3) sudden apprehension, chest discomfort, and dyspnea with findings of cor pulmonale and systemic hypotension. The symptoms occasionally consist of fever, arrhythmias, or refractory congestive heart failure.

59.28.3
Diagnosis

Deep-vein thrombosis is best diagnosed with duplex ultrasonography, which combines pulsed gated Doppler evaluation of blood flow with real-time ultrasound imaging. Other diagnostic tests include x-ray venography, radionuclide venography, radioisotope-labeled fibrinogen, ultrasonography, and impedance plethysmography. Liquid crystal thermography detects increases in skin temperature and is a useful adjunct to ultrasonography or impedance plethysmography.

Ventilation–perfusion (VP) lung scanning is a safe, sensitive means of diagnosing pulmonary embolism. Isotope pulmonary perfusion scan (Q scan) is more specific with inclusion of the isotope ventilation scan (V scan). The definitive diagnosis can be made by pulmonary arteriography, but VP scanning can give a high degree of certainty. Arterial blood gas typically shows reductions in PaO_2 and $PaCO_2$. An electrocardiogram will show tachycardia, but this is best used for ruling out myocardial infarction. Chest x-ray may show basilar atelectasis, infiltrates, pleural effusion, or cardiac dilatation.

59.28.4
Prophylactic Treatment

Low-risk general surgical patients may be treated with graduated compression stockings applied during surgery, early ambulation, and adequate hydration [75]. Keeping the knees flexed on pillows during surgery and avoiding local compression on any areas of the legs are helpful. All patients are treated the same if there are any low-risk factors. The type of surgery does not matter

as long as general anesthesia or intravenous sedation is given. Compression stockings (20–30-mm support hose are adequate) are applied in the operating room, and ambulation is begun when the patient is awake and capable of ambulating with assistance. When the patient is ambulating on a regular basis during the day, the compression stockings can be removed.

For moderate-risk patients, low-dose heparin (5,000 units 2 h before surgery and then every 8–12 h until ambulatory), low molecular weight heparin (LMWH), dextran, or aspirin is recommended. Alternatively, graduated compression stockings or intermittent pneumatic compression started during surgery, used continuously until ambulatory, or a combination of both is recommended [72].

All high-risk patients (unlikely to be encountered in cosmetic surgery) should be treated with low-dose heparin or LMWH and with combined pharmacologic and mechanical methods.

Dextran can result in cardiac overload, and high-dose aspirin (1,000–1,500 mg/day) has limited efficacy in preventing deep-vein thrombosis. In cosmetic surgery the use of aspirin or heparin may result in postoperative bleeding

The best prophylaxis for low-risk cosmetic surgery patients would appear to be mechanical methods, including knee compression stockings and early ambulation. For low-risk patients, the knees should be slightly flexed, and compression of the extremities should be avoided [76].

59.28.5
Hereditary Hypercoagulable States

Patients with a family history of thrombosis, early-onset or recurring thrombosis, thrombosis at unusual sites, or warfarin-induced skin necrosis should be evaluated for possible underlying inherited hypercoagulable disorders.

Antithrombin III (AT-III) is a heparin cofactor that allows heparin to inactivate factor II_a primarily but also factors IX_a, X_a, XI_a, and XII_a [77]. A deficiency in AT-III predisposes to thrombosis by allowing uncontrolled activity of many of the coagulation factors.

Endothelial surfaces have receptors called thrombomodulin that function as anticoagulants because of the ability to neutralize thrombin. The thrombin–thrombomodulin complex activates protein C, a vitamin K-dependent factor that is facilitated by protein S, another vitamin K-dependent factor. Activated proteins C and S metabolize activated factors V and VIII, which results in downregulating of the coagulation system. Patients with protein C deficiency may have recurrent episodes of superficial thrombophlebitis as well as thromboembolism [78]. Patients with protein S deficiency experience more arterial thromboembolism, including stroke [79]. Deficiency in protein C or S may present as neonatal purpura fulminans in the newborn or skin necrosis in adults treated with warfarin, a drug known to cause a sudden fall in protein C or protein S.

Venous thromboembolism occurs in one out of every thousand people with activated protein C resistance (APC-R), responsible for up to 64% of the cases. APC-R is due to a single point mutation in the FV gene for clotting factor V. This mutated FV may be referred to as factor V Leiden (FVL), the FV:Q506 allele, or the APC gene and is less efficiently degraded by APC. A hypercoagulable state results from impairment of the inactivation of factor V by activated protein C (APC). This creates a lifelong increased risk of thrombosis and thromboembolism.

Within the intact vessel, thrombin binds to thrombomodulin on the endothelial cell, acting as an anticoagulant by activating the protein C system. APC, potentiated by cofactor protein S, downregulates the activity of the coagulation system (limits clot formation) by cleaving and inhibiting factors V (FV) and VIII [80–82].

APC testing can be performed with DNA genotyping. This can differentiate acquired from inherited APC-R. Approximately 10% of patients with APC-R phenotype lack the FV mutation (genotype), and the diagnosis of APC-R in these patients will be missed [83]. The combination of phenotype and genotype information aids in establishing prophylactic and therapeutic guidelines.

Asymptomatic patients with APC-R who have never had a thromboembolic event, as well as their family members, should receive counseling regarding the implications of the diagnosis and information concerning the signs and symptoms of venous thromboembolism [84]. Short-term prophylaxis with heparin should be considered when high-risk circumstances are encountered, such as immobilization, surgery, trauma, or obstetric procedures. After a thrombotic event, these patients need extended anticoagulation, balancing the risk of bleeding against the risk of recurrence when therapy is discontinued. Empiric treatment is for at least 1 year after two episodes of thromboembolism and lifelong treatment after three episodes.

59.28.6
Antiphospholipid Syndrome

Antiphospholipid syndrome is an acquired condition that can result in thrombosis.

59.29
Synmastia (Symmastia)

"Syn" means "with, together" (Greek), while "sym" in the dictionary always refers to the Greek "syn." Therefore, both spellings are correct. Synmastia is a fusion of both breasts in the midline; in breast augmentation, it refers to the meeting or near meeting of both prostheses in the midline.

This can be corrected by approaching the midline with the implants removed and suturing the anterior fibrous capsule to the underlying fibrous capsule and fascia or periosteum bilaterally and then doing lateral capsulotomies before replacing the implants. The excess capsule can be excised or electrocoagulated to expose a healing surface. The midline should be compressed for at least 5 days, either with bulky dressings or a garment designed to compress the midline.

59.30
Toxic Shock Syndrome

Toxic shock syndrome has been reported in breast augmentation [85–87]. The syndrome is caused by the exotoxins (superantigens) secreted with infection from *Staphylococcus aureus* and group A streptococci [22]. Knowledge of the criteria for diagnosis is important in order to treat this potentially fatal disease. These criteria include the following [22]:

1. Fever (>102° F)
2. Rash (diffuse, macular erythroderma)
3. Desquamation (1–2 weeks after onset, especially of the palms and soles)
4. Hypotension
5. Involvement of three or more organ systems:
   a) Gastrointestinal (vomiting, diarrhea at onset)
   b) Muscular (myalgia, elevated creatine phosphokinase)
   c) Mucous membrane (conjunctiva, oropharynx)
   d) Renal (BUN or creatinine >2 times normal)
   e) Hepatic (bilirubin, SGOT, SGPT >2 times normal
   f) Hematologic (platelets <100,000)
6. Negative results on the following studies (if obtained):
   a) Blood, throat, or cerebral spinal fluid cultures
   b) Serologic tests for Rocky Mountain spotted fever, leptospirosis, measles

Treatment consists of surgical debridement for necrosis, antibiotics, circulatory and respiratory care, anticoagulant therapy for disseminated intravascular coagulation, and immunoglobulin [23]. Experimental approaches have included the use of antitumor necrosis factor monoclonal antibodies and plasmapheresis.

References

1. Maximovich SP: Transient axillary-upper inner arm subcutaneous fibrous banding following transaxillary subpectoral endoscopic breast augmentation. Plast Reconstr Surg 1996;97(6):1304–1305

2. Young RV: Transaxillary submuscular breast augmentation and subcutaneous fibrous bands. Plast Reconstr Surg 1997;99(1):257

3. Laufer E: Fibrous bands following subpectoral endoscopic breast augmentation. Plast Reconstr Surg 1997;99(1):257

4. Munhoz AM, Fells K, Arruda E, Montag E, Okada A, Aldrighi C, Aldrighi JM, Gemperli R, Ferreira MC: Subfascial transaxillary breast augmentation without endoscopic assistance: technical aspects and outcome. Aesth Plast Surg 2006;30:503–512

5. Dowden RV: Subcutaneous fibrous banding after transaxillary subpectoral endoscopic breast augmentation. Plast Reconstr Surg 1997;99(1):257

6. Shiffman MA: Transient axillary-upper inner arm subcutaneous fibrous banding. Plast Reconstr Surg 1997;99(2):596

7. Botti G: Postoperative self-expansion in augmentation mammaplasty. Plast Reconstr Surg 1994;93(6):1310

8. Signorini M, Grisotti A, Ponzielli G, Pajardi G, Gilardino P: Self-expanding prosthesis complicating augmentation mammoplasties. Aesth Plast Surg 1994;18(2):195–199

9. Robinson OG, Benos DJ: Spontaneous autoinflation of saline mammary implants. Ann Plast Surg 1997;39(2):114–118

10. Ketene M, Saray A, Kara SA: Unilateral osmotic swelling in textured, single-lumen mammary implants: clinical and MRI findings. Aesth Plast Surg 2002;26(3):206–210

11. Chien C-H, Ding Z-Z, Yang Z-S: Spontaneous autoinflation and deflation of double-lumen breast implants. Aesth Plast Surg 2006;30(1):113–117

12. Luke JL, Kalasinsky VF, Turnicky RP, Centeno JA, Johnson FB, Mullick FG: Pathological and biophysical findings associated with silicone breast implants: a study of capsular tissue from 86 cases. Plast Reconstr Surg1997;100(6):1558–1565]

13. Huang TT: Breast and subscapular pain following submuscular placement of breast prostheses. Plast Reconstr Surg 1990;86(2):275–280

14. Lykissa ED, Maharaj SV: Total platinum concentration and platinum oxidation states in bodily fluids, tissue, and explants from women exposed to silicone and saline breast implants by IC-ICPMS. Anal Chem 2006;78(9):2925–2933

15. Rothkopf DM, Rosen HM: Lactation as a complication of aesthetic breast surgery successfully treated with bromocriptine. Br J Plast Surg 1990;43(3):373–375

16. Hartley JH Jr, Schatten WE: Postoperative complication of lactation after augmentation mammaplasty. Plast Reconstr Surg 1971;47(2):150–153

17. Hugill JV: Lactation following breast augmentation: a third case. Plast Reconstr Surg 1991;87(4):806–807

18. Sabbagh WH, Murphy RX Jr, Kucirka SJ, Okunski WJ: Idiosyncratic allergic reaction to textured saline implants. Plast Reconstr Surg 1996;97(4):820–823

19. Widdice L: The effects of breast reduction and breast augmentation surgery on lactation: an annotated bibliography. J Hum Lact 1993;9(3):161–167

20. Hill PD, Wilhelm PA, Aldag JC, Chatterton RT Jr: Breast augmentation and lactation outcome: a case report. MCN Am J Matern Child Nurs 2004;29(4):238–242

21. Hurst NM: Lactation after augmentation mammoplasty. Obstet Gynecol 1996;(87(1):30–34

22. Neifert MR, Seacat JM, Jobe WE: Lactation failure due to inadequate glandular development of the breast. Pediatrics 1985;76(5):823–828

23. Georgiade NG, Serafin D, Barwick W: Late development of hematoma around a breast implant. Plast Reconstr Surg 1979;64(5):708–710

24. Dawl JL, Lewis VL, Smith JW: Chronic expanding hematoma within a periprosthetic breast capsule. Plast Reconstr Surg 1996;97(7):1469–1472

25. Görgü M, Aslan G, Tuncel A, Erdogan B: Late and long-standing capsular hematoma after aesthetic breast augmentation with a saline-filled silicone prosthesis: a case report. Aesthetic Plast Surg 1999;23(6):443–444

26. Hsiao HT, Tung KY, Lin CS: Late hematoma after aesthetic breast augmentation with saline-filled, textured silicone prosthesis. Aesthetic Plast Surg 2002;26(5):368–371

27. Brickman M, Parsa NN, Parsa FD: Late hematoma after breast implantation. Aesthetic Plast Surg 2004;28(2):80–82

28. Veiga DF, Filho JV, Schnaider CS, Archangelo I Jr: Late hematoma after aesthetic breast augmentation with textured silicone prosthesis: a case report. Aesthetic Plast Surg 2005;29(5):431–433

29. Hall v. Rothman, State of South Carolina, County of Greenville, Court of Common Pleas, No. 2005-CP-23

30. Dufour P, Gillet Y, Bes M, Lina G, Vandenesch F, Floret D, Etienne A, Richet H: Community-acquired methicillin-resistant *Staphylococcus aureus* infections in France: emergence of a single clone that produces Panton–Valentine leukocidin. Clin Infect Dis 2002;35(7):819–824

31. Centers for Disease Control and Prevention (CDC): Outbreaks of community-associated methicillin-resistant *Staphylococcus aureus* skin infections—Los Angeles County, California, 2002–2003. MMWR Morb Mortal Wkly Rep 2003;52(5):88

32. Centers for Disease Control and Prevention (CDC): Methicillin-resistant *Staphylococcus aureus* infections among competitive sports participants—Colorado, Indiana, Pennsylvania, and Los Angeles County, 2002–2003. MMWR Morb Mortal Wkly Rep 2003;52(33):793–795

33. Tenover FC, McDougal LK, Goering RV, Killgore G, Projan SJ, Patel JB, Dunman PM: Characterization of a strain of community-associated methicillin-resistant *Staphylococcus aureus* widely disseminated in the United States. J Clin Microbiol 2006;44(1):108–118

34. Chambers HF: The changing epidemiology of *Staphylococcus aureus*? Emerg Infect Dis 2001;7(2):178–182

35. Deresinski S: Methicillin-resistant *Staphylococcus aureus*: an evolutionary, epidemiologic, and therapeutic odyssey. Clin Infect Dis 2005;40(4):562–573

36. Kazakova SV, Hagerman JC, Matava M, Srinivasan A, Phelan L, Garfinkel B, Boo T, McAllister S, Anderson J, Jensen B, Dodson D, Lonsway D, McDougal LK, Aduino M, Fraser VJ, Killgore G, Tenover FC, Cody S, Jernigan DB: A clone of methicillin-resistant *Staphylococcus* among professional football players. N Engl J Med 2005;352(5):468–475

37. Bratu S, Eramo A, Kopec R, Coughlin E, Ghitan M, Yost R, Chpanick EK, Landman D, Quale J: Community-associated methicillin-resistant *Staphylococcus* in hospital and nursery and maternity units. Emerg Infect Dis 2005;11(6):808–813

38. Moran GJ, Krishnadasan A, Gorwits RJ, Fosheim GE, McDougal LK, Carey RB, Talan DA; EMERGency ID Net Study Group: Methicillin-resistant *S. aureus* infections among patients in the emergency department. N Engl J Med 2006;355(7):666–674

39. Holmes A, Ganner M, McGuane S, Pitt TL, Cookson BD, Kearns AM: *Staphylococcus aureus* isolates carrying Panton–Valentine leucocidin genes in England and Wales: frequency, characterization, and association with clinical disease. J Clin Microbiol 2005;43(5):2384–2390

40. Kravitz GR, Dries DJ, Peterson ML, Schlievert PM: Purpura fulminans due to *Staphylococcus aureus*. Clin Infect Dis 2005;40(7):948–950

41. Gillet Y, Issartel B, Vanhems P, Fournet JC, Lina G, Bes M, Vandenesch F, Piemont Y, Brousse N, Floret D, Etienne J: Association between *Staphylococcus aureus* strains carrying gene for Panton–Valentine leukocidin and highly lethal necrotizing pneumonia in young immunocompetent patients. Lancet 2002;359(9308):753–759

42. Francis JS, Doherty MC, Lopatin U, Johnston CP, Sinha G, Ross T, Cai M, Hansel NN, Perl T, Ticehurst JR, Carroll K, Thomas DL, Nuermberger E, Bartlett JG: Severe community-onset pneumonia in healthy adults caused by methicillin-resistant *Staphylococcus aureus* carrying the Panton–Valentine leukocidin genes. Clin Infect Dis 2005;40(1):100–107

43. Waldvogel FA: *Staphylococcus aureus* (including staphylococcal toxic shock). In: Mandell GL, Bennett JE, Dolin R (eds). Principles and Practice of Infectious Diseases, 5th edn. Philadelphia, Churchill Livingstone 2000, pp 2072–2073

44. Hidron AI, Kourbatova EV, Halvosa JS, Terrell BJ, McDougal LK, Tenover FC, Blumberg HM, King MD: Risk factors for colonization with methicillin-resistant *Staphylococcus aureus* (MRSA) in patients admitted to an urban hospital: emergence of community-associated MRSA in nasal carriage. Clin Infect Dis 2005;41(2):159–166

45. Boyce JM: New insights for improving hand hygiene practices. Infect Control Hosp Epidemiol 2004;25(3):187–188

46. Boyce JM, Havill NL, Kohan C, Dumigan DG, Ligi CE: Do infection control measures work for methicillin-resistant *Staphylococcus aureus*? Infect Control Hosp Epidemiol 2004;25(5):395–401

47. Centers for Disease Control and Prevention: Strategies for clinical management of MRSA in the community. March 2006. http://www.ccar-ccra.com/english/pdfs/CAMRSA_ExpMtgStrategies.pdf

48. Gowan JE, Miller LG:Community-acquired methicillin-resistant *Staphylococcus aureus*: right here, right now. ISMR (International Society of Microbial Resistance) Update 2006;1(3):1–12

49. Lee MC, Rios AM, Aten MF, Mejias A, Cavuoti D, McCracken GH Jr, Hardy RD: Management and outcome of children with skin and soft tissue abscesses caused by community-acquired methicillin-resistant *Staphylococcus aureus*. Pediatr Infect Dis 2004;23(2):123–127

50. Llera JL, Levy RC: Treatment of cutaneous abscess: a double-blind clinical study. Ann Emerg Med 1985;14(1):15–19

51. Gorwitz RJ, Jernigan DB, Powers JH, Jernigan JA: Management of MRSA in the community. Centers for Disease Control and Prevention, March 2006. http://www.ccar-ccra.com/english/pdfs/CAMRSA_ExpMtgStrategies.pdf

52. Kollef MH, Micek ST: Methicillin-resistant *Staphylococcus aureus*: a new community-acquired pathogen? Curr Opin Infect Dis 2006;19(2):161–168

53. Fridkin SK, Hageman JC, Morrison M, Sanza LT, Como-Sabetti K, Jernigan JA, Harriman K, Harrison LH, Lynfield R, Farley MM; Active Bacterial Core Surveillance Program of the Emerging Infections Program Network: Methicillin-resistant *Staphylococcus aureus* disease in three communities. N Engl J Med 2005;352(14):1436–1444

54. Miller LG, Tagudar G, Tsui J, et al.: A prospective investigation of risk factors for community-acquired MRSA infection in a non-outbreak setting. Program and Abstracts of the 42nd Annual Meeting of the Infectious Disease Society of America, 29 September–3 October 2004, Boston, abstract LB-7

55. Frazee BW, Salz TO, Lambert L, Perdreau-Remington F: Fatal community-associated methicillin-resistant *Staphylococcus aureus* pneumonia in an immunocompetent young adult. Ann Emerg Med 2005;46(5):401–404

56. Frank AL, Marcinak JF, Mangat PD, Tjhio JT, Kelkar S, Schreckenberger PC, Quinn JP: Clindamycin treatment of methicillin-resistant *Staphylococcus aureus* infections in children. Pediatr Infect Dis J 2002;21(6):530–534

57. Martinez-Aguilar G, Avalos-Mishaan A, Hulten K, Hammerman W, Mason EO Jr, Kaplan SL: Community-acquired, methicillin resistant and methicillin-susceptible *Staphylococcus aureus* musculoskeletal infections in children. Pediatr Infect Dis J 2004;23(8):701–706

58. Chen CJ, Huang YC: Community-acquired methicillin-resistant *Staphylococcus aureus* in Taiwan. J Microbiol Immunol Infect 2005;38(6):376–382

59. Siberry GK, Tekle T, Carroll K, Dick J: Failure of clindamycin in treatment of methicillin-resistant *Staphylococcus aureus* expressing inducible clindamycin resistance in vitro. Clin Infect Dis 2003;37(9):1257–1260

60. Centers for Disease Control and Prevention: Management of multiple-resistant organisms in healthcare settings. http://www.cdc.gov/ncidod/dhgp

61. Chen Z-Y, Wang Z-G, Kuang R-X, Su Y-P: Implant found in thoracic cavity after breast augmentation. Plast Reconstr Surg 2005;116(6):1826–1827

62. Wong L: Pectoralis major myospasm resulting from subpectoral implant. Plast Reconstr Surg 2000;105(4):1571–1572

63. Weaver v. Borsand, No. CV 99–02491, Maricopa County, AZ (1999)

64. Shiffman MA, Mirrafati S: Possible nerve injuries in the axillary approach to breast augmentation surgery. Amer J Cosmetic Surg 2001;18(3):149

65. Maxwell GP, Tornambe R: Management of mammary subpectoral implant distortion. Clin Plast Surg 1988;15:601–611

66. Georgiade NG, Georgiade GS, Riefkohl R: Aesthetic Surgery of the Breast. Philadelphia, Saunders 1990, pp 80–81

67. Osborn JM, Stevenson TR: Pneumothorax as a complication of breast augmentation. Plast Reconstr Surg 2005;116(4):1122–1126

68. Fayman MS, Beeton A, Potgieter E: Barotrauma: an unrecognized mechanism for pneumothorax in breast augmentation. Plast Reconstr Surg 2005;116(6):1825–1826

69. Picha G J, Batra MK: Breast augmentation. In: Achauer BM, Eriksson, E, Guyuron, B, Coleman, JJ III, Russell, RC, Vander Kolk, CA (eds). Plastic Surgery. St. Louis, Mosby 2000, pp 2743–2767

70. Bacilious N, Kulber D, Peters E, Gayle LB, Chen MJ, Harper AD, Hoffman L: Harvesting of the latissimus dorsi muscle: a small animal model for seroma formation. Microsurgery 1995;16(9):646–649

71. European consensus statement of the prevention of venous thromboembolism. Int Angiol 1992;11:151

72. Bick RL, Haas SK: International consensus recommendations: summary statement and additional suggested guidelines. Med Clin N Amer 1998;82(3):613–633

73. Clement DI, Gheeraert P, Buysere M, et al.: Medical patients. In: Bergquist, D, Comerota, AJ, Nicolaides, AN, et al. (eds). Prevention of Venous Thromboembolism. London, Med-Orion 1994, p 319

74. Senior RM: Pulmonary embolism. In: Wyngaarden JB, Smith LH, Jr Bennett, JC (eds). Cecil Textbook of Medicine. Philadelphia WB Saunders 1992, pp 421–428

75. Prevention of venous thromboembolism. International consensus statement: guideline according to scientific evidence. Int Angiol 1997;16:3

76. McDevitt NB: Deep vein thrombosis prophylaxis. Plast Reconstr Surg 1999;104:1923–1928

77. Alving BM: The hypercoagulable states. Hosp Pract 1993;28(2):109–121

78. Bovill EG, Bauer KA, Dickerman JD, Callas P, West B: The clinical spectrum of heterozygous protein C deficiency in a large New England kindred. Blood 1989;73(3):712–717

79. Engesser L, Broekman AW, Briet E, Brommer EJ, Bertina RM: Hereditary protein S deficiency: clinical manifestations. Ann Intern Med 1987;106(5):677–682

80. Zoller B, Hillarp A, Dahlback B: Activated protein C resistance due to a common factor V gene mutation is a major risk factor for venous thrombosis. Annu Rev Med 1997;48:45–58

81. Svensson PJ, Dahlback B: Resistance to activated protein C as a basis for venous thrombosis. N Engl J Med 1994;330(8):517–522

82. Bertina RM, Koeleman BP, Koster T, Rosendaal FR, Dirven RJ, de Ronde H, van der Velden PA, Reitsma PH: Mutation in blood coagulation factor V associated with resistance to activated protein C. Nature 1994;369(6475):64–67

83. Bridgen ML: The hypercoagulable state. Who, how, and when to test and treat. Postgrad Med 1997;101(5): 249–267

84. Ginsberg JS: Management of venous thromboembolism. N Engl J Med 1996;335:1816–1828

85. Olesen LL, Ejlertsen T, Nielsen T: Toxic shock syndrome following insertion of breast prostheses. Br J Surg 1991;78(5):585–586

86. Poblete JV, Rodgers JA, Wolfort FG: Toxic shock syndrome as a complication of breast prostheses. Plast Reconstr Surg 1995;96(7):1702–1708

87. Walker LE, Breiner MJ, Goodman CM: Toxic shock syndrome after explantation of breast implants: a case report and review of the literature. Plast Reconstr Surg 1997;99(3):875–879

Capsular Contracture Following Augmentation Mammaplasty: Etiology and Pathogenesis

60

John A. McCurdy, Jr.

60.1
Introduction

All surgeons who perform augmentation mammaplasty agree that the principal problem associated with this otherwise aesthetically pleasing and popular operation is contraction of the capsule that forms around the implant, firming and often deforming the breast and occasionally causing discomfort—a process commonly known as capsular contracture. This situation occurs so frequently that many surgeons consider it to be an untoward sequela of the operation rather than a complication per se. When considered from a biological standpoint, encapsulation of a foreign body too large to be eliminated by phagocytosis is a normal occurrence. Why this biologically normal capsule around a mammary prosthesis contracts in some cases while remaining stable in others is a perplexing and frustrating question that remains incompletely understood.

Despite numerous clinical studies and laboratory investigations of capsular contracture, its etiology and pathogenesis remain uncertain [1]. Controversy surrounding this condition is so great that most surgeons can agree only on certain general statements concerning the process:

1. Capsular contracture occurs in 0–74% of breast implants depending on the series. (Most contemporary surgeons arbitrarily use a figure of 5–20 % in preoperative patient counseling.)
2. Capsular contracture may occur from several weeks to several years following surgery. Approximately 60% of capsular contracture occurs within 6 months and 90% within 12 months postoperatively.
3. Statistical analysis of capsular contracture suggests that it is a breast-related rather than a patient-based phenomenon, indicating that local rather than systemic factors predominate in its pathogenesis.

While the above observations provide a foundation for the study of capsular contracture, these very characteristics make orderly and objective analysis of the problem difficult and frustrating. Thus, it is not surprising that until recently, little progress was made in elucidat-

ing a comprehensive understanding of this condition and formulating rational plans for its prevention and/or control. During the past 15–20 years, however, application of scientific methods has begun to document reproducible findings applicable to etiology and pathogenesis, particularly on histological, ultrastructural, and molecular levels. Prior to this time, the body of literature on capsular contracture could best be characterized as a collection of largely anecdotal reports, the themes of which could perhaps best be described as variations on a "how I do it" theme. Efforts to isolate variables, collect objective and reproducible measurements, and conduct controlled studies with equivalent cohorts in order to enable evaluation of statistical significance were glaringly lacking.

60.2
Histological Characteristics of Capsules Surrounding Mammary Prostheses

The first studies of the basic histology of breast implant capsules suggested that they were simply collections of laminated collagen with limited cellularity largely consisting of fibroblasts, myofibroblasts, and occasional mononuclear cells and lymphocytes (Fig. 60.1). Muco-

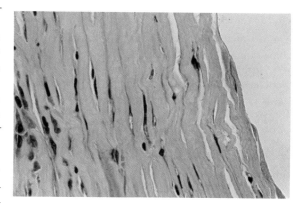

Fig. 60.1 Unsophisticated histological appearance of contracting capsule (circa 1985)

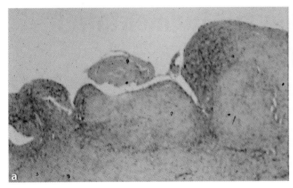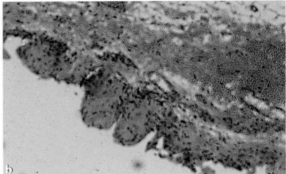

Fig. 60.2 a Histological appearance of BioCell capsule showing villous hyperplasia. **b** BioCell capsule showing hyperplastic configuration

polysaccharides were found in the capsules and presumably constituted a ground substance that "cemented" the latticework of collagen fibers into a cohesive structural unit [2]. Peripheral to this was a less dense membrane that was loosely organized and more vascular and cellular (fibroblasts and mononuclear cells), which blended gradually into the surrounding connective and adipose tissue.

Contemporary analysis of capsules shows a somewhat more sophisticated histological description of a complex structure consisting of three distinct layers [3]. The internal layer adjacent to the prosthesis surface appears to be either single-layered or multilayered, containing macrophages and fibroblasts. The middle layer is composed of loosely arranged connective tissue including an internal vascular supply, while a third layer consists of a dense connective tissue containing an external vascular supply. In approximately 62% of patients, an inner layer of synovial-like metaplasia (Fig. 60.2) composed of mononuclear macrophages with variable numbers of multinucleated giant cells is noted. Capsules tend to become less cellular with time. In approximately 40% of capsular specimens, acute inflammation is noted, and chronic inflammation is found in approximately 90% of capsules [4, 5]. Silicone is present in many, if not most, capsules and is confirmed by vacuolated macrophages containing refractory material. Silicone levels decrease with increasing distance from the surface of the implant, and greater capsular thickness is associated with a greater presence of silicone. Large amounts of silicone are associated with increased local inflammation [4].

Early studies found little correlation between histological characteristics of the capsule around a mammary prosthesis and the class of contracture [6], but more recent studies [4, 5] have shown definite correlations with capsule thickness and clinical firmness of the breast as measured by the Baker classification. A recent suggestion that classification of capsular contracture be based on histological findings, which is consistent with con-

temporary theory that this process is an inflammatory disorder, has been proposed [5], and it has been found that such a histological classification (Table 60.1) correlates well with the clinical classification of Baker. Some investigators are enthusiastic about this correlation, as a precise histological classification is deemed preferable to a more subjective clinical classification when comparing the results of techniques, types of prostheses, and variations of therapeutic interventions.

Silicone has been positively identified in the capsular tissue surrounding both gel- and saline-filled implants. Although initially thought to be a consequence of gel bleed through the elastomer envelope, silicone is also found in macrophages surrounding saline implants. The origin of this material must be frictional, the result of shearing forces on the elastomer envelope similar to shards of material found around other solid silicone implants that do not contain gel [4].

Recent evidence shows that silicone is toxic to macrophages, presumably initiating the release of cytokines,

Table 60.1 Comparison between the Baker (clinical) and Wilflingseder (histological) classification of capsular contracture

Class	Baker	Wilflingseder
I	Prosthesis not visible or palpable	Thin and noncontracted capsule
II	Prosthesis slightly firm but not visible	Constrictive fibrosis; no giant cells
III	Prosthesis firm and visible	Constrictive fibrosis; presence of giant cells
IV	Implant deformation; pain	Inflammatory cells, foreign body granulomas, neovascularization

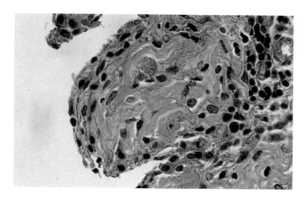

Fig. 60.3 BioCell capsule; note cellularity

leukotrienes and other proinflammatory substances into the milieu surrounding the prosthesis [4].

Other studies suggest that silicone not only induces the formation of laminated collagen and foreign body granulomas but also evokes a strong cellular T-cell-mediated immune response resulting in the infiltration of the activated CD4+ cells [7].

Numerous studies of capsular contracture have examined the influences of implant filler material, surface texture, and position of prosthesis placement as primary variables, generating contradictory results [8–10]. Only one study has shown an increased incidence of capsule contracture around saline versus silicone implants [11].

Prantl et al. [4] demonstrated that the severity of inflammation correlated with greater capsular thickness, which in turn correlated with a higher Baker score. These investigators suggested that the middle capsular layer appears to be the key to the histological changes associated with firming of the contracted capsule, perhaps because of its extensive vascular network. According to Wilflingsender et al., another important etiologic factor in the generation and perpetuation of capsular contracture is the presence of silicone-loaded macrophages [12]. Silicon derivates appear to damage macrophages, inducing them to produce transforming growth factor (TGF)-beta and other proinflammatory substances that stimulate fibroblasts to produce collagen.

Capsules around textured implants are likely to have a palisaded, secretory, and phagocytic multicellular layer devoid of a basement membrane adjacent to the implant, overlaid by a thicker, more disoriented cellular and vascular connective tissue layer attenuating to a loose connective tissue and adipose tissue layer that blends with surrounding breast tissue. Frequently these capsules assume a papillary, hyperplasic appearance (Fig. 60.3). Termed villous hyperplasia, this histology has been reported in approximately 63% of textured capsules up to 5 years old but decreases significantly in capsules with time [13]. Capsular synovium is thought

to be of mesenchymal origin and is believed to be a reaction to movement (micromotion) and shearing forces at the capsule–prosthesis interface. This synovium secretes substances that may lubricate the prosthesis–tissue interface, and there has been speculation that they may help to diminish capsular contracture. The synovial layer tends to diminish over time as noted above, and this may be one explanation of an increase in capsular contracture that some surgeons suspect of textured (as well as smooth) implants as a function of time.

The author's studies [14] of textured implants found a fluid-filled periprosthetic space (bursa) in approximately one-third of specimens (none exhibited tissue adherence to the implant, and all breasts were extremely soft), while the remaining two-thirds of specimens demonstrated tissue adherence without periprosthetic fluid. A characteristic gross as well as histological appearance (Figs. 60.4, 60.5) as well as scanning electron

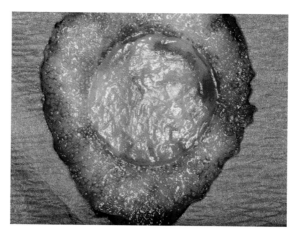

Fig. 60.4 Gross anatomy of BioCell capsule. Note mirror image evidence of tissue adherence and absence on area of capsule over smooth identifying disk on posterior surface of prosthesis

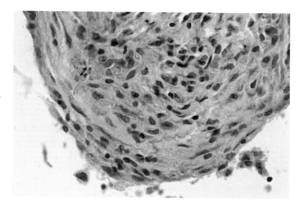

Fig. 60.5 BioCell capsule. Note the polypoid extension

micrographs (Figs. 60.6, 60.7) showing the capsule to be essentially a mirror image of the implant surface were also noted for those prostheses exhibiting tissue adherence. These breasts were firmer (Baker class II) and exhibited a higher incidence of "rippling," although this was rarely of concern to the patient. In contrast, the textured implants reacting with a bursa-like response did not exhibit rippling. This finding suggests that tissue adherence results in micromotion at the capsule–prosthesis interface that may induce a small degree of capsular contracture, while the bursa reaction is not associated with micromotion and thus does not precipitate contracture. Of additional interest is that the "bursal" periprosthetic fluid grossly resembled that commonly found around steroid-treated prostheses. This observation provides additional evidence that capsule-modifying properties of textured prostheses are related to alteration of the inflammatory exudates and cellular reaction induced by these implants (inflammatory milieu).

Current evidence demonstrates that progressive fibrotic disorders affecting the liver, lungs, kidney, heart, and skin are complex and multifactorial processes involving a complicated cascade of cellular, histochemical, and other molecular events, which include leukotrienes, cytokines, and various growth factors initiated by platelet activation [15]. Of significance, therapeutic intervention with inhibitors of inflammatory precursors is currently being explored (see below), which is consistent

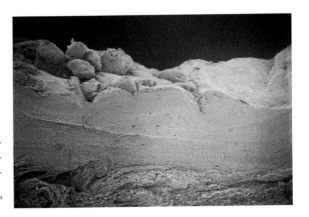

Fig. 60.7 Lateral view of same BioCell capsule segment

with the growing contemporary feeling that the most effective efforts to control capsular contracture may be on the molecular level.

Hyaluronan (also known as hyaluronic acid) is a mucopolysaccharide that comprises a large component of inflammatory exudates, including the ground substance that "cements" the lattice of collagen fibers in capsules forming around breast prostheses. It has been found to be a reliable biomarker correlating with the severity of the degree of fibrosis in fibrotic disorders such as those involving the liver. Prantl et al. [15] studied the relationship between capsular contracture and serum hyaluronan following breast augmentation, correlating the levels of this substance with variables including capsular thickness and histological as well as immunohistochemical evidence of inflammation. Analysis showed that serum levels of hyaluronan are elevated in patients with capsular contracture. A positive correlation was found between serum hyaluronan levels and the severity of capsular contracture as measured by the Baker classification. These investigators suggested that further study was required to determine whether serum hyaluronan levels could serve as biomarkers for predicting capsular contracture preoperatively as well as for selecting patients who might benefit from medical therapy targeting the inflammatory cascade rather than surgical intervention.

60.3
The Enigma of Myofibroblasts

Myofibroblasts—cells that are histologically similar to fibroblasts but contain smooth muscle elements that pharmacologically respond similarly to smooth muscle cells—are found in capsular tissue and have been postulated to be the driving force of the contracture process.

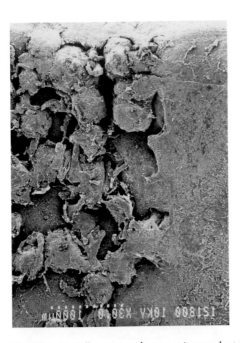

Fig. 60.6 BioCell scanning electron micrograph at junction of textured surface and smooth identifying disk

These cells were first noted in granulation tissue and are responsible for wound contracture, disappearing when a wound has healed. They persist, however, in hypertrophic scars and keloids. Myofibroblasts are also present in disorders characterized by abnormal fibrous tissue proliferation, such as Dupuytren's contracture.

Rudolph et al. [16] found myofibroblasts in 20 of 25 firm capsules, but also found these cells in 16 of 24 soft capsules. Regardless of clinical breast firmness, myofibroblasts were more likely to be found in younger capsules, an observation that is consistent with the life cycle of a myofibroblast in other wounds. A number of other investigators have described and speculated on the significance of myofibroblasts in breast capsules.

Baker et al. [17] studied the pharmacologic response of myofibroblasts and capsular tissue and found that 75% of the tissue specimens responded to smooth muscle contractants and 69% to smooth muscle relaxants. This activity was greater in younger specimens, but there was no correlation between pharmacologic activity and clinical breast firmness. These investigators postulated that myofibroblasts were the cellular elements responsible for contracture of a developing capsule by means of a ratchet-like mechanism involving collagen and cross-linking, the contracting site being maintained by the gluelike properties of mucopolysaccharide ground substance in which a latticework of collagen fibers is imbedded. There has been no explanation, however, of why myofibroblast activity is stimulated in some breasts but not in others. Thus, while this evidence provides a model for the pathogenesis of capsular contracture (Fig. 60.8), there is still little consensus (other than regarding inflammatory processes) concerning the etiologic factors that activate the cellular mechanisms that might be involved in stimulating the contractile properties of myofibroblasts. An excellent review of the structure and reactivity of these cells was published by Coleman et al. [18], who concluded that "capsular contracture is a form of granulation reaction; in vitro contractility correlates with clinical evidence of adverse capsular contracture," and that "these findings support the hypothesis that implant capsules represent a three-dimensional wound around the implant." A schematic of proposed relationships between myofibroblasts and other elements involved in capsular contracture is presented in Fig. 60.8.

60.4 Etiology of Capsular Contracture

Controversy surrounding the etiology of capsular contracture is compounded by the fact that much of the literature concerning this condition is scientifically flawed, largely consisting of subjective and anecdotal testimonials highlighting an individual author's current views on the subject, often related to earlier reports on his or her latest variations in surgical technique. But as noted previously, a number of recent studies have been better designed and provide viable evidence regarding this condition. Because contemporary evidence suggests that the majority of capsular contracture is caused by an inflammatory process or a related foreign body granulomatous reaction, basically any stimulus (or "activator") that precipitated these conditions could be an etiologic factor. At the present time, however, subclinical bacterial infection (or colonization) or a foreign body inflam-

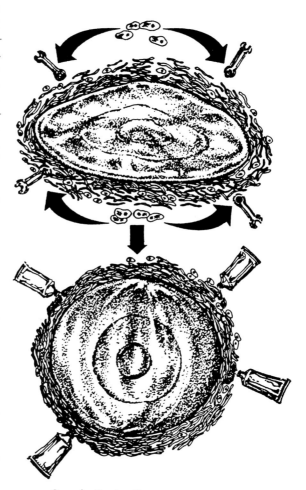

Capsular Contraction

1) Collagen fibers densely laminated by "ratchet action" of myofibroplasts and mucopolysaccharide cement

Fig. 60.8 Proposed mechanism of capsular contracture

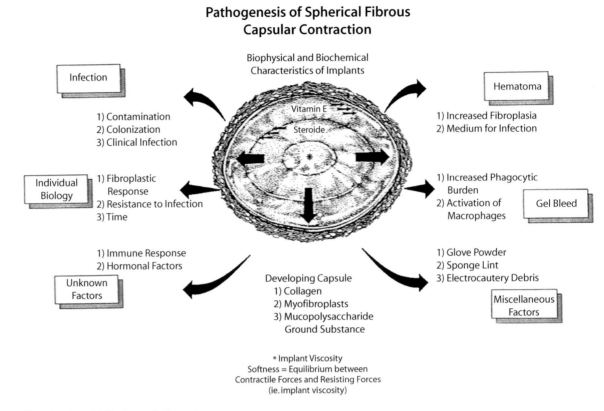

Fig. 60.9 Possible "activators" of capsular contracture

matory stimulus, the major culprit alleged to be silicone droplets or fragments, are the major suspects. Proposed etiologic factors are shown in Fig. 60.9.

60.4.1
Infection

The role of microorganisms and the pathogenesis of capsular contracture has long been a matter of speculation, and increasing evidence supports the possibility that a bacterial contamination (colonization) or subclinical infection of the capsules forming around the implant may stimulate contraction by activating immune processes. A number of investigators have reported a high incidence of positive cultures (predominantly coagulase-negative *Staphylococcus epidermis*) in mammary tissue, nipple secretions, and implant pockets (both before initial implantation and during exploration for capsular contracture), and thus the evidence implicating bacterial contamination as a major cause of capsular contracture has substantial strength. The propensity of bacteria to stimulate fibroplasia and wound contraction is well known. To be fair, it must also be noted that some

studies have found no correlation between cultures of capsular specimens and clinical breast firmness.

The evidence for the relationship between bacteria and capsular contracture is based on the following observations:

1. *S. epidermidis* is readily cultured from breast secretions as well as from apparently normal breast tissue. This organism has been cultured in 55% of dissected implant pockets prior to insertion of the prosthesis and is isolated from 66–95% of fibrous capsules submitted for culture. As noted above, however, isolation from mammary capsules does not always correlate clinically with the subjective assessment of breast firmness in the patient population studied.
2. The ductile system of the breast is traumatized by augmentation mammaplasty, providing a route for introduction of microorganisms from the breast and ductile system into the periprosthetic space.
3. The presence of a foreign body (gel, talc, coagulation debris, etc.) reduces the physiologic threshold for tissue reaction to bacteria.

In a study of 124 augmentation mammaplasties, Burkhart et al. [19] showed that during the first 3 months, the incidence of capsular contracture was seven times higher in a control group compared with mammary pockets irrigated with antibiotics or 5% povidone-iodine solution. Follow-up of the breasts for 24 months showed that the control group had an overall incidence of capsular contracture two times that of the antibiotic/povidone-treated patients, and that the early sevenfold increase in capsular contracture (during the first 3 postoperative months) accounted entirely for the overall decreased incidence of capsular contracture in the irrigation group.

Whether microorganisms can penetrate an established, relatively avascular capsule is a matter of speculation, but if subclinical infection or colonization by S. epidermidis is a prime initiator and perpetuator of capsular contracture, the implications with regard to contracture that develops more than 3 months postoperatively are troubling from a prophylactic and/or therapeutic standpoint. Perhaps the most logical solution to this difficult situation would be to provide some means of reducing the fibroblastic response to the offending agent (bacterial or nonbacterial) regardless of its ultimate etiology. As discussed below, various inhibitors of critical points in the inflammatory cascade are being targeted with pharmacological therapy, in some cases with suggested success:

1. Zafirlukast (Accolate) is a leukotriene inhibitor used successfully to manage the inflammatory aspects of asthma. Initial clinical results were encouraging [20], but subsequent interest by surgeons has been lukewarm at best. Bastos et al. [21] studied the effect of this agent on capsular contracture using a rat model. Capsular analysis involved both histological and immunohistochemical analysis. Noteworthy findings were confined to textured prostheses, for which thinner capsules, decreased collagen density, less vascularity, and smaller numbers of mastocytes and eosinophils were found in comparison with the control group. The investigators encouraged further study of this agent.

2. Cysteinyl leukotriene receptor blockers may interrupt the inflammatory cascade (cycloxygenasic and lipooxygenasic pathways) [22]. These leukotriene receptors populate macrophages and fibroblasts in contracting capsular tissue and mediate such functions as inflammatory activation and regulation, inflammatory cell recruitment, vascular permeability, and fibrosis. Application of agents that modify or block the expression of these receptors requires additional research [23].

3. Regarding sodium 2-mercaptoethane sulfonate (Mesna or the generic uromitexan), Ajmal et al. [24] investigated the ability of Mesna (a thiol used to prevent lesions in the urinary tract caused by anti-

neoplastic agents) to reduce capsular contracture in a rabbit model. Two textured implants were placed into 20 rabbits; 10 ml of 10% Mesna was instilled into one pocket in each rabbit. Sacrifice and histological examination of the capsules was performed at 5 months. The researchers reported that the mean total thickness as well as the thickness of the myofibroblast layer of the Mesna group was approximately one-half that of the control group, and the capsules in the Mesna group were less vascular than those in the control group. These investigators speculated that Mesna acts by changing the inflammatory milieu at the tissue–prosthesis interface by dissolving tissue connections via disrupting disulfide bonds and thus interfering with formation of the extracellular matrix.

In discussing the relationship of capsular contracture to bacterial infection, anecdotal reports have related the onset of capsular contracture to an episode of pain and/or tenderness of the breast following a systemic infection (e.g., cystitis, sinusitis, or, importantly, dental intervention including cleaning), suggesting the possibility of hematogenous spread of microorganisms into the breast. There is, however, no clear evidence to support this observation, although many surgeons advise patients to request a dose of prophylactic antibiotic on the day of a dental visit or other invasive procedure.

Proponents of the infection/capsular contracture scenario postulate that this mechanism may account for the apparently lower incidence of clinically apparent contracture following submuscular implantation, suggesting that the pectoralis muscle may provide a barrier to bacterial contamination through the ductal system. But it should be noted that the inferior aspect of the prosthesis is often in a subglandular and/or subcutaneous location following retromuscular augmentation, and so there is no barrier in this region.

Overt infection, most often requiring prosthesis removal, has a strong correlation with capsular contracture. The current emphasis on the relationship between bacteria and capsular contracture, however, is on subclinical infection and colonization, especially with regard to the ability of such conditions to serve as inflammatory stimuli.

The normal flora of the breast have been shown in vitro to be able to adhere within 2 min to elastomer envelopes and thus to colonize all types of breast implants [25]. They are often located in a "bioslime" film (biofilm) on the surface of the implant, where they exist in a dormant, sessile form (Fig. 60.10) relatively protected from antibiotic action and are thought to be prominent contributors to subclinical infection that may stimulate capsular contracture. Interestingly, there

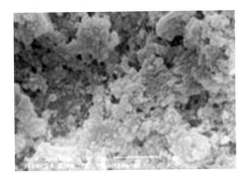

Fig. 60.10 Microorganisms in dormant biofilm on prosthesis surface

is considerable variation in studies on the effect of preoperative and postoperative antibiotics for preventing capsular contracture, although recent studies suggest a protective effect. Bacteria and fungi may enter and thrive inside inflatable implants. These organisms are usually discovered on aerobic and anaerobic culture of implant pockets and capsules and, perhaps surprisingly, are often not involved in clinically apparent postoperative infections.

In general, studies of bacterial interaction with breast prostheses suffer from multiple deficiencies, including the use of variable culture technologies, failure to culture aerobically for a long enough time, or lack of thoroughness in sampling the prosthesis surface or peri-implant tissue.

The differences in frequency of capsular contracture with saline versus gel and textured versus smooth implants are not readily explained by a bacterial theory of causation. Nevertheless, the evidence for a relationship between the presence of bacteria around the implant and capsular contracture, although not conclusive, is certainly suggestive.

As discussed earlier, Burkhardt et al. [19], in a study of 124 augmentation mammaplasties, reported that during the first 3 postoperative months, the incidence of capsular contracture was seven times higher in a control group compared with mammary pockets irrigated with antibiotics or 5% povidone-iodine solution. A 24-month follow-up showed that the control group had an overall incidence of capsular contracture two times that of the irrigated breasts and that the early sevenfold decrease in contracture accounted entirely for the overall decreased incidence in the irrigated group.

These investigators subsequently found some methodological flaws in the study, but Burkhardt and Demas [26] later published a study of the effect of Siltex (small pore) texturing and povidone-iodine irrigation

on capsular contracture, offering additional evidence of the role of bacterial contamination in the etiology and pathogenesis of capsular contracture. A subsequent study [27] of BioCell confirmed that antibacterial pocket irrigation substantially reduced the rate of contracture.

Dobke et al. [25] examined the incidence of bacterial presence on mammary implant surfaces and its relationship to breast firmness. Of 150 explants cultured, 81 were positive (predominately *S. epidermidis*); 76% of the contracted capsules were culture-positive, while 28% of noncontracted capsules were positive.

Pajkos et al. [28] compared clinical breast firmness with microbiological findings in 48 explants, 19 of which demonstrated capsular contracture. Routine cultures were uniformly negative, but the culture broth technique was 50% culture-positive (primarily *S. epidermidis*). Significantly, 17 of 19 breasts with contracture were positive compared with only one of eight from noncontracted breasts. There was no difference in culture positivity between silicone and saline implants. Scanning electron microscopy showed extensive biofilm deposits on prostheses surfaces as well as within capsular tissue, showing inflammatory reactions in a number of instances.

Schreml et al. [29] studied bacterial contamination in contracted capsules, finding a colonization rate of 66.7% around Baker III/IV contractures compared with 0% colonization around Baker II contractures. No significant difference was found between colonization rates of smooth (52.9%) and textured (25.0%) prostheses. These authors postulated that bacterial colonization stimulates and accelerates the inflammatory process, predisposing to fibrosis and capsular contracture.

Animal studies by Darouiche et al. [30] used implants impregnated with minocycline/rifampin. These saline implants were suspended in a bacterial suspension (*S. aureus*) for 30 min, and after drying for 60 min, they were implanted subcutaneously in rabbits. At sacrifice (2 and 4 weeks), impregnated implants were 12 times less likely to be colonized than control prostheses, suggesting that impregnating prostheses with antimicrobial substances may be a way to reduce capsular contracture.

Adams et al. [31] documented a fourfold to fivefold reduction in capsular contracture after augmentation mammaplasty induced by pocket irrigation with a triple antibiotic solution just prior to prosthesis placement. Two mixtures were used: 1) bacitracin, gentamicin, and cephalexin or 2) gentamicin, cefazolin, povidone-iodine. The composition of both mixtures was based on in-vitro analysis of the multiple bacteria potentially involved in capsular contracture. Because this was a prospective study, the "control" group consisted of pre-market approval data from Allergan and Mentor, which found a 9% incidence of capsular contracture after augmentation mammaplasty. Breast pockets irrigated with either antimicrobial mixture subsequently developed contracture in 1.8% of cases at 14 months of follow-up. There was no difference between textured and smooth implants. An interesting and important financial analysis of the benefits of reducing capsular contracture was provided.

60.4.2
Hematoma

Although the etiologic relationship between hematoma (drained or undrained) and subsequent capsular contracture is strong in the opinion of most experienced surgeons, clinical evidence supporting the cause-and-effect relationship is sparse and subjective, while animal studies are either equivocal or not supportive.

If hematoma causes capsular contracture, traces of hemosiderin should be found in contracted capsules. However, Gayou [6] found traces of this substance in both contracted and noncontracted capsules. In an animal study using baboons, hematoma was associated with a marked fibroblastic response; however, it was resolving by the 16th week of the study [32]. Another animal study using micro-implants in mice found that hematoma produced no effect on the thickness, histological appearance, or measured intraluminal pressure of the implants [33].

Because the frequency of clinically apparent hematoma is much lower than that of significant capsular contracture, this complication is, at most, a small contributor to contracture. Human studies of the association between hematoma capsule contracture generally involve very small numbers and thus are not statistically significant, although several studies have found a twofold to threefold increase in the incidence of capsular contracture following hematoma. Undoubtedly, the strong belief among surgeons concerning the relationship between capsular contracture and hematoma is related to the observation that blood precipitates an aggressive fibroblastic response. Also, hematoma provides a fertile medium for bacterial growth.

60.4.3
Position of Implant Placement

Current evidence supports the concept that prosthesis placement in the submuscular plane reduces—in some

studies markedly—the incidence of capsular contracture, particularly severe contraction. Some large studies, however, dispute this contention, finding the incidence of capsular contracture to be similar for submuscular and subglandular prostheses [34, 35]. Postulated mechanisms for decreased firmness of submuscular implants include the following:

1. The contractile activity of the overlying muscle "massages" the implant.
2. The muscle provides a barrier between the implant and the breast parenchyma that protects against bacterial contamination from breast tissue.

Proper implant placement in the submuscular plane usually requires sufficient dissection of the pocket so as to place the inferior aspect of the implant in a subglandular or subcutaneous position, providing a weak link in the proposed barrier function (protection from bacterial contamination) by the pectoralis major muscle. Therefore, it is difficult to conclude that submuscular implants are entirely less prone to infection. There is also no evidence that such implants are in some fashion less sensitive to the effects of silicone droplets or fragments or could benefit from the proposed massaging action of the muscle. Interestingly, some surgeons feel that submuscular placement results in atrophy of the muscle, responsible for its often dramatic thinning after submuscular breast augmentation, which would obviously effectively eliminate massaging activity.

Capsular contracture occurring around submuscular implants is generally more difficult to treat than that occurring around subglandular implants.

60.4.4
Textured Versus Smooth Prosthesis

Textured silicone prostheses have been available since January 1988, and preliminary evaluations by the manufacturer (animal studies as well as clinical trials) suggested a substantial reduction in the incidence of capsular contracture around these implants. The initial enthusiasm of surgeons confirming these lower rates of encapsulation has been somewhat tempered in recent years because of suspicion that the rate of capsular contracture may increase over time around textured implants, as well as because of problems with rippling particularly associated with textured saline implants placed in the subglandular position.

In actuality, however, few studies have analyzed the incidence of capsular contracture around textured prostheses after more than 1 year, but those that have show a continuation of lower rates for up to 7 years postoper-

Table 60.2 Textured prostheses: possible mechanisms of action

1. Random collagen orientation reduces cross-linking, lamination, and additive contractile forces

2. Macrophage inhibition of fibroblasts

3. Obliteration of periprosthetic space by tissue ingrowth and/or adherence

4. Tissue ingrowth reduces "micromotion" at implant/tissue interface, reducing cellular trauma and subsequent inflammation

5. Textured surface allows isolation of microorganisms

6. Bursa effect in nonadherent prostheses alters inflammatory histochemical and cellular milieu

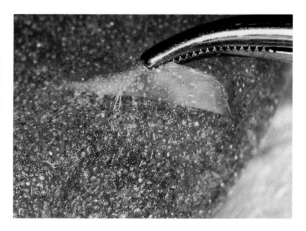

Fig. 60.11 Capsular adherence to BioCell surface

atively [36]. However, after 1 year the "quality or the data deteriorates," and thus the clinical significance of longer-term follow-up is debatable with regard to answering the question of whether textured implants reduce or simply delay the onset of capsular contracture.

The precise mechanism by which textured implants reduce the incidence of capsular contracture remains to be elucidated. Some of the possible mechanisms are listed in Table 60.2. Collagen fibers produced around a smooth implant surface eventually become oriented in only one direction with respect to the implant surface, i.e., parallel to the envelope. Collagen fibers that are oriented in parallel fashion tend to shorten as cross-linking occurs, producing a stronger and more compact scar as these fibers become laminated in mucopolysaccharide ground substance. Myofibroblasts are thought to exert a ratchet-like effect in this cross-linking process, which often results in clinical firmness around a soft, malleable breast prosthesis.

In contrast, collagen fibers produced at the interface of the textured implant demonstrate a random orientation with respect to the implant surface, reducing cross-linking, compaction, and lamination. It is postulated that such random (multilayered) orientation of collagen fibers results in individual capsular segments that are oriented in different directions, thus canceling the contractive forces of each other, in contrast to the theoretically additive contractive forces present around smooth-surfaced prosthesis.

It is further postulated that tissue ingrowth into the implant "pores" stabilizes the implant surface, reducing micromotion between the elastomer surface and fibrous capsule that may theoretically cause continuing cellular trauma and incite continued inflammation and fibroblastic activity. Perhaps even more importantly, this tissue ingrowth and/or adherence

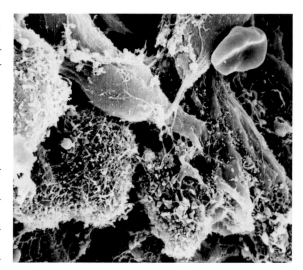

Fig. 60.12 High-power scanning electronic micrograph of BioCell capsule. Note cellularity

(Fig. 60.11) obliterates the periprosthetic space found around smooth implants, which may enhance the ability of cellular defense mechanisms to isolate and destroy microorganisms and other foreign body contaminants on the surface of the textured prosthesis implant. The histological studies (Figs. 60.2–60.5) and scanning electron micrographs previously presented (Figs. 60.6, 60.7, 60.12) show distinct differences in the capsules around textured implants, perhaps correlating with their capsule-modifying properties.

Macrophages persist in great numbers around textured implants surfaces, and because macrophages may eventually inhibit fibroblastic activity (although stimulation of collagenesis is found in the early phases of wound healing), the absolute amount of collagen produced around textured implants may be less than that produced around a smooth implant. Indeed, histological studies of implanted silicone disks having one smooth and one textured surface show that collagen deposition around the smooth surface is thicker than around the textured surface by a ratio of 4:1 (Table 60.2).

The precise physical characteristics of the prosthesis surface appear to be an important factor in the performance of textured implants. Indeed, animal studies show that issue ingrowth around solid implants occurs if a textured surface is constructed such that its indentions or "pores" range in diameter from 100 millimicrons to 1,000 millimicrons [37]. The pores on BioCell implants are 200–800 millimicrons in size, whereas those on the surface of Siltex implants measure 30–70 millimicrons, which is apparently smaller than the range conducive to tissue ingrowth. I have removed numerous BioCell implants and several Siltex textured prostheses and, as described above, noted definite tissue adherence (Fig. 60.11) around two-thirds of the BioCell implants (one-third demonstrated a bursa-like phenomenon characterized by exudate in the periprosthetic space, grossly similar to that found around steroid-containing prostheses) and questionable adherence to the Siltex surface. Histological and scanning electron microscopy of Siltex capsules show distinct differences from BioCell capsules (Figs. 60.13, 60.14).

In final analysis, it appears that the physical characteristics of the prosthesis affect cellular and histochemical reactions (inflammatory milieu) occurring at the tissue–prosthesis interface, thus accounting for the capsule-modifying properties of textured implants. Unfortunately, the phenomenon of rippling that occurs all too frequently around textured saline prostheses, particularly those placed in the subglandular position, has reduced the popularity of textured surfaces.

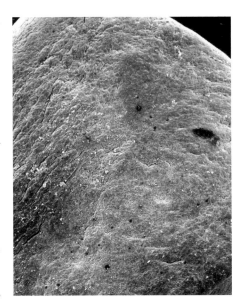

Fig. 60.14 Scanning electron micrograph of Siltex capsule showing undulations incapable of tissue ingrowth

60.5
Miscellaneous Factors

Silicone effects on capsular contracture as a result of gel bleed or fragments of elastomer envelopes apparently sheared from their surfaces have been discussed previously. Some surgeons believe that foreign bodies such as glove talc (which has been shown to cause fibrosis in the abdominal cavity), lint from surgical sponges, or necrotic debris from electrocautery may provide a stimulus for an increased fibroblastic response around a mammary prosthesis.

The immune system, as discussed above, plays a role in capsular contracture by virtue of its intimate association with the inflammatory process. Individual genetic differences in susceptibility to fibroblastic stimuli certainly exist but have not yet been defined.

60.5.1
Steroids

In view of the effects of steroids on wound healing and scar formation, it is not surprising that surgeons have attempted to harness the power of these agents in the struggle against capsular contracture. The use of steroids in conjunction with augmentation mammaplasty is a subject of controversy, but a number of clinical and laboratory studies are available for review by surgeons who wish to objectively evaluate their use. Unfortunately, the dramatic complications that were all too

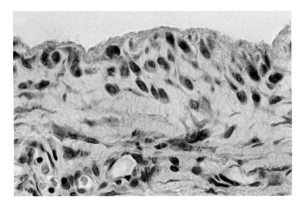

Fig. 60.13 Histological appearance of Siltex capsule showing undulations, not villous morphology

frequently associated with instilling insoluble steroids (triamcinolone) into implant lumens have been experienced only by a small number of younger surgeons. Older and more experienced surgeons are cognizant of these complications and the treatment of such problems. Many such surgeons would agree that treatment of steroid complications is simpler and more effective than treatment of the established capsular contracture, which has a record of generally dismal results (characterized by a high incidence of surgical complications and recurrence), although recently described modifications in technique claim to yield better outcomes (see below).

Numerous investigations have shown that in order to be effective, steroids must be used intraluminally. Periprosthetic instillation of these agents apparently has no discernible effect on the clinical course or histological appearance of the capsule forming around prosthesis. It must be noted, however, that there have been no specific studies of the effect of extraluminal steroids injected into the deeper layers of the dissected pocket.

On the other hand, intraluminal steroids produce a marked effect on both capsule histology and clinical firmness. The histological differences in capsules produced in laboratory animals with and without the use of corticosteroids are summarized in Table 60.3. Biochemical analysis of these capsules shows that while collagenous protein concentration is similar, capsules forming around steroid-containing implants in animals contain smaller concentrations of total protein, suggesting that the mucopolysaccharide component that forms the ground substance cementing the latticework of collagen fibers together (thus accounting for the capsule's structural integrity) is diminished by intraluminal steroids. This hypothesis correlates well with the observed fragility of capsules surrounding steroid-containing implants and also correlates with the histological appearance of

loosely woven, more randomly arranged collagen fibers observed in such capsules. Histological studies of capsules show an absence of myofibroblasts in steroid-treated capsules.

Despite the laboratory evidence documenting the effectiveness of intraluminal steroids on capsule formation, many surgeons are reluctant to use these agents because of the complications reported in the late 1970s [38]. The most severe of these complications are implant ptosis, atrophy of breast tissue and skin, and development of striae associated with the use of triamcinolone, an insoluble steroid that concentrates in the dependent portion of the implant. Reported complications are considerably less frequent and severe in prostheses that contain soluble steroids. Significantly, reports indicate that these complications, except perhaps striae associated with triamcinolone, are reversible by removing the steroid-containing implant and replacing it with an untreated prosthesis.

Shiffman [39] has reported that resolution of steroid atrophy is even more rapid when, in addition to implant replacement, the atrophic area is injected with normal saline. A study by Shumaker et al. confirms this suggestion [40].

Several studies have documented a dose-dependent relationship between soluble steroids, inhibition of capsular contracture, and development of steroid-related complications. These investigations show that if a dose equivalent of methylprednisolone does not exceed 20 mg, the incidence of contracture approximates 10%, whereas steroid-related complications approximate 4%. The authors reported that complications were mild and that few patients even noticed them [41].

A quite graphic and informative demonstration of the dose-dependent relationship between steroids and capsular contracture/steroid complications was provided by

Table 60.3 Histological differences in capsules produced in laboratory animals with and without the use of corticosteroids

	Control	Steroid
Thickness	–	Decreased
Collagen lamination	Uniform-sized fibers oriented parallel to implant surface densely laminated in amorphous mucopolysaccharide ground space substance	Loosely woven nonlaminated fibers of nonuniform size and orientation, increased interfiber
Collagen content	–	Similar
Total protein	–	Less than controls
Mucopolysaccharide content	–	Less than controls

Other findings: Absence of myofibroblasts and failure of ground substance to "cement" collagen fibers

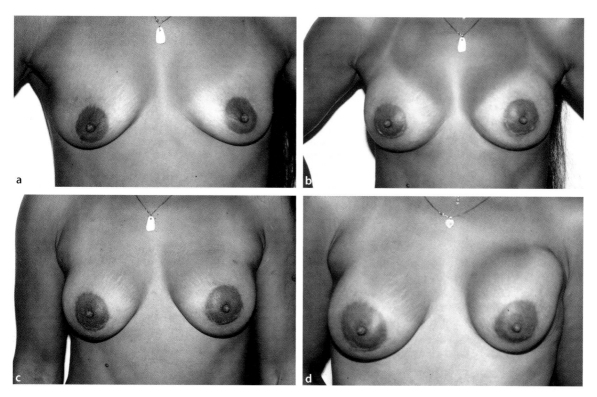

Fig. 60.15 a Preoperative augmentation mammaplasty. **b** Six months postoperative with steroid-containing prosthesis. **c** Bilateral ptosis occurring with the steroid-containing prosthe-sis. **d** Capsular contracture on left developed following prosthesis exchange to non-steroid-containing implant

O'Keefe [42]. Using a specially designed double-lumen implant equipped with a valve allowing percutaneous access to the saline-filled lumen, the effect of methylprednisolone concentration was studied in 224 breasts. A dose of 40 mg/40 cc saline was used at the time of augmentation. Four weeks postoperatively, the steroid concentration was reduced to 10 mg/40 cc in one group, 5 mg/40 cc in a second group, and 0 mg in a third group. The incidence of capsular contracture was dose-related: 7.8% in the first group, 17.6% in the second group, and 23.7% in the group with non-steroid-containing implants. Steroid-related complications were limited to "mild" skin atrophy and implant ptosis. One such breast treated by implant exchange subsequently developed capsular contracture (I have several patients who developed capsular contracture following exchange of steroid-containing implants; see Fig. 60.15). This study suggests that further improvement in the therapeutic ratio for intraluminal steroids is achieved by calculating steroid concentration versus absolute dose, i.e., soluble steroid concentration less than the equivalent of 20 mg methylprednisolone.

A component of the "no-touch" technique described by Mladick [43] that reduced the rate of capsular contracture to 0.6% was inclusion of methylprednisolone in the fill solution.

Although studies do demonstrate a dose–response relationship with steroid use, there is some individuality in the response of each patient. Therefore, proponents of steroid use stress that patients must be followed for an indefinite period of time.

The rate of diffusion of intraluminal methylprednisolone was measured in one animal study, and the steroid concentration was found to be reduced by 30–35% over a 3-month period [44].

In objectively evaluating the effect of steroids on capsular contracture and the problem of steroid-related complications, the following can be concluded:

1. The evidence regarding the efficacy of steroids in preventing capsular contracture is impressive in patients in whom small doses of methylprednisolone are used intraluminally. Additional supporting evidence is the observation that class III/IV contracture develops following the removal of steroid-containing implants in a number of cases (Fig. 60.15). It should be noted that capsular contracture developing around steroid-

containing implants is extremely responsive to closed capsulotomy.

2. The incidence of complications using intraluminal soluble steroids is low if a dose is calculated as a concentration with regard to saline volume. Impending complications (mild atrophy, ptosis) that develop following these doses are unusual but can be easily managed by careful follow-up evaluation and replacement of the implants if they become of concern to the surgeon or patient. This measure, however, appears to be seldom necessary when the dose is calculated as a concentration [45], and in any event, it is considerably easier and more effective than open capsulotomy for treating established capsular contracture.

Critics of steroid use suggest that a decreased incidence of capsular contracture may only delay the contracture process until the intraluminal steroid is depleted. A sophisticated statistical analysis by Ellenbogen and Braun [46], however, suggests that the steroid effect is not merely a temporary phenomenon.

Financial calculations of the savings based on the variables employed by Adams et al. [31] in their analysis of triple antimicrobial irrigation apply to all methods of reducing capsular contracture, including steroid use.

60.5.2
Titanium-Coated Breast Implants

Titanium-coated prostheses manufactured in Europe have been used clinically since 2001. A recent German animal study [47] found decreased tissue integration with these implants, suggesting a potential for a reduction in the rate of capsular contracture. An Australian study involving 3,000 women is planned to test this hypothesis [48].

60.6
Management of Established Capsular Contracture

As all experienced surgeons realize, recurrence of breast firmness is disappointingly high following open capsulotomy, indicating that current methods of treating this condition are less than satisfactory. At least two studies have documented high recurrence rates. Little and Baker [49] reported 40% recurrence after open capsulotomy, while Moufarrege et al. [50] found the recurrence rate to be 54% in patients treated by open capsulotomy.

More recent evidence suggests that recurrence is decreased by total capsulotomy as compared with removal of the anterior dome. Better results are also claimed by leaving the capsule intact and dissecting a new pocket posterior to the existing capsule [51]. The new pocket

can be in the same plane as the original, or it may involve a change in prosthesis position relative to the pectoralis. The most recent suggestion for improved outcome involves "dual-plane" positioning of the implant [52].

Given the generally dismal record of treating established contracture, it must be concluded that redoubled efforts to prevent its occurrence offer the only satisfactory solution to this problem. Attacking the inflammatory cascade is currently the most promising approach, but additional basic research into the etiology and pathogenesis as well as longer-term studies of capsular contracture are necessary if this goal is to be achieved.

In the meantime, the demonstrated reduction in contracture achieved by harnessing the power of corticosteroids, which have been the subject of extensive investigations, should be reevaluated by "doubting Thomases," particularly those "armchair" surgeons who cite and parrot surgical literature without personal experience with the techniques that they condemn [53].

References

1. McCurdy J: Capsular contracture following augmentation mammaplasty: etiology, management and prevention. Amer J Cosmet Surg 1989;6:141–150

2. Smahel J: Histology of the capsules causing constrictive fibrosis around breast implants. Br J Plast Surg 1977;30(4):324–329

3. Rubino C, Mazzarello V, Farace F, D'Andrea F, Montella A, Fenu G, Campus GV: Ultrastructural anatomy of contracted capsules around textured implants in augmented breasts. Ann Plast Surg 2001;46(2):95–102

4. Prantl L, Schreml S, Fichtner-Feigl S, Poppl N, Eisenmann-Klein M, Schwarze H, Fuchtmeiere B: Clinical and morphological conditions in capsular contracture formed around silicone breast implants. Plast Reconstr Surg 2007;120(1):275–284

5. Carpaneda C: Inflammatory reaction and capsular contracture around smooth silicone implants. Aesth Plast Surg 1997;21(2):110–114

6. Gayou R: A histological comparison of contracted and noncontracted capsules around silicone breast implants. Plast Reconstr Surg 1979;63(5):700–707

7. Wolfram D, Rainer C, Niederegger H, Piza H, Wick G: Cellular and molecular composition of fibrous capsules formed around silicone breast implants with special focus on local immune reactions. J autoimmunity 2004;23(1):81–91

8. Poeppl N, Schreml S, Lichtenegger F, Lenich A, Eisenmann-Klein M, Prantl L. Does the surface structure of implants have an impact on the formation of a capsular contracture? Aesthetic Plast Surg. 2007;31(2):133–139

9. Danino D, Basmacioglu P, Saito S, Rocher F, Blanchet-Bardon C, Revol M, Servant JM: Comparison of the capsular response to the BioCell RTV and Mentor 1600 Siltex breast implant surface texturing: a scanning electron microscopic study. Plast Reconstr Surg 2001;108(7):2047–2052

10. Wong C, Samuel M, Tan B, Song C: Capsular contracture in subglandular breast augmentation with textured versus smooth breast implants: a systemic review. Plast Reconstr Surg 2006;118(5):1224–1236

11. Fryzek J, Signorello L, Hakelius,L,. Lipworth L, McLaughlin JK, Blot WJ, Nyren O: Local complications and subsequent symptom reporting among women with cosmetic breast implants. Plast Reconstr Surg 2001;107(1):214–221

12. Wilflingseder P, Probst A, Mikuz G: Constrictive fibrosis following silicone implants in mammary augmentation. Chir Plast (Berl) 1974;2;215–229

13. Wyatt L, Sinow J, Wollman J, Sami D, Miller TA: The influence of time on human breast capsule histology: smooth and textured silicone –surfaced implants. Plast Reconstr Surg 1998;102(6):1922–1931

14. McCurdy J: Relationships between spherical fibrous capsular contracture and mammary prosthesis type; a comparison of smooth and textured implants. Amer J Cosmet Surg 1990;7:235–238

15. Prantl L, Pöppl N, Horvat N, Heine N, Eisenmann-Klein M: Serologic and histologic findings in patients with capsular contracture after breast augmentation with smooth silicone gel implants: is serum hyaluronan a potential predictor? Aesthetic Plast Surg 2005;29(6):510–518

16. Rudolph R, Abraham J, Vecchione T, Guber S, Woodward M: Myofibroblasts and free silicon around breast implants. Plast Reconstr Surg 1978;62(2):185–196

17. Baker JL Jr, Chandler ml, LeVier, RR: Occurrence and activity of myofibroblasts in human capsular tissue surrounding breast implants. Plast Reconstr Surg 1981;68(6):905–1012

18. Coleman DJ, Sharpe DT, Naylor IL, Chander CL, Cross SE: The role of the contractile fibroblast in the capsules around tissue expanders and implants. Br J Plast Surg 1993;46(7):547–556

19. Burkhardt B, Dempsey PD, Schnur PL, Tofield JJ: Capsular contracture: a prospective study of the effect of local antibacterial agents. Plast Reconstr Surg 1986;77(6);919–932

20. Schlessinger S, Ellenbogen R, Desvigne M, Svehlak S, Heck R: Zafirlukast(Accolate): a new treatment of a difficult problem. Aesth Surg J 2002;22:329–336

21. Bastos EM, Neto MS, Alves MT, Garcia EB, Santos RA, Heink T, Pereira JB, Ferreira LM. Histologic analysis of Zafirlukast effect on capsule formation around silicone implants. Aesthetic Plast Surg 2007;31(5):559–565.

22. Riccioni G, Bucciarelli T, Mancini B, Di Ilio C, D'Orazio N: Antileukotriene drugs: clinical application, effectiveness and safety. Curr Med Chem 2007;14(18):1966–1977

23. D'Andrea F, Nicoletti,F Grella,E, Grella R, Siniscalco D, Fuccio C, Rossi F, Maione S, De Novellis V: Modification of cysteinyl leukotriene receptor expression in capsular contracture. Ann Plast Surg 2007;58(2):212–214

24. Ajmal N, Riordan CL, Cardwell N, Nanney LB, Shack RB: The effectiveness of sodium 2-mercaptoethane sulfonate (mesna) in reducing capsular formation around implants in a rabbit model. Plast Reconstr Surg. 2003;112(5):1455–1461

25. Dobke MK, Svahn JK, Vastine VL, Landon BN, Stein PC, Parsons CL: Characterization of microbial presence at the surface of silicone mammary implants. Ann Plast Surg 1995;34(6):563–569

26. Burkhardt BR, Demas CP: The effect of Siltex texturing and povidone-iodine irrigation on capsular contracture around saline inflatable breast implants. Plast Reconstr Surg 1994;93(1):123–128

27. Burkhardt BR, Eades E. The effect of BioCell texturing and povidone-iodine irrigation on capsular contracture around saline-inflatable breast implants. Plast Reconstr Surg 1995;96(6):1317–1325

28. Pajkos A, Deva AK, Vickery K, Cope C, Chang L, Cossart YE: Detection of subclinical infection in significant breast implant capsules. Plast Reconstr Surg. 2003;111(5):1605–1611

29. Schreml S, Heine N, Eisenmann-Klein M, Prantl L: Bacterial colonization is of major relevance for high-grade capsular contracture after augmentation mammaplasty. Ann Plast Surg 2007;59(2):126–13029

30. Darouiche RO, Meade R, Mansouri MD, Netscher DT: In vivo efficacy of antimicrobe-impregnated saline-filled silicone implants. Plast Reconstr Surg 2002:109(4): 1352–1357

31. Adams WP, Rios J, Smith S: Enhancing patient outcomes in aesthetic and reconstructive breast surgery using triple antibiotic breast irrigation: six-year prospective clinical study. Plast Reconstr Surg: 2006;118(7 suppl):46S–52S

32. Williams C, Aston S, Rees T: The effect of hematoma on the thickness of pseudosheaths around silicone implants. Plast Reconstr Surg 1975;56(2):194–198

33. Moucharafeih BC, Wray RC Jr: The effects of steroid instillation and hematomas on the pseudosheaths of miniature breast implants in rats. Plast Reconstr Surg 1977;59(5):720–723

34. Slade C: Subcutaneous mastectomy. Acute complications and long-term follow-up. Plast Reconstr Surg 1984;73(1):84–90

35. Baker J: (Discussion) Augmentation mammaplasty. Plast Reconstr Surg 1999;103(6):1763–1765

36. Tarpila E, Ghassemifar R, Fagrell D, Berggren A: Capsular contracture with textured versus smooth saline-filled implants for breast augmentation. Plast Reconstr Surg 1997;99(7):1934–1939

37. Taylor S, Gibbons D: Effect of surface texture on the soft tissue response to polymer implants. J Biomaterial Res 1983;17(2):205–227

38. Ellenberg A: Marked thinning of the breast skin flaps after insertion of implants containing triamcinolone. Plast Reconstr Surg 1977;60(5):755–758

39. Shiffman MA: New treatment of steroid-induced fat atrophy. Plast Reconstr Surg 2002;109(7):2609–2610

40. Shumaker P, Rao J, Goldman M: Treatment of local, persistent cutaneous atrophy following corticosteroid injection with normal saline infiltration. Dermatol Surg 31 (10): 1340–1343, 2005

41. Cohen I: On the use of soluble steroids within inflatable breast prostheses. Plast Reconstr Surg 1978;62:105–106

42. O'Keefe P: The injection adjustable mammary implant. Ann Plast Surg 1983;11(3):237–241

43. Mladick R: "No-touch" submuscular saline breast augmentation technique. Aesthetic Plast Surg 1993;17(3):183–192

44. Ksander G, Vistnes L, Fogarty D: Experimental effects on surrounding fibrous capsule formation from placing steroid in a silicone bag-gel prosthesis before implantation. Plast Reconstr Surg 1978;62(6):873–884

45. Cohen I, Carrico T: Capsular contracture and steroid related complications in augmentation mammaplasty. Aesthetic Plast Surg 1980;4:267–271

46. Ellenbogen AH, Braun H: A three and one half year experience with double-lumen implants in breast surgery. Plast Reconstr Surg 1980;65(3):307–313

47. Hernandez-Richter T, Wittmann B, Wittmann F, Loehe F, Rentsch M, Mayr S, Jauch KW, Angele MK: Die beschichtung von silikonimplantaten mit titanist nicht effetiv zur vermeidung von infektionen. Zentralbl Chir: 2007;132(1):32–37 (abstract in English)

48. www.news.com.au/story/0,23599,21551073-2,22.html (Aussie women to get metal breast implants.) 13 April 2007. Study leader Dr. Daniel Fleming. Titanium coated breast implants – the Australian study – presentation at ACCS annual conference, Adelaide, 2006

49. Little G, Baker JL Jr: Results of closed capsulotomy for treatment of contracted breast capsules. Plast Reconstr Surg 1980;65(1):30–33

50. Moufarrege R, Beauregard G, Bosse JP, Papillon J, Perras C: Outcome of mammary capsulotomies. Ann Plast Surg 1987;19(1):62–64

51. Baran CN, Peker F, Ortak T, Sensoz O, Baran NK: A different strategy in the surgical treatment of capsular contracture: leave capsule intact. Aesthetic Plast Surg 2001;25(6):427–431

52. Spear SL, Carter ME, Ganz JC: The correction of capsular contracture by conversion to "dual-plane" positioning: technique and outcomes. Plast Reconstr Surg 2006;118(7 suppl):103S–113S

53. Tebbets JB: Conclusions not supported by data: a recurring story in breast augmentation publications. Plast Reconstr Surg 2006;118:563–565

CHAPTER 61

Complications Related to the Implant

Felix-Rüdiger G. Giebler

61.1
Introduction

The silicone controversies in 1992 [1] showed us that there may be complications specifically related to these implants. That is, the silicone shell does not resist very long in the harsh surroundings of a biological environment. We do not know of any material that would not be changed under these conditions. Besides the chemical influence, steady mechanical stress and pressure are placed on the implant by the movements of the muscles and the constriction of the capsule [2].

61.2
History

For thousands of years, humans have tried to change their external appearance for reasons of fashion, rites, and religion. Specifically, the female breast, which is not only a symmetrical feeding organ but a model of female identification and feminine consciousness, has been changed in different ways [3].

The different corsets used in antiquity that represent the function of a push-up bra bettered the cleavage enormously. The augmentation of the pectoral muscle by training and the vacuum suction apparatus of former days did not really augment the breast [4].

At the beginning of the 20th century, physicians tried to augment the breast by putting fat lumps into it [5]. After World War II, "daring" physicians injected free silicone [6] (silicone medical fluid 360; Dow Corning) and paraffin [7] into the breast. Both procedures are no longer acceptable.

The new period of breast augmentation started in 1962 with Cronin and Gerow, who implanted silicone bags into the female breast [8]. The first generation of silicone implants had a smooth outer coat that was filled with soft silicone gel and had Dacron patches on the back sides. In the mid-1970s we had the second generation of silicone implants, which were mostly round, smooth, thin-walled, and had no patches. The filling was made of a less fluid silicone gel with higher viscosity. In the 1980s, with focus on the gel's perme-

ation through the porous silicone shells, a third generation was introduced, which was coated with a double layer of high-performance elastomers with an additional barrier coat of fluorosilicone to reduce ruptures and bleeding. Nowadays, we have the fourth generation of silicone implants, which are made out of cohesive gel, sometimes anatomically formed and sometimes with patches to hamper rotation.

Almost from the beginning of the implantation story there have been implants filled with saline fluid.

It was always clear that these procedures involve a large alloplastic mass implanted into the breast. The foreign body reactions of the female body were and are the biggest challenges to this form of cosmetic surgery [9].

61.3
Techniques

Various techniques exist, and the varied approaches require different implantation materials. By the manifold techniques and the different implants, we have to individualize the augmentation of the female breast. The choice of approach is a prejudgment for a pocket. The tissue coverage is different in each approach, and each of these approaches has its own sequelae.
From the axillary access [10], the implant may be easily placed subglandularly, subfascially, and submuscularly, and prefilled and inflatable implants will fit. With a long-distance approach, lowering of the inframammary fold may be more difficult.

The intraareolar approach involves direct access through the gland, with good surgical overview. It is suitable for all implant placements. The umbilical approach is a long-distance approach that was invented for vascular extraanatomical bypass surgery. With this approach, only the use of inflatable implants is possible. The submammary approach is the one that provides the best surgical overview and allows clear separation of the anatomical structures in order to not leave scars there. From this approach, it is very easy to lower the submammary fold. The submammary access is best for revision operations because of the good overview.

The implant's placement determines the long-term

results for this aesthetic operation. The most natural way to augment the breast is above the muscle because the breast lies above the muscle. Placing the implant beneath the muscle exerts pressure on the implant and on the thorax, with the likelihood of displacement [11]. Submuscular implantation gives partial coverage of the implant with muscle but leaves the lower pole of the implant free of muscle and is covered only with skin and a thin layer of subcutaneous fat. Complete muscle coverage of the implant can be aided with the use of the serratus muscle. Subfascial implantation is between the subglandular and submuscular plane and seems to have certain advantages.

The most important issue in implantation surgery is the tissue coverage. The second most important issue is centering of the implant; the third is lowering of the submammary fold; and the fourth is how to leave a nonvisible scar. The aim of cosmetic breast surgery is an aesthetic, nonoperated appearance. This is not easy to achieve because the long-term results are influenced by the forming of a capsule around the implant.

There should be an aesthetic proportioning between the preoperative and postoperative breast. The larger the implant is in relation to the preexisting breast, the more it will balloon the breast. The telltale signs are the characteristic roundness in the upper and lower poles of the implant. There is a difference in aesthetic taste between those in Europe and the United States; the average implant size in Europe is 200–300 ml, whereas it is 400 ml in the United States.

All implants have a shield of silicone filled with different materials [12] and are manufactured in different forms and styles, from a low round profile to a teardrop shape. The surface of the shield is either smooth or rough (coated or textured), and there are double-lumen implants on the market, some with ports.

Capsular formation is not a sequela, it is a risk. That is, it is a normal reaction to an implanted foreign body. Capsular formation is found in 100% of the cases. The capsule can exert contractile forces and will shrink and tighten around the implant depending on other factors that are still in discussion [13]. The constrictive capsular formation may be the expression of a permanent inflammatory reaction, which can be triggered by infection, hematoma, traumatizing technique, bleeding of an implant, or insufficient tissue coverage. During the early to mid-1970s, there were indications that interrupted implant surfaces (texturing) produced positive results in capsule control by mechanically disrupting the developing collagen matrix and consequently inhibiting the formation of organized parallel fibers that could later become an axis of contraction. However, the textured surfaces led to the ingrowth of tissue associated with rippling and implant immobilization. The problem of constrictive capsular fibrosis seemed only to be delayed.

61.4
Rupture

Constrictive capsular fibrosis (CCF) leads to distortion, extrusion, or rupture [14]. Rupture has become one of the most important issues in cosmetic breast surgery and was the point that led to the silicone controversies in 1989. Implant failure has become one of the most im-

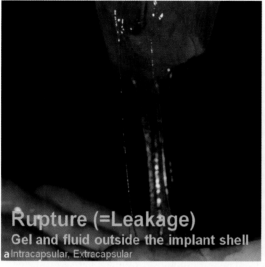
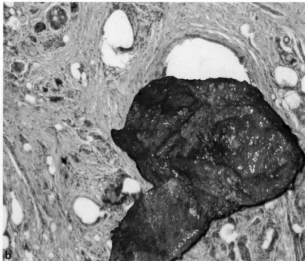

Fig. 61.1 a Intraoperative ruptured capsule. **b** Free droplets of silicone in the soft tissues on microscopic examination. Calcified capsule (*right*)

portant complications for women with breast implants, as well as for physicians, plaintiff attorneys, defense attorneys, and liability insurance companies.

The rupture may be caused through a variety of reasons, by external pressure, or by manufacturing defects (Fig. 61.1). The prevalence of rupture varies with the implant style, type, manufacturer, and implant age. No implant older than 10 years has been found to be intact and in good condition [15]. Peters et al. [16] stated that there is a positive corelationship between the duration of implantation time and the number of ruptured and leaking implants. Rupture (silicone implants) leads clinically to adjacent masses, associated lymph node swelling, asymmetry, and distortion of the breast.

The cases of rupture are corelated for determining the implant's integrity. The physical examination seems to be of little value, whereas surgery gives the utmost proof. Methods of imaging implant rupture have become more and more decisive over the years. Magnetic resonance imaging (MRI) is the most modern and best detector of this failure.

The aim of cosmetic breast surgery is a natural-looking breast both at rest and during movement. For this aim we need an ideal implant that resists mechanical strain, fabricated to the desired form, impervious to tissue fluid, chemically inert, nonirritating, nonallergic, noncarcinogenic, and, if possible, available at a low price. The desired implant is above all defined by the parameters of viscosity, density, molecular mass, pH, physical characteristics, biocompatibility, stability, osmolar activity, and radiolucency.

61.5
Radiolucency

Radiolucency is the numeric factor that allows the penetration of energy, such as x-rays, to a varied extent on the nature of the objectives [17]. The implant's filler material differs enormously regarding the passage of x-rays. The best penetration is allowed by soybean oil. Besides the different radiolucencies of the fillers, mammograms are hampered by scars and adjacent masses. There are different implants on the market with different filler materials regarding radiolucency.

61.6
Silicone

Hyde [18] and McGregor [19] rediscovered and developed silicone. Silicone consists of chains in variable lengths. Silicone rubber, compared to silicone gel, is composed of longer silicone chains and has an increased percentage of cross-linking. Silicone gel consists of two

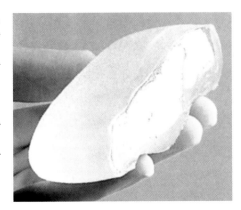

Fig. 61.2 Transected cohesive gel implant shows lack of extrusion of the gel

components: a matrix of long silicone chains cross-linked to each other (the "spaghetti") and non-cross-linked silicone chains filling the spaces surrounding the matrix. The escape of this fluid through the intact implant is called bleeding. When an intact implant is touched, the thin layer of slippery silicone fluid covering the implant's surface is always detectable. Rupture means a broken implant with outflow of gel and fluid (Fig. 61.1). Cohesive gel implants do not flow when broken because of specified variations of cross-linking (Fig. 61.2). Silicone is an excellent and proven biomaterial, essentially inert and highly compatible with human tissue. Silicone is a noncarcinogenic material. In cases of rupture or bleeding, there may be free silicone droplets within the soft tissue. Parts of them are stored in the lymphatic system and the lymph nodes. This lymphadenopathy [20] was the basis for the so-called silicone disease with undefined symptoms that has been of great interest to millions of implanted women. The newer silicone implants filled with cohesive gel have other aesthetic indications than the better adjustable gel implants [21].

61.7
Saline Implants

Saline implants are the most widely used implants in the United States, especially since the silicone controversies. Today approximately 70% of implant surgeons use this type. The saline filler responds to the normal electrolyte range found in blood. There have been reports of infections, even fungal infections, of the filler. Self-augmentations [22] may occur when macromolecules penetrate the shell of the implant. An incidence of 50% deflation in 50% of the cases of the older saline implants has been reported [23, 24].

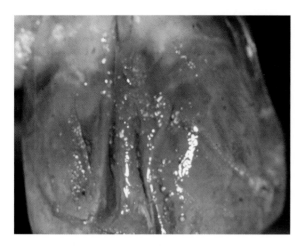

Fig. 61.3 A broken Trilucent implant that resulted in an infection

61.8
Soybean Implants (Triglyceride-Filled)

The soybean (triglyceride-filled) implant was especially invented for reasons of radiolucency, which is the same as breast tissue [25]. It was fabricated with a textured surface and a microchip to control the fate of the implant. Reports of several infections of the biogenic filler material caused it to be taken off the market (Fig. 61.3).

61.9
PVP Implants

The poly(N-vinyl-2-pyrrolidone) (PVP)-filled implant was previously widespread in Europe. Its overall problems were self-augmentation and, in cases of rupture, kidney overload. They were also taken off the market [26].

61.10
Polyurethane-Coated Implants

The idea of coated implants is that the ingrowth of soft tissue hampers the process of CCF (the constriction of myofibrils around the implant). The unknown fate of the breakdown of polyurethane restricted the use of this implant to special cases in Europe, and the Food and Drug Administration in the United States has given no market approval for it [27].

61.11
Titanium-Coated Implants

Titanium-coated implants as well as gold-coated ones had only a short survival on the European market because of unclear results.

61.12
Conclusions

Every implant seems to have its own results profile (Fig. 61.4). The number of available implants, which are different in form, surface, and fillers, indicates that the search for an optimal implantable material will continue. It involves the scientific question of how to control the body's reaction to a foreign material and how to develop materials that are inert or have less reactions.

The challenge in breast implant surgery is to develop a capsule that is thin, pliable rather than thick, fibrous, and potentially contractile. It is very important in implantation cosmetic surgery that the information and explanations given to the patient be crowned by her written consent. Infection plays an important role as a cause of CCF, and infection prevention should be started before the operation. The physician should look for infection in the nasal and throat areas as well as uri-

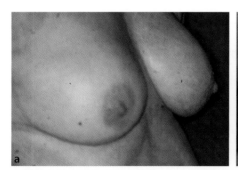
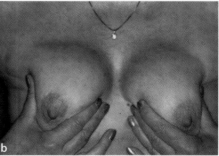

Fig. 61.4 A 60-year-old patient with silicone gel implants inserted 28 years previously (150-ml gel implant, low round profile, smooth). The breasts are still pliable and soft

nary tract infection, express the nipple before the operation, use a nipple shield, try not to cut through the gland, and irrigate the pocket.

Augmentation of the breast is the most desired cosmetic procedure worldwide. Distortion of the breasts by surgery, instead of making them more beautiful, means destruction of the feminine self-image and a catastrophe for the cosmetic surgeon.

References

1. U.S. Food and Drug Administration. Breast implants: an information update. U.S. Food and Drug Administration, Rockville, MD 1997

2. Giebler FRG: Komplikationen und Nebenwirkungen der aesthetisch plastischen Brustchirurgie. In: Mang WL, Bull HG (eds). Aesthetische Chirurgie, Reinbek, Einhorn Presse-Verlag 1995, pp 204–207

3. Birtchnell S, Whitfield P, Lacey JH: Motivational factors in women requesting augmentation and reduction mammaplasty. J Psychosom Res 1990;34(5):509–514

4. Tebbetts JB: Nonsurgical breast enlargement. Plast Reconstr Surg 2001;107(5):1320–1321

5. Czerny V: Plastischer Ersatz der Brustdrüse durch ein Lipom. Zentrabl Chir 1895;22:7

6. Delage C, Shane JJ, Johnson FB: Mammary silicone granuloma. Migration of silicone fluid to abdominal wall and inguinal region. Arch Dermatol 1973;108(1):105–107

7. Paget S: The use of paraffin in plastic surgery. Lancet 1903;1:1354–1357

8. Cronin TD, Gerow FJ: Augmentation mammoplasty: a new "natural feel" prosthesis. In: Transactions of the 3rd International Congress of Plastic Surgery. Amsterdam, Excerpts Medica 1964:41–49

9. Sanchez-Guerrero J, Colditz GA, Karlson EW, Hunter DJ, Speizer FE, Liang MH: Silicone breast implants and the risk of connective-tissue diseases and symptoms. New Engl J Med 1995;332(25):1666–1670

10. Hoehler H: Breast augmentation: axillary approach. Br J Plast Surg 1973;26(4):373–376

11. Strasser EJ: Results of subglandular versus subpectoral augmentation. Aesthetic Surg J 200626(1):45–50

12. Shiffman, MA: Advances in breast implant fillers. Am J Cosmet Surg 1998;15:291–294

13. McCurdy JA: Relationship between spherical fibrous capsular contracture and mammary prosthesis type. Am J Cosmet Surg 1990;7:235

14. Middleton MS, Mattrey R, Dobke MK: Distinguishing breast implant silicone gel leakage from rupture using high resolution MR imaging. Presented at the 12th Annual Meeting of the Society of Magnetic Resonance in Medicine, New York 1993

15. de Camara DL, Sheridan JM, Kammer BA: Rupture and aging of silicone gel breast implants. Plast Reconstr Surg 1993;91(5):828–834

16. Peters W, Keystone E, Smith D: Factors affecting the rupture of silicone gel breast implants. Ann Plast Surg 1994;32(5):449–451

17. Young VL, Diehl GJ, Eichling J, Monsees BS, Destouet J: The relative radiolucencies of breast implant filler materials. Plast Reconstr Surg 1993;91(6):1066–1072

18. Hyde JF: Frame hydrolysis. In: Atkin P, Jones L (eds). Chemistry: Molecules Matter and Change, 3rd edn. New York, WH Freeman 1997

19. McGregor RR: Silicones and Their Uses. New York, McGraw-Hill 1954

20. Lin RP, DiLeonardo M, Jacoby RA: Silicone lymphadenopathy: a case report and review of the literature. Am J Dermatopathol 1993;15(1):82–84

21. Heden P, Jernbeck J, Hober M: Breast augmentation with anatomical cohesive gel implants. The world's largest current experience. Clin Plast Surg 2001;28(3):531–552

22. Robinson OG Jr, Benos DJ: Spontaneous autoinflation of saline mammary implants. Aesthetic Plast Surg 1997;39(2):114–118

23. Price JE: Capsular contracture and deflation associated with inflatable implants. Aesthetic Plast Surg 1983;7(4):257–258

24. Rubin LR: Degradation of the saline-filled silicone-bag breast implant. In: Rubin L (ed). Biomaterials in Reconstructive Surgery. St. Louis, Mosby 1983, pp 260–272

25. Barnett MP: Triglyceride-filled breast implants. Plast Reconstr Surg 1997;99(7):2105–2107

26. Laing JH, Sanders R: The Misti Gold bio-oncotic gel filled breast prosthesis: an acceptable alternative to silicone? Br J Plast Surg 1993;46(3):240–242

27. Sinclair T, Kerrigan C, Buntik R: Biodegradation of the polyurethane foam covering of breast implants. Plast Reconstr Surg 1993;92(6):1003–1013

CHAPTER 62

Imaging Evaluation of Silicone Within the Breast

62

R. James Brenner

62.1
Introduction

With the reintroduction of silicone breast implants into the commercial marketplace following the lifting of a moratorium imposed in 1992 by both HealthCanada and the United States Food and Drug Administration (FDA) except for protocol circumstances (silicone implants were not withdrawn in Europe or Asia), interest in recognizing signs and symptoms of implant failure is likely to reemerge. In the past decade, implants of different strengths, styles, and durability have been manufactured. The range of implants, now produced by only two companies—Mentor and Allergan (formerly Inamed/McGhan)—is beyond the scope of this chapter. The purpose of this discussion is to review the imaging features common to the evaluation of silicone in the breast, especially as it relates to silicone breast implants, with an emphasis on mammography, ultrasound, and magnetic resonance imaging (MRI).

Implants are currently manufactured in a manner that responds to clinical needs for three situations: augmentation, breast reconstruction, and revision. Rates of failure vary both with implant type and indication. All implants maintain a pliable silicone-based outer elastomer shell to provide satisfactory cosmetic appeal, permitting a natural appearing ptosis while maintaining sufficient strength to resist traumatic injury to the device. As such, silicone implants often demonstrate folds, usually called radial folds, which may be sufficiently complex to cause confusion on certain imaging studies and lead to an erroneous conclusion of implant failure.

Implant failure is usually described for silicone implants as intracapsular or extracapsular. Following the placement of a breast implant into either the subglandular or subpectoral location, the body recognizes the implant as a foreign material and develops a fibrous capsule that surrounds the device. The thickness of this capsule is variable and may incite other associated fibrous reactions that result in associated signs and symptoms. The development of a fibrous capsule is therefore a physiologic and anticipated event, although the extent of the reaction is variable (Fig. 62.1)

Silicone compounds have a wide variety of textures and forms. Derived compounds all involve a silicone dioxide bond, with various substitutions made at the methyl groups that are bound to the element silicone (Si). Manufacturing processes are then designed to provide cross-linked geometry, and chemical bonds are designed to achieve the desired degree of solid or liquid consistency in addition to other specific tensile properties. It is the hydrogen proton environment associated with the methyl groups that forms the basis for the MR signals that are imaged and analyzed.

As mentioned, silicone implants may be manufactured in many forms and of different malleable strengths. Historically, most silicone breast implants were designed to have the solid outer elastomer shells with liquid internal contents; recent silicone models have been developed with both a stronger outer shell and a semisolid internal component. Questions remain as to the long-standing status of such internal components under physiologic conditions.

When the silicone envelope or shell fails, it permits the escape of the less solid silicone "gel" beyond the confines of the elastomer solid shell or "envelope." Usually, any future escape is limited by the even stronger fi-

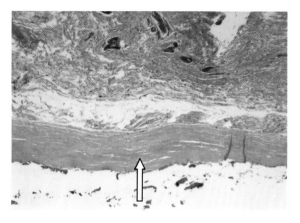

Fig. 62.1 Fibrous capsule surrounding breast implant. Portion of mastectomy demonstrating residual fibrous tissue incited by previous silicone implant (*arrow*)

brous capsule surrounding the implant. This condition is therefore referred to as "intracapsular" rupture or leak. If the fibrous capsule is weak at a specific focus, or violated due to other circumstances such as trauma, the internal silicone gel may escape into the breast parenchyma or other anatomic area, a condition referred to as "extracapsular" rupture or leak. More often than not, the escape into breast parenchyma or other body cavities is not a progressive process, presumably because the body also attempts to confine this new "foreign body." Thus, serial imaging studies often demonstrate an unchanging nature to the observed extracapsular silicone.

Rupture of the silicone elastomer shell surrounding saline implants usually results in rapid decompression of the implant consequent to the rapid resorption of saline. Either by breast self-examination or clinical breast examination, the virtual complete loss of integrity of the deflated saline implant can be detected in most circumstances. Mammographic imaging is usually sufficient to confirm a completely collapsed elastomer shell that has lost saline, a phenomenon that is not observed in silicone implants for the reasons described above.

Many implants have been produced that combine different compartments of silicone and/or saline [1]. All are subject to the above considerations.

Most decisions to pursue explantation are made on clinical grounds and may or may not relate to implant disruption. Indeed, intracapsular leak, without evidence of extracapsular leak or escape of silicone beyond its confined fibrous capsule (usually into breast parenchyma), is often called silent rupture. In the past, when some surgeons would perform closed capsulotomy in an effort to relieve pain or disfigurement from excessive capsular contracture, the knowledge of preexisting intracapsular or silent rupture was more important because such a maneuver risked converting an intracapsular confined rupture to an extracapsular rupture. Extracapsular silicone will elicit a granulomatous reaction, which may manifest as a breast lump and be mistaken for or obscure the detection of breast cancer on clinical examination. Other imaging techniques can often resolve such issues, but not always. Because closed capsulotomy has become increasingly discouraged, the management of intracapsular rupture has invited different commentaries. Nonetheless, knowledge of the status of the silicone breast implant may, of itself, be of value.

Three imaging methods are commonly used to assess the status of a silicone breast implant: mammography, ultrasound, and MRI. Other methods can often detect the condition of the implant; for example, computed tomography (CT) demonstrates signs similar to MRI, but it involves the use of ionizing radiation with no increased accuracy. Of note is the development of new dedicated breast CT units that are likely to afford radiation doses similar to mammograms. If necessary,

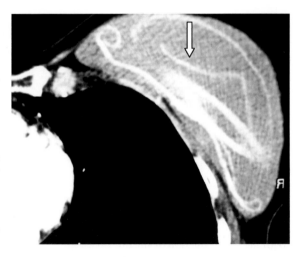

Fig. 62.2 Demonstration of collapse implant on computed tomography (CT). The linguine sign of implant failure is demonstrated on routine chest CT performed for other reasons

however, a CT exam can be performed for implant evaluation in patients in whom metallic implants or other considerations do not permit placement in the strong magnetic field required for MRI. Usually, CT performed for other maladies in the chest or abdomen incidentally identifies implant disruption (Fig. 62.2). Mammography, while using ionizing radiation, is primarily performed for breast cancer detection and evaluation but, given its widespread applicability in screening, may also identify signs of the disrupted implant when there is extracapsular rupture. Ultrasound involves no ionizing radiation and can detect implant rupture, both intracapsular and extracapsular, but with less accuracy than MRI. The clinical evaluation of the implant, except for collapsed saline implants, has relatively poor correlation to imaging findings. The Baker classification of capsular contracture may be helpful when implants cannot be easily displaced, but there are no proven specific imaging findings to correlate with the classification scheme [2].

62.2
Mammographic Imaging

The primary purpose of mammography, including mammography of women who have breast implants, is to detect and evaluate abnormalities with regard to the likelihood of representing breast cancer. However, imaging with x-ray, using either film-screen/analogue methods or full-field digital mammography, will also image breast implants. Specific techniques are required to optimally image both the parenchyma and implant using "implant displaced" and "implant nondisplaced"

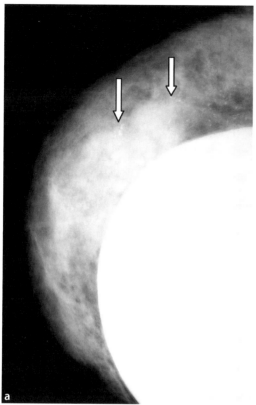

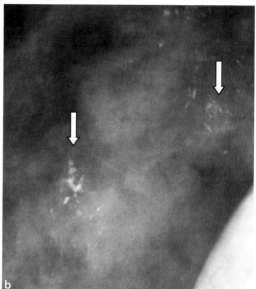

Fig. 62.3 Cluster of calcifications in asymptomatic female with silicone implants. **a** Cluster of calcifications detected. **b** Spot compression magnification view showing pleomorphic particles (*arrows*) representing intraductal and microinvasive carcinoma

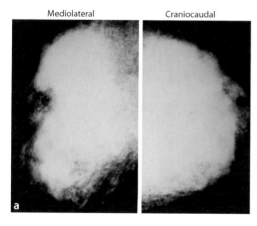

Mediolateral   Craniocaudal

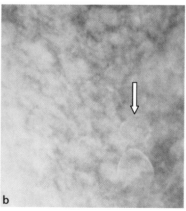

Fig. 62.4 Silicone injections. **a** Craniocaudal and mediolateral mammographic views showing coalesced silicone that forms hard, dense lumps that interfere with x-ray penetration of the breast. **b** Close-up view shows individual silicone cyst (calcified) formation (*arrow*)

views [3]. Implants, by occupying space within the breast, obscuring breast tissue, and compromising implant displaced views when capsular contracture occurs, have been shown to delay diagnosis of breast cancer. However, overall mortality outcomes are unchanged because signs of breast cancer can still be identified and analyzed in such breasts (Fig. 62.3) [4].

Though now illegal, medical practice in the middle of the 20th century included the direct injection of different materials into the breast for purposes of augmen-

tation. Silicone was most commonly employed because it was believed that such an inert substance would elicit a minimal response (Fig. 62.4). However, granulomatous reactions, silicone cyst formation, and hardening of the breast were common untoward complications of this approach. In addition, the ability to detect early breast cancer by mammography was compromised by these foreign substances, which often coalesced to limit both the value of radiographic as well as clinical evaluation of the breast. Both technology development and

Fig. 62.5 Calcified fibrous capsule. **a** Mammography showing "spiculated" projections that represent calcification (*arrow*) of fibrous capsule. **b** Corroborated on computed tomography

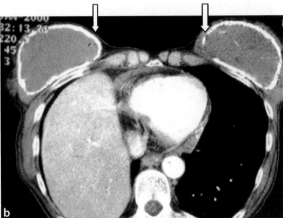

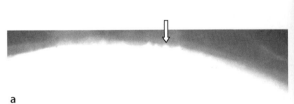

a

b

preference for silicone implant devices coincided with the banning of direct substance injection.

Because silicone within the fibrous capsule appears the same density whether or not it is confined to the silicone elastomer shell, it is not possible to identify intracapsular rupture on mammography. The implant is usually smooth, although a corrugated appearance may sometimes be seen due to calcification of the surrounding fibrous capsule (Fig. 62.5). Occasionally, small indentations can be identified because of fibrous bands extending across the otherwise malleable implant. Likewise, implant folds may frequently be seen.

Rather, extracapsular silicone will often be identified, which, in the absence of a history of prior "reimplantation," necessarily indicates concomitant intracapsular rupture. Silicone within the breast attenuates x-rays more than breast parenchyma or cancer, so its identification as a focus more dense than breast tissue or cancer is usually not a problem Although, as mentioned, silicone rupture into the parenchyma is not a progressive process, with sufficient pressure and manipulation of the breast the silicone can extend and dissect through soft tissue; this process has been identified.

When double-lumen implants are placed with the more common outer component being saline, the saline component, if ruptured, will usually expel the saline into the breast and be quickly resorbed. The evidence of this is the identification of a single-lumen implant (silicone) when the history indicates placement of a double-lumen implant. However, sometimes the saline/silicone interface will rupture, permitting admixture of the two components and providing the uncommon ability to detect intracapsular rupture by radiographic means.

More problematic in terms of radiographic detection of silicone is the presence of small amounts of silicone within lymph nodes, especially intramammary lymph nodes. The dissociation of silicone oils that may osmoti-

cally permeate the elastomer shell membrane provides a situation in which silicone may be transported by the lymphatic system to local–regional lymph nodes. Where those nodes are intramammary, a soft tissue mass may not demonstrate sufficiently high signal to be recognized as silicone and may be the basis for creating a suspicion of malignancy, a situation that may often be reconciled with MRI (Fig. 62.6). Other times, the silicone within the lymph node is sufficiently dense to permit an imaging diagnosis (Fig. 62.7). When sufficient

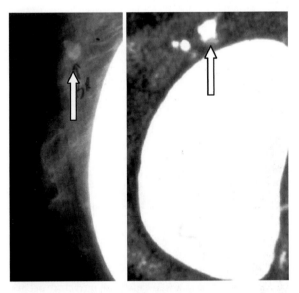

Fig. 62.6 Silicone within intramammary lymph node presenting as soft tissue mass on mammography. *Left:* Small mass on mediolateral oblique mammographic view is denser that soft tissue, but insufficiently dense to be characterized as silicone. *Right:* Magnetic resonance imaging more readily distinguishes the mass as containing silicone signal

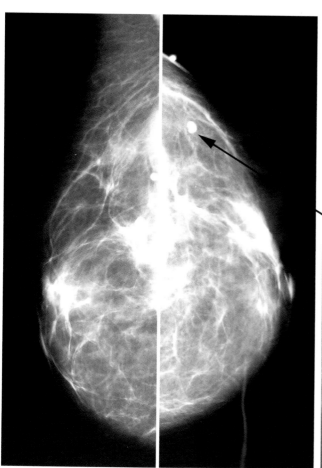

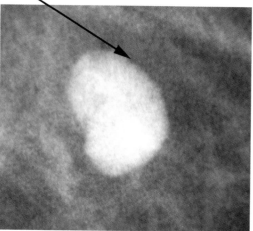

Fig. 62.7 Silicone infiltration of low axillary lymph node characterized by mammography. Following explantation, the remaining lymph node (*close-up on insert*) that has been infiltrated with silicone following prior implant failure has density sufficiently greater than the background breast tissue (or tumor mass) and a lentiform shape, so diagnosis can be made with confidence (*Connecting arrow* relates lymph node in breast to insert close up demonstration)

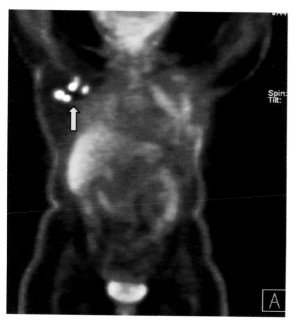

silicone travels to regional lymph nodes such as the axilla, especially following implant failure, an inflammatory response may be incited. Under such circumstances in a patient who has had a mastectomy and silicone implant reconstruction, assessment of the patient for metastatic disease by fluorodeoxyglucose positron emission tomography (FDG-PET) scanning may result in a false-positive image for cancer that actually represents inflammation (Fig. 62.8).

Although the main focus for mammographic detection of silicone implants relates to leakage, another silicone-related problem may be detected, if incompletely resolved, by x-ray. Mammographic depiction of implants may be challenging, especially when multiple im-

◄ **Fig. 62.8** Whole-body positron emission tomography scan with F[18] flouro-deoxyglucose (PET-FDG) for cancer surveillance following mastectomy shows positive uptake of multiple right axillary lymph nodes (*arrow*) that is secondary to inflammation rather than tumor involvement

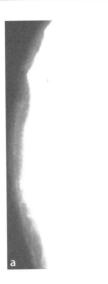

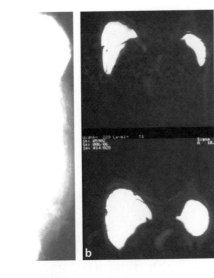

Fig. 62.9 Mammographic image of multiple "stacked" implants. **a** Mammographic craniocaudal and mediolateral views show uninterpretable image of high density. **b** Accompanying magnetic resonance image more clearly demonstrates several implants

Fig. 62.10 Mammographic evidence of herniation of implant following trauma. **a** Mammography demonstrates herniation (*arrow*). **b** Subsequent magnetic resonance imaging shows both the herniation (*arrow*) and its reduction (*double arrow*), without evidence of either intracapsular or extracapsular leak

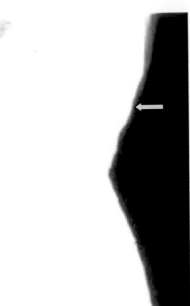

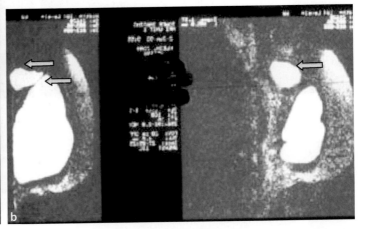

plants are placed in the same breast, sometimes referred to as "stacked" implants. MRI can usually demonstrate more clearly the relationship of such implants to the breast (Fig. 62.9). In addition, although the implant is contained by a fibrous capsule, this capsule may focally weaken, providing the opportunity for the implant to bulge out at such a focus. Thus, both eventration and frank herniation (Fig. 62.10) may occur and may be detected by mammography, but associated implant failure cannot be diagnosed unless there is extracapsular leaking. When such findings occur following trauma, the increased likelihood of implant disruption may prompt another more diagnostic test, such as MRI.

As discussed, because most intracapsular leaks cannot be detected by mammography, rupture is diagnosed primarily on the basis of extracapsular silicone (Fig. 62.11). Thus, the sensitivity of mammography for rupture is variable but generally low (11–81%), and for the same reason, the specificity is high (89–100%) [5].

62.3
Ultrasound

Evaluation of breast implants by detecting differential propagation of sound waves through both the breast

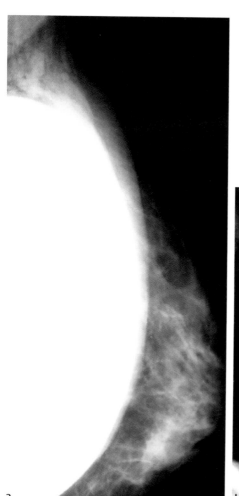

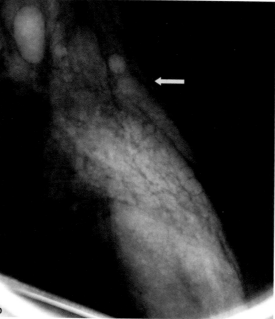

Fig. 62.11 Extracapsular silicone demonstrated on mammography. **a** Lateral mammographic view. **b** Spot compression magnification (*arrow* shows extracapsular silicone)

a

b

and silicone implants has demonstrated the ability to detect both intracapsular and extracapsular leak. Sound transmission through the breast is a complicated process. Technologic adaptations such as harmonic imaging and spatial compounding, which may demonstrate breast lesions to advantage, have not been reported to improve silicone detection. First described in 1983 [6], a normal ultrasound image of an implant—limited considerably by wavelength and resolution capability if the implant is placed behind the pectoral muscle, but better seen in subglandular implants—depicts a fluid-filled structure (for liquid silicone implants) that is usually accompanied by a variable number of radial folds seen as echogenic lines extending to the surface of the implant (Fig. 62.12). A smooth interface between the anterior portion of the implant and the surrounding breast parenchyma is seen, but the posterior component of the implant cannot be well resolved. Textured implants may create a more multilayered echogenic interface.

Commonly, reverberative anterior echoes may be seen due to the differential sound transmission between the breast and the implant, but usually these are readily recognized. Saline implants will contain valves that are also easily identified, but they may be confused with a lump during physical examination; under such circumstances, ultrasound may be very helpful because of its real-time capabilities of correlating the palpable finding to the imaging demonstration of the valve (Fig. 62.13).

Radial folds are seen as thick echogenic lines that can be traced to the outer elastomer shell. As mentioned above, fibrous bands or nonradial folds may be associated with implants that are not meant to be maximally distended (for cosmetic reasons) and can occasionally be confused with both radial folds and, more importantly, failing implants [7–9]. In like manner to mammography, eventration and herniation may be suspected with focal and abrupt changes in the peripheral outline of the implant, creating a contour deformity.

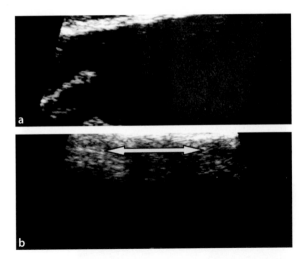

Fig. 62.12 Ultrasound view of normal breast silicone implant. **a** Smooth anterior surface is noted at anterior margin of implant where device abuts fibrous capsule. Linear echo represents normal radial fold. **b** Normal reverberative artifact can be seen (*double-sided arrow*)

Unlike mammography, the sonographic characteristics of extracapsular silicone may vary in part depending on the length of time the silicone has been within the breast. The presence of granuloma formation, associated with free silicone, may vary its sonographic appearance [9]. Free silicone within the breast is quite specific when a focal, clearly defined anterior echogenic line is seen, posterior to which is a strong reverbera-

tive artifact [10]. This is attributed to the admixture of silicone droplets with granulation tissue and a resulting disruption and discoherence of the ultrasound beam [11, 12]. This is often referred to as a "snowstorm" appearance (Fig. 62.14).

When silicone is taken up into a lymph node by means of intramammary lymphatics, a highly echogenic focus is seen, distinctly different from the hypoechoic foci usually associated with breast cancer (Fig. 62.15) [13]. Thus, in a case where a mass is identified mammographically but is insufficiently dense to recognize silicone infiltration, ultrasound may provide the distinguishing features required for diagnosis.

Depending on the age and degree of granuloma formation, silicone nodules within the breast may at times be hypoechoic and difficult to distinguish from cancer. Ultrasound imaging, being highly operator dependent, should be performed by qualified personnel who will attempt to carefully interrogate the echogenic parallel lines of the elastomer shell to evaluate for discontinuity or disruption. The presence of a hypoechoic nodule adjacent to the implant can represent extracapsular silicone or a tumor. In addition, suboptimal scanning of fat lobules can further complicate the analysis [14]. This phenomenon may, if seen as an isolated finding, raise the suspicion of malignancy (Fig. 62.16). Fine needle aspiration biopsy will often not show the silicone because the material may be dissolved by chemical fixation. However, the presence of foreign body giant cells containing large vacuoles within the cytoplasm where the silicone resided following phagocytosis is usually indicative of this situation. These circumstances may

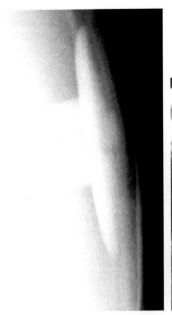

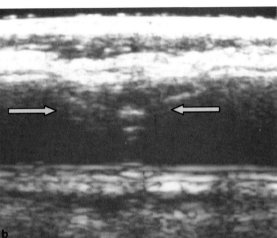

Fig. 62.13 Normal expander valve corresponding to palpable finding. **a** Mammogram shows valve. **b** Ultrasound that can be performed while palpating area in real-time imaging circumstances demonstrates correlation to valve (*between arrows*)

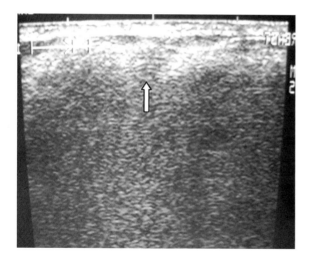

Fig. 62.14 Ultrasound showing extracapsular silicone. Focal intense reverberative echogenic artifact (*arrow*) begins immediately posterior to thick echogenic line indicating evidence of abrupt transition of breast tissue to silicone deposit within the parenchyma, known as the "snowstorm" appearance

be complicated when the implant contains prominent infoldings beyond the usual radial folds commonly encountered.

Ultrasound is far less costly and more accessible than MRI for implant evaluation, but it has a lower sensitivity for detecting implant failure. Some of the signs of intracapsular leak are similar [15]. When the implant collapses upon itself so that the elastomer shell is floating within a collection of free silicone, a series from anterior to posterior of long echogenic lines can be seen, often referred to as the "stepladder" sign [11]. These can usually be distinguished from radial folds by the longer length, abundant number, and array from anterior to posterior (Fig. 62.17). However, most implant ruptures, for reasons that will be clarified during the discussion of MRI, do not result in complete infolding of the implant, and thus the stepladder sign has been reported in less than half of surgically proven ruptures [16]. Instead, what may be observed are focal echogenic collections, sometimes called "heterogeneous aggregates," that have no specific anatomic or chemical correlate at explantation (Fig. 62.18). This is one of the reasons that diagnosis of intracapsular rupture is not as high for most operators as MRI [8, 9, 15, 16].

With the newer implants that contain a more cohesive gel prior to implantation, ultrasound signs of failure may vary. This has not been the case for MRI, but too few of the newer implants have been studied and reported at the present time to form conclusions. If, however, the historic signs of rupture that are seen in MRI

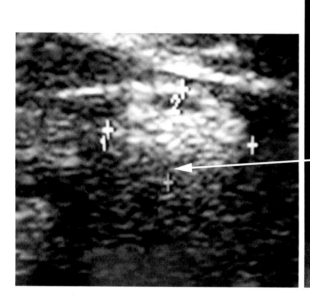

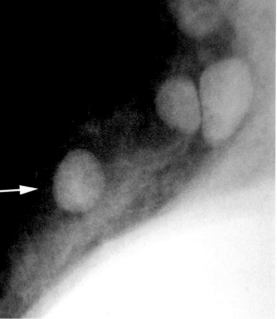

Fig. 62.15 Ultrasound demonstration of lymph node infiltrated with silicone. Sonographic features show recapitulated lentiform morphology with increased echogenicity characteristic of silicone infiltration, corresponding to mammographic evidence of silicone infiltration (*double arrow* correlating sonographic and mammographic demonstration of lymph node)

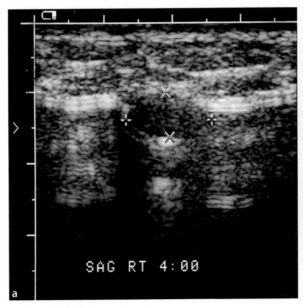

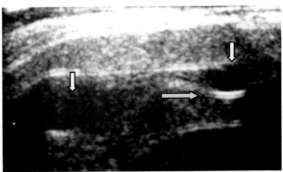

Fig. 62.16 Suboptimal ultrasound scan incorrectly suggesting breast mass or extracapsular silicone. **a** Poor scanning technique suggests hypoechoic nodule considered suspicious for silicone or breast mass. **b** Repeat scan demonstrates intact implant, with "mass" representing a normal fat lobule (*double arrow*). *Single arrow* points to normal fold

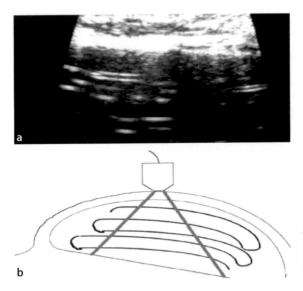

Fig. 62.17 Ultrasound appearance of collapsed silicone implant, "stepladder sign," showing multiple horizontal lines depicting collapsed elastomer shell floating within a free bed of silicone confined by the fibrous capsule. **a** Ultrasound image (image courtesy of Dr. Nannette DeBruhl). **b** Schematic

Fig. 62.18 Ultrasound appearance of collapse silicone implant: "heterogeneous aggregates." Posterior to fibrous capsule are clumps of echogenicity (*small arrows*) interrupted by sharp echogenic lines (*single arrow*) representing infolding of the elastomer envelope

studies of more current implants are demonstrated by ultrasound studies, then general accuracy rates should be expected to be similar.

Ultrasound is ineffective in breasts that have undergone direct silicone injections. The extensive and coalescent reverberative artifacts virtually prevent sound waves from penetrating and returning to the ultrasound transducer in a manner that allows the beams to form an anatomic image (Fig. 62.19) [15–17]. The appearance is similar to the "snowstorm" appearance of extracapsular silicone for the same reasons [11]. This is an important restriction when trying to assess an implant that has been placed subsequent to a history of injections. It is also an issue when MRI performed for tumor detection identifies a focus for which targeted ultrasound is often performed to corroborate a specific lesion. Indeed, this problem is particularly severe for patients with silicone injections in whom screening mammography is less effective and contrast-enhanced MRI is performed.

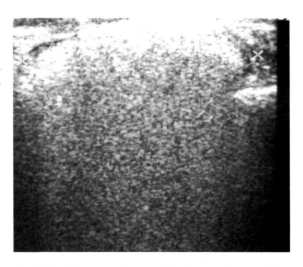

Fig. 62.19 Ultrasound of breast with silicone injections. Widespread reverberative artifacts caused by the repeated interfaces between breast tissue and silicone injections obscure the sonographic anatomy, obviating the depiction of discreet abnormalities

62.4
Magnetic Resonance Imaging

MRI is based on the differential resonant frequencies created in a strong magnetic field when radiofrequency (RF) pulses are propagated into tissue. The speed at which different atoms relax from the temporary excited state created by the RF pulse depends on their chemical structure and local environment. Hydrogen has been the main atomic element studied with MRI because of its abundance and the need to obtain sufficient signal following an RF pulse within a short period of time.

Evaluation of breast implants by MRI requires no intravenous contrast injection, the latter being necessary for tumor evaluation. In this context it should be noted that MRI examinations tailored to silicone implants, although performed on the same machine, involve acquisition protocols distinctly different and not applicable to tumor evaluation. Although implant and tumor evaluation studies may be performed sequentially, they are separate exams, and one protocol is not suitable for both. Unlike ultrasound and mammography, the study is performed in the prone position (like all breast MRI studies) to avoid compression of the implant upon itself. Small amounts of pleural fluid or even fluid surrounding the implant may be seen and are normal variants. Sometimes fluid is injected into the silicone-containing implant, so small droplets of fluid are not considered evidence of rupture.

The physics associated with the production of MRI signals is complex, and the interested reader is referred to other sources for further discussion [18, 19]. A preliminary working understanding may be obtained by appreciating that in the breast, signals from hydrogen found in three different environments need to be distinguished, namely, hydrogen associated with silicone, fat, and water. Because fat and silicone resonate at similar frequencies under most magnetic fields [e.g., at 1.5 Tesla (T), there is only a 110-MHz difference], a number of image acquisition strategies have been developed to separate the two. Water resonates at a frequency sufficiently different from silicone and fat (220-MHz difference at 1.5 T), so its signal can be "chemically suppressed" by electronic spoiling without significantly affecting the signals from fat and silicone. By manipulating the conditions and time at which the relaxing protons are sampled, high-contrast and high-resolution images may be obtained.

Although the prior discussion noted that ultrasound evaluation is a real-time examination that is therefore, unlike x-ray examination, operator dependent, it should be noted in this context that acquisition schemes and technical parameters play a controlling influence on images that are produced for MRI. For example, magnet strengths vary from 0.3 T to 3 T (higher-strength magnets are under current investigation); the strength of the received signal will be a product of magnet power, which in turn will impact the ability to resolve signals among different tissues. Signals are received by coils that are designed to anatomically adapt to the organ system being imaged, and thus improve resolution. The geometry of the coils is also a variable that impacts image quality. Indeed, some studies have reported results

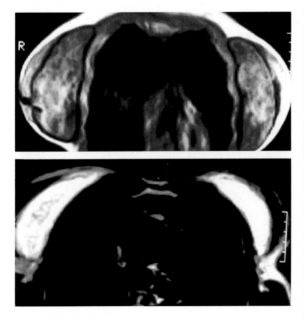

Fig. 62.20 Whole-body magnetic resonance imaging of breast with silicone implants. Although the implants can be identified, internal detail is poor, preventing proper evaluation of possible intracapsular rupture

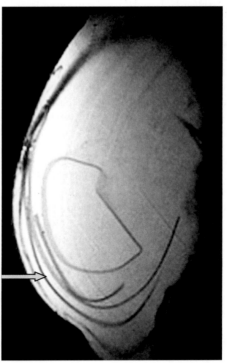

Fig. 62.21 Magnetic resonance imaging demonstration of intracapsular rupture as "linguine sign." Collapsed silicone envelope appears as multiple wavy lines, representing the elastomer shell floating in a bed of free silicone, confined by the fibrous capsule (*arrow*)

using coil technology unsuitable for optimal visualization of the breast, such as "whole body" coils (Fig. 62.20). The difference may be analogized to attempting to listen to a radio close to the transmitter (dedicated breast coil) compared to hearing it at a distance (general body coil). In general, higher-field magnets (1 T or greater) are recommended, as are dedicated breast coils. A number of techniques have been successfully used in the acquisition of information. Poor MRI results for silicone implant rupture are often, if not usually, a reflection of suboptimal techniques [20, 21].

The signs relating to breast implants as detected by ultrasound are detected in a more accurate manner by MRI. However, MRI is more expensive and less accessible than ultrasound or mammography. By providing cross-sectional images in virtually any plane of section, the entire implant may be imaged, subject to technical limitations (for example, incomplete suppression of fat signal may introduce artifacts that obscure the image due to the nature of the way in which the information is processed and reconstructed). Types of implants—single, double, triple—can be better assessed, as can the determination of multiple or "stacked" implants that may be present within a given capsule (Fig. 62.9) [1].

Extracapsular silicone can be detected, especially when not present for an extended length of time (due to change of signal from granuloma formation), as a focus of silicone signal outside the dark fibrous capsule. As

noted above, the image appearances of fat and silicone may be similar due to their similar resonant frequencies when stimulated by a given RF frequency within a magnetic field. Therefore, to detect the silicone as a bright signal, the similar bright signal from fat must be suppressed. A common method for imaging the outside of the fibrous capsule to distinguish silicone from fat involves a technique called inversion recovery, which is a technical trick to obtain signal from silicone at a specific time when the recovery of fat stimulation is such that it has no signal. Thus, the bright signal of silicone is the only high signal that will be seen within the breast.

However, the age of the extracapsular deposit will affect its MR signal. The body, recognizing a foreign substance, will initiate a granulomatous process that will affect the signal of silicone because it is the entire area of deposit that is being imaged; the postinflammatory granulation tissue will be imaged together with the silicone and may decrease the overall silicone-specific signal. In like manner, silicone that may have been transferred by the lymphatic system to intramammary or axillary lymph nodes may also be identified by MRI, with the same considerations applying.

Identifying extracapsular silicone without evidence of an intracapsular rupture raises the presumption that a prior explanted implant operation left some of the silicone within the breast. Implants that are ruptured often do not lend themselves to easy enucleation of the entire implant device, which may become fragmented. Therefore, silicone may remain in the breast prior to the implantation of a new device. Anecdotal instances of identifying extracapsular silicone without intracapsular rupture have been noted, in part recognizing that MRI is very accurate but imperfect for identifying all intracapsular ruptures. No published reports have provided an estimate for how often this occurs.

Intracapsular rupture is most reliably defined by MRI, compared to both clinical examination and other routine imaging technologies. When an implant with internal liquid-state silicone collapses entirely, the fragments of the elastomer shell float within the free silicone that has escaped the shell but is still confined within the outer fibrous capsule. In ultrasound this was noted as the stepladder sign. In MRI, this is referred to as a "linguine" sign because its appearance is similar to the pasta (Fig. 62.21) [22]. However, more often than not, the entire shell does not collapse upon itself be-

cause dissociated oils of the original molecule that have permeated the shell may cause adhesion to the fibrous capsule. Thus, if a rent or violation of the capsule occurs, the silicone will begin to exude from inside to outside the envelope, but the entire envelope will fail to collapse into the cavity because of the adhesions. Instead, the silicone will transit outside the envelope but still be confined within a stronger fibrous capsule, causing an involution that, due to its appearance, has been referred to as the inverted-loop sign; other terms used include the keyhole or hang-noose sign (Fig. 62.22) [23]. When this involution occurs over a broad base, the term often applied is "subcapsular sign," caused by a dark signal from the elastomer shell paralleling the dark signal of the fibrous capsule.

Excessive dissociation of silicone oils, which have an MR signal indistinguishable from silicone, may lead to focal accumulations that may mimic small inverted loops. This phenomenon has been referred in the past as "gel bleed," although it is not the gel that is crossing the semipermeable membrane of the envelope [24]. Both situations may cause the implant to feel sticky at explanation surgery, and close inspection is often required to determine whether this clinical presentation is due to excessive oil dissociation that can be confused on MRI for the inverted-loop sign of intracapsular rupture.

Although most radial folds are easily recognized, the nondistended implant may on occasion fold into itself in such a manner that the appearance can be confusing on MRI, similar to the situation discussed above with ultrasound. By following the image throughout its manifestation on all images, both the absence of implant discontinuity and more specific signs of intracapsular rupture may help reconcile this phenomenon. Sometimes a diagnosis of complex fold versus intracapsular leak cannot be distinguished with certainty (Fig. 62.23).

As mentioned earlier, there is little value added in performing MRI of saline implants that have collapsed, a phenomenon that is usually suspected quickly on clinical grounds and can be validated with x-ray mammography (Fig. 62.24). However, clinical history is sometimes elusive, and when there is a bona fide question regarding the type of implant present, MRI may help clarify the issue (Fig. 62.24).

62.5
Expected Outcomes of Imaging Implants

The presence of extracapsular silicone in a patient who has only undergone one implantation procedure necessarily infers intracapsular rupture and thus implant failure. This may be due to trauma following implantation, trauma during the implantation surgery, or unrecognized factors relating to aging and patient-specific

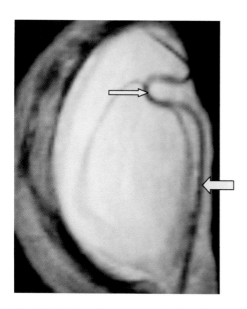

Fig. 62.22 Magnetic resonance imaging demonstration of inverted-loop and subcapsular signs. Saggital view demonstrates involution of elastomer shell without a wide base (which would be more indicative of a fold; *thin arrow*), indicating the inverted-loop sign. Broader base infolding (*wide arrow*) characterizes the subcapsular sign

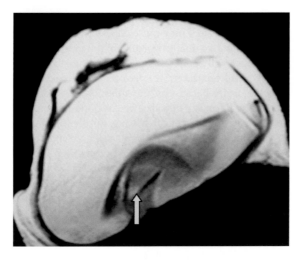

Fig. 62.23 Complex fold on magnetic resonance imaging. Oblique and overlapping complex folds simulate but do not conform to accepted signs of implant disruption. No discontinuity of the implant was identified on multiple section review

conditions. Current implant manufacturing has emphasized the importance of creating stronger elastomer shells and internal contents that begin as a more solidified structure. The history of implant development has

been described [25]. For this reason, mammography is a reasonably accurate and specific way to detect extracapsular silicone and implant failure associated with this condition. Because it cannot detect intracapsular failure (except where an outer saline component admixes with an inner silicone component), ultrasound and MRI are required. In fact, because MRI has shown the highest accuracy for detecting implant failure, it is the method the FDA has designated for studying the long-term durability of current implants, the failure of which may not be clinically detectable.

Experimental work on rabbits provides a theoretical basis for comparing mammography, ultrasound, and MRI. In a study of 40 single-lumen silicone implants surgically placed in 20 rabbits (one intact and one ruptured implant), five radiologists reviewed images for all three modalities. Receiver operating characteristic (ROC) analysis showed MRI values of 0.95 (CT had a value of 0.91) compared to mammography and ultrasound, which had ROC values of 0.77; this was of statistical significance ($p<.05$) [26]. Ultrasound was more comparable to MRI if an experienced radiologist did the ultrasound examination. One investigator reported the comparative accuracy of MRI and ultrasound to be 84% and 49% respectively, although a later report by the same group suggested the sensitivity and specificity to be 65% and 57%, respectively [27, 28]. A more compre-

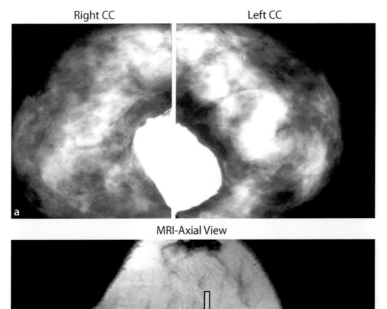

Fig. 62.24 Collapse of saline implant. **a** Craniocaudal and mediolateral oblique mammographic images demonstrate collapsed saline implant consistent with clinical examination. **b** Magnetic resonance imaging demonstrates collapsed silicone envelope folding upon itself, but adds little to the diagnostic impression

hensive comparison of mammography, ultrasound, and MRI in the evaluation of 32 patients and 63 implants showed that relative sensitivities for these three methods of imaging were 23%, 59%, and 95%, with respective specificities of 98%, 79%, and 93% [29].

62.6
Conclusions

Prior studies reflecting on the prevalence and incidence of silicone implant failure were restrained by the absence of clear clinical history, early-generation silicone implants, and a self-selection bias attendant to which patients were being imaged. Newer-generation implants have been prospectively studied by direction of the FDA. In addition, serial studies of newer-generation implants have provided a basis for estimating current rates of rupture prevalence.

Based on empiric observation of implant rupture in Denmark, which maintains an unusually comprehensive national health database, the rupture rate at 2 years was estimated to be 2% and at 10 years to be 15% if the implant was intact at 3 years [30].

As can be inferred from the above discussion, MRI is the most accurate manner of evaluating implant failure, especially for intracapsular rupture. The study can be performed without intravenous contrast, and most protocols require about 20–30 min of scanning time. Both sensitivities and specificities, when proper techniques are applied and experienced readers are interpreting the studies, should be expected to exceed 95%. Ultrasound, thought to be more accessible and less expensive, will detect both extracapsular and intracapsular leak but with a lower accuracy than MRI. Finally, mammographic evaluation of implant leak is generally confined to the detection, with high sensitivity, of extracapsular silicone.

References

1. Middleton MS: Breast Implant Classification. In: Gorczyka DP, Brenner RJ (eds). The Augmented Breast. Thieme, New York 1997, pp 27–34
2. Bostwick J III: Plastic and Reconstructive Breast Surgery, vol 1. St Louis, Quality Medical Publishing 1990, p 181
3. Eklund GW, Busby RC, Miller SH, Job JS: Improved imaging of the augmented breast AJR 1988;15:469–473
4. Miglioretti DL, Rutter CM, Geller BM, Cutter G, Barlow WE, Rosenberg R, Weaver DL, Taplin SH, Ballard-Barbash R, Carney PA, Yankaskas BC: Effect of breast augmentation on the accuracy of mammography and cancer characteristics. JAMA 2004;291(4):442–450
5. Gorczyca DP, Debruhl ND, Ahn CY, Hoyt A, Sayre JW, Nudell P, McCombs M, Shaw WW, Bassett LW: Silicone breast implant ruptures in an animal model: comparison of mammography, MR imaging, US, and CT. Radiology 1995;190(1):227–232
6. Cole-Beuglet C, Schwartz G, Kurtz A, Patchefsky AS, Goldberg BB: Ultrasound mammography for the augmented breast. Radiology 1983;146(3):737–742
7. Berg WA, Caskey CI, Hamper UM, Kuhlman JE, Anderson ND, Chang BW, Sheth S, Zerhouni EA: Single and double lumen silicone breast implant integrity: prospective evaluation of MR and US criteria. Radiology 1995;197(1):45–52
8. Ahn CY, DeBruhl DN, Corczyca DP, Shaw WW, Bassett LW: Comparative silicone breast implant evaluation using mammography, sonography, and magnetic resonance imaging: experience with 59 implants. Plast Reconstr Surg 1994;94(5):620–627
9. Debruhl ND, Gorczyka DP, Ahn CY, Shaw WW, Bassett LW: Silicone breast implants: US evaluation. Radiology 1993;189(1):95–98
10. Cruz G, Gillooley JF, Waxman M: Silicone granuloma of the breast. NY State J Med 1985;85(10):599–601
11. Harris KM, Ganott MA, Shestak K, Losken HW, Tobon H: Silicone implant rupture: detection with US. Radiology 1993;187(3):761–768
12. Rubin JM, Helvie MA, Adler RS, Ikeda D: US appearance of ruptured silicone breast implants (letter). Radiology 1994;190(2):583–584
13. Hausner RJ, Schoen FJ, Mendex-Fernandez MA, Henly WS, Geis RC: Migration of silicone gel to axillary lymph nodes after prosthetic mammoplasty. Arch Path Lab Med 1981;105(7):371–372
14. Steinbach BG, Hardt NS, Abbitt PL, Lanier L, Caffee HH: Breast implants, common complications, and concurrent breast disease. Radiographics 1993;13(1):95l–118
15. Harris KM: Ultrasonographic evaluation of the failing implant. In: Gorczyka DP, Brenner RJ (eds). The Augmented Breast. Thieme, New York 1997, pp 74–110
16. Caskey CI, Berg WA, Anderson ND, Sheth S, Chang BW, Hamper UM: Breast implant rupture: diagnosis with ultrasonography. Radiology 1994;190(3):819–823
17. Leibman AJ, Sybers R: Mammographic and sonographic findings after silicone injection. Ann Plast Surg 1994;33(4):412–414
18. Gorczyca DP, Schneider E, DeBruhl ND, Foo TK, Ahn CY, Sayre JW, Shaw WW, Bassett LW: Silicone breast implant rupture: comparison between three-point Dixon and fast spin-echo imaging. AJR Am J Roentgenol 1994;162(2):305–310
19. Monticciolo DL, Nelson RC, Dixon WT, Bostwick J, Mukundan S, Hester TR: MR detection of leakage from silicone breast implants: value of a silicone-selective pulse sequence. AJR Am J Roentgenol 1994;163(1):51–56

20. Scaranelo AM, Marques AF, Smialowski EB, Lederman HM: Evaluation of the rupture of silicone breast implants by mammography, ultrasonography and magnetic resonance imaging in asymptomatic patients: correlation with surgical findings. Sao Paulo Med J 2004;122(2):41–47

21. Cher DJ, Conwell JA, Mandel JS: MRI for detecting silicone breast implant ruptures: meta-analysis and implications. Ann Plast Surg 2001;47:367–380

22. Gorczyka DP, Sinha S, Ahn CY, DeBruhl ND, Hayes MK, Gausche VR, Shaw WW, Bassett LW: Silicone breast implants in vivo: MR imaging. Radiology 1992;185(2):407–410

23. Gorczyka DP: Magnetic resonance imaging of the failing implant. In: Gorczyca DP, Brenner RJ (eds). The Augmented Breast. Thieme, New York, 1997, pp 121–142

24. Brody GS: Fact and fiction about breast implant bleed. Plast Reconstr Surg 1977;60(4):615–616

25. Brenner RJ, Gorczyca DP: The silicone controversy: a brief history of the problem. In: Gorczyca DP, Brenner RJ (eds). The Augmented Breast. Thieme, New York, 1997, pp 1–5

26. Gorczyca DP, DeBruhl ND, Ahn CY: Silicone breast implant ruptures in an animal model: comparison of mammography MR, imaging, US and CT. Radiology 1994;190:227–232

27. Berg WA, Caskey CI, Hamper UM, Anderson ND, Chang BW, Sheth S, Zerhouni EA, Kuhlman JE: Diagnosing breast implant rupture with MR imaging, US, and mammography. Radiographics 1993;13(6):1323–1328

28. Berg WA, Caskey CI, Hamper UM, Kuhlman JE, Anderson ND, Chang BW, Sheth S, Zerhouni EA: Single- and double-lumen silicone breast implant integrity: prospective evaluation of MR and US criteria. Radiology 1995;197(1):45–52

29. Everson LI, Parantainen H, Detlie T, Stillman AE, Olson PN, Landis G, Foshager MC, Cunningham B, Griffiths HJ: Diagnosis of breast implant rupture: imaging findings and relative efficacies of imaging techniques. AJR Am J Roentgenol 1994;163(1):57–60

30. Holmich LR, Vejborg I, Conrad C, Sletting S, McLaughlin JK: The diagnosis of breast implant rupture: MRI findings compared with findings at explantation. Eur J Radiology 2005;53(2):213–225

Treatment of Capsule Contracture with Endoscopic CO_2 Laser

63

Franck Landat

63.1
Introduction

With the insertion of a breast implant, of whatever type, the organism reacts and develops a scarring phenomenon around the implant, forming a capsule. This reaction is important and may have an impact on the breast. Baker [1] established a classification of capsule contracture that is used in this study:

Stage 1: Inspection and palpation of the normal breast; the implant is unnoticeable (Fig. 63.1)

Stage 2: Palpation of the implant is possible (Fig. 63.2)

Stage 3: The breast is slightly deformed, and the implant is easily palpable (Figs. 63.3, 63.4)

Stage 4: The breast hurts, is deformed, or both (Fig. 63.5)

The fibrous capsule created after breast implant insertion can become more or less hard and painful, and deformation of the breast may occur. Repair methods have included approaching the capsule through incisions around the areola or through the mammary fold. A large opening is used to cut the fibrous capsule. This can be inconvenient because of new scarring, a risk of

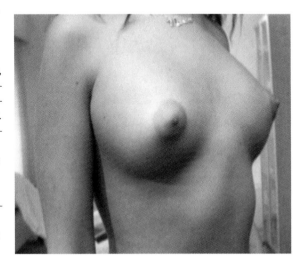

Fig. 63.2 Stage 2 Baker classification of capsular contracture

damaging the implant, or irregular sectioning of the fibrous capsule.

The author has devised a new technique that links the advantages of the endoscope and the laser.

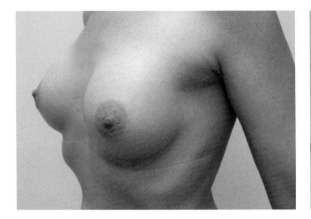

Fig. 63.1 Stage 1 Baker classification of capsular contracture

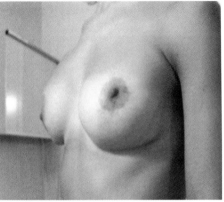

Fig. 63.3 Stage 3 Baker classification of capsular contracture

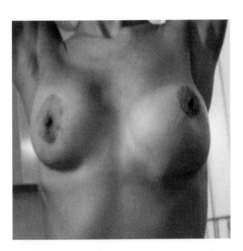

Fig. 63.4 Stage 3 Baker classification of capsular contractures plus distortion of the prosthesis

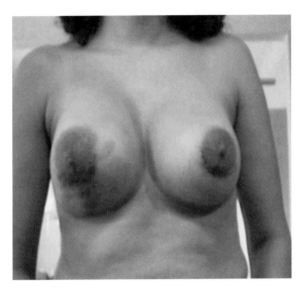

Fig. 63.5 Stage 4 Baker classification of capsular contracture

63.2
Technique

The intervention is carried out using neuroleptanalgesia. With the patient standing, the incisions to be made internally are marked (Fig. 63.6):

- A lower circular incision
- A midway circular incision
- Separate radial incisions 3 cm long

A pericapsular injection of 250 ml saline (0.9%) plus a bottle (50 ml) of 2% Xylocaine with epinephrine is used. After waiting 20 min, a 1-cm incision is made at the level of the areola in the lower part at the midway level.

Dissection is continued up to the implant with the CO_2 laser. The CO_2 laser is coupled to a "laparoscopy endoscope" linked to an adapter. There is no bleeding. After the capsule is opened 2 cm, the endoscope is introduced between the implant and the capsule (Fig. 63.7).

Before starting the laser incisions, it is necessary to lift the prosthesis from the capsule. This is made easier with the endoscope with the help of a foam-covered lifter. It is necessary to lift the entire superficial part of the implant. Only after this important and absolutely necessary step, the section as such may be carried out according to the drawings marked preoperatively. This step is easy to carry out with the endoscope and does not present specific difficulties. Visualization is clear

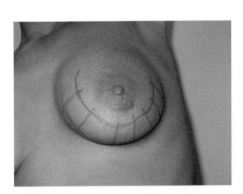

Fig. 63.6 Marking for the capsulotomy

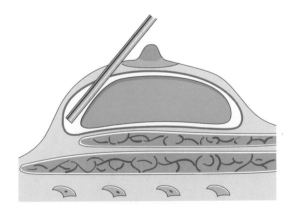

Fig. 63.7 Diagram of the endoscope placement between the capsule and the implant

with the absence of bleeding and use of fume aspiration. There is no risk of damage to the implant as it is pushed back by the endoscope. The end of the endoscope is in contact with the fibrous capsule. Only a single pass of the laser is necessary. After all the incisions are made, it is necessary to check the integrity of the implant and feel the breast to see whether it has gained back its softness and ideal form.

Before closing, the cavity is abundantly rinsed with 0.9% saline. No drainage is necessary because no bleeding or seromas were encountered. Subcutaneous skin closure is done with Vicryl 3-0. The skin incision is closed with Prolene 4-0 and covered with Steri-Strips. After the operation, it is not necessary to use special bandages. A normal bra is left in place night and day for 10 days.

Nevertheless, massage and early mobilization of the implants are necessary. The breast massage, vertically and laterally, can be done by the patient herself twice daily for 1 month.

63.3
Results

This study was based on 159 interventions with follow-up over a period of 4 years, with checks after 1 year and 4 years. Eighty percent of the patients were an average of 32 years old. Sixty percent of the implants were in the subglandular position, and 75% of the implants were smooth.

Twenty percent of the capsular contractures were located on only one breast, with the contralateral breast being totally normal. Twenty percent of the patients operated on were at Baker stage IV, and 80% were at stage III.

The immediate results were excellent (Figs. 63.8, 63.9). No patient suffered from pain even without taking analgesics when the effects of the local anesthesia wore off. No pain was noted in the first 24 h or in the following days.

There were no seromas, hematomas, or infection.

The medium-term and long-term results, at 1 year, 2 years, and 4 years, showed that the patients were happy with the breast form. The index of satisfaction was excellent even for the cases of stage IV capsular contracture.

63.4
Discussion

The necessity to solve the problem of capsular contracture after breast implant placement has led the author to find a new method of treatment; a change of implants and the consequences thereof will not definitely avoid recurrences [2–4]. Baran et al. [5] have recommended the systematic change of prostheses.

The classic intervention leads to either a larger periareolar incision or an incision on the inframammary fold. On very dark skin, this technique may be a handicap. Some authors have attempted closed compression capsulotomy with cases of bleeding or implant rupture [6], and Collis and Sharpe [7] carried out a comparative study on the recurrence of subglandular breast implant capsular contracture.

The endoscope allows the surgeon to make sections of the fibrotic capsule in a very precise manner and without apparent risk to the prosthesis. The use of the endoscope allows control of the state of the implants.

The use of the CO_2 laser with 6 watts of power leads

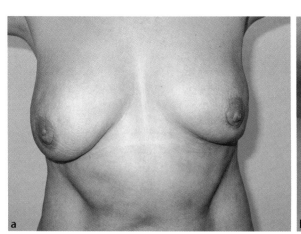
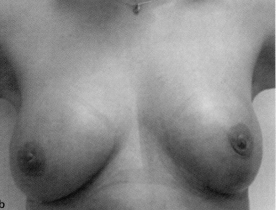

Fig. 63.8 a Left breast with Baker stage 4 before surgery. The breast is painful, and distortion can be seen. **b** Three months postoperatively, the left breast is soft

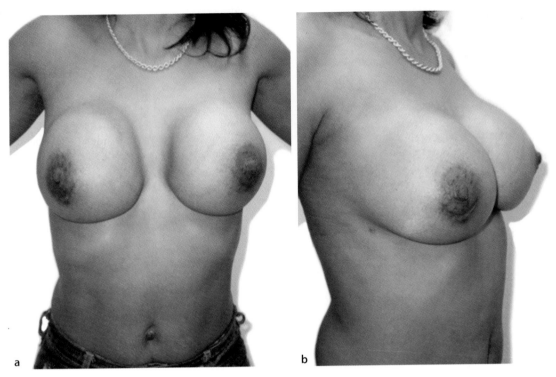

Fig. 63.9 a Baker stage 3 in the right breast of a patient with dark skin. **b** Six months postoperatively, and no problem with pigmentation

to unequaled safety compared with the classic method, which depends on the skill of the surgeon. There is regularity of the incising of the capsule, precision that is necessary to avoid any damage to the prostheses or the skin. Herrmann [8] had previously described this method with the Nd:YAG laser.

Independent of the Baker stage, continuous power of only 6 watts is sufficient but necessary. Power of less than 6 watts requires a second and maybe a third pass and thus extends the duration of the treatment. Power of more than 6 watts could lead to a section above the fibrosis and harm the skin internally.

Results obtained with other lasers seem to be of less quality. If the integrity of the implant is not respected during the operation, the implant must be changed. Sections of the capsule may be removed after removal of the implant in much more easily, as during normal surgery.

In any case, incising with the CO_2 laser is painless and much faster than the classic methods. As per Kompatscher [9], before any intervention on capsular contractures, mammography or magnetic resonance imaging (MRI) is necessary.

The only examples the author had to deal with were all Baker stage III with textured-shell prostheses—no

Baker stage IV with textured surface or silicone gel implants.

The most significant difficulties were with persons of phototype IV and Baker stage IV with round and smooth implants filled with saline. The fibrosis not only was very thick and hard, but the contracture deformed the implant. Incising the fibrosis with a CO_2 laser at 6 watts, continuous, was sufficient to gain back a flexible and nondeformed breast.

If damage to the integrity of the prosthesis is noted during the operation, the implant must be changed. The endoscope is then no longer indicated. This can be avoided by preoperative mammography or, if necessary, MRI in case of doubt.

63.5 Conclusions

Treatment of capsular contractures with the CO_2 laser with the endoscope is an easy-to-use technique with no risk to the implant or the breast. Surgical outcomes are without pain or hematoma. The use of the endoscope allows minimal incisions and maximum vision with high precision and security.

The use of the CO_2 laser at a medium power level allows physicians to solve any cases of capsular contraction, in accordance with the Baker classification, on all types of skin. Short-, medium-, and long-term results meet with patient satisfaction for this type of surgery, which does not require a general anesthetic.

References

1. Baker JL Jr: Augmentation mammaplasty. In: Owsley J, Peterson R (eds). Symposium on Aesthetic Surgery of the Breast, vol. 18. St. Louis, Mosby 1978

2. Vasquez B, Given KS, Houston GC: Breast augmentation: a review of subglandular and submuscular implantation. Aesth Plast Surg 1987;11:101–102

3. Moufarrege R, Beauregard G, Bosse JP, Papillon J, Perras C: Outcome of mammary capsulotomies. Ann Plast Surg 1987;19:62–64

4. Cairns TS, de Villiers W: Capsular contracture after breast augmentation—a comparison between gel- and saline-filled prostheses. S Afr Med J 1980;57:951–953

5. Baran C, Peker F, Ortak T, Sensoz O, Baran N: A different strategy in the surgical treatment of capsular contracture: leave capsule intact. Aesth Plast Surg 2001;25:427–431

6. Baker JL, Bartels RJ, Douglas WM: Closed compression technique for rupturing a contracted capsule around a breast implant. Plast Reconstr Surg 1976;58:137–138

7. Collis N, Sharpe DT: Recurrence of subglandular breast implant capsular contracture: anterior versus total capsulectomy. Plast Reconstr Surg 2000;106:792–796

8. Herrmann U: Endoscopic capsulotomy by means of laser: a new therapeutic method in cases of capsular contracture. Endoscop Surg Allied Technol 1995;3:112–114

9. Kompatscher P: Endoscopic capsulotomy of capsular contracture after breast augmentation: a very challenging therapeutic approach. Plast Reconstr Surg 1992;90:1125–1126

CHAPTER 64

Hammock Capsulorrhaphy

Richard Moufarrège

64.1
Introduction

Among all the retropectoral dissection limits in preparing the pocket to receive the breast augmentation prosthesis, only the development of the inferior limit of the dissection remains uncertain. In very experienced hands, it is easy to limit the extension of muscular disinsertion medially toward the sternum, laterally to the anterior axillary line, or even superiorly. Concerning the superior dissection, one can even elevate the prosthesis over the desirable limit. But even there, it is very easy, through an inferior capsulotomy and especially with a smooth prosthesis, to correct the prosthesis position. But there is still a problem controlling the inferior level.

64.2
Physiopathology

The submuscular plane must not be dissected too far inferiorly, and the blunt or instrument dissection has to be performed medially toward the sternum, with muscular disinsertion superiorly and laterally. In experienced hands, it is easy to limit medial or lateral dissection in order to avoid exaggerated medial or lateral displacement. These would oblige us ultimately to position correctly by capsulorrhaphy, with or without a compensatory opposite capsulotomy.

There is another way to avoid displacing the prosthesis in all directions, consisting primarily of correctly selecting a prosthesis of reasonable volume, "*primum non nocere.*" This will have a less wide diameter than the available prethoracic space. If the measurement not respected, there is a serious risk of axillary displacement out of the desirable final space.

Regardless of the care taken, a certain number of prostheses will succeed in downward migration, developing the typical deformity shown in Fig. 64.1.

64.3
Etiology

The spontaneous inferior dissection of the prosthesis is secondary either to the effect of the weight of the pros-

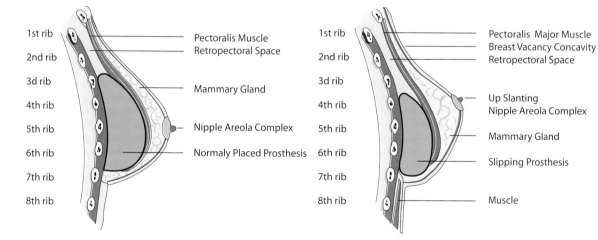

Fig. 64.1 a Normal position of prosthesis. **b** Inferior descent of prosthesis

thesis or the centripetal force applied downward on the prosthesis from all sides: from the top by muscle contraction, from the lateral and medial sides by an incomplete disinsertion, or simply because of a pocket that is too small for a prosthesis that is too big (Fig. 64.2).

In this study we present a way to correct the descent of the prosthesis. Such migration is often difficult to predict, especially when all the criteria from prosthesis selection to introduction technique have been observed.

In our series, we use 3% as the percentage of downward prosthesis displacement of one of the two breasts without any evident reason.

64.4
Anatomic Features

Inferior descent of the prosthesis is accompanied by its surrounding capsule. The migration is premuscular because the muscular fibers under the incision are not noted without a concentrated surgical effort, and they consist mainly of rectus abdominis fibers (Fig. 64.1).

64.5
Technique

The principle of capsulorrhaphy consists of an incision of an inferior crescent of the capsule with its posterior and anterior components (Fig. 64.3). This is performed through the inframammary augmentation incision. With the help of the assistant holding tissues elevated with hooks after exteriorization of the prosthesis through the elliptical excision of the scar, the cautery tool is used to make incisions in the posterior arch and the anterior corresponding arch. These arches are curved lines with a superior concavity, and their extremities will reach the dead ends constituted by the encounter of the posterior and anterior walls of the capsular pocket medially and laterally. The height and limit of such arches constitute the inferior limit of the future desired prosthesis pocket. This sequestrated crescent is always easy to reevaluate by referring to the skin lines drawn preoperatively on the patient in a sitting position. The anterior wall incision will correspond to the posterior capsular wall incision; that is, the incisions are at the same level and communicate together at the dead ends.

With a resorbable continuous suture (Dexon 2/0), closure is performed from the lateral to the medial dead ends of the free edges of the sequestrated lower crescent of the pocket capsule. This suture will contain the capsule wall, the surrounding muscular tissue, and all surrounding soft tissue that will develop into a hammock-

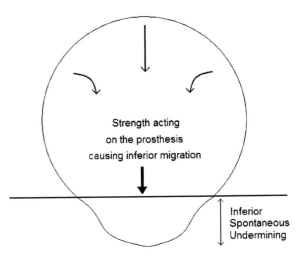

Fig. 64.2 Descent of prosthesis is secondary either to the effect of the weight of the prosthesis or the centripetal force applied downward on the prosthesis from all sides (from the top by muscle contraction, from the lateral and medial sides by an incomplete disinsertion, or simply because of a pocket that is too small for a prosthesis that is too big)

shaped "sausage" with an upper concavity, constituting a solid vault that will resist any downward pressure of the prosthesis (Fig. 64.4).

The prosthesis is then put back in its final position, and with a wide retractor protecting the prosthesis, the anterior and posterior inferior edges of the capsular wall are sutured together, maintaining the prosthesis in the main upper capsular pocket (Fig. 64.5). The skin is then closed as usual.

64.6
Results

We have seen no recurrence of inferior prosthesis migration in over 18 capsulorrhaphies. A 1-cm overcorrection is necessary, which will resume a final normal position between 1 and 3 months after surgery.

64.7
Conclusions

The hammock-style capsulorrhaphy constitutes a very efficient way to treat all prosthesis migrations. Its execution is simple and does not add any additional scar.

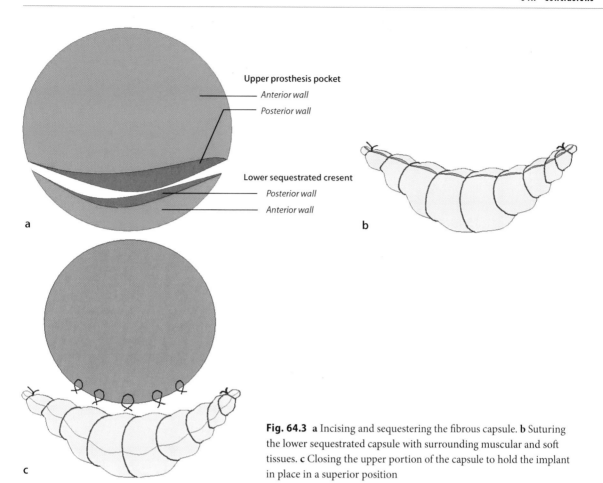

Fig. 64.3 a Incising and sequestering the fibrous capsule. **b** Suturing the lower sequestrated capsule with surrounding muscular and soft tissues. **c** Closing the upper portion of the capsule to hold the implant in place in a superior position

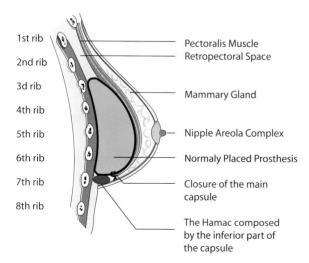

Fig. 64.4 The hammock-shaped "sausage" with an upper concavity, constituting a solid vault that will resist any downward pressure of the prosthesis

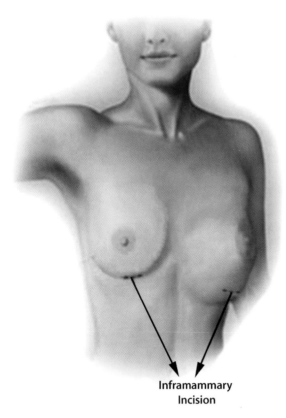

Inframammary Incision

Fig. 64.5 Left breast pretreated with descended prosthesis. Right breast following the hammock procedure

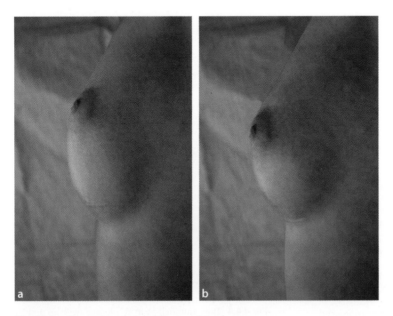

Fig. 64.6 a Pre-op lateral view. **b** Post-op lateral view

CHAPTER 65

Breast Implant Malposition: Prevention and Correction

65

Christine A. DiEdwardo, Shawkat A. Sati

65.1 Introduction

Although patient satisfaction is thought to be quite high after breast augmentation, the incidence of secondary procedures leads one to believe that suboptimal results occur more frequently than is documented [1]. This is evidenced by the number of patients who pursue revisional surgery. Hidalgo's review encompassed a total of 63 secondary cases over a 7-year period [1]. Gabriel et al. quoted an overall local complication rate of 12% at 5 years in a review of patients undergoing cosmetic breast augmentation [2]. These complications included capsular contracture, rupture of the implant, hematoma, leakage, and wound healing problems.

Displacement of the implant has been noted as the second most frequent complication following augmentation mammaplasty, after capsular contracture [3]. In Howard's series of 96 consecutive patients undergoing augmentation via a transaxillary approach, implant malposition in particular was documented to occur in 8.6% of patients. This was reduced to 2% when endoscopic techniques were used [4]. Overly aggressive medial pocket dissection and placement of excessively large implants can lead to synmastia [7]. Capsular contracture, particularly Baker grades III and IV, may result in breast asymmetry and implant malposition [5]. In addition to complaints of firmness, patients may notice that the breast has a rounder shape, and the implant may become displaced in the vertical or horizontal dimension. Mild contracture may result in an "uplifted" appearance, whereas greater degrees result in excessive tightening and distortion of the breast [6]. The treatment of the severe forms may involve addressing the capsule with either capsulotomy or total capsulectomy, placement of a textured surfaced implant, pocket reassignment, or administration of antibiotics [6].

Data obtained from premarket approval studies over a period of two and a half decades revealed a reoperation rate after breast augmentation of 15–20% [8]. These data reflect both reoperative procedures (breast biopsies, change of implant size, scar revisions, and subsequent mastopexies) and revisional surgeries (implant malposition, infection, extrusion, and capsular contracture). Averaged data from Mentor and McGhan reported an overall average reoperation rate of 17% following breast augmentation with saline implants over a 3-year follow-up period, with a 2% reoperation rate for implant malposition [9].

Tebbetts reported his results of a 12-year follow-up of 1,414 patients (2,828 breasts) who underwent breast augmentation. The overall reoperation rate for these cases was 3% of patients (or 1.5% of breasts) [9]. Two reoperations were performed for implant malposition (0.14% of patients, 0.07% of breasts). Tebbetts notes that key factors resulting in a low reoperation rate include an appropriate surgical plan dictated by a thorough preoperative analysis and meticulous surgical technique.

Correction of implant malposition requires a thorough understanding of the etiology. Multiple variables are involved in the art of breast augmentation. These include the anatomic features of the patient's breast and chest wall as well as the surgeon's aesthetic goals, intraoperative approach, and implant selection. A critical evaluation of the specific complication in the light of each of these factors must be delineated before proceeding with secondary surgery. In addition, the patient's desires must also be clearly outlined to obtain a result that is satisfactory to her as well as to the surgeon. It is imperative for the patient to understand that asymmetry is always present to some degree. The patient therefore must have realistic expectations.

65.2 Preoperative Analysis

Preoperative evaluation of the patient should focus on preventing implant malposition. During this evaluation, attention must be given to the chest wall's anatomic features. Breast volume, shape, base width, inframammary fold position, and glandular density each play an important role in outcome. A breast mound that is positioned laterally on the chest wall and a wide cleavage particularly pose a challenge in creating medial fullness. Skeletal deformities—most importantly, scoliosis, pectus excavatum, and pectus carinatum—affect the positioning of the implant relative to the chest wall. Asymmetries should be documented because they may be magnified after augmentation.

Rohrich et al. [10] performed a retrospective study to evaluate the incidence of breast and chest wall asymmetry in patients who underwent breast augmentation. They found that 88% of the women had some degree of asymmetry, and 65% had more than one parameter of asymmetry. These included nipple–areola complex asymmetry (24%), nipple position (53%), mound asymmetry (44%), base constriction (29%), inframammary fold position (30%), and ptosis (29%). These data substantiate the importance of a thorough systematic evaluation to detect preoperative breast and chest wall asymmetries that should be addressed to obtain an optimal postoperative result. Rohrich et al. recommend several steps for preoperative analysis. First, identify chest wall abnormalities; second, assess for the presence and degree of breast ptosis; third, identify breast asymmetries (breast mound volume, presence of base diameter constriction, asymmetry of nipple–areolar size and position); and fourth, note discrepancies of the inframammary fold position and base width of the breast. Finally, assess each quadrant of the breast intraoperatively for symmetry [10].

Aesthetic goals must be clearly delineated preoperatively. Correcting volume asymmetries by adjusting fill volume, releasing or altering the inframammary fold, and improving nipple–areola complex position by means of a mastopexy might be appropriate to consider. Patients with ptosis, especially if it is asymmetric, pose special challenges. Improvement of breast shape in these patients is influenced by pocket position, adjustment of the skin envelope [11], or a combination of these two approaches.

65.3 Operative Technique

The operative approach is dictated by careful preoperative evaluation and consideration of the aesthetic goals for the particular patient. Breast shape and volume and areolar size are important influencing factors in choosing the incision location: inframammary, areolar, axillary. An inframammary approach is preferred in a patient with ptosis in whom the scar will be somewhat concealed. If the inframammary fold needs to be raised, lowered, or released, as in a patient with tubular breast deformity, an areolar incision has advantages. Thin patients with minimal or no ptosis may be best suited with

an axillary approach to avoid a noticeable scar on the breast. Spear et al. have presented a comprehensive algorithm to guide incision location based on the characteristics of the breast [12].

The choice of implant type and size is determined primarily by the natural base width of the breast and the desires of the patient. Choosing an implant that is larger than the base width may result in synmastia or an implant that lies too far laterally on the chest wall. Pocket plane selection—i.e., subglandular versus partial or complete submuscular—is determined by breast volume, the thickness and distribution of breast parenchyma, and the presence and degree of breast ptosis. For saline implant placement, we most often prefer a partial submuscular position for the implant. If there is lower-pole hypoplasia, subglandular release of the breast tissue from the pectoral fascia may prevent a double-bubble deformity [11]. Certain patients may benefit from a "dual-plane" technique to maximize soft tissue coverage and allow for maximal expansion of the lower pole [9]. This involves dissection in the retromammary plane to a certain degree in addition to partial retropectoral augmentation.

The technical issues involved in developing the pocket are also important. We prefer to mark the region of the proposed pocket dissection with the patient in an upright position preoperatively. The midsternal line is marked in a vertical orientation from the substernal notch to the xyphoid. A line 1.5 cm from the midline is then marked. The pocket dissection will not pass medial to this line in an attempt to prevent synmastia. The outline of the implant pocket is drawn on the patient (Fig. 65.1a, b). The procedure begins with identification of the lateral border of the pectoralis major muscle. The submuscular plane is defined, and dissection proceeds medially, and then superiorly under direct vision. Care is taken to remain in a plane superficial to the pectoralis minor muscle. Lateral dissection over the serratus anterior muscle is initially limited to prevent lateral migration of the implant and to maximize medial fullness and cleavage definition. The pectoralis major muscle is then completely divided with the electrocautery tool perpendicular to its fibers along the inferior attachments to the chest wall. Tebbetts recommends dividing the muscle 1 cm above the origin to leave a "shelf" that may prevent inferior migration of the implant and lowering of the inframammary fold [9]. This proceeds from the lateral pectoral border medially to the level where the inframammary fold meets the sternal border (Fig. 65.2). Pectoralis fibers cephalad to this along the sternal border are not divided because this may result in synmastia. The implant volume can be adjusted to correct mound asymmetry. The incision is closed in two layers. It is

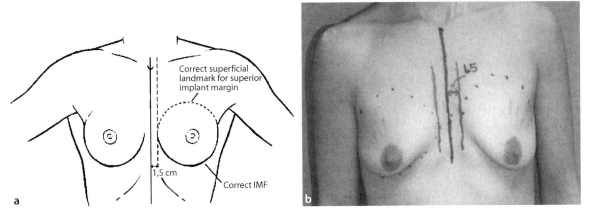

Fig. 65.1 a The patient is marked preoperatively with a vertical line 1.5 cm from the midline. **b** With the patient in a standing position, the planned pocket dissection is drawn

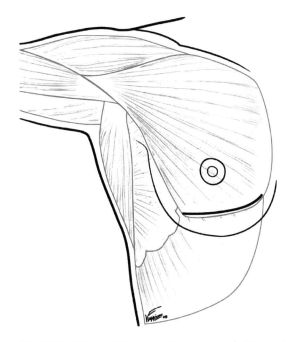

Fig. 65.2 Release of the pectoralis major muscle is important during submuscular augmentation and is performed under direct vision with electrocautery. Fibers along the inferior attachment to the chest wall are divided from the lateral pectoral border to the sternal border. Fibers cephalad to this along the sternal border are not divided because this may result in synmastia

important to place the patient in the erect position (as close as possible to sitting at 90°) to evaluate implant position and symmetry of the breast mound, nipple–areolar position, and inframammary fold.

65.4 Postoperative Management

Patients are informed that the final position of the implants evolves over the first 6 months. We instruct patients to begin displacement exercises, which are performed twice a day beginning in the immediate postoperative period.

65.5 Correction of Implant Malposition

When an implant malposition is detected in the postoperative period, it is important to focus on the patient's chief complaints. Analysis of the preoperative photos can assist in identifying preexisting anatomic factors that may have contributed to the malposition. Quite frequently, in retrospect one can identify preoperative asymmetry that may have initially gone unnoticed [13]. The relationship of the implant to the breast parenchyma and to the sternum as well as assessment of the implant volume give valuable information required in planning a corrective procedure.

Established implant malposition is most often addressed by either pocket reassignment or pocket dimension adjustment using capsulorraphy sutures, with or without changing the implant. Malposition of the implant can occur in the vertical or horizontal plane. If the implant is too high with resulting superior fullness, further dissection of the pocket in a lower plane will correct the problem. When the implant is too low, a double-bubble deformity or altered inframammary fold may result. Tebbetts reported in his review of 90 transaxillary augmentation procedures that the most common complication was asymmetry resulting from

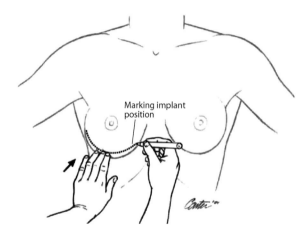

Fig. 65.3 Preoperative planning for a laterally displaced implant includes placing markings for the proposed capsulorrhaphy. This is accomplished by manual displacement of the implant to the new desired position

discrepant level of the inframammary folds in 9% of the patients [14].

In our experience, the most common presentation for implant malposition has been lateral displacement of one or both implants with resultant wide-set breast cleavage, which is unsatisfactory to both the surgeon and patient. We have found that factors contributing to this complication of lateral displacement include either a wide-set breast cleavage preoperatively or excessive lateral dissection of the pocket plane. In our experience, closure of the lateral aspect of the pocket by suture capsulorrhaphy is often helpful to correct this type of mal-

position. The technique of breast capsulorrhaphy was previously described by Spear and Little in 1988 [15] and Parsa in 1990 [16]. Troilius has also published his technique for suture correction of the lateral aspect of the capsule via a percutaneous approach [3].

The patient is marked preoperatively in an upright position. In addition to marking the inframammary fold, the implant is manually displaced to the desired new position. This proposed position of the correction sutures is marked on the skin (Fig. 65.3). The pocket is approached via the previous inframammary or periareolar incision, and the capsule is opened. The implant is removed, and the skin markings for the proposed pocket adjustment are used to guide the placement of interrupted 3-0 Prolene or PDS sutures to close the desired aspect of the capsule (Figs. 65.4, 65.5). The pocket is irrigated with antibiotic solution, the implant is replaced, and the wound is temporarily closed. The patient is placed in an upright position, symmetry is assessed, and then the wounds are closed in two layers.

65.6 Conclusions

The adage "an ounce of prevention is worth a pound of cure" applies to breast implant malposition. The most crucial time to avoid implant malposition is preoperatively by conducting a thorough assessment of each patient's anatomic factors and developing a surgical plan that addresses these issues. When malposition is detected postoperatively, adequate treatment includes addressing each type of malposition in light of the patient's concerns. The surgeon should consider performing a pocket readjustment using the capsulorrhaphy

LATERAL DISPLACEMENT

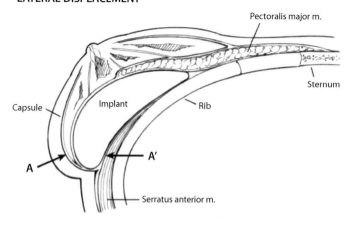

Fig. 65.4 Capsulorrhaphy is performed with either a single or double row of interrupted 3-0 Prolene sutures

AFTER CAPSULORRHAPHY

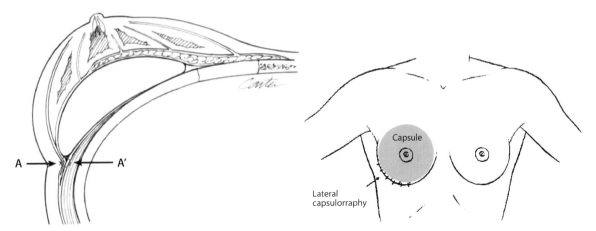

Fig. 65.4 Capsulorrhaphy is performed with either a single or double row of interrupted 3-0 Prolene sutures

Fig. 65.5 Capsulorrhaphy for lateral implant displacement includes placing sutures along the inferior and lateral margins of the capsule

technique described, along with replacing the implant if necessary.

Case 1: A 34-year-old woman presented with bilateral micromastia. Her chest wall was notable for a long torso with slight scoliosis. Her breast base width was 12.3 cm. Bilateral retropectoral breast augmentation was performed via a transaxillary incision. Smooth round implants with a base width of 11.6 cm and a fill volume of 300 ml were used. The postoperative result showed a wide cleavage plane that was partly related to her preoperative anatomy (Fig. 65.6a–e). Endoscopic-assisted transaxillary augmentation allows more precise control of pectoralis major muscle release and can be used in this type of patient for accurate placement of the implant and improved consistency of the desired result.

Case 2: A 31-year-old woman presented with breast asymmetry and, in particular, a constricted breast deformity of both breasts. The right breast was more severe than the left. She underwent partial retropectoral breast augmentation via an infraareolar incision. Smooth round implants were used and filled to 335 ml on the right and 350 ml on the left. Postoperatively, the patient was found to have lateral displacement of the right implant. In addition, she desired a larger volume and more superior fullness as well as medial repositioning of the right implant. Revision augmentation was then performed, which included inferior and lateral capsulorrhaphy with 3-0 Prolene sutures. A smooth round 450-ml saline implant was inserted, and the in-

framammary fold was raised. The left implant was also changed to a 450-ml implant, which was placed after a lateral capsulorrhaphy was done. Postoperatively, the patient's goals of increased volume and improved cleavage definition were obtained (Fig.65.7a–i).

Case 3: A 37-year-old woman presented with glandular ptosis and capsular contracture with superiorly displaced implants. She had asymmetric nipples that were high on the breast mound. She had undergone a Wise-pattern mastopexy 8 years prior and augmentation mastopexy 3 years prior, both at another institution and by different surgeons. The implants were smooth, round Mentor high-profile implants filled to 210 ml on the left and 275 ml on the right (to account for a previous glandular asymmetry). The implants were in a partial retropectoral position. Her main concerns were superior fullness (particularly in the upper outer quadrants) and the "sagging" appearance of her breasts. She was not bothered by the nipple asymmetry or wide areolar scars. Revision augmentation was performed, which included resection of an ellipse of skin at the level of the inframammary fold to shorten the vertical distance from the nipple–areola complex to the inframammary fold. Partial capsulectomy was performed inferiorly, followed by capsulorrhaphy in the upper outer quadrants using interrupted 2-0 PDS sutures. Mentor smooth round moderate-profile saline implants were placed with a 160-ml fill on the left and 225 ml on the right (Fig. 65.8a–k).

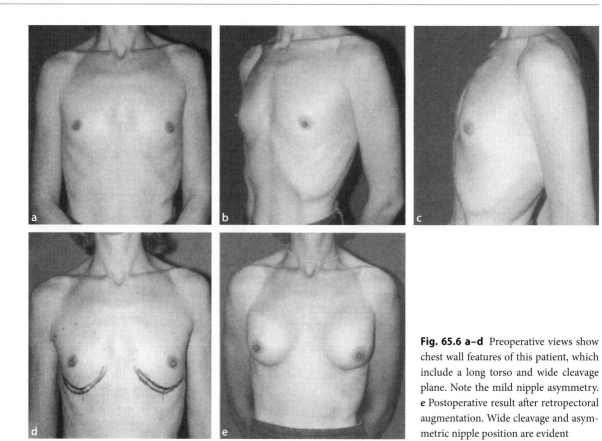

Fig. 65.6 a–d Preoperative views show chest wall features of this patient, which include a long torso and wide cleavage plane. Note the mild nipple asymmetry. **e** Postoperative result after retropectoral augmentation. Wide cleavage and asymmetric nipple position are evident

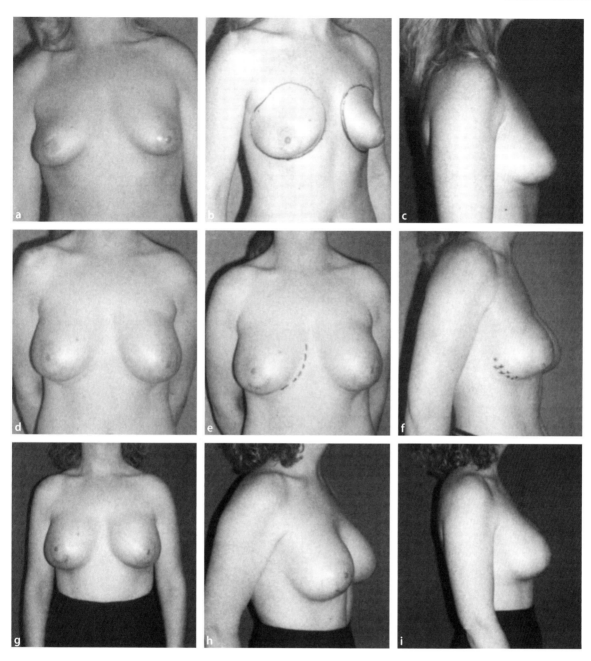

Fig. 65.7 a–c Preoperative views of this patient with breast asymmetry and a mild constriction deformity. Retropectoral augmentation was performed. **d** The patient was dissatisfied with the postoperative result. Lateral displacement of the right implant was evident. In addition, she desired increased breast volume. **e, f** Revision augmentation was performed. The patient was marked preoperatively by displacing the implant supero-medially to the new desired position. The planned lateral capsulorrhaphy sutures were marked on the skin. **g–i** Results after correcting the implant malposition. Inferior and lateral capsulorrhaphy were performed with a double row of interrupted 3-0 Prolene sutures. The inframammary fold was also raised, and larger implants were placed bilaterally. The goals of increased volume and improved cleavage definition were achieved

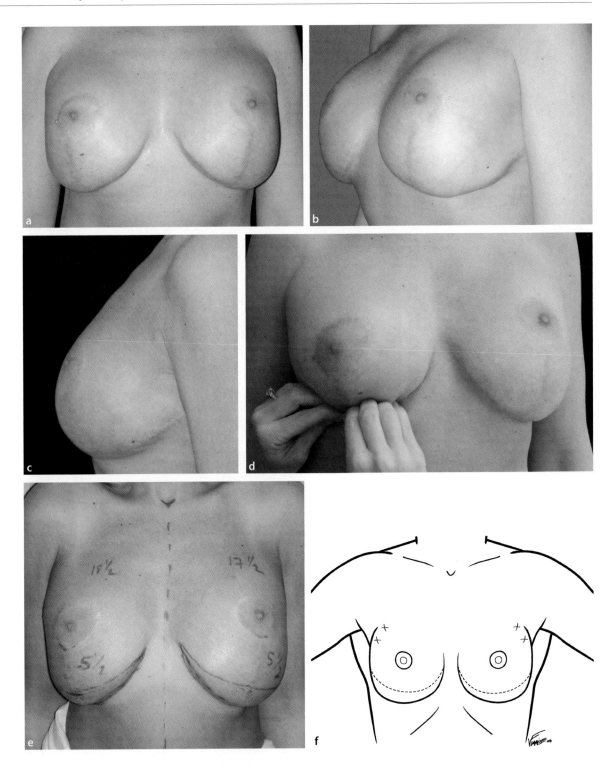

Fig. 65.8 a–c Preoperative views of a patient who presented with complaints of excessive fullness of the upper outer quadrants of her breasts following retropectoral augmentation mastopexy, which was performed by another surgeon. She also disliked the "sagging and boxy appearance" of the lower poles of her breasts. Exam revealed glandular ptosis and capsular contracture with superiorly displaced implants. The areola-to-inframammary distance was 8 cm. She also had asymmetry of the nipple–areola complex and wide scars, which were not bothersome to her

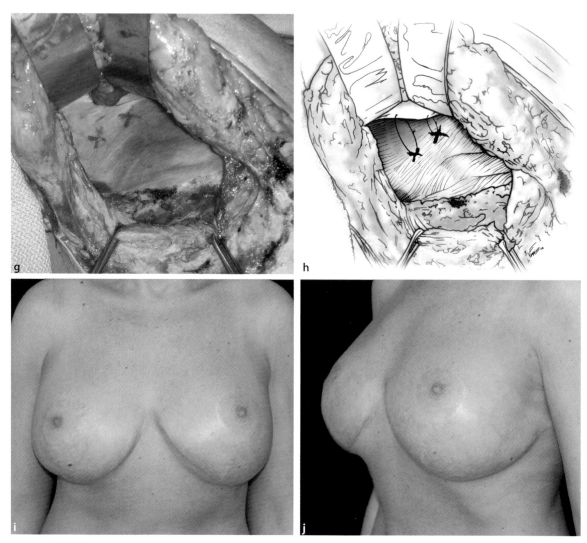

Fig. 65.8 *(continued)* **d–f** Revision augmentation was performed. The patient was marked preoperatively. The implant was displaced inferomedially to the new desired position, and the position of the planned location for the capsulorrhaphy was marked on the skin. Markings were also placed for the planned skin resection along the inframammary fold to achieve a 5.5-cm distance from the areola to the inframammary fold. Manually tightening the proposed skin excision resulted in a rounder breast with an improved nipple–areolar position relative to the breast mound. **g, h** Intraoperative capsulotomy and placement of a single row of capsulorrhaphy sutures (3-0 PDS) in the proposed position. **i–j** Postoperative results. High-profile Mentor saline implants were removed, and smaller Mentor moderate-profile saline implants were placed. The goals of decreased volume and improved contour were achieved

References

1. Hildalgo D: Breast augmentation: choosing the optimal incision, implant, and pocket plane. Plast Reconstr Surg 2000;105:2202–2216

2. Gabriel SE, Woods JE, O'Fallon WE, et al.: Complications leading to surgery after breast implantation. N Engl J Med 1997;336:667–682

3. Troilius C: Correction of implant ptosis after transaxillary subpectoral breast augmentation. Plast Reconstr Surg 1996;889–895

4. Howard P: The role of endoscopy and implant texture in transaxillary submuscular breast augmentation. Ann Plast Surg 1999;42:245–248

5. Vinnik CA: Spherical contracture of fibrous capsules around breast implants. Prevention and treatment. Plast Reconstr Surg 1976;58:555–560

6. Hammond D, Hidalgo D, Slavin S, et al.: Revising the unsatisfactory breast augmentation. Plast Reconstr Surg 1999;104:277–283

7. Spear SL: Synmastia after breast augmentation. Plast Reconstr Surg 2006;118 (suppl):168S–171S

8. Adams WP, Teitelbaum ST, Bengston BP, Jewell ML, Tebbetts J, Spear S: Breast augmentation roundtable. Plast Reconstr Surg 2006;118 (suppl):175S–187S

9. Tebbetts JB: Dual plane breast augmentation: optimizing implant-soft tissue relationships in a wide range of breast types. Plastic Recontr Surg 2006;118 (suppl): 89S–102S

10. Rohrich RJ, Hartly W, Brown S: Incidence of breast and chest wall asymmetry in breast augmentation: a retrospective analysis of 100 patients. Plast Reconstr Surg 2006;118 (suppl):7S–12S

11. Brink R: Evaluating breast parenchymal maldistribution with regard to mastopexy and augmentation mammaplasty. Plast Reconstr Surg 2006;106:491–496

12. Spear SL, Bulan EJ, Venturi ML: Breast augmentation. Plast Reconstr Surg 2006;118(suppl):188S–196S

13. Spear SL: Discussion: incidence of chest wall asymmetry in breast augmentation: a retrospective analysis of 100 patients. Plast Reconstr Surg 2006;118 (suppl):15S–17S

14. Tebbetts JB: Transaxillary subpectoral augmentation mammaplasty: long term followup and refinements. Plast Reconstr Surg 1984;74:636–647

15. Spear SL, Little JW III: Breast capsulorrhaphy. Plast Reconstr Surg 1988;81:274–279

16. Parsa FD: Breast capsulopexy for capsular ptosis after augmentation mammaplasty. Plast Reconstr Surg 1990;85:809–812

CHAPTER 66

Aesthetic Outcome of Breast Implant Removal 66

David T. Netscher, Asaad Samra

66.1
Introduction

Since the silicone breast implant controversy in the early 1990s, distance and time have lent perspective to what was then a crisis that saw increasing numbers of women with breast implants return to plastic surgeons for advice on how to manage real or imagined problems with their implants. The large number of women seen during that time gave surgeons an opportunity to review their own techniques, to evaluate the efficacy and safety of breast implant devices, and also to gain experience in dealing with complications. Although some of the anxieties were media-driven, patients did have significant problems specifically related to implant rupture, development of severe capsular contracture, and, less commonly, periprosthetic infection and extreme thinning of soft tissues over the implant. At the time of the U.S. Food and Drug Administration moratorium on silicone breast implants, many patients had their breast implants removed because of personal safety fears alone. Going forward from that experience to today, we can learn from the past [1–3]. It would seem that systemic complications, risk of developing breast cancer, and immune disorders are unlikely to be related to breast implants [4–6]. Nonetheless, recent studies show that local complications are fairly common and that reoperation is not infrequent [7, 8]. On occasion, the only option remaining for such patients is to remove their implants.

Over the years there has been a variety of implant types, with differences in shell thickness, filler material, surface texturing, and implant configuration. However, most local complications are common to all breast implants. The aesthetic outcome following implant removal and the secondary reconstructive options offered to patients will vary according to a number of circumstances, but patients will essentially fall into two large categories depending on whether their implants were initially placed for either reconstructive or cosmetic purposes.

66.2
Reasons for Implant Removal

Implant malposition generally requires replacing the implant in conjunction with internal capsulorrhaphy, capsule modifications, and mastopexy. These conditions may lead to such severe problems that they preclude implant replacement, although in many cases treatment will involve replacement of the implant. Various pathologic situations may require implant removal (Fig. 66.1).

66.2.1
Implant Rupture

The incidence of saline-filled implant rupture has not been fully evaluated, but that of silicone-filled rupture appears to be related to the duration of implant placement. This rupture rate is also clearly related to the generation and type of gel implant [9]. The overall rupture rate of silicone gel implants is about 50%, and the median life span of silicone gel implants from a meta-analysis of more than 1,099 implants was 16.4 years [10]. Neither anatomic placement of breast implants (prepectoral or subpectoral) nor the reason for implantation (reconstruction or cosmetic augmentation) appears to be related to implant rupture.

When a saline-filled breast implant ruptures, implant deflation occurs, with a noticeable decrease in breast size and volume. The deflated shell may be palpated as a mass. Deflation may occur due to leakage at a fill-valve or seam, or it may occur at a true fold flaw, often secondary to underinflation of the implant. An external force may on occasion be sufficiently great to directly rupture the implant. In contrast, most silicone gel implant ruptures remain intracapsular and may be more difficult to diagnose clinically. Extracapsular rupture may result in a breast parenchymal granuloma that may be confused with a breast tumor, or the silicone may follow the course of least resistance and be squeezed up

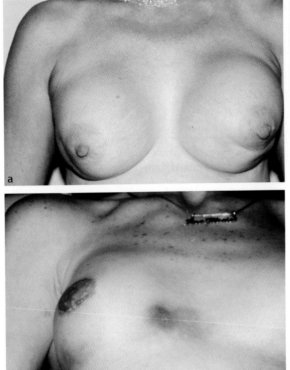

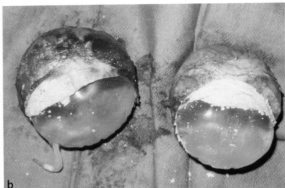

Fig. 66.1 a Patient with severely deforming painful capsule contracture. She desired implant removal. **b** Hard calcified capsules around implants that were removed. **c** Patient with periprosthetic infection who required implant removal

toward the axilla, leading to visible and palpable breast deformity (Fig. 66.2). Mammograms can also reveal unexpected findings with silicone that is not clinically palpable but is visible mammographically (Fig. 66.2b).

The authors do not, however, believe that any of the breast imaging techniques play a routine role in preoperative evaluation of a patient who is to have an implant removed [11–13]. It is not fully clear what to advise the asymptomatic patient who has an apparent intracapsular gel implant rupture that was diagnosed by one of the various imaging techniques, although most would advise removing such a ruptured implant (Figs. 66.3, 66.4). The sensitivity and specificity of ultrasound and magnetic resonance imaging (MRI) for detection of implant rupture are not sufficient to recommend routine screening ultrasound or MRI evaluation for this potential problem, even in patients who have had implants in place for over 10 years (the rupture rate of gel implants may be over 50%) [14, 15] if these patients are clinically asymptomatic. The potential incidence and rate of implant rupture with the newer generation of silicone gel implants remains to be evaluated.

66.2.2
Capsular Contracture

The incidence of symptomatic capsular contracture that causes significant breast deformity and/or pain (Baker grades III and IV) has been reported to be between 0% and 50% (Fig. 66.1) [16–18]. Contracture rates for implants vary according to implant type: the old sponge types, 100%; gel-filled with a patch, 70%; patchles gel-filled, 55%; saline inflatable, 35%. Saline-filled implants seem to reduce the incidence of contracture in nearly every study. The incidence of capsular contracture, in most studies, follows an initial rapid rise to about 30% in the early years after implantation, followed by a more gradual increase over time. A limitation of most studies on capsular contracture is that data interpretation is difficult because of changes in implant design over time.

Another factor that seems to influence capsular contracture is the anatomic placement of the implant. A prosthesis placed in a subcutaneous pocket after subcutaneous mastectomy has a significantly higher risk of capsular contracture than an implant placed in the subpectoral plane. However, this finding of subpectoral placement reducing the incidence of capsular contracture following cosmetic augmentation has not been borne out by all studies [14].

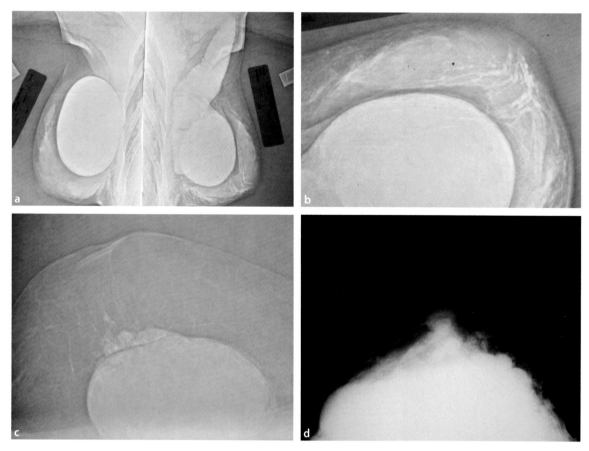

Fig. 66.2 **a** Ruptured silicone gel implant showing extrusion of silicone up toward the axilla on the patient's right. **b** Mammogram shows apparently intact gel implant but probability of silicone in the lactiferous ducts deep to the nipple. **c** Silicone granuloma on the anterior surface of a ruptured gel implant. **d** Silicone injections bilaterally into the breasts that led to masses of silicone granulomas totally obscuring the mammographic evaluation of breast parenchyma

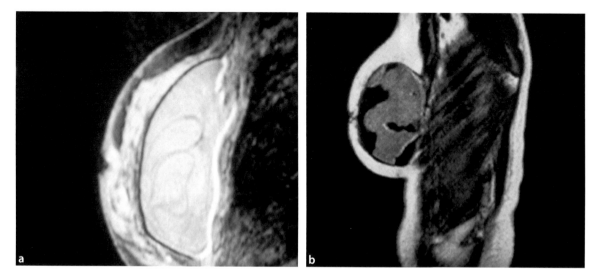

Fig. 66.3 **a** Intracapsular rupture of breast implant showing the "linguini" sign on magnetic resonance imaging (MRI). **b** The implant folds can sometimes be confused for implant rupture, as seen with MRI

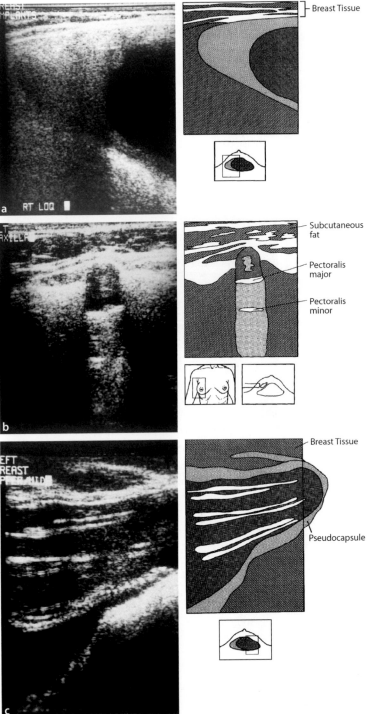

Fig. 66.4 a Ultrasound with diagrammatic explanation for retained intracapsular silicone gel implant rupture. **b** Ultrasound with diagrammatic explanation for silicone extravasation and granuloma formation. **c** Ultrasound with diagrammatic representation of intracapsular rupture of a gel implant with resulting inward collapse of the implant shell showing the parallel lines of the characteristic "stepladder" sign

Subclinical bacterial colonization in mammary implants appears to be etiologically related to the development of capsular contracture [19]. Experimental studies with irrigation of antiseptic solutions and antibiotic impregnation appear to be helpful in this regard [18, 20, 21]. However, whether these measures interfere with the mechanical integrity of breast implants has not been fully investigated.

66.2.3
Periprosthetic Infection

Infection occurs in 1–4% of cases following augmentation mammoplasty [22, 23]. Symptoms are usually present within a week following surgery, but delayed infections may occur. The risk of infection is unrelated to location of the operative incision, surface characteristics of the implant, filler material, or implant position (submammary or subpectoral) [24]. Most infections are caused by gram-positive organisms, usually *Staphylococcus aureus*, *Staphylococcus epidermidis*, and streptococci types A and B. Less frequently, such organisms as *Pseudomonas aeruginosa* or even atypical *Mycobacterium* cause infections.

If the process is localized and superficial, such as a suture abscess, simply opening, irrigating, and packing the wound and administering appropriate antibiotics may be sufficient. However, if the periprosthetic space is involved, eradication of infection is impossible unless the implant is removed (Fig. 66.1c). The contralateral implant, even if unaffected, may have to be removed as well for aesthetic reasons. Heroic efforts to salvage an infected implant with intravenous antibiotics and pocket irrigation are unjustified because they are very inconvenient, costly, and at best meet with unfavorable results with hard capsular contracture and at worst lead to disastrous results with tissue loss and permanent deformity.

66.2.4
Implant Extrusion

Augmentation mammoplasty patients may occasionally present with impending or overt extrusion of the implant, which was more common when steroids were instilled into the surgical pocket. This caused soft tissue atrophy and thinning of the skin in the dependent part of the breast. The most conservative approach is removal of the implant with reimplantation at a later date. However, if there is significant soft tissue loss, a local rotation flap may be required for adequate soft tissue coverage, or the physician may even resort to autogenous tissue reconstruction.

66.2.5
Implant Malposition

Breast deformities may result from excessively lateral dissection of the breast pockets, loss of symmetry of the inframammary creases, or synmastia with confluence of the breasts in the midline. These problems are generally handled by a variety of techniques, including capsu-lorrhaphy, changing the plane of the implant, replacing a smooth implant with a textured implant, creating a sling for the implant with a muscle flap (such as latissimus dorsi), or with a decellularized human cadaveric dermis (such as Alloderm, LifeCell, Branchburg, NJ, USA). Occasionally, especially in those who have had multiple prior breast operations, the tissues may be so thin and atrophic that it is best to perform the repair in two stages—the first stage to remove the implant and at least part of the capsule to allow tissue surfaces to adhere together, and the second stage to perform a secondary implant placement (usually in a different plane from before). In rare cases, one may have to resort to autogenous tissue reconstruction.

66.2.6
Implant Palpability and Rippling

Implant palpability and rippling may be a late problem that is very unsettling to the patient and is more likely to occur if there is an unusually thin layer of breast tissue covering the implant, which is more common in small-breasted or thin women. This is generally improved by placing the implant under the muscle, providing more padding over the upper half of the implant, adding more saline to the prosthesis if it seems underfilled, or replacing with a silicone gel device. Rippling seems to be more common with textured implants than with smooth ones, and with saline-filled than with gel-filled prostheses [25]. Thin individuals who have previously been advised of this potential problem may simply desire removal of the implants.

66.2.7
Patient Desire

Occasionally, a patient may desire removal of implants for no apparent cosmetic problem. She may be concerned about no longer wanting prosthetic material in her body, or the original reasons for having implants may simply have passed. Whatever the reasons may be, the plastic surgeon should listen to the patient sympathetically, and if she has realistic expectations and understands the potential complications, it would seem reasonable to comply with the patient's request to remove the implants. It is for this very reason that one should avoid excessively large breast augmentation and not be coerced by the body-dysmorphic patient to place implants that are too large, since at a later date, removal of very large implants that have stretched the skin excessively may create a variety of reconstructive problems.

66.3
Implant Removal and Timing of Any Reconstructive Options

The authors believe that the surgical technique used for implant removal is important to overall enhanced outcome. We generally perform implant removal with a total capsulectomy. There is a slightly increased risk of a contained postoperative seroma if the capsule is retained. Retained implant capsules may also result in a spiculated mass suspicious for carcinoma, or dense calcifications that obscure neighboring breast tissue on subsequent imaging studies [26]. There may be increased risk of creating a pneumothorax if the posterior capsule is removed in a subpectoral implant, so leaving a small disk of posterior capsule against the chest wall may be prudent.

Removal of a thickened capsule leaves behind a more pliable breast envelope that more easily drapes over a new implant and molds more readily for a mastopexy. Finally, extracapsular dissection enables one to contain an unrecognized intracapsular rupture of a gel implant and thus minimize the risk of silicone spillage into the surrounding breast tissue, with consequent avoidance of potential future silicone granulomas. Meticulous hemostasis must be achieved when the capsulectomy is done. Care is taken to remove the capsule only by dissecting within the easily defined extracapsular surgical plane so as not to remove any breast parenchymal tissue.

When an implant is removed in a patient who has previously had a mastectomy, and no further attempt at reconstruction is made, it is obvious that there will be significant chest wall deformity (Fig. 66.5). If reconstruction is not performed in such a patient, the only option available to her is to wear a prosthetic bra, which for some may be a suitable solution (Fig. 66.5). However, when breast implants are removed in the patient with a previous cosmetic augmentation, there will be changes in both breast volume and shape, but these are harder to predict. In a patient of thin body build and a previous augmentation mammoplasty, implant removal reveals the expected appearance with an exaggerated degree of ptosis and loss of upper breast pole cleavage (Figs. 66.6, 66.7). For the patient who is to have breast implant removal, it is often difficult to explain the results of implant removal alone without photographic examples for the patient to review. Potential surgical options following implant removal in the cosmetic patient are then dependent on the patient's needs, her aesthetic desires, and the plastic surgeon's advice. The problem is how best to predict which patients will return most closely to their preaugmentation state and which will develop the worst of these deformities when implants are removed, requiring consideration of additional reconstructive procedures. On occasion, removal of implants may unmask previously unrecognized breast asymmetry (Fig. 66.8).

In both previously reconstructed and augmented patients, it is better to minimize deformities at the time of implant removal than to attempt to correct them at a later date, for both technical and economic reasons.

A patient who had previously had implants placed

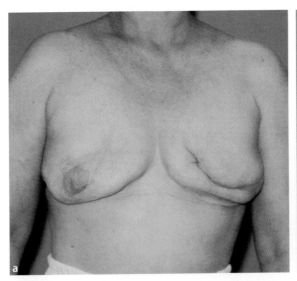 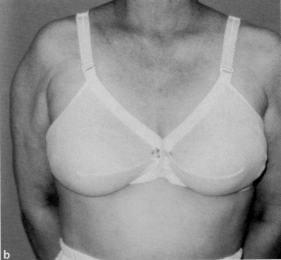

Fig. 66.5 a A patient with previous breast reconstruction had her implants removed, leaving an unaesthetic appearance, even though she was happy to no longer have pain from her hard capsular contracture. **b** She did not desire autologous tissue reconstruction and was willing to disguise the appearance with a prosthetic bra

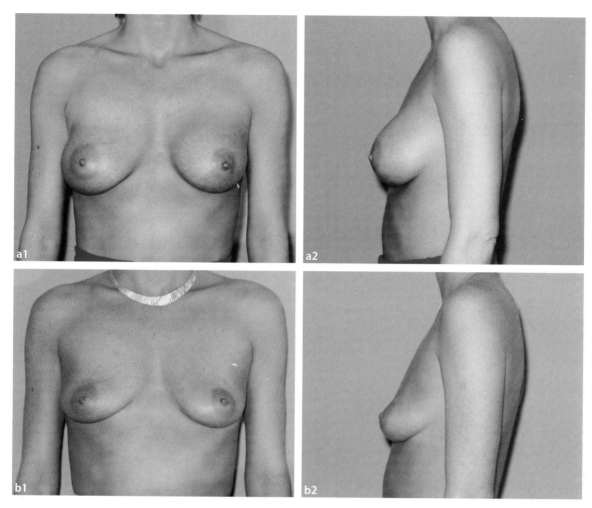

Fig. 66.6 a *1* Patient with previous silicone gel breast augmentation. *2* Lateral view. **b** *1* Loss of upper breast fullness and sagging is noted once the implants were removed without further augmentation. *2* Lateral view

for reconstructive reasons (Fig. 66.9) for previous subcutaneous mastectomies presented with severe, painful capsular contractures. She initially underwent implant removal alone. Subsequently, she desired autogenous tissue reconstruction. The reconstructive result following bilateral transverse rectus abdominis musculocutaneous (TRAM) flaps was suboptimal, largely because of the difficulty in recreating a smoothly contoured skin envelope. Once contracture of the skin envelope has developed over time following implant removal, reconstruction becomes more complex and may even require pre-expansion. In a previously reconstructed patient who has had implants removed, it may be very difficult to redrape the skin. It is our contention that the result is far more favorable if one can use the existing skin envelope immediately following implant removal and capsulectomy.

In a patient who previously had a cosmetic augmentation and is now unhappy with the breast shape and form once implants have been removed, the problem may be financial rather than technical. Often the aesthetic problem can be readily solved by simple reaugmentation, but the patient may now be unable to afford a second operation. While financial concern should not impede one's surgical judgment, whenever it is surgically prudent, one should simultaneously combine the removal of implants in the cosmetic patient with some form of reconstruction, such as mastopexy or reaugmentation. Conversely, in a patient who is initially opposed to implant replacement or when it is discovered intraoperatively that a mastopexy is simply not possible, it may be more prudent to back out, let the patient evaluate her "new" appearance, and then jointly make a decision about the need for any further surgical management.

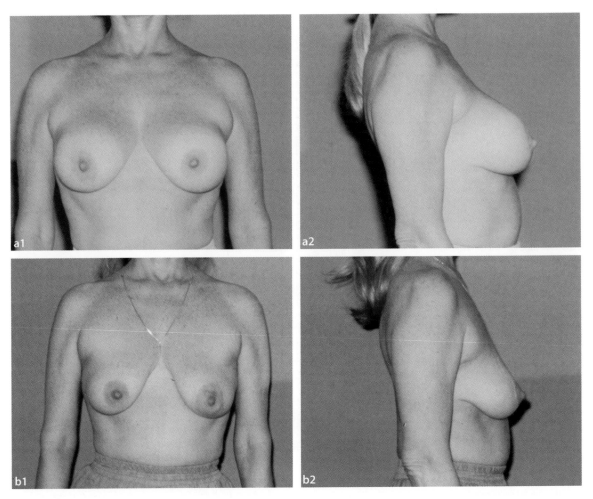

Fig. 66.7 a *1* Thin patient with augmentation mammaplasty. *2* Lateral view. **b** Predicted result following implant removal above, showing loss of upper breast cleavage. *2* Lateral view

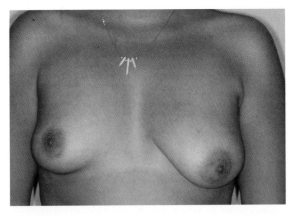

Fig. 66.8 Breast asymmetry that was "unmasked" by removal of implants previously apparently placed for cosmetic purposes

If a mastopexy is selected in a cosmetic patient who has implants removed but does not desire them to be replaced, a tailor-tacking type of mastopexy is planned. This enables the surgeon to adjust the markings and place temporary sutures to evaluate the efficacy of the mastopexy intraoperatively before committing to incisions (Fig. 66.10). If the patient enters the explantation surgery with the knowledge that the surgeon may discover intraoperatively that a mastopexy may not be in her aesthetic best interest, this leaves the option open to the surgeon. The patient can then, over the following months, determine whether a reaugmentation should be performed.

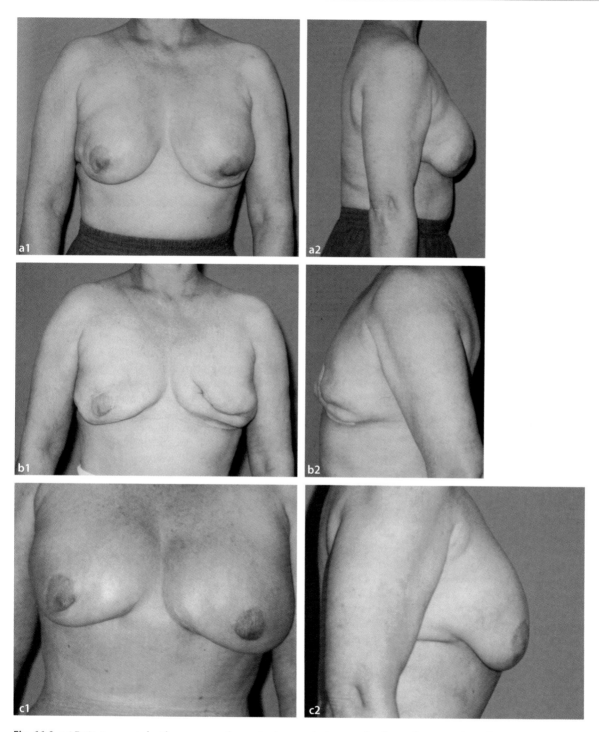

Fig. 66.9 a *1* Patient presented with severe capsular contracture around implants that were previously placed for breast reconstruction. *2* Lateral view. **b** *1* Appearance following bilateral im-plant removal and capsulectomy. *2* Lateral view. **c** *1* Appearance after delayed autogenous tissue reconstruction. *2* Lateral view

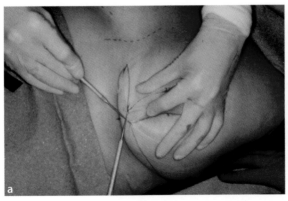
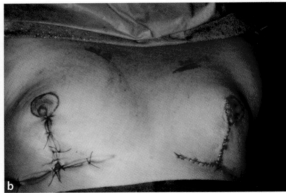

Fig. 66.10 Intraoperative view showing placement of tailor-tacking sutures (**a**), before committing to actual skin incisions (**b**)

66.3.1
Goals for Reconstruction Following Implant Removal

The goals for reconstruction are the following:
1. Minimize the breast contour deformity.
2. Restore the breast volume, shape, and aesthetic appearance.
3. Create skin flaps to accommodate the appropriate breast volume.
4. Resolve any infection.
5. Minimize external scars.
6. Provide emotional support to the patient.

66.3.2
Diagnostic Studies and Preoperative Evaluation

To achieve the best reconstructive outcome and to satisfy the patient's requirements, the clinical examination must highlight a number of features [27, 28]. These will help the physician preoperatively predict what the potential outcome might be following implant removal alone or with any of the possible reconstructive options. This is especially important in the previously aesthetically augmented patient when reconstruction is planned simultaneous with implant removal. The following evaluations are important:
1. Estimation of current volume of breast tissue: The change in bra cup size following prior augmentation, record of the implant size, and previous photographs are helpful to determine how much breast tissue will remain after an implant is removed. Mammography may also help determine the volume of breast tissue relative to implant size (Fig. 66.11). In the patient represented in Fig. 66.12, who had multiple prior breast implant surgeries and in whom it was apparent that very little breast tissue would remain even

though she had a prior cosmetic augmentation, surgery was undertaken to remove the implants in the full knowledge that autogenous tissue reconstruction would be immediately undertaken.
2. Skin elasticity: If the breast skin is elastic, it is more likely that implant removal alone will mimic the preaugmentation state. However, patient age, presence of striae, number of prior pregnancies, and degree of existing breast ptosis are all helpful in evaluating the potential appearance after breast implant removal. If one anticipates that there will be an excessive degree of postoperative breast ptosis, and the patient does not desire reaugmentation, then implant removal accompanied by a mastopexy will almost certainly be necessary.

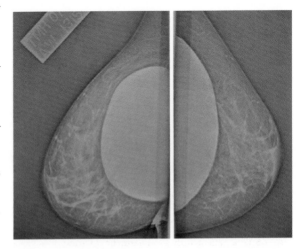

Fig. 66.11 Preoperative mammogram shows that this patient will have adequate breast parenchyma remaining once implants are removed

3. Breast asymmetry: Removal of breast implants may unmask previously existing breast asymmetry. The patient's history may report a significant degree of existing asymmetry that may indeed have been the original reason for the breast augmentation. Breast asymmetry may have been present before the breast augmentation, or it may have been acquired as a result of multiple breast biopsies, infections, ruptured gel implants, or multiple capsulectomies. In patients with true extracapsular implant rupture resulting in extrusion of silicone into the breast tissue with granuloma formation, removal may result in loss of breast tissue as well.

4. The patient's view of breast aesthetics: The patient may now have personal desires that are totally different from those when she first sought breast augmentation. Acceptance of additional scars, especially those of mastopexy, and willingness to receive a new implant must therefore all be evaluated. The patient may now have also gained additional weight since

her original augmentation was performed in her younger years. This may actually lead to increased soft tissue within the breast, and therefore on some occasions there is surprisingly little influence on the aesthetic outcome with breast implant removal alone.

In the patient who has saline-filled implants and desires removal, it is possible to deflate the implants in the office by simply puncturing the implant percutaneously and attaching the needle to wall suction. This will allow one to determine, the day before surgery, whether the added volume of a new implant will be necessary.

5. The role of breast imaging techniques: As a rule, breast imaging (mammography, MRI, and ultrasonography) does not play a significant role in the preoperative evaluation of a patient who is planning to have implants removed. However, when a screening mammogram is indicated to evaluate breast parenchymal disease, it should be done preoperatively.

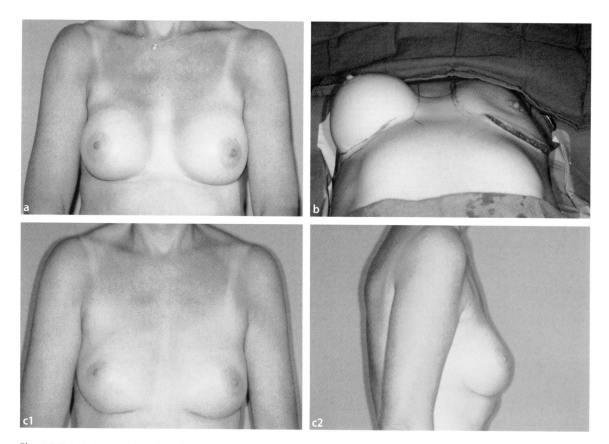

Fig. 66.12 a Patient with good aesthetic appearance but who had multiple previous surgeries to remove ruptured implants and treat capsular contracture. **b** Intraoperative view showing very little breast tissue remaining once implants are removed, even though she had an initial cosmetic augmentation. **c** *1* Following autogenous tissue reconstruction with deepithelialized (transverse rectus abdominis myocutaneous) TRAM flaps. *2* Lateral view

Mammography may sometimes be helpful in giving an idea of the volume of breast tissue relative to implant size. Mammography may also occasionally detect extracapsular silicone gel implant rupture in the presence of palpable masses. For some cases in which rupture is uncertain, MRI remains the most accurate diagnostic tool.

66.4
Technique and Results

66.4.1
Management Options

Management options, once the decision is made to remove an implant, depend on both the patient's desires and, especially, correct analysis of the problem by the surgeon. These options must be clearly outlined to the patient. They are fourfold:
1. Implant removal alone
2. Implant removal with surgical adjustments to include capsule modification, resuspension of the breast superiorly up to the chest wall, and mastopexy
3. Implant removal and replacement with a new (and possibly different) implant
4. Reconstruction with autogenous tissue

66.4.2
Management of the Patient Previously Reconstructed with Implants

A patient who has previously had subcutaneous mastectomy and has either a ruptured implant or deforming capsular contracture, but whose skin envelope is noncontracted and has a well-defined inframammary crease, is an ideal candidate for implant removal and simultaneous implant replacement. A very favorable outcome can be achieved with simultaneous replacement of implants. Some might use contoured implants, but we have had good results with replacement of round saline or gel-filled implants, generally placed in a subpectoral plane in these patients.

When body habitus allows, autogenous tissue reconstruction using deepithelialized flaps gives good results in the patient with prior subcutaneous mastectomy and implant reconstruction, since the skin envelope and inframammary crease are already formed. Bilateral TRAM flaps may be used. The ideal patient for such an autogenous tissue reconstruction is one in whom the removed implant is of similar volume to that which would be achieved from a unilateral TRAM flap.

If there is a sufficient adipose roll in the back and flank region, then deepithelialized extended latissimus dorsi flaps tend to give good results as the sole form of reconstruction, especially in patients who have had prior abdominal surgeries or when the patient is unwilling to risk abdominal weakness [29]. A deepithelialized transverse crescent of skin is taken bilaterally with extended fat dissection. Back scars and contour deformity after this type of reconstruction may be adverse (Fig. 66.13).

On occasion, chest soft tissue may be excessively thin, or autogenous tissue from the abdomen or back may be insufficient to provide bilateral breast reconstruction alone. Providing that the patient is willing to accept an implant, a reasonable reconstructive option would be to use latissimus dorsi flaps in association with a smaller implant. In a patient unwilling to accept an implant, bilateral free microvascular TRAM flaps can often yield more lower abdominal soft tissue than can be safely achieved with a pedicle TRAM flap, or perhaps a microvascular free-tissue transfer from other anatomic sites such as the gluteal region may help salvage the previously reconstructed patient who now presents with severe problems and breast implants [30].

The majority of these patients previously reconstructed with implants often have had their prior implants placed in a subpectoral location. For optimal aesthetic results, when autogenous reconstruction is planned with a deepithelialized flap to provide breast volume fill, a new breast pocket must be created in a subcutaneous plane.

66.4.3
Management of the Patient with Previous Cosmetic Breast Augmentation

It is reassuring to know that even among those who choose to have their implants removed without replacing them, patients are generally satisfied with the outcome with regard to general health, vitality, and also appearance, even though the plastic surgeon may feel that there is room for aesthetic improvement [31]. Indeed, with implant removal alone, some patients may actually experience improvement of a deformity that had resulted from deforming encapsulation while they had the implants [1]. Furthermore, when blinded observers graded outcomes, the overall breast aesthetics for implant removal alone in the patient who had previously undergone cosmetic augmentation was still acceptable, but was nonetheless generally somewhat downgraded from the preoperative appearance (prior to implant removal) [1]. Patients who did not desire implant replacement but who had an associated mastopexy gener-

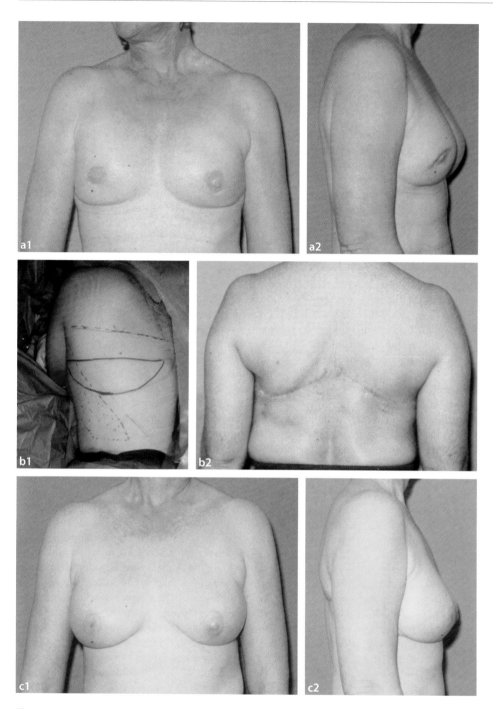

Fig. 66.13 **a** *1* Symptomatic capsular contracture in a patient previously reconstructed with breast implant. *2* Lateral view. **b** Crescent deepithelialized and extended latissimus dorsi pedicle flaps are used bilaterally (*1*) but leave obvious donor site scars (*2*). **c** *1* Favorable breast reconstruction using only autogenous tissue. *2* Lateral view

ally fared better cosmetically than those with implant removal alone.

It is in this group of previously augmented patients that a high degree of clinical skill is required on the part of the plastic surgeon. The problem must be correctly diagnosed in order to institute the appropriate surgical treatment.

Autogenous tissue reconstruction following implantation in the previously cosmetically augmented patient is often impractical because of the expense and extent of the surgery involved. On a few occasions we have performed bilateral TRAM flaps in patients who have not had prior mastectomies. These have included patients with chest wall asymmetry such as Poland's syndrome and for whom the original reason for breast implant placement was to disguise such an asymmetry. The authors have likewise used autogenous tissue in the previously augmented patient who has had several surgeries for excision of silicone granulomas due to implant rupture. Removal of implants in these patients is known to leave very little remaining breast tissue (Fig. 66.12). A favorable result under such circumstances is achieved by "augmentation" using bilateral deepithelialized TRAM flaps.

If the patient is reaugmented and the breast is soft (such as following implant rupture or deflation), an implant of similar size to that previously used would be appropriate. However, if the breast now represents a Baker III or IV capsular contracture associated with skin striae and ptosis, then the new implant should preferably be slightly larger. This is because once the contracted capsule is excised, the skin envelope will expand and require additional fill volume. We also generally recommend treating a patient with severe capsular contracture by placing the new implant in the "dual-plane" position [32].

If a patient does not desire replacement of an implant, or if the plastic surgeon deems replacement medically unwise, then one is faced with the dilemma of whether to perform an associated mastopexy. In one study [1] that questioned woman who had breast implants removed after prior cosmetic augmentation, when they were specifically asked about external scarring, this fact alone did not adversely affect perceived outcome in those who had implant removal together with a mastopexy.

One of the more technically challenging body types for breast augmentation is the thin patient with severe breast hypoplasia. Because of the paucity of available soft tissue, the implant itself predominantly affects breast shape postoperatively. An error would be to choose an implant that is too wide for the existing base diameter of the breast. The skin envelope has only a limited ability to stretch, so an excessively large implant will create a distorted breast with excessive upper-pole fullness. Also, with time, the weight of a large implant may result in inferior migration of the device and create a "bottomed-out" distortion. Problems such as these must be identified preoperatively in planning implant removal or when revising an unsatisfactory breast augmentation [33].

Based on the preoperative evaluation and on the results of previously published outcome studies [1], if the patient does not desire reaugmentation or is unsuitable for reaugmentation, we are able to advise patients as follows.

Older, thin patients who have breast striae are more likely to experience adverse aesthetic outcomes when implants are removed without further surgery. Even in slender patients with a small amount of breast tissue and inelastic skin, a pleasing breast shape can be achieved with mastopexy despite the loss of breast volume (Fig. 66.14).

In contrast, in the full-framed, full-breasted patient who has previously undergone only modest augmentation and who might have gained weight since her initial cosmetic surgery, and who may also have a mild degree of capsular contracture with minimal ptosis, a good aesthetic outcome can be anticipated following implant removal alone. Similarly, for youthful women with thin body build and elastic skin, no prior pregnancies, no evidence of striae, and who previously had only modest augmentation, good results can be expected following implant removal only, and they can be expected to closely resemble their preaugmentation state (Fig. 66.15). The ideal candidate for mastopexy associated with implant removal is one with a relatively full frame, a substantial amount of breast tissue, and breast ptosis with skin striae (Fig. 66.16).

Mastopexy should not rely on reshaping the skin alone or on the resulting dermal suspension. The breast parenchyma and skin flaps are appropriately undermined, and parenchymal shaping sutures are used. Additionally, the breast parenchyma can be undermined and suspended superiorly by suturing to the chest wall. The mastopexy technique is modulated by the degree of breast ptosis and the size of the areola. The skin incisions range from a periareolar mastopexy, to vertical short-scar mastopexy, to a full Wise-pattern incision [2]. Use of an interlocking purse-string Gore-Tex suture around the areola helps fixate the areola at the desired dimension and greatly facilitates completion of the mastopexy [34]. Occasionally, it might be advisable to perform a delayed mastopexy, either because of patient wishes or because of a potential increased risk of vascular compromise to the nipple–areola complex, such as in a patient who is a heavy smoker or a patient with significant breast ptosis who requires substantial nipple elevation [2].

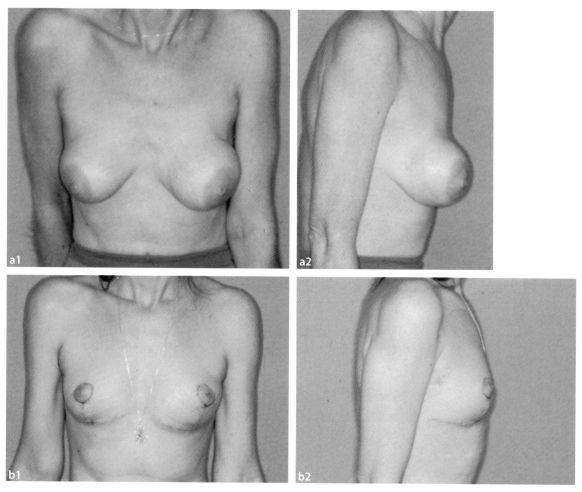

Fig. 66.14 a *1* Thin patient who had prior augmentation mammaplasty presenting with deforming capsular contracture. *2* Lateral view. **b** *1* A favorable result was obtained with implant removal and simultaneous mastopexy. She did not desire implant replacement. *2* Lateral view

66.5
Conclusions

In the previously augmented patient who has reason for implant removal, autogenous tissue reconstruction is indicated in only a few special circumstances. Implant reaugmentation generally provides favorable results. However, one must beware of the contracted, ptotic breasts with stretch marks. Such a patient may require a larger implant to be placed in a different surgical plane. We have become increasingly liberal with our indications for mastopexy when reaugmentation is not performed. Tailor-tacking mastopexy helps define the breast form before committing to an incision.

If a patient has been previously reconstructed with implants, autogenous tissue reconstruction generally gives uniformly good results, although one is often limited in volume for bilateral breast reconstructions. Recourse to free-tissue transfer may be required.

A patient who is to have her breast implants removed emphasizes the importance of the surgeon's taking the time to understand the aesthetic problem and determine what the patient wants. Finally, this situation illustrates the necessity of practicing the art of medicine—even if we are sometimes still lacking in the science, we continue to strive for improved implant design and techniques [35].

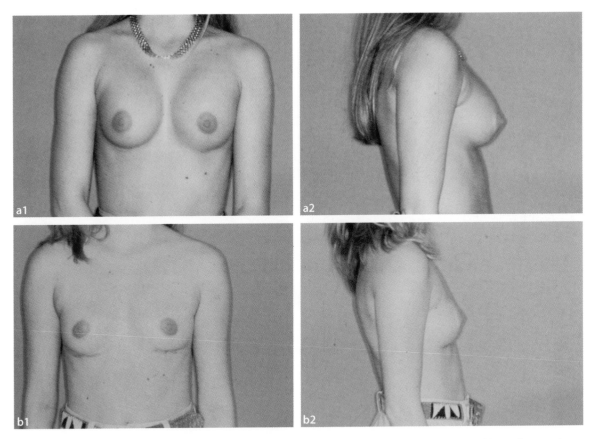

Fig. 66.15 a *1* Thin patient with capsular contracture who desired implants to be removed. *2* Lateral view. **b** *1* In a youthful patient, a favorable aesthetic result can be achieved by implant removal alone, albeit with the anticipated loss in breast volume. *2* Lateral view

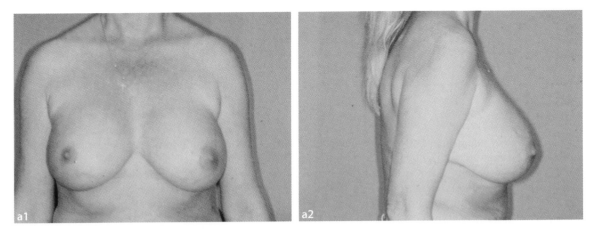

Fig. 66.16 **a** *1* Patient with full body frame has capsular contracture, breast ptosis, and skin striae. *2* Lateral view

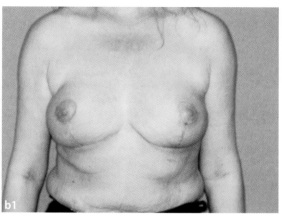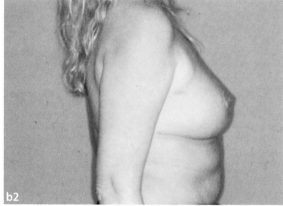

Fig. 66.16 *(continued)* **b** *1* Postoperative after breast implant removal and simultaneous mastopexy. *2* Lateral view

References

1. Netscher DT, Sharma S, Thornby J, Peltier M, Lyos A, Fater M, Mosharrafa A: Aesthetic outcome of breast implant removal in 85 consecutive patients. Plast Reconstr Surg 1997;100(1):206–219

2. Rohrich RJ, Beran SJ, Restivo RJ, Copit SE: Aesthetic management of the breast following explantation, evaluation and mastopexy options. Plast Reconstr Surg 1998;101(3):827–837

3. Melmed VP: A review of explantation of 240 symptomatic women: a description of explantation and capsulectomy of reconstruction using a periareolar technique. Plast Reconstr Surg 1998;101(5):1364–1373

4. Silicone breast implants do not cause chronic disease, but other complications are of concern (news release). Washington, D.C.:National Academy of Sciences Institute of Medicine, June 21, 1999

5. Schusterman MA, Kroll SS, Reece GP, Miller MJ, Ainslie N, Halabi S, Balch CM: Incidence of autoimmune disease in patients after breast reconstruction with silicone gel implants versus autogenous tissue: a preliminary report. Ann Plast Surg 1993;31(1):1–6

6. Gabriel SE, O'Fallon WM, Kurland LT, Beard CM, Woods JE, Melton LJ 3rd: Risk of connective tissue diseases and other disorders after breast implantation. N Engl J Med 1994;330(24):1697–1702

7. Gutowski KA, Mesna GT, Cunningham DL: Saline-filled breast implants: A Plastic Surgery Educational Foundation multicenter outcome study. Plast Reconstr Surg 1997;100(4):1019–1027

8. Gabriel SE, Woods JE, O'Fallon M, Beard CM, Kurland LT, Melton LJ III: Complications leading to surgery after breast implantation. N Engl J Med 1997;336(10):677–682

9. Peters W, Smith D, Lugowski S: The life-span of silicone gel breast implants and a comparison of mammography, ultrasonography, and magnetic resonance imaging in detecting implant rupture: a meta-analysis. Ann Plast Surg 1999;43(1):97–99

10. Goodman CM, Cohen B, Thornby J, Netscher D: The life-span of silicone gel breast implants and a comparison of mammography, ultrasonography, and magnetic resonance imaging in detecting implant rupture: a meta-analysis. Ann Plast Surg 1998;41(6):577–585

11. Ahn CY, Shaw WW, Narayanan K, Gorczyca DP, Sinha S, Debruhl ND, Bassett LW: Definitive diagnosis of breast implant rupture using magnetic resonance imaging. Plast Reconstr Surg 1993;92(4):681–691

12. Debruhl ND, Mgorcezyca, DP, Ahn CY, Shaw WW, Bassett LW: Silicone breast implants: US evaluation. Radiology 1993;189(1):95–98

13. Netscher DT, Weizer G, Malone RS, Walker LE, Thornby J, Patten BM: Diagnostic value of clinical examination and various imaging techniques for breast implant rupture as determined in 81 patients having implant removal. South Med J 1996;89(4):397–404 de Camara DL, Sheridan JM, Kammer BA: Rupture in 18 silicone gel breast implants.

14. Plast Reconstr Surg 1993;91(5):828–834

15. Netscher DT, Walker LE, Weizer G, Thornby J, Wigoda P, Bowen D: A review of 198 patients (389 implants) who had breast implants removed. J Long-Term Eff Med Implants 1995;5(1):11–18

16. Burkhardt BR: Capsular contracture, hard breasts, soft data. Clin Plast Surg 1998;15(4):521–532

17. Hakelius L, Ohlsen L: A clinical comparison of the tendency to capsular contracture between smooth and textured gel-filled silicone mammary implants. Plast Reconstr Surg 1992;90(2):247–254

18. Burkhardt BR, Demas CP: The affect of Siltex texturing and povidone-iodine irrigation on capsular contracture around saline inflatable breast implants. Plast Reconstr Surg 1994;93(1):123–128

19. Netscher DT, Weizer G, Wigoda P, Walker LE, Thornby J, Bowen D: Clinical evidence of positive breast periprosthetic cultures without overt infection. Plast Reconstr Surg 1995;96(5):1125–1129

20. Adams WP, Conner CH, Barton FE Jr, Rohrich RJ: Optimizing breast pocket irrigation: an in vitro study in clinical implications. Plast Reconstr Surg 2000;105(1):339–343

21. Darouiche RO, Netscher DT, Mansour I, Meade R: Activity of antimicrobial-impregnated tissue expanders. Ann Plast Surg 2002;49(6):567–571

22. Courtiss EH, Goldwyn RM, Anastasi TW: The fate of breast implants with infections around them. Plast Reconstr Surg 1979;63(6):812–816

23. Freedman A, Jackson I: Infections in breast implants. Infect Dis Clin North Am 1989;3(2):275–287

24. Handel N, Jensen JA, Black Q, Waisman JR, Silverstein MJ: The fate of breast implants, a critical analysis of complications and outcomes. Plast Reconstr Surg 1995;96(7):1521–1533

25. Hetter GP: Satisfactions and dissatisfactions of patients with augmentation mammoplasty. Plast Reconstr Surg 1979;64(2):151–155

26. Hardt NS, Yu L, LaTorre G, Steinbach B: Complications related to retained breast implant capsules. Plast Reconstr Surg 1995;95(2):364–371

27. Netscher DT: Management of breast implant complications. In: McCarthy JG, Galiano RD, Boutros SG (eds). Current Therapy in Plastic Surgery. Philadelphia, Saunders Elsevier 2006, pp 397–402

28. Netscher DT, Walker LE, Spira M: Avoidance and treatment of breast contour deformities encountered with implant removal. Perspectives Plast Surg 1998;11(2):35–54

29. 29. McCraw JB, Patt CT: Latissimus myocutaneous flap: "fleur-de-lis" reconstruction. In: Hartramf CR (ed). Breast Reconstruction with Living Tissue. Norfolk, VA, Hampton Press 1991, pp 211–248

30. Shaw WW, McCraw JB, Beegle PH: The gluteal flap. In: Hartramf CR (ed). Breast Reconstruction With Living Tissue. Norfolk, VA, Hampton Press 1991, pp 269–291

31. Rohrich RJ, Kenkal JM, Adams WP, Beran S, Conner WC: A prospective analysis of patients undergoing silicone breast implant explantation. Plast Reconstr Surg 2000;105(7):2529–2537

32. Spear SL, Carter ME, Ganz JC: The correction of capsular contracture by conversion to "dual-plane" positioning: technique and outcomes. Plast Reconstr Surg 2003;112(2):456–466

33. Hammond DC, Hidalgo D, Slavin S, Spear S, Tebbetts J: Revising the unsatisfactory breast augmentation. Plast Reconstr Surg 1999;104(1):277–283

34. Hammond DC: Augmentation mastopexy: general considerations. In: Spear SL, Willey SC, Robb GL, Hammond DC, Nahabedian MY (eds). Surgery of the Breast: Principles and Art, 2nd edn. Philadelphia, Lippincott Williams & Wilkins 2006, pp 1403–1416

35. Slavin SA, Goldwyn RM: Silicone gel implant explantation: reasons, results, and admonitions. Plast Reconstr Surg 1995;95(1):63–69

Inframammary Fold Elevation and External Synmastia Repair: Morgan–Metcalf Method

67

Robert Yoho

"Raising the IMF: it's the hardest thing in breast surgery."
Peter Cheski, MD

67.1
Introduction

After several hundred cases using the transumbilical approach to breast augmentation, the author found that overdissection of the cleavage area and sometimes the inframammary crease led to an occasional complication of low inframammary fold or synmastia. Taping these areas with foam tape secured with tincture of benzoin or other tape adherent under a supportive bra sometimes yielded good results, but other times it did not. Of additional help was an inframammary crease garment invented by Metcalf and perfected in 2006 by Design Veronique™ [1]. Although the Veronique™ garment is truly a significant improvement on anything we have had before, and it can sometimes correct a problematic dissection if the patient is compliant (wearing it for 1–3 weeks), it does not work every time, and sometimes it will "ride up" to make an inframammary crease that is too high.

Opening the breast and suturing a mature capsule from the inside is the time-honored approach to this problem. However, the following method works well and avoids an additional scar load on a breast for the right candidate. As with most surgeries, the patient's ability to heal properly and thus produce a durable result is clearly related to her nutritional and health status. This is particularly important when trying to ensure a smooth, round contour around a foreign body, the implant.

67.2
Synmastia

Synmastia is often related to inadequate lateral breast pocket dissection, which puts pressure on the medial

aspect of the implant. The admonition to be conservative with the lateral dissection of any breast implant pocket is well taken, for obvious reasons: the importance of avoiding manipulation of the 4th intercostal nerve, and the ease with which overdissection is often, unfortunately, accomplished. The best policy is to dissect only what is needed for implant fit— no more and no less. Great cleavage, which is a desirable feature of breast implants, is always a trade-off between the rate of synmastia and how many of a surgeon's cases have too much space between the implants centrally. The ideal is to choose the implant diameter that allows a finger's width between the breasts yet shows implant centering side to side under the nipple–areola complex. Using only the (less expensive) regular-profile implants is not a good approach, for the surgeon often cannot meet the above requirements and still satisfy the patient's volume/cup size desires. For example, for a size 34–36 chest, the most appropriate implant is a medium-profile implant, unless unusually large size and projection are desired, in which case the high-profile implant may be best.

67.3
Technique

The surgeon should always obtain consent for incision and open surgery in case the implant is accidentally punctured or if other complications necessitate repair from the inside.

Prep and drape the patient in sterile fashion. Mark the new contour of the breast carefully. Using number 1 Prolene or nylon on a curved needle, and with the assistant holding the implant away from the area being sutured, perform a running submerged suture (Fig. 67.1). The suture can either be run both ways and the ends tied to each other, or it can be tied at each end. Pull it tight to submerge the suture points where entry is affected. There is little danger of invading the thorax because as the curved needle is passed through the deep tissues, and possibly even the periosteum, it is kept parallel to

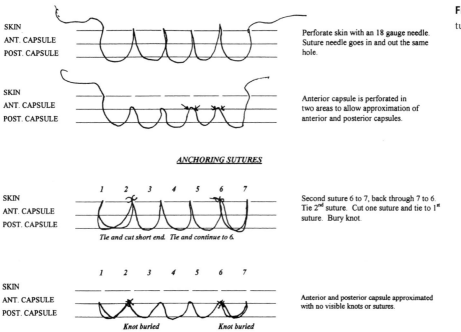

SKIN
ANT. CAPSULE
POST. CAPSULE

Perforate skin with an 18 gauge needle.
Suture needle goes in and out the same
hole.

SKIN
ANT. CAPSULE
POST. CAPSULE

Anterior capsule is perforated in
two areas to allow approximation of
anterior and posterior capsules.

ANCHORING SUTURES

SKIN
ANT. CAPSULE
POST. CAPSULE

1 2 3 4 5 6 7

Tie and cut short end.   Tie and continue to 6.

Second suture 6 to 7, back through 7 to 6.
Tie 2nd suture. Cut one suture and tie to 1st
suture. Bury knot.

SKIN
ANT. CAPSULE
POST. CAPSULE

1 2 3 4 5 6 7

Knot buried   Knot buried

Anterior and posterior capsule approximated
with no visible knots or sutures.

Fig. 67.1 Subcuticular suture technique

the chest wall. In the technique originally described by Metcalf [2], an 18-gauge needle is used to allow the knot and puncture points to submerge. It is useful to slightly dilate the puncture wounds with iris scissors. As the suture is passed with the large curved needle, the overlying skin can be manipulated so the holes are only 1–1.5 cm apart.

The lateral/superior dissection must have previously been adequate, or this technique will not work long term because of the extra tension at the suture line, causing breakdown of the repair.

Results have been durable, and skin changes have resolved nicely (Figs. 67.2, 67.3).

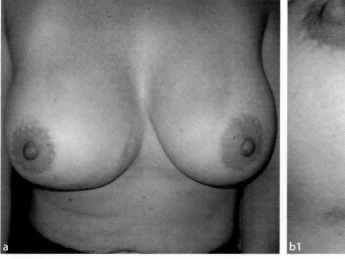
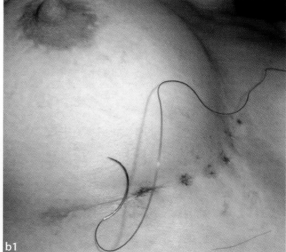

Fig. 67.2 a Patient with overdissected medial aspect of the right breast. **b** *1* Correction with the continuous suture technique. *2* Sutures not visible

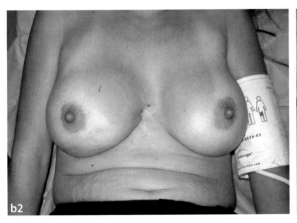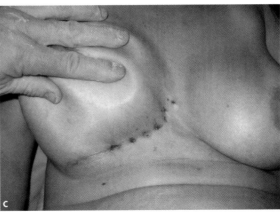

Fig. 67.2 *(continued)* **b** *1* Correction with the continuous suture technique. *2* Sutures not visible. **c** Three weeks following the procedure. The result was excellent, although irregularities of the inframammary crease were seen; these had almost disappeared a few months later

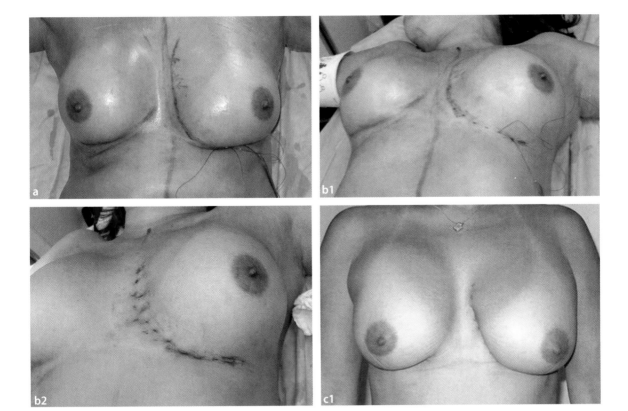

Fig. 67.3 a Overdissected medial aspect of the left breast. **b** *1* Using number 1 Prolene or nylon on a curved needle, and with the assistant holding the implant away from the area being sutured, a running submerged suture is performed. *2* Suture site. **c** *1* Results 3 weeks after the procedure. *2* Suture site

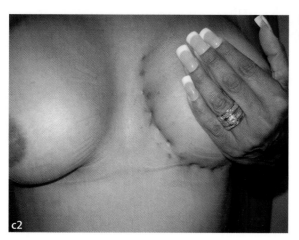

Fig. 67.3 *(continued)* **c** *1* Results 3 weeks after the procedure. *2* Suture site

---

References

1. Design Veronique home page. http://www.designveronique.com. Accessed 29 May 2008
2. Metcalf D: Breast implant complications. Presented at the 18th Annual Meeting of the American Society of Cosmetic Breast Surgery, Newport Beach, CA, 8 June 2002

Intracapsular Allogenic Dermal Grafts for Periprosthetic Breast Implant Problems

68

Richard A. Baxter

68.1
Introduction

Techniques for breast augmentation surgery have improved tremendously, as have designs and manufacturing techniques for both saline and silicone gel implants. Among these specific improvements are a greater variety of implant profiles [1], allowing for better tailoring of the implant dimensions to the patient's individual anatomic constraints while maintaining some flexibility of choice in volume. Methods for assessing the adequacy of the soft-tissue envelope have also been advanced [2], facilitating greater predictability in maintaining stable implant–tissue relationships. Antibiotic irrigation [3] and other refinements have reduced the incidence of capsular contracture.

In the wake of these advances, however, the previously underappreciated problem of periprosthetic atrophy has emerged. An inadequate capsular envelope is the common denominator contributing to a variety of problems. These include visible rippling, "bottoming out," implant malposition, and perhaps symmastia. Although a thin capsule is not always the sole cause of these problems, recognizing it as an element of the underlying pathophysiology holds the key to correcting it.

Periprosthetic capsular atrophy is likely due to a variety of contributing factors. Tissue expansion typically results in a degree of tissue thinning. Gravity, pressure from an oversized implant relative to tissue elasticity, and involution of breast tissue related to aging may all accelerate capsular atrophy. Some patients simply have too little subcutaneous fat, a condition made more challenging with postmastectomy reconstruction using implants. Bottoming out may be caused primarily by pectoral muscle activity pushing down on the implant or by lax lower-pole support, but the result in either case is thinning of the lower pericapsular tissues as the implant migrates downward. Overzealous medial release of the pectoralis muscle may also result in an unsupported medial capsule, allowing for implant migration and symmastia.

Options for capsular reinforcement have been extremely limited. Generally, these include muscle flaps, which may be appropriate for reconstruction patients but difficult to recommend for the aesthetic augmentation patient. Conversion to submuscular placement may be an option, but there is typically insufficient muscle available for the lower and lateral quadrants. Acellular allogenic dermal grafts (Alloderm, LifeCell, Branchburg, NJ, USA) have proven to be a reliable option for many cases of periprosthetic atrophy [4, 5]. Use of Alloderm in reconstruction with implants has proven useful as well [6, 7].

68.2
Technique

The patient is marked prior to surgery to identify the targeted areas of capsular thinning. Generally this is done in the upright position, although sometimes a forward-leaning posture will better reveal the problem areas. Alloderm grafts are supplied in specific sizes and thicknesses, so the markings should correspond to the dimensions of the grafts to be used. It is generally best to use fewer large grafts rather than several smaller ones and thereby avoid seams and overlaps, but the grafts need to be placed so as to prevent folds and wrinkles. For capsular onlay grafting, the thick (0.79–1.78 mm) size usually works best; the "ultrathick" (1.55 mm+) is too rigid.

Access for graft placement is usually through scars from previous surgery, though some may be impractical. Exposure needs to be adequate for orienting and suturing the material, typically an incision of 4 cm or more. Any trimming of the grafts is most easily done with scissors prior to hydration. The grafts are bathed in saline according to the manufacturer's recommendations while operative exposure is gained. They are then positioned in an onlay fashion and secured with 3-0 or 2-0 polyglactin (e.g., Vicryl) sutures spaced no more than 1 cm apart.

The most common orientation for the grafts is around the periphery, with the posterior margin of the graft along the junction of the anterior and posterior portions of the capsule. For repair of symmastia due to excessive medial muscle release, the graft acts as a sort of muscular aponeurosis bridging the dehisced muscle edge and the chest wall. It may be similarly deployed to correct bottoming out when the dual-plane technique has been used; in this instance, the muscle spans between the inferior margin of the pectoral muscle where it fuses with the anterior capsule, and the chest wall at the inframammary fold. For visible implant rippling, only grafts to the anterior capsule may be required, but this is uncommon.

Because the graft is sandwiched between the implant and the capsular surface, good apposition against the capsule is needed for graft survival by vascular ingrowth. Suction drains are usually indicated to prevent fluid collections that may interfere with graft adherence.

68.3
Results

Graft survival has been evident up to 4 years of follow-up. However, relapse of bottoming out has occurred in some cases, and repeat grafting has been beneficial in instances of severe atrophy in order to build up a thicker capsule.

Periprosthetic atrophy can follow multiple previous operations (Fig. 68.1). In Fig. 68.1, the patient presented with severe rippling with smooth round subpectoral implants (McGhan style 20, 425 cc), and recurrent bottoming out after two attempts at correction with capsulorrhaphy. Correction was done with a repeat capsulorrhaphy, reinforced with 4×7-cm Alloderm grafts inferolaterally and superomedially. The 6-month follow-up results are shown (Fig. 68.1). Although some rippling is still apparent, her condition is much improved.

The tissue expansion–implant sequence in reconstruction following bilateral mastectomy can result in implant malposition and poor aesthetic results (Fig. 68.2). In Fig. 68.2, this thin patient presented with implant malposition and poor aesthetics despite submuscular placement. A series of Alloderm grafts were placed around the periphery for capsular reinforcement and to smooth the transitions from the chest wall into the breast mound. This patient has been followed for more than 4 years with stable results.

A graft after 6 months becomes well-incorporated into the capsule, with no apparent loss of volume (Fig. 68.3).

68.4
Complications

There have been two cases in which the graft did not take. One of these was an attempt to shore up the implant position in a patient with severe chest wall asymmetry and pectus excavatum; the graft spanned across a tissue gap where it did not have a surface of healthy tissue for support. In both of these cases of non-take, the material had disintegrated and appeared to liquefy, and it could have been mistaken for an abscess. However, cultures were negative, and there were no systemic indications of infection in either case, so graft non-take appears to be a benign condition. There have been no cases of capsular contracture or infection following intracapsular Alloderm grafting.

When the thicker grafts (ultrathick) became available, they were tried in two cases in which maximal correction was indicated. These relatively unyielding grafts initially appeared to worsen rippling, although in both instances this condition self-corrected after several months.

68.5
Discussion

Breast implant–tissue interaction is a dynamic and ongoing process. Regardless of the care with which implant dimensions are optimized relative to the soft-tissue envelope, periprosthetic atrophy may develop. Intracapsular Alloderm grafting provides one option for capsular reinforcement. Clinical experience confirms graft longevity, and histologic evaluation at 6 months shows vascular ingrowth and active fibroblasts without inflammatory markers [4]. As long as there is one surface of healthy tissue apposing the graft, graft take is reliable. The author has not used the grafts with primary augmentation, but in cases of reconstruction with implants, the material can be used to cover the areas where muscle is inadequate or unavailable.

68.6
Conclusions

Intracapsular Alloderm grafting provides a versatile option for capsular reinforcement in cases of periprosthetic atrophy. Although it is not especially challenging technically, precise planning and execution are required for optimal results. The grafts are long-lasting and appear to pose minimal risk.

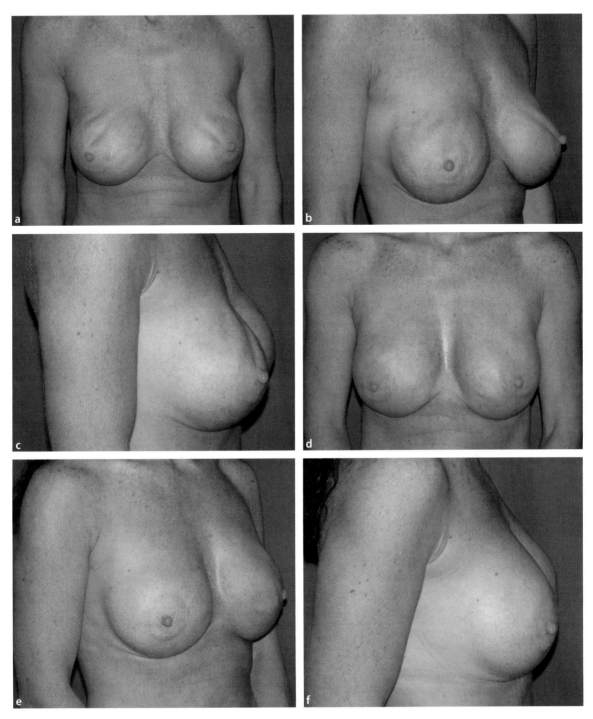

Fig. 68.1 a–c The patient had severe rippling with smooth round subpectoral implants and recurrent bottoming out after two attempts at correction with capsulorrhaphy. **d–f** Six months after repeat capsulorrhaphy, reinforced with 4×7-cm Alloderm grafts inferolaterally and superomedially. Although some rippling is still apparent, her condition is much improved

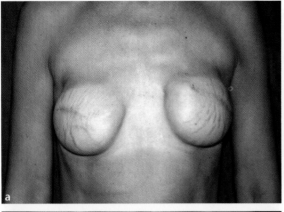

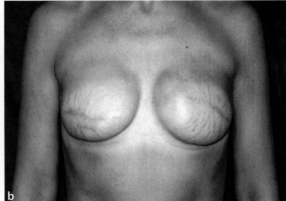

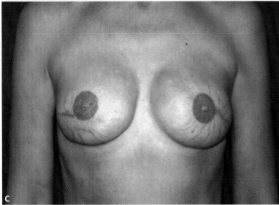

Fig. 68.2 a This thin patient had implant malposition and poor aesthetics despite submuscular placement after reconstruction. **b** Following a series of Alloderm grafts placed around the periphery for capsular reinforcement and to smooth the transitions from the chest wall into the breast mound, with stable results. **c** Four years postoperatively after nipple–areola replacement

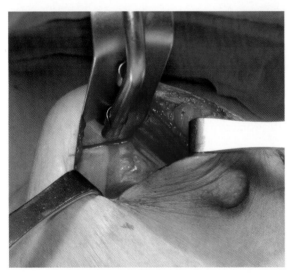

Fig. 68.3 A graft after 6 months becomes well incorporated into the capsule, with no apparent loss of volume

References

1. Baxter R: Indications and practical applications for high-profile saline implants. Aesthetic Surg J 2004;24(1):24–27
2. Tebbetts JB: Breast implant selection based upon patient tissue characteristics and dynamics: the TEPID system. Plast Reconstr Surg 2002;109(4):1396–1409
3. Adams WP, Rios JL, Smith SJ: Enhancing patient outcomes in aesthetic and reconstructive breast surgery using triple antibiotic breast irrigation: six-year prospective clinical study. Plast Reconstr Surg 2006;117(1):30–36
4. Baxter R: Intracapsular allogenic dermal grafts for breast implant-related problems. Plast Reconstr Surg 2003;112(6):1692–1696
5. Dowden DI: Correction of implant rippling using allograft dermis. Aesthetic Surg J 2001;21:81–84
6. Breuing KH, Warren SM: Immediate bilateral breast reconstruction with implants and inferolateral Alloderm slings. Ann Plast Surg 2005;55(3):232–239
7. Gamboa-Bobadilla GM: Implant breast reconstruction using acellular dermal matrix. Ann Plast Surg 2006;56(1):22–25

Chapter 69

Submammary Flap for Correction of Severe Sequelae from Augmentation Mammaplasty

69

José Juri, Maria Fernanda Valotta, Susana Létiz

69.1
Introduction

Augmentation mammaplasty is a simple procedure that needs to be performed by an experienced plastic surgeon. This is because, as with almost all surgical procedures, the ability to manage complications requires experience and expertise. Infection, the most feared complication, must be solved quickly. The surgeon must be aware of the onset of symptoms such as fever, abnormal swelling, erythema, local pain and tenderness, and increased warmth of the implanted breasts. In this difficult situation, the decision to surgically remove the implant is mandatory, together with culture of the liquid present in the cavity, profuse irrigation with saline and antibiotic solutions, and empiric systemic antibiotic treatment until culture results are obtained. If these measures are taken, after a period of 6 months to allow the inflammation to subside and the tissues to soften, a new implant can be inserted without compromising the final aesthetic result [1, 2].

Our experience in solving permanent disfigurement of breast tissue is based in patients with a history of a 6–8-month attempt to salvage the infected implant with measures such as dressings of the exposed implant together with prolonged antibiotic treatment, with the usual appearance of side effects. Prolonged infection leads to total atrophy of fat and glandular tissue and permanent loss of skin, especially in the lower pole of the breast, because of the force of gravity. The final result of this process, after late removal or spontaneous extrusion of the implant, is severe deformity with scar retractions.

These emotionally distressed patients are very difficult to treat. They chose an elective aesthetic procedure to enhance their body image and ended up with severe disfigurement. After several months of carrying an open and painful secreting wound, with dressing changes several times a day and expensive and prolonged antibiotic treatment, their level of compliance is low. The surgeon has to offer these patients a simple solution with the best aesthetic results, with minimal or inconspicuous donor site scars.

Because it is a local flap, the submammary flap provides tissue that equals breast tissue regarding skin texture and color match. The donor site scar is located at the level of the inframammary fold. Being an axial flap, medially or laterally based, vitality is guaranteed. No undermining is needed for closure of the donor site, minimizing complications. For this reasons, the submammary flap is our procedure of choice for treating severe sequelae from augmentation mammaplasty.

69.2
Historical Background

The first description of the use of the hypogastric region for mammary reconstruction dates back to 1959 when Pierer [3] described a laterally based transverse epigastric flap located at the projection of the midclavicular line in the submammary region, with the tip of the flap crossing the midline. Closure of the donor site was achieved primarily. Chardot and Carolus in 1961 [4] were the first to describe a medially based pedicled flap in this region. In 1972 Bohmert [5] described the use of a "triangular rotation flap" that was based medially, to add tissue to a mastectomy site. Closure of the donor site was achieved by extensive undermining of the abdominal wall. In 1974 Tai and Hasegawa [6] described a large abdominal flap that needed skin grafting to achieve closure of the donor site. They used it for reconstruction of large chest wall defects created by extensive resection of recurrent breast cancer. Whereas Bohmert's flaps were 14 cm in width and 16 cm in length, the flaps described by Tai and Hasegawa were much larger and reached the posterior axillary line. Vascularization of the flap is compared with the deltopectoral flap described by Bakamjian et al. [7]. Vessels of the medially based flaps were well described by Bohmert in 1979 [8]. A cadaver study was performed along with selective preoperative and postoperative angiography in patients. An

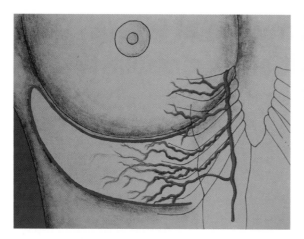

Fig. 69.1 Cutaneous perforators of the internal mammary and superior epigastric artery emerge at the level of the lateral border of the rectus muscle to provide vascular supply of the medially based flap. This is why the base of the flap is designed at this level

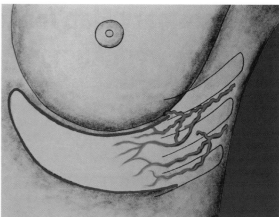

Fig. 69.2 The intercostal perforators are responsible for vascularization of the laterally based flap. They emerge at the level of the midaxillary line

axial pattern was found by means of the lateral branch of the superior epigastric artery and three to four muscular perforators emerging at the lateral border of the rectus muscle. Bohmert described the axial territory as extending to the midaxillary line. Since then, this flap has been used extensively for mammary reconstruction [9, 10]. In 2004, Juri et al. [11] were the first to describe the use of a submammary flap to correct severe sequelae from augmentation mammaplasty. This publication collected 24 years of experience with this flap, as the first procedure performed dates back to 1980.

69.3
Anatomic Considerations

A considerable amount of loose skin and subcutaneous fat is usually present below the submammary fold and can be used for reconstructive purposes. The flap is designed horizontally in this region. It can be medially or laterally pedicled, depending on the location of the defect. When medially based, the perforating branches of the epigastric artery or the distal part of the internal mammary artery, well described by Mathes and Nahai [12], supply the flap (Fig. 69.1). The number of branches included in the flap can range from one to six, depending on the width of the pedicle. When laterally based, the intercostal perforators emerging at the level of the anterior axillary line are responsible for the axial pattern of the flap (Fig. 69.2) [13]. This area is described as number 15 on Manchot's map of cutaneous perforators (Fig. 69.3). Manchot, when he was still in medical school, created an outstanding work by mapping the

dorsal and ventral sides of the entire body, excluding the face, describing in detail all areas of the skin nourished by cutaneous perforators. Following this map's guidelines, surgeons were able to design flaps throughout the entire body [14].

69.4
Timing of the Operation

When a patient with active infection with or without exposure of the implant comes for consultation, we surgically remove the device, using profuse irrigation of the

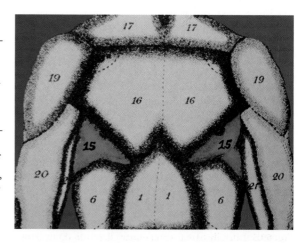

Fig. 69.3 The area labeled as *15* on Manchot's map corresponds to the area of the laterally based flap, nourished by the intercostal perforators

cavity, culture, and antibiotic treatment. Exposure occurs mainly in the inferior pole but can also be seen in the medial quadrant. After this primary approach, we wait for clinical remission of the infection (2–3 months) to address the extent and type of missing tissue (skin and/or glandular tissue) and decide whether a flap is required. The dimensions of the flap are determined according to the reconstructive needs.

69.5
Step-by-Step Surgical Technique

69.5.1
Flap Design

The first issue to be addressed is the choice of pedicle. This depends on the location of the missing tissue. In most instances, the medial pedicle is used. The superior border of the flap is designed slightly higher than the inframammary fold. The inferior border is placed 4–7 cm from the upper border, depending on tissue requirements, measured at the base of the flap. This line narrows gradually as it reaches the tip of the flap that can go as far as the end of the fold.

69.5.2
Flap Harvest

All subcutaneous tissue is included in the flap. The undermining starts at the tip of the flap. If the pedicle is medial, the undermining reaches the lateral border of

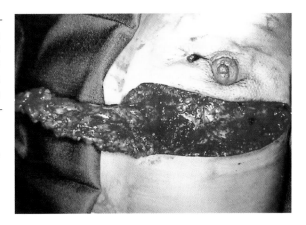

Fig. 69.4 Dissection of the flap starts from the tip and includes all subcutaneous tissue. The aponeurosis is left intact. In the medially based flap, as shown, dissection stops at the lateral border of the rectus muscle

the rectus muscle (Fig. 69.4). If it is laterally based, the dissection stops at the anterior axillary line (Fig. 69.5).

69.5.3
Preparation of the Recipient Site

A subglandular pocket is created to allow for insertion of the flap. In cases of full-thickness tissue loss, cicatricial retractions are removed, and the missing skin is provided by the flap.

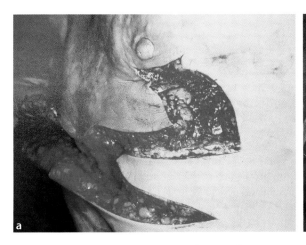

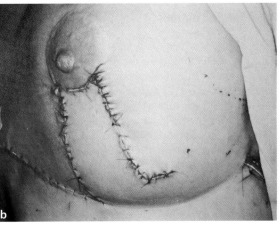

Fig. 69.5 Laterally based submammary flap. **a** In this patient a cicatricial retraction has been resected in the lower pole of the breast. The base of the flap can be situated between the center of the submammary fold and the anterior axillary line, depending on the location of the defect to be reconstructed. **b** The flap is transposed, and the donor site is sutured first. A small back-cut at the base of the flap corrects the dog-ear deformity resulting from flap transposition

69.5.4
Donor Site Closure

In almost all cases the donor site can be closed with no undermining. This can be done because a great amount of laxity is present at this level. In this way, complications such as hematoma and seroma formation are avoided. The resulting scar is inconspicuous and hidden by the inframammary fold.

69.5.5
Flap Transposition

Usually the proximal portion of the flap replaces missing skin and soft tissue. The tip of the flap is undermined and buried beneath the areola, since some degree of areolar retraction is almost always present (Fig. 69.6). The tip of the flap is sutured to the remaining glandular tissue (Figs. 69.7, 69.8). The flap is not fixed to the thoracic wall. When no skin is needed, the flap can be fully deepithelialized and used as tissue bulk only.

In some cases an island flap can be designed, according to tissue requirements (Fig. 69.9).

69.5.6
Implant Placement

When needed, after a minimum of 6 months to allow for tissue softening and scar maturation, a mammary implant with a textured surface can be inserted with no additional risks.

69.6
Other Surgical Options

Other methods widely used for mammary reconstruction are the latissimus dorsi flap [15, 16], the transverse rectus abdominis musculocutaneous flap described in 1982 by Gandolfo [17] and Hartrampf et al. [18], and microsurgical flaps such as the deep inferior epigastric perforator flap [19]. However, these operations are major procedures and must be avoided as much as possible in this group of patients. The disadvantages of the dorsal flap are the resulting scar in the donor site and the different color and skin texture, resulting in a notorious "patch defect." It could be useful in selected patients with undernourishment and large defects in whom tissue would be insufficient for the submammary flap.

The transverse rectus abdominis musculocutaneous flap has no indication in this situation because if infraumbilical redundancy exists, it is present in the submammary region as well. The only time this flap

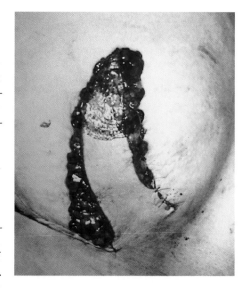

Fig. 69.6 Medially based flap. The tip of the flap is deepithelialized and used to add tissue bulk beneath the areola. The tip is not fixed to the thoracic wall; instead, it is sutured to the remaining gland

may have some indication is in the presence of damage to both medial and lateral pedicles from scarring. The only advantage this flap has over the submammary flap is that it provides a sufficient amount of tissue, thus avoiding the need for an implant. We believe this advantage does not justify the morbidity of the procedure and the high incidence of abdominal wall complications. Microsurgical flaps such as the deep inferior epigastric perforator flap avoid abdominal wall complications but are not justified in this kind of patient because, even leaving behind the procedure's cost and complexity, these patients simply cannot afford the risk of flap failure.

69.7
Conclusions

It is a well-known plastic surgery principle that the best aesthetic result is obtained by local flaps. These flaps should be the first choice when feasible, for reconstruction of any area of the face and body. This is because no distant tissue equals local tissue regarding skin texture and color match. If we add to this advantage the simplicity of the operation, the minimal donor site morbidity, and the safety of the procedure due to its excellent blood supply (no necrosis has been seen in our experience), the submammary flap becomes the procedure of choice for correcting severe sequelae from augmentation mammaplasty.

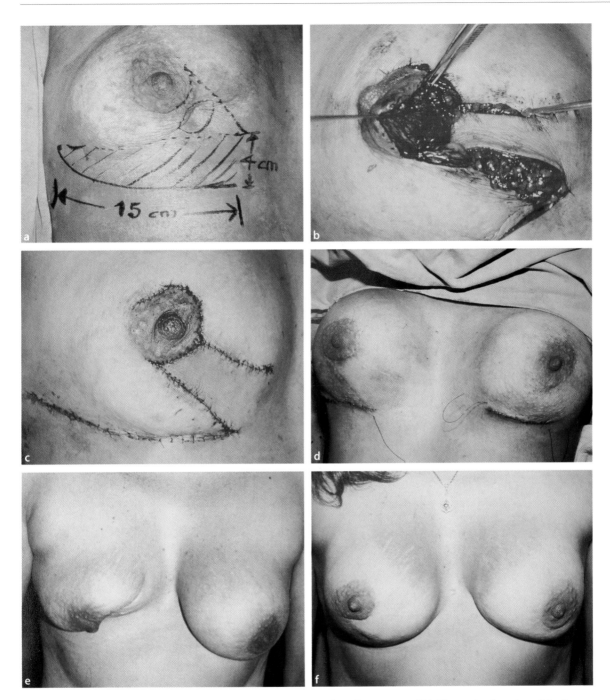

Fig. 69.7 a A medially based flap is designed to correct a cicatricial retraction in a 38- year-old with tissue loss in the inferomedial pole of the breast due to a history of 3-month postoperative infection and spontaneous extrusion of a breast implant. The *diagonal dotted line* indicates the superior level of the tissue to be resected. **b** The tip of the flap is deepithelialized and buried beneath the areola. **c** The donor site is closed and lies hidden in the inframammary fold. The proximal portion of the flap replaces the full-thickness tissue loss. **d** After 6 months, a 220-cc round textured implant is placed. The contralateral implant is replaced at this setting. **e** Preoperative view of the deformed breast. **f** Postoperative view 6 months after placement of the implants. Symmetry was restored, and an excellent result has been achieved

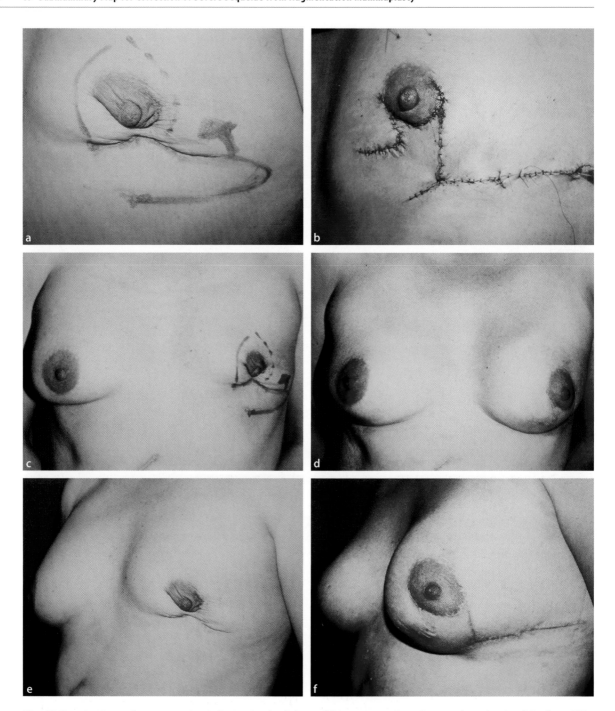

Fig. 69.8 a A 12-month postoperative infection in the left breast in a 35-year-old patient left a significant cicatricial retraction at the lower pole. In this case, the superior border of the flap is marked at the inferior limit of the retraction. **b** Donor site sutured and flap transposed. The tip was deepithelialized to add tissue bulk beneath the areola. **c** Preoperative view. The *dotted line* corresponds to the site where the tip of the flap will be buried. **d** Eight months after the initial procedure and 2 months after placement of a round textured 255-cc silicone implant, with implant replacement in the contralateral side. **e** Preoperative. **f** Postoperative

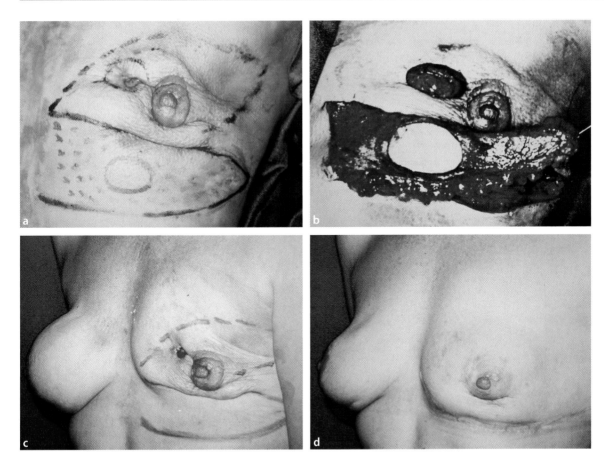

Fig. 69.9 a Severe disfigurement that compromises the whole breast in a 50-year-old patient after 8 months of a suppurative process with exposure of the implant during the previous 3 months. A medially based flap is planned, with an island of skin that will replace the full-thickness defect in the medial pole. The *dots* in the flap represent the area to be deepithelialized. The *dashed line* corresponds to the future position of the flap inside the pocket. **b** The flap has been dissected and deepithelialized, preserving an island flap to replace the full-thickness defect resulting from extrusion of the implant. Notice the adequate tissue bulk provided by this flap. **c** Preoperative. **d** Postoperative at 3 years. This patient required no further augmentation

References

1. Rudolph R: Unfavorable results of augmentation mammaplasty. In: Noone RB (ed). Plastic and Reconstructive Surgery of the Breast. Philadephia, Mosby Year Book 1991
2. Handel N: Managing local implant-related problems. In: Spear SL (ed). Surgery of the Breast: Principles and Art. Philadelphia, Lippincott-Raven 1998
3. Pierer H: Probleme der plastischen Deckung bei Operationen des Mamakarzinoms und Lokalrezidiven. Klin Med Osterr Z Wiss Prakt Med 1959;14:598–604
4. Chardot C, Carolus JM: La prévention des infections ou la prophylaxie du ¨gros bras¨ dans le traitement du cancer du sein. Ann Chir Plast 1961;6:195–202
5. Bohmert H: Personal method for reconstruction of the female breast following radical mastectomy. Transactions of the Sixth International Congress of Plastic and Reconstructive Surgeons. Paris, Masson 1976, p 542
6. Tai Y, Hasegawa, H: A transverse abdominal flap for reconstruction after radical operations for recurrent breast cancer. Plast Reconstr Surg 1974;53(1):52–54
7. Bakamjian VY, Culf NK, Bales HW: Versatility of the deltopectoral in reconstruction following head and neck cancer surgery. Transactions of the 4th International Congress of Plastic and Reconstructive Surgeons. Amsterdam, Excerpta Medica 1967, p 808
8. Bohmert H: Reconstrucción con el colgajo toracoepigástrico. In: de la Plaza R, da Mata A, Die Goyares D (eds). El Cáncer de Mama y su Reconstrucción. Madrid, Altalena, 1983, pp 175–177

9.   Cronin TD, Upton J, McDonough JM: Reconstruction of the breast after mastectomy. Plast Reconstr Surg 1977;59(1):1–14

10. Bostwick J, Vasconez L, Jurkiewicz MJ: Breast reconstruction after a radical mastectomy. Plast Reconstr Surg 1978;61(5):682–693

11. Juri J, Valotta F, Létiz S: Submammary flap for correction of severe sequelae from augmentation mammaplasty. Plast Reconstr Surg 2004;114(2):567–574

12. Mathes SJ, Nahai F: Clinical Applications for Muscle and Musculocutaneous Flaps. St. Louis, Mosby 1982, p 111

13. Testut L, Latarjet A: Tratado de Anatomía Humana. Barcelona, Salvat 1960, pp 316, 352

14. Manchot C: Die Hauarteterien des Menschlichen Köpers. Leipzig, Verlag von Vogel 1889. Reprinted in Rev Arg Cir Plast 1991;1:67

15. Olivari N: The latissimus flap. Br J Plast Surg 1977;29(2):126–128

16. Muhlbauer W, Olbrisch R: The latissimus dorsi myocutaneous flap for breast reconstruction. Chir Plast 1977;4:27

17. Gandolfo E: Nueva técnica para reconstrucción de mama. Rev Arg Cir Plast 1982;6:54

18. Hartrampf CR, Scheflan M, Black PW: Breast reconstruction with a transverse abdominal island flap. Plast Reconstr Surg 1982;69(2):216–225

19. Allen RJ, Treece P: Deep inferior epigastric perforator flap for breast reconstruction. Ann Plast Surg 1994;32(1):32–38

Idiosyncratic Allergic Reaction: A Rare Complication of Augmentation Mammoplasty

Robert X. Murphy, Jr.

70.1
Introduction

The year 1992 was a landmark year in the history of medical implantable biomaterials in the United States. It was in that year that the U.S. Food and Drug Administration (FDA) placed a moratorium on silicone gel breast prostheses because of questions concerning their safety [1, 2]. These concerns would result in 15 years of unprecedented controversy, a national class-action lawsuit, and ultimately, the financial ruin of one of the leading U.S. manufacturing companies of its day.

To that point in time, silicone enjoyed great success in the medical community. Silicone is the second most abundant element on Earth. Silicone, in combination with oxygen, makes up 75% of the earth's crust. Although the ratio of silicone to carbon is about 250:1 in the earth's crust, it is approximately 1:5,000 in mammals [3]. In both free injectable and device form, silicone was used widely throughout the world. As an implantable biomaterial, silicone was considered a privileged inert substance, the complications of which were heretofore considered limited and acceptable. After all, silicone gel breast prostheses had been used in the United States since 1962 [4]. It was later estimated that the total number of U.S. women with silicone breast implants in 1989 was 815,700, for a prevalence rate of eight per 1,000 women, and by 1992 the estimated prevalence of breast implants had risen to approximately 11–12 per 1000 women [5]. During that 30-year period, the major post-implantation concerns of the surgical community had been capsular contracture, implant failure, and interference with mammography [6–10].

However, by 1991 enough pressure was brought to bear on the FDA by legal, women's rights, and media communities that silicone gel implants were withdrawn from the cosmetic, but not reconstructive, market. The literature was replete with reports of women with conditions ranging from fatigue and myalgias, to systemic autoimmune diseases, to even brain cancer [11–20], which they attributed to their silicone gel implants.

Studies addressing women's satisfaction at the time of this controversy were few. One survey conducted in 1992 queried 174 women who had undergone reconstruction after mastectomy and found that 34% would be "completely unlikely" to have silicone implants again [21]. In that same year, the Surveillance Program of the National Cancer Institute collaborated with the Postmarket Product Management of the FDA to survey women who had reported local or systemic issues after breast implant surgery to the Problem Repository Program of the FDA. Coon and her associates [22] later conducted telephone interviews with a cohort of these women who reported self-perceived problems with their implants as part of this program. They found that a full 99% of these women had heard of problems with silicone gel prostheses, with the main source of their information being television, newspapers, and magazines, but not the physicians, manufacturers, or the FDA [23–25]. Sixty-five percent of those surveyed reported being dissatisfied with their implants. In this report, some of the dissatisfactions in this self-selected cohort of patients were fear, anger, and perceived disability [22].

What is most interesting, however, is that despite the involvement of patients, the plaintiff's bar, the government, and physicians, the issue of simple allergy never arose. Arguably the most ubiquitous reactive response of the human being to all manner of agents—be they airborne, contact, ingested, or injected—allergic reaction was never raised as a significant issue. A single paper cited self-limited acute urticarial reactions to textured breast implants, but it failed to characterize these as true allergic reactions [6].

70.2
Case Reports

In 1995, Kirwan [26], in a letter to the editor in *Plastic and Reconstructive Surgery*, reported his experience with two cases of apparent allergy to silicone breast implants. In one scenario, a 45-year-old woman, who had had augmentation mammoplasty 10 years prior and a first-stage reconstruction of a scar contracture with tissue expander placed 2 months previously, developed a cervical rash. The rash persisted after the expander was removed. The breast implants were exchanged with new gel implants because of rupture of the prostheses several months later. However, the rash did not resolve until the breast implants were removed and the patient underwent bilateral reconstruction using transverse rectus abdominis myocutaneous (TRAM) flaps. The second patient experienced a much stormier course. Five months after silicone gel implant mammoplasty, she developed a rapidly evolving rash of her breasts and axillae. The right implant was removed due to rupture and replaced. The rashes continued, ultimately resulting in angioneurotic edema and anaphylactic shock. Both implants were removed, with complete resolution of the patient's symptoms. Notably, a rash recurred several months later after placement of a silicone Port-a-Cath, requiring removal of that device.

One year later, with my colleagues, I reported a case of an allergic reaction to saline implants with textured shells [27]. Five months after undergoing a one-stage bilateral breast reconstruction using Siltex Becker tissue expander mammary prostheses (Mentor, Santa Barbara, CA, USA), the patient began complaining about a painful, pruritus rash of the scalp, chest, and arms, which did not respond to topical or oral steroids. Examination revealed erythematous papules and pustules on her chest and arms. Cultures did not document any pathologic bacteria. These lesions gradually spread to her neck, chin, and cheeks. A biopsy of these lesions documented perivascular lymphohistiocytic infiltrate consistent with a drug reaction, photodrug reaction, or polymorphous light eruption. In order to document a potential allergic etiology of this condition, representative materials were obtained from the Mentor Corporation. Patch testing was performed using the injection port, as well as the inner and outer aspects of the implant. The patient noted an itching and burning sensation within 15 min. Urticarial plaques developed exclusively under the textured shell patch without any reaction noted at the port or smooth surface of the implant test sites after 30 min. Reluctantly, the patient underwent removal of the textured-shell prostheses and, at her insistence, replacement with smooth-shell saline implants. Her symptoms resolved almost immediately. It was hypothesized that the process of vulcanization of the textured implant shell may have been responsible for her allergic reaction, since textured devices are cured at a higher temperature than smooth wall implants to texture the silicone (Mentor Corporation, personal communication, 1994).

A report of the Implant Awareness Society, published in the *Israel Journal of Occupational Health* in 1999 [28], studied eight breast implant patients who were referred for occupational medicine assessment in 1993 because of respiratory symptoms, rhinorrhea, and pruritus. Although the focus of this study was respiratory and pulmonary symptomatology, patients had some measure of urticaria, characterized as being intermittent to "intolerable pruritus," and rashes. However, in only one case was it documented that the rash and breast pain resolved when the implants were removed.

70.3
Discussion

For the last 25 years, innumerable reports have appeared in the literature either positing or refuting a causative role for silicone breast prostheses in the evolution of a myriad of medical conditions. The questionable uniqueness of silicone breast implants in this phenomenon has always been an issue because silicone polymers are widely used in other implantable biomedical devices, such as shunts, pacemakers, artificial valves, penile implants, chin implants, nasal struts, finger and toe joints, tendon replacement devices, tissue expanders, ear pinna, pectoral and calf muscle implants, intraocular lenses, scleral bands, ophthalmic bands, silicone sheeting for replacement of inguinal and other hernias and dura mater of the brain, antireflux devices, bariatric devices, facial implants, and breast implants [29].

An exhaustive review of the literature failed to reveal any study that was able to definitively link silicone breast prostheses with connective tissue disease [17, 19, 30–44], neurologic disease [36, 45], perinatal problems [46, 47], congenital deformities, lactation of silicone in breast milk [43, 48], breast cancer [49–51], brain cancer [52], or other health issues [33, 53, 54]. The body of scientific literature led the Institute of Medicine to release its landmark 440-page report in 2000, the report summary of which stated that "a review of 17 epidemiological reports of connective tissue disease in women with breast implants was remarkable for the consistency in finding no elevated relative risk or odds ratio for an association of implants with disease" [55].

Other studies have examined the durability of silicone prostheses and the potential role of extracapsular or free silicone as an etiologic agent of disease. Marotta et al. [56] conducted a large cohort meta-analysis of failure data for silicone gel prostheses based on literature reports while also investigating shell and gel properties from explanted silicone gel breast implants. They postulated that implant failure would occur in a time-dependent manner. Brandon et al. [57] noted silicone implants that were intact for 32 years and suggested that shell degradation was not a primary mechanism for implant failure. Assuming this to be true, one would expect a subpopulation of those women with silicone gel prostheses to have free silicone either within or outside the breast capsule. Although a high incidence of self-reported fibromyalgia was noted [19, 20], no conclusive evidence was found to support the hypothesis that silicone contributed in any way to any disease state [35, 36, 58–61].

Of course, if true allergic reactions to silicone breast implants were a significant issue, one would expect that one's immune system and the classic antigen–antibody reaction would play a significant role. Studies from around the world have investigated this phenomenon without defining a cause-and-effect relationship.

Studies in Denmark examined two different facets of the antibody issue and its potential role in the silicone breast implant controversy. First, the Danes developed a new assay to evaluate antipolymer antibody (APA) levels in women with silicone breast implants [62]. Their study concluded that women with silicone breast implants did not have higher levels of APAs than women without silicone breast implants. They used this assay to compare silicate antibody levels in women with and without silicone breast implants and to correlate this information with those who carried the diagnosis of "muscular rheumatism." The authors determined that there was absolutely no correlation between silicate antibody levels and symptom severity scores [62].

The British literature contains a report based on four matched cohorts of 20 women each: those with silicone breast implants, those without silicone breast implants, those with documented seropositive autoimmune disease, and anonymous controls. These authors were not able to demonstrate a significant difference in antibody levels between silicone breast implant patients and women without silicone breast implants, but they did document a statistically significant difference in levels of patients with silicone breast implants and those without silicone breast implants but with autoimmune disease [63].

Numerous studies on this topic also appeared in the U.S. literature. Holmich and colleagues [59] identified a random population of 271 patients with silicone breast implants and obtained baseline magnetic resonance imaging (MRI) scans. Two years later, a cohort of these women who had not undergone explantation of their silicone breast implants were again evaluated by MRI. This identified a subset of 64 women who had untreated, confirmed ruptures of their silicone breast implants. Among other variables, comparisons were made for differences in serum values of antinuclear antibodies, rheumatoid factor, and cardiolipin antibodies immunoglobulin G and immunoglobulin M. Interestingly, there was no increase in levels of autoantibodies during the study period in either of the groups of those with intact or ruptured implants [60].

Finally, in a study appearing in the *Journal of Rheumatology* [64], serological testing was performed on 298 women with silicone breast implants, 298 women without silicone breast implants, and 52 diabetic patients who had presumed silicone exposure due to needles. In 14 of 16 serologic tests, there was no statistically significant difference among the three groups. A difference was detected between implanted patients and those without silicone breast implants, with small decreased levels of C_3 and C_4 in those patients with silicone breast implants. These results seemed to indicate that there was little evidence of immune system activation in breast implant patients.

70.4 Conclusion

The human immune system is a very highly refined mechanism of defense. Although charged with mounting an antibody response to any unrecognized antigen threat, it must also possess enough checks and balances to not cause unwarranted host-versus-host reactions. Silicone exists naturally in all mammals. An exhaustive search of the literature seems to indicate that silicone, as it exists in the current forms of implantable biomedical devices including breast implants, is an immunologically privileged and inert material. It remains incumbent for the medical practitioner, however, to consider an idiosyncratic reaction as a diagnosis of exclusion in a differential diagnosis for an individual with a history of a bioimplantable device and an unusual allergic response beginning after device implantation. Appropriate confirmatory evaluation, including patch testing, is recommended. If this diagnosis is supported, explantation of the device is curative.

References

1. Dunn KW, Hall PN, Khoo GTK: Breast implant materials: sense and safety. Br J Plast Surg 1992;45(4):315–321
2. Brody GS, Conway DP, Deapen DM, Fisher JCU, Hochberg MC, LeRoy EC, Medsger TA Jr, Robson MC, Shons AR, Weisman MH: Consensus statement on the relationship of breast implants to connective tissue disorders. Plast Reconstr Surg 1992;90(6):1102–1105
3. WGBH Educational Foundation. Silicone: a brief history. www.pbs.org/wgbh/pages/frontline/implants/corp/history.html

4. Freeman BS: Subcutaneous mastectomy for benign breast lesions with immediate or delayed prosthetic replacement. Plast Reconstr Surg 1962;30:676–682

5. Cook RR, Delongchamp RR, Woodbury M, Perkins LL, Harrison MC: The prevalence of women with breast implants in the United States—1989. J Clin Epidemiol 1996;48:519–525

6. Burkhardt BR: Capsular contracture: hard breasts, soft data. Clin Plast Surg 1988;15(4):521–532

7. U.S. Food and Drug Administration. Important information on breast implants. Washington, DC, U.S. Government Printing Office 1991. DHHS publication no. BG91-6.1

8. Goldberg EP, Widenhouse C, Marotta J, Martin P: Failure of silicone gel breast implants: analysis of literature data for 1652 explanted prostheses. Plast Reconstr Surg 1997;100(1):281–284

9. Hovi SL, Hemminki E, Swan SH: Cosmetic and postmastectomy breast implants: Finnish women's experiences. J Womens Health Gend Based Med 1999;8:933–939

10. Marotta JS, Widenhouse CW, Habal MB, Goldberg EP: Silicone gel breast implant failure and frequency of additional surgeries: analysis of 35 studies reporting examination of more than 8,000 explants. J Biomed Mater Res 1999;48(3):354–364

11. Varga J, Schumacher R, Jimenez SA: Systemic sclerosis after augmentation mammoplasty with silicone implants. Ann Intern Med 1987;111(5):377–383

12. Spiera H: Scleroderma after silicone augmentation mammoplasty. J Amer Med Assoc 1988;260(2):236–238

13. Brozena SJ, Fenske NA, Cruse CW, Espinoza CG, Vasey FB, Germain BF, Espinoza LR: Human adjuvant disease following augmentation mammoplasty. Arch Dermatol 1988;124(9):1383–1386

14. Hirmand H, Latrenta GS, Hoffman LA: Autoimmune disease and silicone breast implants. Oncology 1993;7(7):17–24; discussion 24, 28, 30

15. Weiner SR, Pauley HE: Chronic arthropathy occurring after augmentation mammoplasty. Plast Reconstr Surg 1986;77(2):185–192

16. Slavin SA, Goldwyn RM: Silicone gel implant explantation: reasons, results and admonitions. Plast Reconstr Surg 1995;95(1):63–69

17. Bridges AJ: Rheumatic disorders in patients with silicone implants: a critical review. J Biomater Sci Polym Ed 1995;7(2):147–157

18. Brinton LA, Lubin JH, Burich MC, Colton T, Hoover RN: Mortality among augmentation mammoplasty patients. Epidemiology 2001;12(3):321–326

19. Brown SL, Duggirala HJ, Pennello G: An association of silicone-gel breast implant rupture and fibromyalgia. Curr Rheumatol Rep 2002;4(4):293–298

20. Brown SL, Pennello G, Berg WA, Soo MS, Middleton MS: Silicone gel breast implant rupture, extracapsular silicone, and health status in a population of women. J Rheumatol 2001;28(5):996–1003

21. Winer EP, Fee-Fulkerson K, Fulkerson CC, Georgiade G, Catoe KE, Conaway M, Brunatti C, Holmes V, Rimer BK: Silicone controversy: a survey of women with breast cancer and silicone implants. J Natl Cancer Inst 1993;85(5):1407–1411

22. Coon SK, Burris R, Coleman EA, Lemon SJ: An analysis of telephone interview data collected in 1992 from 820 women who reported problems with their breast implants to the Food and Drug Administration. Plast Reconstr Surg 2002;109(6):2043–2051

23. Burke W, Olsen AJ, Pinsky LE, Reynolds SE, Press NA: Misleading presentation of breast cancer in popular magazines. Eff Clin Pract 2001;4(2):58–64

24. Kahn C: How the media influences women's perceptions of health care. Mark Health Serv 2001;21(1):12–17

25. Dobias KS, Moyer CA, McAchran SE, Katz SJ, Sonnad SS: Mammography messages in popular media: implications for patient expectations and shared clinical decision-making. Health Expect 2001;4(2):127–135

26. Kirwan L: Two cases of apparent silicone allergy. Plast Reconstr Surg 1995;96(1):236–237

27. Sabbagh WH, Murphy RX Jr, Kucirka SJ, Okunski WJ: Idiosyncratic allergic reaction to textured saline implants. Plast Reconstr Surg 1996;97(4):820–823

28. Harbut MR, Churchill BC: Asthma in patients with silicone breast implants. Report of a case series and identification of hexachloroplatinate contaminant as a possible etiologic agent. Israel J Occup Health 1999;3:73–82

29. Arepalli SR, Bezabeh S, Brown SL: Allergic reaction to platinum in silicone breast implants. J Long Term Eff Med Implants 2002;12:299–306

30. Bar-Meir E, Eherenfeld M, Shoenfeld Y: Silicone gel breast implants and connective tissue disease—a comprehensive review. Autoimmunity 2003;36(4):193–197

31. Blackburn WD Jr, Everson MP: Silicone-associated rheumatic disease: an unsupported myth. Plast Reconstr Surg 1997;99(5):1362–1367

32. Blackburn WD Jr, Grotting JC, Everson MP: Lack of evidence of systemic inflammatory rheumatic disorders in symptomatic women with breast implants. Plast Reconstr Surg 1997;99(4):1054–1060

33. Brinton LA, Buckley LM, Dvorkinam O, Lubin JH, Colton T, Murray MC, Hoover R: Risk of connective tissue disorders among breast implant patients. Am J Epidemiol 2004;160(7):619–627

34. Brown SL: Epidemiology of silicone-gel breast implants. Epidemiology 2002;13(3):S34–S39

35. Duffy MJ, Woods JE: Health risks of failed silicone gel breast implants: a 30-year clinical experience. Plast Reconstr Surg 1994;94(2):295–299

36. Englert H, Joyner E, McGill N, Chambers P, Horner D, Hunt C, Makaroff J, O'Connor H, Russel N, March L: Women's health after plastic surgery. Intern Med J 2001;31(2):77–89

37. Friis S, Mellemkjaer L, McLaughlin JK, Breiting V, Kjaer SK, Blot W, Olsen JH: Connective tissue disease and other rheumatic conditions following breast implants in Denmark. Ann Plast Surg 1997;39(1):1–8

38. Gabriel SE, O'Fallon WM, Kurland LT, Beard CM, Woods JE, Melton LJ III: Risk of connective-tissue diseases and other disorders after breast implantation. N Engl J Med 1994;330(24):1697–1702

39. Janowsky EC, Kupper LL, Hulka BS: Meta-analysis of the relation between silicone breast implants and the risk of connective-tissue diseases. N Engl J Med 2000;342(11):781–790

40. Jensen B, Bliddal H, Kjoller K, Wittrup H, Friis S, Hoier-Madsen M, Rogind H, McLaughlin JK, Lipworth L, Danneskiold-Samsoe B, Olsen JH: Rheumatic manifestations in Danish women with silicone breast implants. Clin Rheumatol 2001;20(5):345–352

41. Lipworth L, Tarone RE, McLaughlin JK: Breast implants and fibromyalgia: a review of the epidemiologic evidence. Ann Plast Surg 2004;52(3):284–287

42. Sanchez-Guerrero J, Colditz GA, Hunter DJ, Speizer FE, Liang MH: Silicone breast implants and the risk of connective-tissue diseases and symptoms. N Engl J Med 1995;332(25):1666–1670

43. Semple JL, Lugowski S, Baines CJ, Smith DC, McHugh A: Breast milk contamination and silicone implants: preliminary results using silicone as a proxy measurement for silicone. Plast Reconstr Surg 1998;102(2):528–533

44. Tugwell P, Wells G, Peterson J, Welch V, Page J, Davison C, McGowan J, Ramroth D, Shea B: Do silicone breast implants cause rheumatologic disorders? A systematic review for a court-appointed national science panel. Arthritis Rheum 2001;44(11):2477–2484

45. Winther JF, Friis S, Bach FW, Mellemkjaer L, Kjoller K, McLaughlin JK, Lipworth L, Blot WJ, Olsen JH: Neurological disease among women with silicone breast implants in Denmark. Acta Neurol Scand 2001;103(2):93–96

46. Hemminki E, Hovi SL, Sevon T, Asko-Seljavaara S: Births and perinatal health of infants among women who have had silicone breast implantation in Finland, 1967–2000. Acta Obstet Gynecol Scand 2004;83(12):1135–1140

47. Signorello LB, Fryzek JP, Blot WJ, McLaughlin JK, Nyren O: Offspring health risk after cosmetic breast implantation in Sweden. Ann Plast Surg 2001;46(3):279–286

48. Kjoller K, Friis S, Signorello LB, McLaughlin JK, Blot WJ, Lipworth L, Henriksen TF, Jorgensen S, Bittmann S, Olsen JH: Health outcomes in offspring of Danish mothers with cosmetic breast implants. Ann Plast Surg 2002;48(3):238–245

49. Brinton LA, Lubin JH, Burich MC, Colton T, Brown SL, Hoover RN: Breast cancer following augmentation mammoplasty (United States). Cancer Causes Control 2000;11(9):819–827

50. National Institutes of Health. Breast implants: status of research at the National Institutes of Health, amended report, 24 March 2005. http://orwh.od.nih.gov/pubs/rev305breastimplantsreport.pdf

51. Strom SS, Baldwin BJ, Sigurdson AJ, Schusterman MA: Cosmetic saline breast implants: a survey of satisfaction, breastfeeding experience, cancer screening, and health. Plast Reconstr Surg 1997;100(6):1553–1557

52. McLaughlin JK, Lipworth L: Brain cancer and cosmetic breast implants: a review of the epidemiologic evidence. Ann Plast Surg 2004;52(2):115–117

53. Kjoller K, Holmich LR, Fryzek JP, Jacobsen PH, Friis S, McLaughlin JK, Lipworth, L, Henriksen TF, Hoier-Madsen M, Wiik A, Olsen JH: Self-reported musculoskeletal symptoms among Danish women with cosmetic breast implants. Ann Plast Surg 2004;52(1):1–7

54. Breiting VB, Holmich LR, Brandt B, Fryzek JP, Wolthers MS, Kjoller K, McLaughlin JK, Wiik A, Friis S: Long-term health status of Danish women with silicone breast implants. Plast Reconstr Surg 2004;114(1):217–226; discussion 227–228

55. Bondurant S, Ernster V, Herdman R (eds): Safety of Silicone Breast Implants. Washington, DC, Institute of Medicine, National Academy Press 2000

56. Marotta JS, Goldberg EP, Habal MB, Amery DP, Martin PJ, Urbaniak DJ, Widenhouse CW: Silicone gel breast implant failure: evaluation of properties of shells and gels for explanted prostheses and meta-analysis of literature rupture data. Ann Plast Surg 2002;49(3):227–242; discussion 242–247

57. Brandon HJ, Jerina KL, Wolf CJ, Young VL: Biodurability of retrieved silicone gel breast implants. Plast Reconstr Surg 2003;111(7):2295–2306

58. Austad ED: Breast implant-related silicone granulomas: the literature and litigation. Plast Reconstr Surg 2002;109 (5):1724–1730; discussion 1731–1732

59. Holmich LR, Kjoller K, Fryzek JP, Hoier-Madsen M, Vejborg I, Conrad C, Sletting S, McLaughlin JK, Breiting V, Friis S: Self-reported diseases and symptoms by rupture status among unselected Danish women with cosmetic silicone breast implants. Plast Reconstr Surg 2003; 111(2):723–732; discussion 733–734

60. Holmich LR, Vejborg IM, Conrad C, Sletting S, Hoier-Madsen M, Fryzek JP, McLaughlin JK, Kjoller K, Wiik A, Friis S: Untreated silicone breast implant rupture. Plast Reconstr Surg 2004;114(1):204–214; discussion 215–216

61. Noone RB: A review of the possible health implications of silicone breast implants. Cancer 1997;79(9):1747–1756

62. Jensen B, Wittrup IH, Wiik A, Friis S, Bliddal H, Thomsen B, McLaughlin JK, Danniskiold-Samsoe B, Olsen JH: Antipolymer antibodies in Danish women with silicone breast implants. J Long Term Eff Med Implants 2004;14:14(2):73–80

63. Oliver D, Walker MS, Walters AE, Chatrath P, Lamberty BG: Anti-silicone antibodies and silicone containing breast implants. Br J Plast Surg 2000;53(5):410–414

64. Karlson EW, Lee IM, Cook NR, Buring JE, Hennekens CH, Bloch KJ: Serologic evaluations of women exposed to breast implants. J Rheumatol 2001;28(7):1523–1530vv

Chapter 71

Complications of Silicone Gel Implants

71

Antonino Araco

71.1
Introduction

There are many risks and complications of using breast implants for breast augmentation. Some of these risks are specifically related to silicone gel implants.

71.2
Seroma

Seroma is the excessive accumulation of clear or blood-stained fluid in the periprosthetic space during the early postoperative period (Fig. 71.1). The overall incidence is about 1%. Its cause is unknown. There is no difference in incidence of seroma with implant position or surgical access, and smoking does not seem to be associated with the condition. The hypothesis is that some unknown microbiological agent or immunological factor overstimulates the inflammation process. This result is overproduction of fluid that accumulates in the closed periprosthetic space. No specific pathogens or immunological agents that correlate with the condition have been found in the serum. The rationale of a postoperative surgical drain is to keep the periprosthetic space dry, but so far no scientific evidence indicates that use of a drain may reduce the risk of seroma. A recent meta-analysis of 51 randomized controlled trials reported no risk factor for seroma formation in breast surgery [1], but there is a moderate evidence to support the risk in individuals with heavier body weight and greater drainage volume in the initial 3 postoperative days.

Generally, one breast or, rarely, both breasts become significantly more swollen than expected. The patient does not complain of pain as long as the swelling does not increase, and it can remain untreated. Tenderness may be present, but the skin is not ecchymotic. Clear blood-stained fluid may leak from the surgical wound. Bacteriological swab is generally negative.

On physical examination a fluid wave may be elicited. Diagnosis can be confirmed by ultrasonography. Treatment depends on the entity of the seroma: If moderate swelling is present and the discomfort is mild, the treatment is conservative and consists of rest and avoiding movement of the upper extremity on the affected

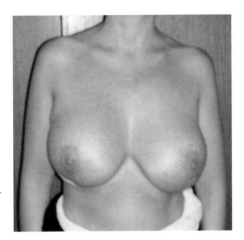

Fig. 71.1 Seroma of the right breast 6 days postoperative

side. A surgical bandage must remain in place day and night for at least 1 week; this will ease reabsorption of the fluid. The seroma will usually resolve within a few weeks.

If the swelling is severe, the patient complains of pain, or conservative treatment has not been effective, the surgical option is favored. This consists of opening the wound, irrigating the pocket, replacing the implant, and leaving a drain for at least 24 h. A surgical bandage and immobilization are mandatory. In very rare cases of recurrent seroma, it may be necessary to explant the implant and wait a reasonable period of time, after which the implant can be replaced, possibly in a different position such as submuscular pocket for previous subglandular or vice versa. There is no scientific evidence that seroma increases the risk of infection, delayed contracture, or other complications. Breast asymmetry may result from a seroma if it is not treated properly.

71.3
Hematoma

Hematoma after breast augmentation has a reported frequency in the range of 1–2% (Fig. 71.2) [2, 3]. Cigarette smoking, medications such as aspirin and antico-

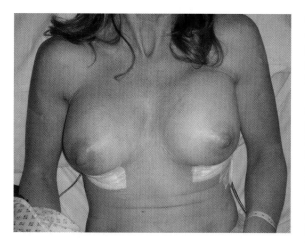

Fig. 71.2 Hematoma of the left breast 12 h postoperative

the pocket and drain the hematoma. In the majority of cases, a point of bleeding is not identified. Accurate hemostasis is necessary. The pocket is irrigated with normal saline, and the implant is replaced. A surgical drain is recommended to keep the implant pocket dry.

When blood remains in the periprosthetic space, it may be a field for pathogens to start an infection. It is proven that infection is an increased risk after hematoma, so antibiotic coverage is recommended. The inflammatory reaction may be overreactive, becoming a chronic condition leading to scarring; this may be the basis for later capsular contraction. Retrospective studies have demonstrated that hematoma is a risk factor for delayed capsular contracture, even though these studies must be confirmed in prospective randomized trials [4, 5].

agulants, and some food products such as mushrooms must be discontinued for 4 weeks before and 4 weeks after the operation. To the best of our knowledge, no study has reported a statistically different incidence of bleeding rate associated with implant position (subglandular, subfascial, or submuscular), the use of drains, or the surgical access site. Generally there is a slightly higher risk of bleeding when a submuscular pocket is prepared. This may be due to incising of the pectoralis major muscle and disconnection from the ribs, or it may occur when drains are not used, as is common practice of many surgeons for the subglandular and subfascial positions. Typical hematoma is characterized by swelling of the affected breast, pain, tenderness, and ecchymosis. The breast is hard and painful when palpated.

Treatment depends on the severity of the hematoma. When minimal swelling and pain are present, conservative treatment may be initiated. This consists of observation, immobilization of the affected upper limb, and surgical bandaging. If a drain is present, it becomes easier to monitor the evolution of the bleeding and the effectiveness of the conservative treatment. If a drain is not present, physical evaluation must guide any further action. If the patient's condition remains stable and the severity of the bleeding does not progress, the swelling will eventually go down within days or weeks. Antibiotic therapy is advisable to prevent infection. Many surgeons do not favor the conservative approach because of the evidence of increased risk of infection, delayed seroma, and capsular contracture [4].

When a significant accumulation of blood produces moderate to severe swelling, mild to severe pain, or whenever the patient's clinical condition worsens after conservative treatment, it becomes necessary to explore

71.4
Infection

Infection following breast augmentation is reported in 1–4% of cases in different studies (Fig. 71.3, 71.4) [6, 7]. Many risk factors have been correlated with breast infection. General conditions such as obesity, diabetes, immunodeficiency, and cigarette smoking are associated with an increased risk of infection [8–10]. Randomized studies have not reported a statistically different incidence of breast infection for different incision locations (inframammary, periareolar, or axillary), implant characteristics (smooth versus textured or saline versus silicone), position of the implants (submammary or submuscular), or drain use [11, 12]. Preoperative intravenous antibiotic and periprosthetic pocket irrigation using one or more antibiotics are shown to be as-

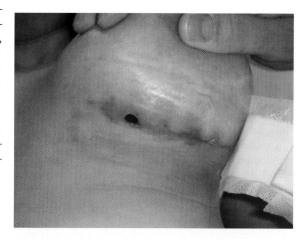

Fig. 71.3 Infection of the left breast 13 days postoperative. Implant exposure

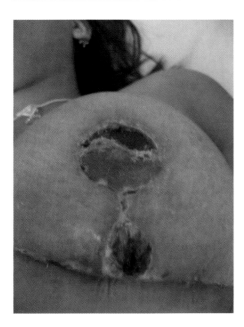

Fig. 71.4 Mastopexy with augmentation 22 days postoperative with infection and necrosis of the left breast, which was treated with intravenous antibiotics for 8 days

sociated with a reduced incidence of infection and capsular contraction [13]. Generally the infection is caused by gram-positive organisms; the most common are *Staphylococcus aureus*, *Staphylococcus epidermidis*, and streptococcus types A and B. Less commonly, enteric bacteria such as *Pseudomonas aeruginosa* or even atypical *Mycobacterium* are the causative agents [14, 15].

Symptoms of infection usually manifest during the first 2 postoperative weeks, but delayed infections may occur months or even years after the operation. The patient complains of tenderness or pain that is moderate to severe. It may also radiate to the shoulder and in severe cases may limit arm movement on the affected side.

Physical examination shows abnormal swelling and erythema. The breast is warm and painful when soft pressure is applied. Sometime pus leaks out of the incision, or an open wound with implant exposure may be present. The axillary lymph nodes may be enlarged and tender, and systemic manifestations such as fever, chills, and elevated leukocyte count are occasionally present. Diagnosis may be confirmed with echography. Wound exudate, when available, must be sent for microbiological culture and sensitivity.

The treatment for breast infection must be immediate. When the infection is localized to the wound, it may present in different grades of severity, from a suture ab-

scess to superficial or deep wound infection. Treatment consists of opening the wound, eventually draining the abscess, irrigating with saline and antibiotic solution, and applying serial surgical dressings. If mild to moderate cellulitis is present, oral antibiotics become necessary and in most cases are effective. Broad-spectrum antibiotics are started when the cellulitis is severe, when oral antibiotics fail, or when the process is more generalized.

If the implant (periprosthetic space) is involved, the best treatment consists of removing the implant, irrigating the breast pocket with normal saline or antibiotic solution, leaving a drain for at least 24 h, and starting systemic antibiotics. Surgical debridement is sometimes required. Efforts to salvage the implant with periprosthetic antibiotic irrigations and systemic antibiotics have proven to be ineffective and dangerous. After a momentary improvement, the symptoms reappear when the treatment is discontinued. This may lead to continuous inflammation and tissue destruction, causing extensive tissue loss and permanent breast deformity.

After a minimal period of 3 months, when the inflammation has subsided and tissues have softened, a new implant can be inserted. Breast asymmetry may result after breast infection because of the thickness of the breast tissue and scars in the periprosthetic pocket. Skin incision at the time of infection from the surgical operation and new skin incisions when the implant is replaced give extra chances of asymmetry. The patient must be informed that breast implant replacement after several weeks may lead to significant breast asymmetry.

71.5
Capsular Contracture

A capsule of scar tissue forms around the implant when an implant is placed either in the subglandular or submuscular pocket (Figs. 71.5–71.7). At first, this membrane is thin, soft, pliable, and has little effect on the contour of the breast. But over the years, the scar undergoes progressive thickening, hardness, and shrinkage that can affect the contour of the breast and produce symptoms such as tenderness or pain. This process is known as capsular contraction [16]. The implant is deformed in spherical configuration, and the breast becomes progressively hard and firm. Capsular contracture affects all breast implants, and it is just a matter of time for the condition to become symptomatic. It is clear that the capsule is scar tissue that is the end result of the inflammatory process. We hypothesize that whenever inflammation is exuberant or chronic because of local or systemic conditions, this may lead to overproduction of scar tissue.

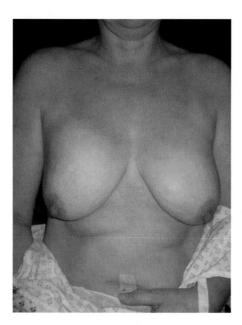

Fig. 71.5 Capsular contracture, submuscular breast enlargement in 1999. Baker grade 3 right breast

Two different pathologic theories are current: the microbiological and the immunological. According to the former, microbiological agents present in the periprosthetic space are responsible for subclinical infection and chronic inflammation. Their pathogenicity is not severe enough to lead to a symptomatic breast infection, but they instead produce mild chronic inflammation and scarring. This theory is supported by the evidence of bacterial biofilm contamination around the implant [17–19], and contracture has an increased

incidence after breast infection or hematoma [5]. Opposing this theory is the evidence that microbiological investigations have usually failed to systematically and constantly identify microbiological agents in the periprosthetic space. Protocols of preoperative and postoperative courses of antibiotics have failed to reduce the incidence of capsular contraction, and when symptoms first appear, antibiotics do not reduce progression of the condition.

According to the immunological theory, systemic or local humoral factors are responsible for initiating and maintaining chronic inflammation [20]. Progressive fibrotic tissue will form in the periprosthetic space. The serum fibrosis indexes hyaluronan, the amino terminal propeptide of procollagen type III (PIIINP), matrix metalloproteinases (MMPs), and tissue inhibitor of metalloproteinases (TIMPs) correlate well in several studies with inflammation grade and fibrosis in patients with fibrotic disorders [21]. Many studies [22, 23] have reported significant elevation in these humoral factors in patients with capsular contracture after breast augmentation, and there is also a positive correlation with stage of the contracture. No major histocompatibility complex pattern has been associated with capsular contraction, and no study has reported systemic or local variation of cytokine pattern.

A main role in the formation and progressive increase of scar tissue must certainly be played by the extracellular matrix. Fibroblasts overproduce components of the connective tissue (collagens, hyaluronic acids, fibronectin, etc.) or, probably, specific isoforms of them. Further scientific studies must address these extracellular matrix components.

Shell characteristics such as a textured surface, a low-bleed elastomer shell, and filler material such as saline seem to decrease the rate of capsular contracture, as

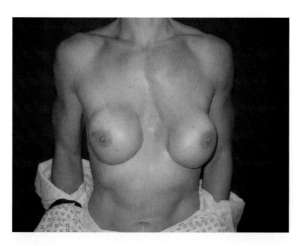

Fig. 71.6 Capsular contracture, subglandular breast enlargement in 1994. Baker grade 4

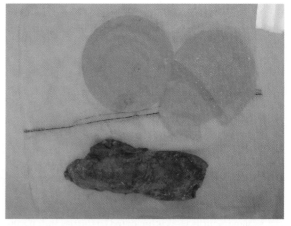

Fig. 71.7 Capsular contracture; capsulectomy performed

scientific studies suggest [24–28]. A recent meta-analysis of randomized trials demonstrates the superiority of textured over smooth breast implants for decreasing the rate of capsular contracture [29]. The submuscular position does not seem to reduce the incidence of contracture as opposed to subglandular or subfascial positioning of the implant, but clinical evidence is delayed. This may be due to the muscular layer covering the scar tissue.

The Baker classification [30] is the most widely used subjective system of staging breast contracture. Grade 1 is assigned to breasts that are soft to palpation and easily compressible, a normal outcome of breast implant. Grade 2 is assigned to breasts having greater firmness than desired but no visible deformity. This condition does not necessitate treatment. Grade 3 is applied when external deformity is apparent, usually manifested as a spherical appearance. The breast is firm and tender when touched. Grade 4 contracture is characterized by extreme firmness, marked deformity, pain, and sometimes coolness.

Treatment is reserved for Baker grades 3 or 4 contracture. Antibiotics, steroids, and vitamins A and E have been shown to be ineffective in treating or even reducing progression of the contraction. Although capsular contraction is a multifactor process, one common denominator in the successful treatment of this complication is believed to be the abatement of inflammation. Leukotriene antagonists have recently emerged as effective prophylactic agents for reactive airway diseases [31]. Anecdotal reports indicate that zafirlukast and montelukast may reduce pain and breast capsule distortion for patients with long-standing contracture who either are not surgical candidates or do not wish to undergo surgery [32]. Randomized clinical trials are currently ongoing. So far, the use of Accolade should not be recommended for treating capsular contraction because its side effects and effectiveness have not yet been proven.

For many years a maneuver used for capsular contraction was the closed capsulotomy. The breast was firmly grasped and manually compressed in an effort to break the capsule's scar tissue. This practice must be avoided because of the risk of rupturing the implant shell and causing leakage of silicone or uncontrolled rupture of the scar with formation of a "pseudoherniation" causing abnormal breast shape.

Baker grades 3 and 4 contractures are suitable for surgical intervention. The patient must be informed that having the implant removed without replacement is actually the only certain way to avoid further problems or recurrence of contracture. If explantation without replacement is indicated, complete capsulectomy by removing the anterior and posterior scar tissue capsule will enable the potential space to heal. When complete resection of the capsule is not possible, it may be useful to score and cut the capsule in order to promote tissue adherence. The cosmetic result depends on the amount of skin excess and ptosis that follow the empty and atrophic breasts. Mastopexy may be indicated at the same time as explantation or afterward.

Surgical treatment for capsular contraction is open capsulotomy or capsulectomy, and whenever possible, a change in the position of the implants. The treatment must be personalized according to the grade of capsular contraction, the position of the implants, and the needs and desires of the particular patient. Capsulotomy consists of circumferential and longitudinal cuts in the capsule to break the thick and strong scar envelopment that deforms the implant, thus making the breast softer. Serial openings to the capsule facilitate reattachment of the tissue.

Generally, the implants are changed in position from the subglandular to the submuscular plane. Mastopexy may be necessary to correct the excess skin that often results from the change of position. The subpectoral plane is indicated because it gives more soft tissue padding over the implant, especially superiorly, and because of the evidence of a lower risk of recurrent contracture. This position also facilitates mammographic investigation. If the patient is active in sports, the submuscular position is a disadvantage. The implant could be replaced in the subglandular position, but the risk of recurrent contracture is high.

When the implant is already in the submuscular position, capsulotomy is indicated. The posterior wall of the capsule lies on the ribs, and the risk of pneumothorax is high when trying to remove it. The implant is usually replaced in the same submuscular position and rarely is placed in a new submammary position. In most cases, there is not enough tissue to cover the implant, and the risk of rippling is very high.

Capsulectomy consists of removing the implant with its entire surrounding capsule by keeping it in the periprosthetic plane. When the capsule is eliminated, the tissue becomes softer, and the breast deformation improves. The advantage of staying outside the capsule is that many older gel implants have significant gel bleed and sometimes frank rupture. By keeping the entire dissection extracapsular, there is little chance of leakage and contamination of the wound with silicone. When it is not technically possible to remove the implant and capsule as a single entity, the implant should be removed, avoiding rupture and material leakage. Afterward, by applying traction on the scar tissue capsule, it is possible to dissect it off the adjacent structures by using dissecting scissors or electrocautery. If the posterior capsule is densely adherent to the chest wall (particularly when the pocket is in the subpectoral position), there may be a risk of penetrating the intercostal space and injuring the parietal pleura, resulting in pneumothorax. In such cases, a portion of, or the entire, posterior scar capsule may be left behind.

If the implant is in the subglandular position, it is generally replaced in the submuscular position. If skin excess is present, mastopexy may be considered. If the implant is in the subpectoral position, capsulotomy is recommended, and the implants are replaced in the same submuscular position.

References

1. Kuroi K, Shimozuma K, Taguchi T: Evidence based risk factors for seroma formation in breast surgery. Jpn J Clin Oncol 2006;36(4):197–206

2. Rheingold LM, Yoo RP: Experience with 326 inflatable breast implants. Plast Reconstr Surg 1994;93(1):118–122

3. Gabrial SE, Woods JE: Complications leading to surgery after breast implantation. N Engl J Med 1997;336(10):718–719

4. Williams C, Aston S, Rees TD: The effect of hematoma on the thickness of pseudosheaths around silicone implants. Plast Reconstr Surg 1975;56(2):194–198

5. Handel N, Cordray T, Gutierrez J: A long term study of outcomes, complications and patient satisfaction with breast implant. Plast Reconstr Surg. 2006;117(3):757–767

6. Pittet B, Montandon D, Pitted D: Infection in breast implants. Lancet Infect Dis 2005;5(8):462–463

7. Freedman A, Jackson I: Infections in breast implants. Infect Dis Clin North Am 1989;3(2):275–287

8. Krueger JK, Rohrich RJ: Clearing the smoke: the scientific rationale for tobacco abstention with plastic surgery. Plast Reconstr Surg. 2001;108(4):1063–1073

9. van Adrichem LN, Hoegen R, Hovius SE, Kort WJ, van Strik R, Vusevski VD, van der Meulen JC: The effect of cigarette smoking on the survival of free vascularized and pedicled epigastric flaps in the rat. Plast Reconstr Surg 1996;97(1):86–89

10. Chang LD, Buncke G, Slezak S, Buncke HJ: Cigarette smoking, plastic surgery, and microsurgery. J Reconstr Microsurg 1996;12(7):467–474

11. Handel N, Jensen JA: The fate of breast implants: a critical analysis of complications and outcomes. Plast Reconstr Surg 1995;96(7):1521–1533

12. Araco A, Gravante G, Araco F, Delogu D, Cervelli V, Wilgenbach K: A retrospective analysis of 3000 primary aesthetic breast augmentations: postoperative complications and associated factors. Aesthetic Plast Surg 2007;31(5):532–539

13. Adams WP, Rios JL, Smith SJ: Enhancing patient outcomes in aesthetic and reconstructive surgery using triple antibiotic breast irrigation: six year prospective clinical study. Plast Surg 2006;117(1):30–36

14. Brand KG: Infection of mammary prosthesis: a survey and the question of prevention. Ann Plast Surg 1993;30(4):289–295

15. Vinh DC, Rendina A, Turner R: Breast implant infection with Mycobacterium fortuitum group: report of case and review. J Infect 2006;52(3):63–67

16. Vinnik CA: Spherical contracture of fibrous capsules around breast implants. Plast Reconstr Surg 1976;58(5):555–560

17. Virden CP, Dobke MK, Stein P: Subclinical infection of the silicone breast implant surface as a possible cause of capsular contracture. Aesthet Plast Surg. 1992;16(2):173–179

18. Pajkos A, Deva AK, Vickery K: Detection of subclinical infection in significant breast implant capsules. Plast Reconstr Surg 2002;11(5):1605–1611

19. Netscher DT: Subclinical infection in breast capsules. Plast Reconstr Surg 2004;114(3):818–280

20. Granchi D, Cavedagna D, Ciapetti G, Pizzoferrato A: Silicone breast implants: the role of immune system on capsular contracture formation. J Biomed Mater Res 1995;29(2):197–202

21. Ulrich D, Repper D, Pallua N: Matrix metalloproteinases, tissue inhibitors of metalloproteinases, aminoterminal propeptide of procollagen type III, and hyaluronan in sera and tissue of patients with capsular contracture after breast augmentation with Trilucent breast implants. Plast Reconstr Surg 2004;114(1):229–236

22. Prantl L, Poppl N, Horvat N, Heine N: Serologic and histologic findings in patients with capsular contracture after breast augmentation with smooth silicone gel implants: is serum hyaluronan a potential predictor? Aesthet Plast Surg 2005;29(6):510–518

23. Prantl L, Angele P, Schreml S, Ulrich D: Determination of serum fibrosis indexes in patients with capsular contracture after breast augmentation with smooth silicone gel implants. Plast Reconstr Surg 2006;118(1):224–229

24. Hakelius L, Ohlsen L: A clinical comparison of the tendency to capsular contracture between smooth and textured gel-filled silicone mammary implants. Plast Reconstr Surg 1992;90(2):247–254

25. Fagrell D, Berggren A, Tarpila E: Capsular contracture around saline-filled fine textured and smooth mammary implants: a prospective 7.5-year follow-up. Plast Reconstr Surg 2001;108(7):2108–2112

26. Caffee HH: The influence of silicone bleed on capsular contracture. Ann Plast Surg 1986;17(4):284–287

27. Wong CH, Samuel M, Tan BK: Capsular contracture in subglandular breast augmentation with textured versus smooth breast implants: a systematic review. Plast Reconstr Surg 2006;118(5):1224–1236

28. McKiney P, Tresley G: Long-term comparison of patients with gel- and saline-filled mammary implants. Plast Reconstr Surg 1983;72(1):27–31

29. Barnsley GP, Sigurdson LJ: Textured surface breast implants in the prevention of capsular contracture among breast augmentation patients: a meta-analysis of randomized controlled trials. Plast Reconstr Surg 2006;117(7):2182–2190

30. Little G, Baker JL: Results of closed compression capsulotomy for treatment of contracted breast implant capsules. Plast Reconstr Surg 1980;65(1):30–33

31. D'Andrea F, Nicoletti GF, Grella E, Grella R, Siniscalco D, Fuccio C, Rossi F, Malone S, De Novellis V: Modification of cysteinyl leukotriene receptor expression in capsular contracture: preliminary results. Ann Plast Surg 2007;58(2):212–214

32. Scuderi N, Mazzocchi M, Fioramanti P, Bistoni G: The effects of zafirlukast on capsular contracture: preliminary report. Aesthet Plast Surg 2006;30(5):513–520

CHAPTER 72

Aesthetic Management of the Breast Capsule After Explantation

72

Greg Chernoff

72.1
Introduction

In the past 10 years, over one million women have undergone breast augmentation, and nearly half a million underwent breast reconstruction in the United States [1]. After implantation, a fibrovascular capsule forms around the implant.

Many consider this capsule to be a static structure, an effective barrier to the egress of foreign material. Even the less severe capsule formation can cause a feeling of discomfort because the breast starts to be fixed to the rear chest wall, thus resulting in a feeling of slight tightening. In extreme cases, a painful, distorted knot appears, which can immobilize the patient and result in the development of the so-called tennis ball deformity [2]. During this period of time, a lower rate of contracture of these capsules has been seen, in the order of 2–3% [3]. The development of a soft, thin, but strong capsule that neither distorts the shape of the breast nor fixes the breast to the rear chest wall is much more frequent.

Patients with recurrent capsular contracture often do not want replacement with a new prosthesis but desire maintenance of their breast volume with a safe alternative [4]. Citing evidence that breast-implant-related capsules resolve uneventfully, some surgeons elect to leave the capsules in place when implants are removed because capsulectomy adds morbidity and expense to the procedure [5]. But clinical and histopathologic evidence suggests that uneventful resolution is not always the case, and several potential problems may arise from retained capsules after removal of the implant. Retained implant capsules may result in a spiculated mass suspicious for carcinoma, dense calcifications obscuring adjacent breast tissue on subsequent imaging studies, cystic masses due to persistent serous effusions, expansile hematoma, and encapsulated silicone cysts. Retained capsules are also a reservoir of implant-related foreign material that can promote tissue ingrowth, as with silicone and textured implants [6].

Reoperation rates for new implants remain remarkably high in the United States. Some reports show rates of up to 13% for saline and 21% for silicone [6]. Explantation remains a common procedure, with more than 200,000 patients undergoing this in the past 5 years in the United States [7, 8].

72.2
Histology

The histology of capsular tissue is well described in the literature. Several studies have compared smooth to textured implant capsules, saline to silicone capsules, and implant age-related capsules. Most studies assess the following histology features: synovial-like metaplasia, villous hyperplasia, density of the collagenous capsule, alignment of collagen fibers within the capsule, presence of foreign material, and presence of a foreign body reaction.

The following trends have been described [9]: With smooth implants, increasing implant duration is associated with a decrease in synovial-like metaplasia and villous hyperplasia. There are no significant differences regarding the presence of a dense collagenous capsule, the orientation of the collagen fibers, or the presence of a foreign body reaction. An increase in foreign material has been observed.

With textured implants, increasing implant duration is associated with a decrease in synovial-like metaplasia, villous hyperplasia, dense collagenous architecture, and parallel orientation of collagen fibers. An increase in foreign material and the presence of a foreign body reaction have been observed.

There is no statistically significant difference between smooth and textured implants with respect to development of capsular contracture. The severity of capsular contracture shows a positive linear correlation with the degree of local inflammatory reactions, independent of the implant surface.

72.3
Discussion

Many options exist for the patient faced with capsular contracture and explantation. The "implant fear" of the 1990s has generally been alleviated through numerous excellent epidemiologic and rheumatologic studies. These studies demonstrated no association between silicone breast implants and any connective tissue diseases [10–15].

Currently, most women facing explantation will choose implant exchange, typically smooth saline placed in the subpectoral plane. Another common choice is exchange with mastopexy. This differs again from the 1990s when most women seemed to choose not to replace their implants. In the group of women today who chose implant exchange, those who chose silicone previously will replace with silicone.

An option always open to the patient is explantation without breast contouring or capsule modification. This has the advantage of simplicity and perceived safety to the patient. While this may yield acceptable cosmetic results in some patients, the resulting breast contour is usually not acceptable. Most of the time this yields significant ptosis and volume deficiency, especially in the upper pole.

The majority of patients opt for implant exchange after explantation. This gives the patient the best chance of breast volume and contour restoration. Open capsulotomy and implant exchange are sufficient in simple cases of implant rupture or leakage. Capsular contracture requires capsulectomy. A subglandular contracture requires a complete capsulectomy with conversion to the subpectoral plane. Subpectoral contractures can be treated with total or anterior capsulectomy; replacement is then in the same plane.

The retained capsule can be problematic if the patient chooses not to replace the implant. With ongoing aging and the resultant continued breast hypoplasia, palpability of the retained capsule may be an issue that should be reviewed in the informed consent. The corollary is sculpting of the capsule, which will further decrease volume, adding potential deformity to the remaining breast tissue. Again, this must be addressed in the informed consent.

Patients with advanced ptosis may opt for implant replacement with mastopexy. The additional scarring involved as well as the increased potential for complications sometimes dissuades patients from opting for this combination. Rohrich and Parker [3] have presented an excellent algorithm for mastopexy and explantation. They stage mastopexy if the nipple requires elevation greater than 4 cm.

The most challenging patient situation is the choice to explant, not replace, and to then have mastopexy alone. The ideal candidate has grade 2–3 ptosis and adequate parenchymal tissue, and requires less than 4 cm of nipple elevation. Because of a higher risk of flap necrosis, smokers and patients requiring greater than 4 cm elevation of the nipple should be staged, undergoing explantation first and waiting a minimum of 4 months for the mastopexy.

The type of mastopexy chosen is based on patient assessment. Implant position and size, degree of ptosis, areola size, skin elasticity, and amount of parenchyma help the surgeon decide on the appropriate operation.

Wedge resection is an excellent procedure for patients with pseudoptosis. This provides enhanced projection of the breast and is suitable when no nipple elevation is required. Up to 4 cm of tissue can be safely resected.

Vertical "short-scar" mastopexy can be used for patients with moderate ptosis. This would include those patients requiring up to 2 cm of nipple elevation. Although circumareolar mastopexy can be utilized, especially with large areolas, flattening of the breasts can yield less than satisfactory results.

The Wise-pattern mastopexy is employed for patients requiring up to 4 cm of nipple elevation. This "workhorse" procedure, while increasing scarring, affords the greatest versatility for contouring.

72.4
Conclusions

The treatment of breast hypotrophy continues to be challenging. Even in the best of hands and with the most reliable of prostheses, the major risk of a fibrous capsule still persists. As a result, one of the most beautiful operations is often doomed to failure, with unacceptable morphological and psychological implications.

Retained capsules can cause further problems and should be addressed. Open communication and proper informed consent are paramount when dealing with breast surgery. Although augmentation mammaplasty is a popular procedure, it is associated—perhaps more than any other cosmetic procedure—with a relatively high rate of revisional surgery. A sound knowledge of options and patient selection should never be overlooked.

References

1. American Society of Plastic Surgeons. Procedural statistics, 2006. http://www.plasticsurgery.org. Accessed 6 June 2007
2. Szemerey IB: The fasciocapsular flap in capsular herniation. Aesthetic Plast Surg 2006;30(3):277–281

3. Rohrich RJ, Parker TH III: Aesthetic management of the breast after explantation. Plast Reconstr Surg 2007;120(1):312–315

4. Spear S, Carter M, Ganz JC: The correction of capsular contracture by conversion to "dual plane" positioning: technique and outcomes. Plast Reconstr Surg 2003;112(2):456–466

5. Hardt N, Yu L, LaTorre G, Steinbach B: Complications related to breast implant capsules. Plast Reconstr Surg 1995;95(2):364–371

6. Tebbetts J: Dual plane breast augmentation. Plast Reconstr Surg 2001;107(5):1255–1272

7. Mladick R: "No-touch" submuscular saline breast augmentation technique. Aesthetic Plast Surg 1993;17(3):183–192

8. Rohrich RJ: A prospective analysis of patients undergoing silicone breast implant explantation. Plast Reconstr Surg 2000;105(7):2529–2537

9. Wyatt LE, Sinow D, Wollman JS, Sami DA, Miller TA: The influence of time on breast capsule histology: smooth and textured silicone-surfaced implants. Plast Reconstr Surg 1998;102(6):1922–1931

10. Peters W, Smith D, Fornasier V, Lugowski S, Ibanez D: An outcome analysis of 100 women after explantation of silicone gel breast implants. Ann Plast Surg 1997;39(1):9–19

11. Rohrich RJ: Safety of silicone breast implants: scientific validation/vindication at last. Plast Reconstr Surg 1999;104(6):1786–1788

12. Netscher DT: Aesthetic outcome of implant removal in 85 consecutive patients. Plast Reconstr Surg 2004;113(3):1057–1059

13. Rohrich RJ, Coberly DM, Krueger JK, Brown SA: Planning elective operations on patients who smoke: survey of North American plastic surgeons. Plast Reconstr Surg 2002;109(1):356–357

14. Krueger J: Clearing the smoke: the scientific rationale for tobacco abstention with plastic surgery. Plast Reconstr Surg 2001;108(4):1063–1073

15. Rohrich RJ: Cosmetic surgery and patients who smoke: should we operate? Plast Reconstr Surg 2000;106(1):137–138

CHAPTER 73

Complications of the Transumbilical Approach   73

Melvin A. Shiffman

73.1
Introduction

The transumbilical approach to breast augmentation has a few complications that differ from those with approaches from the axilla, areola, or inframammary regions. Although the literature may seem to suggest that using the endoscope is essential, many experienced surgeons using the transumbilical approach do not rely on the endoscope to check for bleeding or implant position.

73.2
Reports of Complications

Johnson and Christ [1] studied 91 patients with the transumbilical approach for submammary breast augmentation. One patient had excessive bleeding at the time of surgery and required an inframammary incision to control the vessel. Implant deflation occurred in one patient, and two patients had subpectoral implantations that were corrected through submammary incisions.

Vila-Rovira [2] reported on 145 patients using the transumbilical approach. There were no cases of hematoma or infection. Postoperative pain was described as mild. Some cases of postoperative edema occurred. Twenty percent of patients had capsule contracture, with 75% being Baker grade I, 15% grade II, 6% grade III, and 4% grade IV. Rippling occurred in 30% of patients (saline implants were used in all 145 patients, 80% smooth and 20% textured). Some patients had asymmetry, but some of this was due to undetected preexisting anatomical deformities. Areolar sensory changes were transitory. A fibrous cord along the tunnel tract was detectable in two cases but resolved after 6–8 weeks.

Caleel [3] reported on 513 patients. One patient had bleeding, two patients had postoperative hematoma, one patient had implant leak, and three patients had inadequate implant pocket dissection.

Sudarsky [4] operated on 90 patients, of whom 70 had follow-up. One patient had accidental submuscu-

lar entry into the pocket, and there were four capsule contractures.

Songcharoen [5] treated 93 patients with the transumbilical approach. There were no infections; 1% of patients had hematoma at the tunnel area, 3% had implant leakage, and 4% had unequal breast size.

73.3
Incorrect Implant Pocket Position

Usually, the tunnel extending lateral to the nipple with the breast not elevated will place the dissector in the submammary plane on blunt dissection. If the tunnel is placed medial to the nipple while the breast is lifted, the pocket is usually in the subpectoral plane. Certainly it is a known complication of the transumbilical approach to put the implant in the incorrect plane by accident.

The problem of positioning the implant in the correct plane, submammary or subpectoral, may be accidental or due to inexperience, or endoscopic examination may have fooled the surgeon. When the implant pocket is placed in the submammary position, the endoscope will show visible fat superficially (anteriorly), and the pectoralis major muscle will be visible posteriorly. However, when a subpectoral pocket is formed, there is usually a layer of fat under the muscle that may be mistaken for the fat under the breast tissue. When viewed posteriorly, the pectoralis minor muscle may not be distinguished from the pectoralis major muscle since it arises from the upper margins of the 3rd, 4th, and 5th ribs and from the aponeuroses covering the intercostal muscles. The muscle fibers pass upward and laterally and converge to form a flat tendon that inserts into the coracoid process of the scapula. The endoscopic examination is not perfect for determining implant pocket position.

An instrument to change implants from the subglandular to the subpectoral position was described by Rey [6]. This instrument can be used without a separate incision by developing the correct pocket (submuscular) with the bullet dissector, inserting the implant into the subpectoral space, and then removing the implant from the false pocket. Rey developed another instrument to lift the pectoralis muscle via the umbilical incision and then place the implant into the correct pocket.

73.4
Implant Postoperatively too High

An implant that is too high postoperatively may occur because the inframammary fold portion of the pocket was not dissected low enough, or, with a well-developed low pocket, the implant may not have migrated downward enough to fill the inframammary fold. This complication is more frequent with the inexperienced surgeon and is a well-known complication of the transumbilical approach.

73.5
Capsule Contracture

The capsule contracture rate for Baker grades II–IV is 5% with saline implants in the submammary position [2]. According to the Inamed Aesthetics statistics [7], the capsule contracture rate with saline implants for Baker grades III/IV is 7.2% for 1-year cumulative occurrence and 8.7% for 3-year cumulative occurrence.

The causes of capsule contracture include the patient's biophysiology, infection, bleeding, silicone oil leakage, and foreign bodies (talc from gloves, perhaps dust). The umbilical approach has very little bleeding [8–11] compared with other approaches, and this may be the reason for the lower capsule contracture rate.

References

1. Johnson GW, Christ JE: The endoscopic breast augmentation: the transumbilical insertion of saline-filled breast implants. Plast Reconstr Surg 1993;92(5):801–808
2. Vila-Rovira R: Breast augmentation by an umbilical approach. Aesthet Plast Surg 1999;23(5):323–330
3. Caleel RT: Transumbilical endoscopic breast augmentation: submammary and subpectoral. Plast Reconstr Surg 2000;106(5):1177–1182
4. Sudarsky L: Experience with transumbilical breast augmentation. Ann Plast Surg 2001;46(5):467–472
5. Songcharoen S: Endoscopic transumbilical subglandular augmentation mammaplasty. Clin Plast Surg 2002;29(1):1–13
6. Rey RM Jr: Transumbilical breast augmentation: a new instrument for changing implants from the subglandular to the subpectoral position. Plast Reconstr Surg 2001;107(5):1310–1311
7. Inamed Aesthetics: BioCell® Textured and Smooth Saline-Filled Breast Implants package insert, 2005
8. Baccari ME: Dispelling the myths and misconceptions about transumbilical breast augmentation. Plast Reconstr Surg 2000;106(1):195–196
9. Dowden R: Breast augmentation by umbilical approach. Aesthetic Plast Surg 2000;24:71
10. Dowden R: Dispelling the myths and misconceptions about transumbilical breast augmentation. Plast Reconstr Surg 2000;106(1):190–194
11. Johnson GW, Dowden RV: Breast augmentation: umbilical approach. In: Ramirez OM, Daniel RK (eds). Endoscopic Plastic Surgery. New York, Springer 1995, pp 156–175

CHAPTER 74

Subfascial Breast Augmentations: Complications

74

Melvin A. Shiffman

74.1
Introduction

The subfascial approach to breast augmentation has had very good results with few complications. Surgeons planning to perform the procedure should first observe the technique and, better yet, get hands-on training. The inexperienced surgeon is more likely to have complications. The usual risks and complications following breast augmentation should be discussed with the patient prior to the surgery as well as the risk of misplacing the implant below the pectoralis major muscle instead of above it.

The purpose of the subfascial pocket is to have less capsule contracture and rippling while avoiding the submuscular problem of distortion with muscle tension.

74.2
Difficulty Dissecting the Pocket

Parsa et al. [1], without having been trained in this procedure, performed subfascial pocket dissection in three patients. They had difficulties with the dissection, shredded the fascia, found it time-consuming, and had increased blood loss. However, experienced, trained surgeons have no difficulty dissecting the pocket, have little difficulty with bleeding, and can perform the surgery in the same or less time than it takes to do a submammary or subpectoral pocket.

74.3
Incorrect Pocket

It is possible to place the prosthesis is a subpectoral pocket accidentally instead of in the intended submammary pocket. This can occur with blind dissection or even with the endoscope. Endoscopically, in the subpectoral pocket the anterior muscle may not be visible through the fat layer under the muscle and may appear to be the fat under the breast. Posteriorly, the pectoralis major muscle should be visible if submammary, and the ribs should be visible if subpectoral, but the pectoralis minor muscle, which arises from the 3rd, 4th, and 5th ribs and inserts into the coracoid process of the scapula, may be mistaken for the pectoralis major muscle.

74.4
Reported Complications

Stoff-Khalili et al. [2] described the complications in 69 patients having the subfascial approach. Baker grade III capsule contracture occurred in 2.6% and Baker grade IV in 0.0%. Rippling was noted in 1.5% of patients, and there were no patients with hematoma or seroma.

Graf et al. [3] reported on 263 patients with the endoscopic transaxillary subfascial approach. Six patients had grade II capsule contracture (2.3%), three patients had unilateral hematoma (1.1%), and eight patients had implant malposition requiring surgical intervention (3%). There were no patients with implant distortion from muscle contraction.

Ventura and Marcello [4] had 63 patients who received subfascial placement. Two patients (2%) had Baker grade II capsule contracture, and one patient had excess drainage that required surgical exploration. There were no seromas or infections, and there was less edema and faster recovery than with submuscular or subglandular placement.

Munhoz et al. [5] saw no capsule contractures in 42 patients with the subfascial approach who were followed for 16 months.

74.5
Discussion

Others have reported on subfascial placement of prostheses [6–8]. Duman et al. [9] performed research on rabbits that showed that the capsule formed was thinner and less cellular in the fascia-covered implant group than in the control group without fascia covering. Fascial tissue may decrease capsule formation and, probably, capsule contraction.

Capsule contracture occurs less often with the subfascial pocket than with submuscular implant placement, without the problem of the pectoralis major muscle causing distortion with contraction.

74.6
Conclusions

The subfascial placement of implants has fewer complications than some of the other approaches. Training is necessary to perform the procedure properly.

References

1. Parsa FD, Parsa AA, Hsu A: Subfascial periareolar augmentation mammaplasty. Plast Reconstr Surg 2006;117(2):681–682
2. Stoff-Khalili MA, Scholze R, Morgan WR: Subfascial periareolar augmentation mammaplasty. Plast Reconstr Surg 2004;114(5):1280–1288
3. Graf RM, Bernardes A, Rippel R, Araujo LRR, Costa Damasio RC, Auersvald A: Subfascial breast implant: a new procedure. Plast Reconstr Surg 2003;111(2):904–908
4. Ventura OD, Marcello GA: Anatomic and physiologic advantages of totally subfascial breast implants. Aesth Plast Surg 2005;29:379–383
5. Munhoz AM, Fells K, Arruda E, Montag E, Okada A, Aldrighi C, Aldrighi JM, Gemperli R, Ferreira MC: Subfascial transaxillary breast augmentation without endoscopic assistance: technical aspects and outcome. Aesth Plast Surg 2006;30(5):503–512
6. Barbato C, Pena M, Triana C, Zambrano MA: Augmentation mammoplasty using the retrofascial approach. Plast Reconstr Surg 2004;28(3):148–152
7. Graf RM, Bernardes A, Auersvald A, Costa Damasio RC: Subfascial endoscopic transaxillary subfascial augmentation mammoplasty. Aesthet Plast Surg 2000;24:216–220
8. Benito-Ruiz J: Subfascial breast implant. Plast Reconstr Surg 2004;113(3):1088–1089
9. Duman A. Dincler M, Findik H, Uzunismail A: Further advantages of using the subfascial implant in terms of capsular formation. Plast Reconstr Surg 2005;115(3):950–952

CHAPTER 75

Complications of Autologous Fat Transfer to the Breast

Melvin A. Shiffman

75.1
Introduction

There are few statistics on the actual rate of complications in patients with fat transfer to the breast area for augmentation. The present method of injecting fat into the subpectoral, intrapectoral, and submammary regions rather than into the breast reduces the problem of breast calcifications. However, inadvertent injection into the breast tissue can occur.

The patient should always be counseled as to the possible risks and complications of breast augmentation with autogenous fat. These include asymmetry, loss of fat over several months, fat necrosis, calcifications, infection, injection of fat into the breast tissue, and bleeding. Repeat injections of fat may be needed.

75.2
Reported Complications

Da Silveira [1] reported on 31 patients with hypomastia, asymmetry, postgestational involution, and the need for finishing touches postmammaplasty who had fat transfer to the breast. He stated that edema resolved after 3–4 weeks and resorption ended around the 3rd or 4th month. Complications included resorption, steatonecrosis, one case of calcification in a cyst wall, and one case with microcalcifications characteristic of benign disease.

Castello et al. [2] reported on a patient with a painful mass (giant liponecrotic pseudocyst) after breast augmentation with fat, which required lumpectomy, breast reconstruction, and bilateral breast augmentation with prostheses.

Vakdetta et al. [3] noted one case of bilateral mammary abscesses with sepsis after autologous fat transfer to the breast.

Kwak et al. [4] described fat necrosis in the right breast and a solid inflammatory mass in the left breast of one patient. These areas were biopsied for confirmation.

75.3
Discussion

The commonest complication of injection of autologous fat into the area of the chest wall is the occurrence of oil cysts, which may cause some discomfort and may be palpable as a mass. The fat cyst may become calcified if left for a prolonged period of time, resulting in round or curved calcifications. If there is fat necrosis and small calcifications, these are almost always round and easily distinguished by an experienced mammographer from malignant calcifications. Similar calcifications have been seen in breasts that have had breast reduction surgery.

Some mammographers are inexperienced with seeing mammography of fat injected into areas of the chest and may be confused by the dark areas under the pectoralis major muscle, in the muscle, and over the muscle; these areas are the fat deposits.

References

1. Da Silveira JW: Breast augmentation with autologous lipograft. Am J Cosmet Surg 1998;15(2):109–115
2. Castello JR, Barros J, Vazquez R: Giant liponecrotic pseudocyst after breast augmentation with fat. Plast Reconstr Surg 1999;103(1):291–293
3. Vakdetta L, Thione A, Buoro M, Tuinder S: A case of life-threatening sepsis after breast augmentation by fat injection. Aesthet Plast Surg 2001;25(5):347–349
4. Kwak JY, Lee SH, Park, HL, Kim JY, Kim SE, Kim EK: Sonographic findings in complications of cosmetic breast augmentation with autologous fat obtained by liposuction. J Clin Ultrasound 2004;32(6):299–301

Part VIII
Miscellaneous

CHAPTER 76

Breast Conservation Therapy After Augmentation Mammaplasty

J. Arthur Jensen

76.1 Introduction

In April 2005, the Fifth International Consensus Conference of the Breast Health Institute was convened in Milan. Experts in breast cancer representing multiple disciplines discussed various issues of breast conservation therapy. A consensus statement that developed from the conference [1] specifically addressed the question of breast cancer in patients with prior augmentation mammaplasty. The group of experts agreed that prior augmentation mammaplasty was not a contraindication for breast conservation therapy. However, the experts agreed that radiation therapy can be expected to result in a higher risk of capsular contracture, and the breast will not be the same as it was prior to treatment. Women who understand these facts are candidates for breast conservation.

The use of breast conservation for augmented patients has been evaluated in two significant studies in the United States. Both studies reported significant complications with this approach and concluded that conservation techniques might not be optimal in the augmented patient.

An international consensus conference recommends breast conservation in all patients who have been told about the risk of capsular contracture. Clinical experience demonstrates high reoperation rates and cosmetically unsatisfactory results.

How should augmentation patients be treated when they are found to have breast cancer?

This chapter carefully reviews the studies that have cast doubt on the conventional wisdom that breast augmentation patients can be routinely treated with breast conservation techniques. By understanding these data, a plastic surgeon can more intelligently advise patients about the likely outcomes of various choices of breast cancer management.

76.2 Definition

Breast conservation therapy can be defined as complete removal of a breast tumor with a concentric margin of healthy tissue performed in a cosmetically acceptable manner and followed by radiation therapy. The dose of radiation to treat the entire breast is 45–50.4 Gy delivered over approximately 5 weeks. In addition, most North American radiation oncologists use a "boost" of radiation for the tumor site plus a 1–2-cm margin of surrounding tissue. The tumor bed is therefore treated with 60–66 Gy. In the United States, most axillary lymph nodes are evaluated using sentinel node techniques. If the sentinel node is positive, completion axillary dissection is performed.

76.3 Oncologic Consultation: Treatment Alternatives

Each patient who presents with breast cancer must be informed about the treatment alternatives. At one time, women were taken to the operating room with an undiagnosed breast mass and could emerge from the operating room with a mastectomy. Fortunately, such a practice is now outside the standard of care. All women must be told about the choices they have for local management of breast cancer.

The controversy regarding how breast cancer should be managed has raged for at least 50 years. Halsted popularized the radical mastectomy in the United States for cancers that frequently recurred in the pectoral muscles and in the skin overlying the breast. With improvements in medical technology and delivery, breast cancers were discovered earlier in their course. Lumpectomy was proposed as a less mutilating procedure with equivalent survival rates, but this alternative was not without its skeptics. Removing almost all the breast using mastectomy resulted in low recurrence rates within the breast tissue (because so little breast tissue was left), but the patient was left with a mutilating postoperative defect.

Leaving a large percentage of the breast using lumpectomy resulted in higher local recurrence rates, but often left almost a normal appearing breast. Adding radiation therapy to lumpectomy further reduced the chance that cancer would develop or recur in the preserved breast, but this left some aesthetic changes secondary to the radiation therapy.

Did mastectomy produce improved long-term survival at the cost of a mutilating cosmetic defect? This question was tested directly in the National Surgical Adjuvant Breast and Bowel Project (NSABP) B-06 protocol, the results of which have recently been reported with 20 years of follow-up [2].

These results are very important because this study and other European studies like it [3] have revolutionized the surgical management of breast cancer. After 20 years, no survival advantage was found for any of the approaches. Survival was the same for lumpectomy, lumpectomy with radiation therapy, and modified radical mastectomy. If survival is the same for lumpectomy and mastectomy, why would anyone choose to have a mastectomy for breast cancer?

Several peculiarities of the B-06 study make the study difficult to extrapolate to clinical practice. First, the study was an "intention to treat" study. If a patient was randomized to lumpectomy but was found to have positive margins, she was converted to mastectomy but was followed in the original lumpectomy group. Second, if cancer recurred in the breast following lumpectomy, the study did not consider the recurrence to be a local failure. The rationale for this practice was that the mastectomy group did not have a breast in which such a recurrence could appear, so such a comparison would be unfair.

It is important to realize that if a patient developed a recurrence in the preserved breast at a later time, she was treated with a mastectomy but continued to be followed in the originally assigned group. Therefore, to achieve equivalent survival rates as were reported in the B-06 study, patients who develop in-breast recurrences following lumpectomy must be treated with immediate mastectomy. Obviously, the longer that cancer grows in a preserved breast, the greater the chance that such a cancer might seed metastatic disease. B-06 did not study lumpectomy versus mastectomy for 20 years; it studied lumpectomy as a first "intention to treat" versus mastectomy with lumpectomies being converted to mastectomies when cancer recurred or margins were positive. Therefore, surveillance of the preserved (lumpectomy) breast is mandatory. If cancers develop in the preserved breast, patients must be treated with mastectomy so that the cancers have less time to seed the body with metastases or to mutate to cancers that have a better chance of becoming metastatic.

76.4
Lumpectomy: Effect of Breast Implants on Mammography

Mammography is the most commonly used radiological test for discovering early breast cancers. Unfortunately, mammography is impaired in the setting of augmentation mammaplasty. In a series of 99 known invasive breast cancers in augmented women [4], mammography was normal in 43%. In contrast, mammography was normal in only 5% of women without implants. Although other studies [5] have concluded that cancers discovered in augmented patients are of similar prognostic characteristics as cancers discovered in nonaugmented patients, it is indisputable that breast implants impair the diagnostic efficiency of mammography. However, because small breast cancers are more easily palpated in women with breast implants, breast implants have not been demonstrated to have a negative survival effect.

Certainly contributing to the reduction in mammographic efficiency in patients with breast implants is capsular contracture. Capsular contracture has been found to severely limit the ability of mammograms to detect breast cancer [6]. Radiation therapy is well known to increase the incidence of capsular contracture.

Patients with breast implants who have chosen to have breast conservation must be informed that they have a risk of new cancer and also of recurrent cancer in their treated breast. Because they are at relatively high risk for such recurrent and new cancers, they should be screened using magnetic resonance imaging (MRI). MRI has been demonstrated to be more effective than mammography in discovering early breast cancers [7]. Therefore, patients who elect breast conservation treatment should understand that mammography is impaired in the setting of breast implants and that they will need to be followed with MRI scans for surveillance of their treated breasts.

76.5
Lumpectomy: Effect of Radiation on Rate of Capsular Contracture

Radiation therapy is almost always done in cases of lumpectomy to prevent early recurrence of breast cancer. But how does radiation affect the patient's cosmetic result?

Radiation therapy is well known to have effects on normal tissue that are not desirable but are frequently seen. For instance, the irradiated skin can become inflamed and later develop pigmentation changes. In addition, radiation is known to cause fibrosis of normal

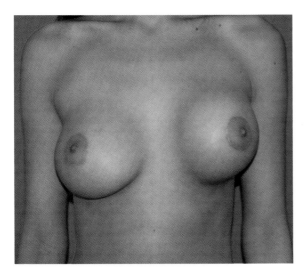

Fig. 76.1 Capsular contracture is caused by fibrosis of the capsule around a breast implant and results in a firm, superiorly displaced, and often painful breast implant. The chance of capsular contracture is much higher if the breast is treated with radiation therapy

tissue. Radiation of a normal breast following lumpectomy can result in loss of volume of the breast and some superior retraction of the breast. The superior retraction might actually improve the appearance of a ptotic breast. However, the fibrosis around a breast implant does not improve the cosmetic result of augmentation mammaplasty. Capsular contracture results in a more palpable implant that might become hard to the touch. If this process is progressive, a firm implant can become tender or painful for the patient. The fibrosis around the implant can also result in thinning of the tissues

and displacement of the implant. Distorted, painful, hard breasts are commonly seen in women who have radiation therapy after augmentation mammaplasty (Figs. 76.1, 76.2).

76.6
Lumpectomy and Radiation Versus Glandular Replacement Therapy

The B-06 study was initiated in the 1970s when mastectomy without reconstruction was the standard of care. The study demonstrated that doing lumpectomy as an "intention to treat" a patient with an early breast cancer was a reasonable alternative because if the patient developed a local recurrence and needed a mastectomy, she was able to enjoy an almost normal breast until such a recurrence developed. The most important finding of the study was that starting with breast conservation techniques did not result in a worse prognosis for the patient: Survival rates at 20 years were the same. Since the 1970s, breast reconstruction has improved dramatically. Tissue expansion allows a much more reliable approach to breast reconstruction than was available earlier. The latissimus dorsi myocutaneous flap and the transverse abdominal myocutaneous flap emerged as workhorses of breast reconstruction. How do these technologies affect the management of breast cancer?

The aesthetic outcome of breast reconstruction depends significantly on what needs to be reconstructed. With advanced cancers, wide excision of breast skin is required. While flap reconstruction of a large skin defect allows a more aggressive oncologic approach than could be obtained if the surgeon were attempting primary closure, reconstructions requiring a large skin paddle rarely produce aesthetically pleasing results. But

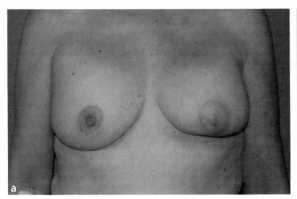

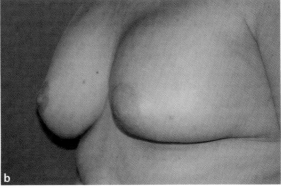

Fig. 76.2 Previously augmented patients who are treated for breast cancer with lumpectomy and radiation therapy often fail conservative therapy. This patient complained that her breast implant on the treated side had become hard and superiorly displaced. In addition, she was found to have recurrent ductal carcinoma in situ near the site of her lumpectomy

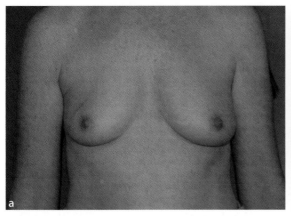
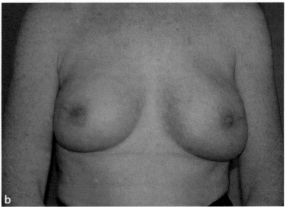
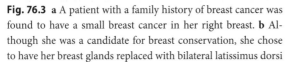

Fig. 76.3 a A patient with a family history of breast cancer was found to have a small breast cancer in her right breast. **b** Although she was a candidate for breast conservation, she chose to have her breast glands replaced with bilateral latissimus dorsi flaps and breast implants. This alternative must be discussed with patients with prior augmentation mammoplasty because breast conservation is much more complicated in the setting of previously placed breast implants

if the skin envelope can be preserved, a much more cosmetically pleasing reconstruction is possible [8].

Studies of breast conservation have also clarified the safety of performing nipple-sparing mastectomies. If leaving the nipple, as is done routinely in lumpectomy patients, gives the same survival outcome as removing the nipple, as is done routinely in mastectomy patients, then removing the nipple offers no survival benefit [9]. Nipple-sparing mastectomies were advocated as early as the 1960s, but concerns about the impact of nipple recurrence on patient survival limited the practice. With the realization that nipple sparing does not affect survival, new interest in this technique has emerged [10, 11].

If almost complete skin-preserving and nipple-sparing mastectomy is performed, cosmetic results can very closely simulate breast conservation. Thus, improvements in mastectomy and reconstruction might very well change a woman's decision about whether to "preserve" her breast [12]. A patient might be resistant to the mutilating image of a mastectomy but be much more interested in the notion that her breast gland can simply be replaced. Glandular replacement therapy might very well be a better choice for augmented patients than lumpectomy and radiation therapy because such patients would not be so concerned about in-breast recurrence, the adverse effects of implants on mammographic detection of recurrence (or new cancer), or increased incidence of capsular contracture. An improved alternative to breast conservation must also be considered by any patient who is trying to weigh her surgical choices.

76.7
Breast Conservation Therapy in the Augmented Patient: Clinical Experience

The first large study [13] to report on the treatment of breast cancer in augmented women was done at the Van Nuys Breast Center from 1981 to 1994. Of the 66 augmented women with primary breast cancer, 27 had modified radical mastectomy, three chose alternative treatments, three (all cases of ductal carcinoma in situ) had lumpectomy alone, and 33 had lumpectomy with radiation therapy. Capsular contracture was evaluated using the Baker classification.

Because all of the augmented women had unilateral breast cancer, radiation therapy in this population represents the best evaluation available in the literature of the effect of radiation therapy on breast augmentation. Baker grade was evaluated before treatment on both sides prior to the unilateral radiation therapy and was reevaluated after radiation treatment. The average Baker grade at the beginning of the study was 1.19 on the cancerous side and 1.15 on the opposite, normal side. After the radiation therapy, the average Baker grade on the radiated side was 3.08 while the opposite, nonradiated side was found to have an average Baker grade of 1.73. Altogether, 17 patients developed a significant increase in contracture on the treated side. In five patients there was no change in the Baker grade. Of the 17 patients with significant increase in capsular contracture, eight had undergone corrective surgery at the time of the report.

The most important conclusion from this study is that almost two-thirds of patients with prior breast augmentation will develop capsular contracture. While the decision to treat such patients with surgery depends on many variables, according to this reported experience at least half of patients with radiation treatment involving a breast implant will require operative intervention.

A second large study [14] of patients with prior augmentation mammaplasty who were found to have primary breast cancer was conducted at the UCLA Breast Center from 1991 to 2001. Of the 58 patients treated, 32 underwent modified radical mastectomy. In this study population, 28 patients underwent breast conservation therapy, but six of the 22 had their implants removed prior to radiation therapy. The remaining 22 women were radiated. Eleven of the 22 patients later underwent completion mastectomies with implant removal. Four of the 22 had positive margins, five had local recurrences of breast cancer, and two had implant complications. Of the remaining 11 patients, nine developed capsular contracture, erosion, pain, or rupture of the implant.

An important point to emerge from this study is that nine of the 22 patients who underwent lumpectomy with radiation therapy had either positive margins or early local recurrence of breast cancer. Patients who undergo augmentation mammaplasty are motivated because their breasts are smaller than they would like them to be. Assuming that the breast cancers that are discovered in the augmentation population are the same size as those in the normal population and assuming that augmentation patients have less breast tissue than women in the normal population, treatment for breast cancer in the augmented population must necessarily remove a greater percentage of a woman's breast than in the normal population. Surgeons trying to spare the smaller amount of breast tissue possessed by these women might be tempted to get by with smaller margins than in a patient with more breast tissue. However, smaller margins might lead to higher recurrence rates.

76.8 Conclusions

Patients with breast augmentation are at higher risk to fail an attempt at breast conservation therapy for several reasons. First, breast implants interfere with mammographic detection of recurrent or new breast cancers. Surveillance of the breast for such cancers is an important goal in patients with potentially curable early breast cancer. MRI scans are recommended for augmented patients who have had breast conservation therapy. Second, radiation therapy increases the chance of capsular contracture. Capsular contracture renders the breast firm and sometimes painful and can also distort the appearance of the breast. Creating an aesthetic breast is part of the definition of breast conservation therapy. Third, because of the option of nipple sparing and improvements in breast reconstruction, replacing the gland is a much more attractive alternative than was possible in the days of mutilating, skin-sacrificing mastectomies without reconstruction. Patients with early breast cancer must be fully advised concerning the effects of radiation fibrosis in the setting of breast implants.

Despite reservations, plastic surgeons who work closely with oncologic breast surgeons know that implants can be well tolerated by patients who have chosen to conserve their breasts. Patients who do develop capsular contractures can frequently be treated with open capsulectomies, and long-term satisfactory results can be achieved. Because capsulectomy is generally much less involved than flap transfer, many patients might choose to have breast conservation and simply take the increased risks associated with this treatment alternative. Such patients might logically reason that flap technology can be used if undesirable complications are realized (Fig. 76.4).

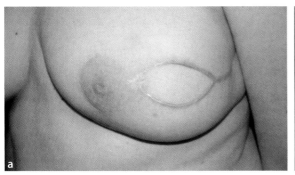
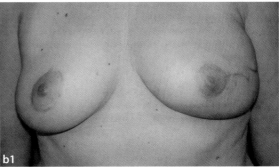

Fig. 76.4 a This patient (preoperative photographs shown in Fig. 76.2) underwent an open capsulectomy on the right side and a nipple-sparing mastectomy on the left side. **b** *1* Replacing the breast gland and breast implant with a muscle-sparing free transverse rectus abdominis myocutaneous flap gave her a much softer breast with a lower risk of recurrent ipsilateral cancer. *2* Lateral view

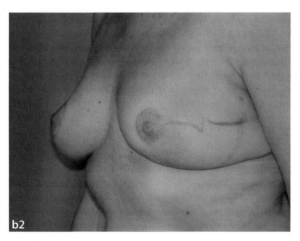

Fig. 76.4 *(continued)* **b** *1* Replacing the breast gland and breast implant with a muscle-sparing free transverse rectus abdominis myocutaneous flap gave her a much softer breast with a lower risk of recurrent ipsilateral cancer. *2* Lateral view

Like many other questions of cancer treatment and aesthetic surgery, this question must ultimately be resolved by patient choice. Although the patient can be enlightened by discussions with her doctors, only she can choose her treatment as she weighs the above considerations in combination with many other variables known only to her.

References

1. Schwartz GF, Veronesi U, Clough KB, Dixon JM, Fentiman IS, Heywang-Kobrunner SH, et al.: Consensus conference on breast conservation. J Am Coll Surg 2006;203(2):198–207
2. Fisher B, Anderson S, Bryant J, Margolese RG, Deutsch M, Fisher ER, Jeong JH, Wolmark N: Twenty year follow-up of a randomized trial comparing total mastectomy, lumpectomy, and lumpectomy plus irradiation for the treatment of invasive breast cancer. N Engl J Med 2002;347(16):1233–1241
3. Veronesi U, Casinelli N, Mariani L, Greco M, Saccozzi R, Luini A, Aguilar M, Marubini E: Twenty year follow-up of a randomized study comparing breast-conserving surgery with radical mastectomy for early breast cancer. N Engl J Med 2002;347(16):1227–1232
4. Skinner KA, Silberman H, Dougherty W, Gamagami P, Waisman J, Sposto R, Silverstein MJ: Breast cancer after augmentation mammoplasty. Ann Surg Oncol 2001;8(2):138–144
5. Miglioretti DL, Rutter CM, Geller BM, Cutter G, Barlow WE, Rosenberg R, et al.: Effect of breast augmentation on the accuracy of mammography and cancer characteristics. J Amer Med Assoc 2004;291(4):442–450
6. Handel N, Silverstein MJ, Gamagami P, Jensen JA, Collins A: Factors affecting mammographic visualization of the breast after augmentation mammaplasty. JAMA 1992;268(14):1913–1917
7. Kriege M, Brekelmans CT, Boetes C, Besnard PE, Zonderland HM, Obdeijn IM, et al: Efficacy of MRI and mammography for breast-cancer screening in women with a familial or genetic predisposition. N Engl J Med 2004;351(5):427–437
8. Freeman BS: Subcutaneous mastectomy for benign breast lesions with immediate or delayed prosthetic replacement. Plast Reconstr Surg 1962;30:676–682
9. Jensen JA: When can the nipple–areolar complex safely be spared during mastectomy? Plast Reconstr Surg 2002;109(2):805–807
10. Crowe J, Kim JA, Yetman R, Banbury J, Patrick RJ, Baynes D: Nipple-sparing mastectomy: technique and results of 54 procedures. Arch Surg 2004;139(2):148–150
11. Margulies AG, Hochberg J, Kepple J, Henry-Tillman RS, Westbrook K, Klimberg VS: Total skin sparing mastectomy with preservation of the nipple–areola complex. Am J Surg 2005;190(6):907–912
12. 12. Jensen JA: Should improved mastectomy and reconstruction alter the primary management of breast cancer? Plast Reconstr Surg 1999;103:1308–1310
13. Handel N, Lewinsky B, Jensen JA, Silverstein MJ: Breast conservation therapy after augmentation mammaplasty: is it appropriate? Plast Reconstr Surg 1996;98(7):1216–1224
14. Karanas YL, Leong DS, Da Lio A, Waldron K, Watson JP, Chang H, Shaw WW: Surgical treatment of breast cancer in previously augmented patients. Plast Reconstr Surg 2003;111(3):1078–1083

Serologic and Histologic Findings in Capsule Contracture Patients with Silicone Gel Implants

Lukas Prantl

77.1
Introduction

Since 1962 when the first silicone implants were developed in the United States, they have been widely used for reconstruction after breast amputation to correct breast malformations, dysplasia, and aplasia and for aesthetic breast augmentation. Local and systemic reactions of the body to implants are still under discussion and are the subject of intensive research to improve biocompatibility [1–3].

To decrease the rate of local complications caused by implants, such as progressive shrinking of the capsule (so-called capsular contracture) and penetration of silicone gel (so-called gel bleed) through the intact implant shell, silicone implants have undergone further development. The incidence of capsular contracture varies in the literature from less than 1% up to 74% [4, 5]. The high variability of the stated capsular contracture rate by various authors depends on many factors. An objective assessment of the degree of capsular contracture is difficult. The severity is mainly assessed by the purely clinical classification according to Baker [6]. This palpation method is largely dependent on the experience and sensitivity of the clinician. Often the studies are hardly comparable because different implant types of different implant generations were used. In addition, every implant company uses its own production process and its own editing. This demonstrates the importance of an study in which the mentioned variables (implant-specific factors) in addition to the individual factors are kept very small.

77.2
Investigations, Results, and Discussion

In prospective studies the author has tried to hold these variables very low. The author has also done long-term studies of the last implant generation with highly cohesive gel [4, 5, 7]. Histologic investigations of the capsular tissue are generally not comparable in previous studies because uniform histologic criteria are absent in the classification of the degree of capsular contracture. Such a classification was described by Wilflingseder and colleagues in 1983 [8], but this soon fell into oblivion.

On the basis of morphological investigations of implant capsules in support of the work of Wilflingseder and colleagues, the author set up a histologic classification of capsular contracture that correlates with clinical findings. It takes the pathogenetic mechanism into consideration and serves as a basis for further studies (Fig. 77.1) [7].

Histologically, the fibrous capsule shows a three-layer composition:
1. The internal layer abutting the silicone surface appears to be single-layered or multilayered containing macrophages and fibroblasts. In some cases, a pseudoepithelial cellular layer at the implant/capsule interface (synovia-like metaplasia) is found.
2. The middle layer consists of loosely arranged connective tissue including the internal vascular supply.
3. The outer layer is formed by dense connective tissue with the external vascular supply (Fig. 77.2a,b,c).

Semiquantitative analysis of samples of capsular tissue with regard to silicone content and the cellular inflammatory reaction was performed according to the above mentioned classification pattern. In implants with high gel cohesiveness, vacuolated macrophages with microcystic structures containing silicone and silicone particles are present in the capsular tissue. Silicone-charged macrophages in the form of foam cells could be found, preferably close to the implant, in 66.6%. Silicone deposits in the capsule were frequently surrounded by foam cells, giant foreign body cells, and other inflammation cells, representing siliconomas (Fig. 77.3). These distinctive silicone enrichments were demonstrated in 54.2% of the patients.

Grade	Baker	Wilflingseder
I	Implant shell not palpable and not visible	Thin and uncontracted capsule
II	Implant shell slightly firm, but not visible	"Constrictive fibrosis" no giant cells
III	Implant shell clearly firm and implant visible	"Constrictive fibrosis" giant cells present
IV	Implant shell very firm, implant dislocation and deformation	Inflammatory cells, foreign body granulomas, neovascularization, neuromas possible

Fig. 77.1 Clinical classification (Baker score) and histological classification (Wilflingseder score) of capsular contracture

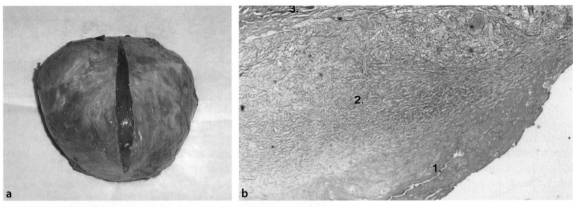

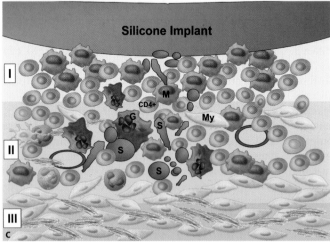

Fig. 77.2 **a** Fibrous capsule around the silicone implant. **b** Three-layer composition of the fibrous capsule. *1* Inner layer toward the implant. *2* Middle layer. *3* Outer layer. **c** The different cells of the tree-layer of the fibrous capsule

A positive correlation exists between the number of silicone particles and the degree of capsular contracture. High silicone content in the tissue is associated with a reinforced local inflammatory reaction and greater capsular thickness. Recently, it has been documented that silicone gel induces the activation of human macrophages, which leads to increased production of interleukin-1 (IL-1). IL-1, a proinflammatory cytokine,

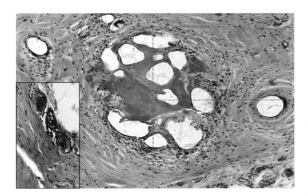

Fig. 77.3 Typical siliconoma: extracted silicone, foam cells, foreign body giant cells, and other inflammation cells

has an important regulatory effect on fibroblast proliferation and protein synthesis [9]. High levels of transforming growth factor beta (TGF-β), which stimulates fibroblasts to produce collagen, have been detected in peri-implant capsules. The author has hypothesized that the degree of capsular contracture is directly related to the inflammatory reaction and also to increased secretion of TGF-β [4, 7].

No correlations were found between the patient's age, time of implantation, or duration of implantation and the appearance of capsular contracture.

Periprosthetic bacterial contamination is also discussed as a potential cause of capsular contracture [10, 11]. None of the previous studies has demonstrated a relationship between bacterial contamination of the implant pocket and the degree of capsular contracture (Baker I–IV). In total, 16 (35.6%) of 45 capsules in the author's study showed positive swabs [12]. Coagulase-negative staphylococci (33.3%) were found most frequently, followed by *Propionibacterium acnes* (21.8%), *Staphylococcus aureus* (8.3%), *Escherichia coli*, and beta-hemolyzing streptococci colonies (4.2%). Interestingly, no colonization was detected in Baker I/II contractures, whereas the colonization rate in Baker III/IV contractures was 66.7%, showing a highly significant difference between the two groups. Current studies show an upregulation of toll-like receptor 2 (TLR-2), which induces activation of fibroblasts by *Propionibacterium acnes*. Other fibrosing diseases such as liver cirrhosis have also been reported to be associated with TLR-2 activation, so this mechanism should be investigated further to clarify its role in the process of capsular contracture [13].

The influence of surface texture (smooth versus textured), surface coating (polyurethane), implant filler (saline versus silicone), manner of insertion (inframammary, axillary, periareolar, or transareolar), and implant placement (subglandular, submuscular, subfascial) in the development of capsular contracture are discussed controversially in various studies. Although several studies showed an advantage of the textured implants after they were introduced, this advantage is not longer confirmed by long-time studies [1, 5, 14].

Besides silicone expression and subclinical bacterial colonization of implants, there must be additional individual factors that are independent of the implant bearers. According to other studies, a lymphoplasmacellular inflammation exists with some capsules without evidence of bacterial colonization or silicone extravasation. These findings suggest a need to search for serological fibrosis and immune stimulation parameters.

Serum hyaluronic acid (HA), the amino-terminal propeptide of procollagen type III (PIIINP), collagen type IV (CIV), and the matrix metalloproteinases (MMPs) as well as their natural inhibitors, the tissue inhibitors of metalloproteinases (TIMPs), play an important role in various fibrous tissue diseases [15]. Serum HA, PIIINP, and CIV can be tested for an accurate diagnosis of hepatic fibrosis at various stages, and serum levels of these markers correlate with the degree of fibrosis.

In 1934, Meyer and Palmer [16] described a procedure for isolating a novel glycosaminoglycan from the vitreous of bovine eyes. Today this macromolecule is most frequently referred to as hyaluronan. Its polymeric chemical structure consists of a sequential alignment of disaccharides, which are formed by D-glucuronic acid and D-N-acetylglucosamine. Hyaluronan is present in all vertebrates. It is a major constituent of extracellular matrices, and it is also found in blood, coming from the lymphoid circulation of peripheral tissues. The major biological function of hyaluronan is still unclear, and a variety of functions have been suggested for it. The presence of the polysaccharide itself seems to be of vital importance, since no inherited diseases lacking hyaluronan are known today. The production of hyaluronan is increased during inflammation, and generally, the viscous solutions seem to inhibit cellular activities. Hyaluronan seems to increase phagocytosis in monocytes and granulocytes, but the importance of this phenomenon is unknown [16].

In the author's study, the serum hyaluronan concentration of patients with capsular contracture after augmentation with smooth silicone breast implants was analyzed with an enzyme-linked immunosorbent assay (ELISA; Chugai, France) and compared with sera from 20 healthy female patients without capsular contracture. There was a significantly higher level ($p < 0.05$) of hyaluronan serum concentration in patients with capsular contracture (26 ± 14 µg/l) compared with control subjects (12 ± 6 µg/l). There was a positive correlation between the grade of capsular contracture (Baker grades I–IV) and hyaluronan serum concentration (Baker II, 15±3 µg/l; Baker III, 34±13 µg/l; Baker IV 42±11; r^2=0.73; $p<0.05$; Figs. 77.4, 77.5) [15].

Several studies have shown that PIIINP serves as a marker for the extent of skin fibrosis after major burn injury and for the risk of new severe fibrotic reactions after scar correction [17], but the author could not find a correlation between serum concentration of PIIINP and capsular contraction.

To clarify the role of single nucleotide polymorphisms (fibronectin 1/HSP60) that could be important in the development of capsular contracture, 30 patients were investigated with severe capsular contracture (Baker degree III/IV). An evaluation of these 30 patients and 66 controls showed no significant difference, so the study was temporarily interrupted.

The question of whether silicone implants can induce an autoimmune response and trigger a mixed image in musculoskeletal pain syndrome, partially connected with chronic states of exhaustion, lymphadenopathy, Reynaud's phenomenon, and neurological symptoms for

which the term "human adjuvant disease" or silicone-related (unclassified) connective tissue disease was chosen, has not been clarified yet [2, 18]. In 1999 the Institute of Medicine of the National Academy of Sciences published a comprehensive review on the safety of silicone breast implants to clarify the controversial relationships between silicone breast implants and systemic side effects [2]. Based on the data available, the Scientific Advisory Board concluded that there was no convincing evidence to support clinically significant immunologic effects of silicone or silicone breast implants. Although some silicones have adjuvant activity, the committee stated that there is no evidence that this has any clinical significance. After rigorous scientific review, in 2006 the U.S. Food and Drug Administration (FDA) approved the marketing of silicone-gel-filled breast implants made by two companies (Allergan and Mentor) for breast reconstruction in women of all ages and for breast augmentation in women ages 22 and older.

Nevertheless, most studies show that the controversy still persists regarding the ability of silicone materials to induce a specific immune reaction versus a nonspecific

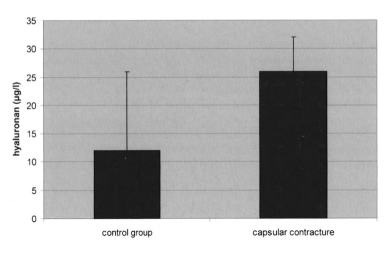

Fig. 77.4 Hyaluronan serum concentration in patients with capsular contracture (26±14 µg/l) compared with control subjects (12±6 µg/l), ($p<0.05$)

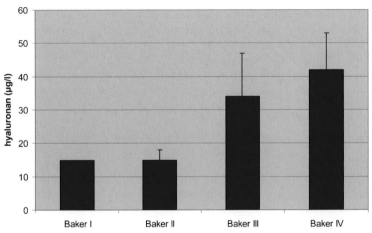

Fig. 77.5 Correlation between the grade of capsular contracture (Baker grade) and hyaluronan serum concentration (Baker grade II 15±3 µg/l; Baker grade III 34±13 µg/l; Baker grade IV 42±11; r^2=0.73, $p<0.05$)

inflammatory response. In the author's study, there was no difference in the distribution of peripheral lymphocyte subsets in patients with breast implants compared with normal controls (Fig. 77.6) [19]. In further studies the author would like to determine the immunological potential of peripheral blood lymphocytes regarding their cytokine production (e.g., IL-6, IL-8, IL-13, monocyte chemotactic protein-1). The ratio of proinflammatory, anti-inflammatory, and profibrotic cytokines might show in more detail whether implanted silicone material has a stimulating effect on the immune system. We want to specifically investigate the pivotal role of macrophages and mast cells in the inflammatory phase and scar formation to understand the effect of the

drugs that are already being used (leukotriene receptor antagonists) and to develop this further [20–22].

77.3 Conclusions

If we better understand the etiopathogenesis of severe capsular fibrosis, we may be able to reduce the number of patients who require surgical intervention (Fig. 77.7). New strategies might include the development of implants to reduce silicone extravasations, implant coatings that contain novel immunosuppressive agents [e.g., mammalian target of rapamycin (mTOR) inhibitors or

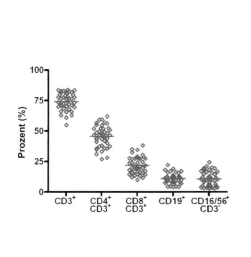

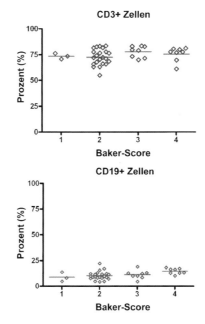

Fig. 77.6 Peripheral blood lymphocyte populations in patients with capsular contracture (*n*=41) compared with normal values (**a**) and in correlation with the Baker score (**b,c**)

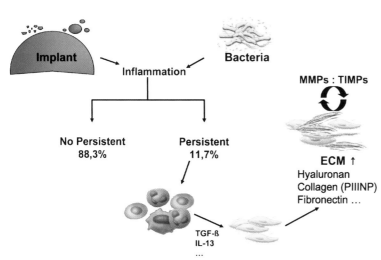

Fig. 77.7 Pathogenetic mechanism of the capsular contracture. Fibrosis is the end result of chronic inflammatory reactions induced by silicone and/or bacterial contamination of the implant. In our patients in 11.7 % the inflammation persisted and lead to increased production of cytokines (Il-13, TGF-ß) with activation of myofibroblasts, the key cellular mediators of fibrosis. The deposition of ECM (collagen) increase. The net amount of collagen deposited by fibroblasts is regulated continuously by collagen synthesis and collagen catabolism. The turnover of collagen and other ECM proteins is controlled by various MMPs and their inhibitors (tissue inhibitors of metalloproteinases) TIMPs

TLR antagonists] in combination with intraluminal antibiotics or antibiotic coatings, and new drugs to reduce or prevent the inflammatory reaction and thus fibrosis. At the moment there are many different recommendations for preventing or treating capsular contracture, including breast massage, external ultrasound, preintervention prophylactic single-dose antibiotics, papaverine (to relax the smooth-muscle-like fibers), vitamin E (to soften the collagen strands), leukotriene receptor antagonists, and, finally, surgical intervention. It may be possible to modify the leukotriene receptor antagonists so as to alter the inflammatory cascade, thereby preventing a severe fibrotic reaction.

References

1. Handel N, Cordray T, Gutierrez J, Jensen JA: A long-term study of outcomes, complications, and patient satisfaction with breast implants. Plast Reconstr Surg 2006;117(3):757–767

2. Bondurant S, Ernster V, Herdman R (eds): Safety of Silicone Breast Implants. Committee on the Safety of Silicone Breast Implants, Division of Health Promotion and Disease Prevention, Institute of Medicine. Washington, DC, National Academy Press 1999

3. Adams WP Jr, Haydon MS, Raniere J Jr, Trott S, Marques M, Feliciano M, Robinson JB Jr, Tang L, Brown SA: A rabbit model for capsular contracture: development and clinical implications. Plast Reconstr Surg 2006;117(4):1214–1219; discussion 1220–1221

4. Prantl L, Schreml S, Fichtner-Feigl S, Pöppl N, Roll C, Eisenmann-Klein M, Hofstädter F: Histologische und immunhistochemische Untersuchungen bei Kapselkontraktur nach glatten Brustimplantaten. Handchir Mikrochir Plast Chir 2006;38(4):224–232

5. Prantl L, Pöppl N, Horvat N, Heine N, Eisenmann-Klein M: Serologic and histologic findings in patients with capsular contracture after breast augmentation with smooth silicone gel implants: is serum hyaluronan a potential predictor? Aesthet Plast Surg 2005;29(6):510–518

6. Spear SL, Baker JL Jr.: Classification of capsular contracture after prosthetic breast reconstruction. Plast Reconstr Surg 1995;96(5):1119–1123

7. Prantl L, Schreml S, Fichtner-Feigl S, Pöppl N, Eisenmann-Klein M, Schwarze H, Füchtmeier B: Clinical and morphological conditions by capsular contracture formed around silicone breast implants. Plast Reconstr Surg 2007;120(1):275–284

8. Mikuz G, Hoinkes G, Propst A, Wilflingseder P: Tissue reactions with silicone rubber implants (morphological, microchemical, and clinical investigations in humans and laboratory animals). In: Hastings GW, Ducheyne P (eds). Macromolecular Biomaterials. Boca Raton, FL, CRC Press 1983, pp 239–249

9. Tavazzani F, Xing S, Waddell JE, Smith D, Boynton EL: In vitro interaction between silicone gel and human monocyte-macrophages. J Biomed Mater Res A 2005;72(2):161–167

10. Pittet B, Montandon D, Pittet D: Infection in breast implants. Lancet Infect Dis 2005;5(2):94–106

11. Pajkos A, Deva AK, Vickery K, Cope C, Chang L, Cossart YE: Detection of subclinical infection in significant breast implant capsules. Plast Reconstr Surg 2003;111(5):1605–1611

12. Schreml S, Eisenmann-Klein M, Prantl L: Bacterial infection is of major relevance for high-grade capsular contracture in breast implants. Ann Plast Surg 2007;59(2):126–130

13. Jugeau S, Tenaud I, Knol AC, Jarrousse V, Quereux G, Khammari A, Dreno B: Induction of toll-like receptors by *Propionibacterium acnes*. Br J Dermatol 2005;153(6):1105–1113

14. Poeppl N, Schreml S, Lichtenegger F, Lenich A, Eisenmann-Klein M, Prantl L: Does the surface structure of implants have an impact on the formation of a capsular contracture? Aesthet Plast Surg 2007;31(1):133–139

15. Prantl L, Angele P, Schreml S, Ulrich D, Pöppl N, Eisenmann-Klein M: Determination of serum fibrosis indexes in patients with capsular contracture after augmentation with smooth silicone gel implants. Plast Reconstr Surg 2006;118(1):224–229

16. Meyer K, Palmer JW: The polysaccharide of the vitreous humor. J Biol Chem 1934;107:629–634

17. Ulrich D, Noah EM, von Heimburg D, Pallua N: TIMP-1, MMP-2, MMP-9, and PIIINP as serum markers for skin fibrosis in patients following severe burn trauma. Plast Reconstr Surg 2003;111(4):1423–1431

18. Janowsky EC, Kupper LL, Hulka BS: Meta-analyses of the relation between silicone breast implants and the risk of connective-tissue diseases. N Engl J Med 2000;342(11):781–790

19. Prantl L, Fichtner-Feigl S, Hofstädter F, Lenich A, Eisenmann-Klein M, Schreml S: Flow cytometric analysis of peripheral blood lymphocyte subsets in patients with silicone breast implants. Plast Reconstr Surg 2008;121(1):25–30

20. Niessen FB, Spauwen PH, Schalkwijk J, Kon M: On the nature of hypertrophic scars and keloids: a review. Plast Reconstr Surg 1999;104(5):1435–1458

21. Schlesinger SL, Ellenbogen R, Desvigne MN, Svehlak S, Heck R: Zafirlukast (Accolate): a new treatment for capsular contracture. Aesth Surg J 2002;22:329–335

22. Scuderi N, Mazzocchi M, Fioramonti P, Bistoni G: The effects of zafirlukast on capsular contracture: preliminary report. Aesthet Plast Surg 2006;30(5):513–520

CHAPTER 78

Medical-Legal Aspects of Breast Augmentation   78

Melvin A. Shiffman

78.1
Introduction

Medical malpractice suits are upsetting, depressing, and frustrating for surgeons in cosmetic breast surgery who have done the "best they can" and still encounter complications or a dissatisfied patient. Surgeons must understand the medical-legal consequences of their practice, especially when elective cosmetic surgery is performed and litigation follows.

78.2
Requirements for Medical Negligence

The plaintiff's attorney must establish all four aspects of negligence in order to pursue a case of medical negligence.

78.2.1
Duty

When the physician establishes a relationship with a patient, the physician has a duty of due care in the care and treatment of that patient.

78.2.2
Breach of Duty

The physician may breach that duty by not using adequate skill and knowledge in treating a patient. This breach may be established by an expert witness testifying to the opinion that the defendant failed to follow the standard of care. The type of breaches may also include lack of informed consent. A lay jury may establish the standard if the facts are within the knowledge and experience of laypersons. This can best be seen in a case in which a foreign body (sponge, instrument) was left in the surgical wound.

78.2.3
Injury

An injury, physical or mental, to the plaintiff must be shown by the facts of the case, usually through the medical records.

78.2.4
Causation

Causation requires that the injury be caused by the breach of duty. For example, the breach of the standard of care may have been failure to place a breast implant under the muscle on the right side, but the injury was capsule contracture on the left side.

78.3
Standard of Care

The standard of care is what a reasonably prudent (careful) physician would do under the same or similar circumstances. The court considers expert testimony to establish the standard of care in most instances except if the circumstances are in the purview of a layperson. Also, the court may consider what a responsible minority of physicians would do under the same or similar circumstances. The medical literature may help establish the standard of care.

The standard can also be what a reasonably prudent physician in a responsible minority would do under the same or similar circumstances.

78.4
Informed Consent

78.4.1
Definition

The patient has the absolute right to receive enough information about his or her diagnosis, proposed treatment, prognosis, and possible risks of proposed therapy and alternatives to enable him or her to make a knowledgeable decision. The patient is the one who makes all the decisions, in opposition to the old paternalistic view that gave the physician complete control over all decisions. A physician would now have to prove that the decision he or she made was because of the patient's inability to make the decision or because there was an extreme emergency.

Other requirements of the informed consent doctrine in law require that a complication that was not explained to the patient did in fact occur and that the patient would not have agreed to have the surgery if he or she had been informed of that particular risk or complication.

78.4.2
Legal Definition

In terms of surgical procedures, the surgeon must have explained to the patient the nature and purpose of any proposed operation or treatment, any viable alternatives, and the material risks and benefits of both. All of the patient's questions must have been answered.

In order for the plaintiff to succeed in a complaint for lack of informed consent, he or she must show 1) that the risk or complication, which was not explained to the plaintiff, did indeed occur, and 2) that if the plaintiff had been informed of that particular risk, he or she would not have consented to the surgical procedure.

There are different means of proof at trial depending on the jurisdiction (state). The opinion as to which risks are "material" to the patient in order to make his or her decision under the same or similar circumstances can be that of:

1. A reasonably prudent physician: This allows a physician to testify as to what is material.
2. A reasonably prudent patient: This allows the jury to decide what a reasonably prudent patient would consider material risks.
3. The plaintiff patient: This places the onus on the plaintiff to decide what the material risks would be. The cosmetic surgery patient may be unique because cosmetic surgeries are elective procedures and not medically required except, perhaps, for the patient's mental well-being.

78.5
Patient Rapport

There is nothing as important as a good doctor–patient relationship before performing cosmetic breast surgery. This requires careful discussion between the patient and the doctor or another caring, empathetic staff person about the surgical procedure proposed, viable alternatives, and the potential risks and complications of each. The surgeon must, at the very least, give the patient the opportunity to ask questions of him or her to allow the patient to feel more comfortable with the person doing the surgery. Be careful when the patient is first seen by the surgeon on the day of surgery—this is not a good idea if ultimate litigation is to be avoided. If a patient is coming from a long distance or another state, a consultation can usually be done at least the day or night before surgery.

There should be strict control of all staff persons involved in the patient's care so that incorrect information is not given to the patient and that the patient is not told, "Don't worry." This requires detailed training of each of the office staff, from receptionist to scrub tech and registered nurse, on what to say and what not to say to patients and how to respond to patients' problems.

No one should get angry with a patient or appear rushed. The patient should be treated with respect and dignity. Questions must be answered and phone calls returned in a timely fashion.

78.6
Complications

If a complication occurs, the surgeon should be available to talk to the patient, examine the wound, and explain how long it will take for the complication to subside. Every complication seen by the office personnel should be reported to the surgeon, and the surgeon should decide what to do.

Any complication can lead to a lawsuit, even if it appears minor, because the patient may think it is major. Remember that the cosmetic surgery patient, despite all the warnings about possible complications, believes that there will be no complications and that she or he will look much better than before the surgery.

78.7
The Angry Patient

If a patient shows anger, whatever the cause, the surgeon should try to handle the problem in an expeditious manner. That means speaking with the patient to find out the cause of the anger and figure out ways to satisfy the patient. Avoiding this type of patient after surgery will frequently lead to litigation. Therefore, the physician should answer all phone calls in a timely fashion, show a truthful and caring attitude, and see the patient frequently enough to satisfy the patient's needs.

78.8
Medical Record

Handwriting that cannot be deciphered should be avoided. Not only is this irritating to the attorneys and expert witnesses, but the state medical board may find this to be inadequate record-keeping and thus unprofessional conduct, and loss of medical license may ensue. Handwritten notes are a continuous problem especially when, years later, the doctor who wrote the note cannot read it.

Typewritten notes are easy to read and usually contain much more information than written notes. This author dictates all of the medical record notes. The cost to get a microcassette for dictation and hire someone to transcribe the dictation will save the surgeon time at minimal cost, including maintaining his or her medical license.

78.9
Legal Aspects

The first thing an attorney thinks is that a bad result was the surgeon's fault because of a negligent act. This may include claims of poor training, lack of skill, or inattention during surgery. The attorney will seek out an "expert witness" to show a breach in the standard of care. The standard of care is essentially a legal term referring to what a reasonably prudent (careful) physician would do under the same or similar circumstances. The defendant surgeon's attorney will try to find an expert witness to show that there was no breach in the standard of care. The surgeon should be realistic because everyone makes mistakes, and the expert witness should not be biased and should give an honest opinion as to whether or not the standard of care was breached.

78.10
The Misinformed Expert Witness

There are times when the expert witness in medical malpractice litigation is not aware of advances made in breast augmentation or what the standard of care really means. When this happens, misinformation is provided to the court that may be difficult to refute. There are also instances in which different training and experience come into play.

For instance, the rate of capsule contracture has been different between the smooth and the textured implant (i.e., more capsule contracture with smooth implants). Implants have changed over the past 20 years, and prior information may not be the same. For instance, Fragen

[1] stated in 2007 that the rate of capsule contracture was 4% (eight out of 200 patients) with smooth implants. This is comparable to the contracture rate of textured implants. There is now controversy about whether there is a difference in capsule contracture rate when the implant is placed under or over the pectoralis muscle. Previous reports stated that the contracture rate was higher in the submammary position compared with the subpectoral position, but more recent discussions have described similar contracture rates with proper examination since the implant under the muscle is more difficult to palpate in order to feel the contracture.

Experts have stated that inadvertent placement of an implant under or over the muscle is below the standard of care, even in a blind dissection from the axillary or umbilical incision. But there is no such standard of care because inadvertent placement is accidental and not necessarily from poor technique, lack of training, lack of skill, or lack of knowledge. The use of an endoscope is not a requirement for either of these access incisions but is useful for the beginner to appreciate the problems of dissection.

78.11
Legal Cases

McMillan v. Dow Corning Corp.; Rosenfeld; New York (NY) Supreme Court, Index No. 26858/92. In: Med Malpr Verdict Settlements Experts 2005;21(5):36–37

The 30-year-old plaintiff had breast augmentation and mastopexy. The plaintiff claimed that too much pressure was placed on the tissue, leading to excessive scarring, that her nipples were raised, and that too much tissue was removed. The defense argued that the plaintiff had good results, that her nipples were properly raised and repositioned, and that the plaintiff had had a tattoo placed on her chest after the procedure, an action that countered the plaintiff's argument that she was embarrassed by her appearance. There was a confidential settlement with the manufacturer and a jury verdict for the defense.

Comment: The defendant lost the case against the surgeon by lying about her embarrassment, and the scar was a known complication of the procedure.

Zaika v. Swartz; Cook County (IL) Circuit Court, Case No. 01L-7146. In: Med Malpr Verdicts Settlements Experts 2005;21(1):41

The 29-year-old plaintiff had breast augmentation in June 1999. The right breast appeared too high and too lateral compared with the left, so a second surgery was performed in October 1999. The right breast remained too high and lateral. The plaintiff claimed that the defendant negligently created implant pockets that were asymmetrical and in the wrong location. The defendant maintained that the plaintiff developed capsule contracture that caused the breast to shift or displace and that this is a known complication of the surgery. There was a jury verdict for $1,000,000.

Comment: Capsule contracture and asymmetry are known complications of breast augmentation, and the award should not have been as high as it was, which leads to the presumption that something else was going on at trial such as an arrogant defendant or misrepresentations by the plaintiff's expert. There is no way to determine what actually happened.

Houston v. Carli; Los Angeles County (CA) Judicial Arbitration Mediation. In: Med Malpr Verdicts Settlements Experts 2005;21(11):41–42

The 37-year-old plaintiff had breast augmentation through an axillary approach. She developed left brachial plexus injury with severe pain in the arm. The plaintiff claimed that the defendant was negligent for failing to guard the brachial plexus. The defendant denied negligence and argued that the injury occurred while trying to secure a bleeder. There was an arbitration award of $291,089.

Comment: There is very little excuse for a brachial plexus injury in an axillary approach to breast augmentation, although this is a known complication of the procedure. Great care should be taken when trying to secure a bleeder in the axilla. The surgeon should not use cautery or a hemostat on tissue unless all the vessels and nerves in the area can be visualized.

Schubert v. Dolsky; Philadelphia County (PA) Common Pleas Court, Case No. 940803583. In: Med Malpr Verdicts Settlements Experts 2005;21(11):42

The 22-year-old plaintiff had breast augmentation with polyurethane-coated silicone-gel-filled implants in 1985 by the defendant. In 1992 the defendant ordered a mammogram, which did not indicate any problems. In 1993 the defendant performed a breast examination and noted firmness on the left breast representing the palpable edge of the implant. An ultrasound was done that indicated that both implants were ruptured. At explantation surgery, the right implant was noted to be intact although there was a large amount of free silicone in the pocket. The plaintiff claimed that she did not receive the information necessary to give an informed consent because the defendant did not advise her of the risk that the implants could wear out and break and that the defendant was negligent in delaying the diagnosis of implant rupture. The plaintiff also claimed that the silicone caused multiple medical problems, including neurologic deficits, disfigurement, and sleeplessness. The defendant denied that any of the plaintiff's prob-

lems were related to silicone leakage. There was a jury verdict for the defendant.

Comment: Ultimately it has been shown that silicone does not cause autoimmune disease. Deflation or rupturing of implants is a known risk of breast augmentation surgery. The delay in diagnosis of the rupture did not result in any injury except for continued medical symptoms, but it is not known whether the plaintiff's symptoms cleared up after removal of the implants.

Douthitt v. Basselberg; U.S. District Court, District of Maryland, Case No. 1:03-CV-01741. In: Med Malpr Verdicts Settlements Experts 2005;21(12):42

The 40-year-old plaintiff had breast augmentation after which she had the appearance of a "double breast" on each side, with the implants appearing to have shifted downward and the nipples having transmigrated down. The plaintiff claimed that the wrong size of implants was used and that the situation could not be corrected because there would be double scarring. The defendant failed to appear for trial, and his carrier denied coverage due to lack of cooperation. The jury awarded the plaintiff $622,500.

Comment: There is never an excuse for a physician to fail to appear at his or her trial for malpractice. Insurance coverage depends on the defendant's ability to help in his or her own defense. The claim that the implants were the wrong size would depend on what the defendant would say as far as informed consent and what was told to the plaintiff before surgery. Correction of the deformity should have been easy with one surgical procedure despite the excuse of a possibility of a double scar, since scars can be concealed very nicely in the areola.

Mitchell v. Chu; Chautauqua County (NY) Supreme Court, Index No. 1000168/04. In: Med Malpr Verdicts Settlements Experts 2006;21(11):41

The 21-year-old plaintiff had asymmetry of the breast that was corrected by insertion of a single breast implant and bilateral mastopexy. The plaintiff complained that the procedure did not correct the asymmetry, that there were severe residual scars, that the right breast had a deformity resembling an extra nipple, that the defendant failed to obtain informed consent by failing to explain that the mastopexy would move her nipples and decrease their size, and that the defendant was negligent in performing the surgery. The defendant acknowledged that he did not recall the specific information he had addressed but contended that he typically discusses all aspects of the procedure being considered, that the scars were not optimal, and that the plaintiff's smoking impaired healing. There was a jury verdict for $553,826.

Comment: The patient's chart did not contain enough information to show that the informed consent discussion was held or what was discussed. Mastopexy almost always results in significant scarring, and it should be obvious, even to a layperson, that a breast lift will move the nipples upward.

Swanson v. Widenhouse; U.S. District Court, District of South Carolina at Charleston, Case No. 2:03-CV-03938. In: Med Malpr Verdicts Settlements Experts 2006;21(11):42

The 49-year-old plaintiff had a breast augmentation and postoperatively was slow in healing. The plaintiff claimed that there was permanent scarring, breast pain, and misshapen breast and that the defendant used a substandard surgical technique. The defendant argued that the plaintiff's complications were due to poor wound healing and were known complications of the surgery. There was a defense verdict.

Comment: Scarring and breast deformity are known risks of breast augmentation. There was no statement in the record that the patient was a smoker, which would have been a probable cause of the delayed wound healing.

Zien v. Stompro; Contra Costa County (CA) Superior Court, Case No, CIV-MSC-03-00701. In: Med Malpr Verdicts Settlements Experts 2007;23(1):43

The 31-year-old plaintiff had implant replacement by the defendant. The surgery was necessary because one implant was leaking, and both implants were too far lateral. The defendant agreed to replace the implants with a type of implant (Silimed) that was less likely to leak or move laterally. The defendant had difficulties placing the implants through the areolar incision and after 3 h used a different set of implants. The next day the defendant and plaintiff agreed to attempt replacement of the desired implants without charge. This time an inframammary incision was used. The plaintiff claimed that she never consented to the placement of the implants used in the initial surgery. The defendant argued that the placement had consented to placement of either type of implant and that the surgery had been performed properly. There was a judgment for $51,600.

Comment: The problem with using a new type of implants is that the full risks and complications may not be known to the surgeon. The manufacturer, even with the sales representative present at the time of surgery, may not have informed the surgeon about similar previous problems encountered, or the problem faced by the surgeon may never have occurred before. The jury believed the plaintiff and not the defendant.

Allis v. Boemi; Collier County (FL) Circuit Court, Case No. 94-0031-35. In: Med Malpr Verdicts Settlements Experts 2007;23(5):41

The plaintiff had a breast lift and augmentation, followed by intense pain in her breasts. The nipple and areola as well as some of the breast tissue bilaterally became necrotic. The plaintiff underwent 13 surgeries to repair the wounds and reshape the breasts. The plaintiff's expert stated that the breast lift and breast augmentation should not have been performed in the same surgery. The plaintiff claimed that the implants were used without consent. The defendant claimed that the procedure was proper and that the unfortunate result had nothing to do with how the surgery was performed. There was a verdict for $8,250,000.

Comment: The plaintiff's claim that the implants were used without consent could very well have convinced the jury that the damages suffered were from a battery ("a touching without consent") and may have been influential in the verdict, or the jury could have felt sorry about the number of surgeries necessary to repair damage. The use of implants at the same time as a mastopexy may result in slightly more complications, but most patients prefer to have one surgery rather than two. Most surgeons perform both procedures at the same time, and this would not be below the standard of care.

Storme v. Baeke, Jr.; Johnson County (KS) District Court, Case No. 03CV07684. In: Med Malpr Verdicts Settlements Experts 2007;23(6):41

The plaintiff underwent breast augmentation by the defendant, following which surgery the implants rotated and were moveable by the patient. Two revisional surgeries were necessary. The plaintiff alleged that her before-and-after photos were used on the defendant's Web site without her permission. The defendant claimed that the plaintiff initially gave consent, but later withdrew the consent. There was a $36,000 verdict for invasion of privacy. The manufacturer, Mentor, had a confidential settlement.

Comment: The use of a patient's photos without consent is actionable even if the patient gave consent initially but withdrew the consent later.

Lukyan v. Swarz; Cook County (IL) Circuit Court, Case No. 01-L-007146. In: Med Malpr Verdicts Settlements Experts 2005;21(9):46

The 29-year-old plaintiff had breast augmentation by the defendant. Following the procedure, the breast became asymmetrical and necessitated a second procedure on the right breast. The procedure was unsuccessful and resulted in permanent disfigurement. The plaintiff alleged that the defendant negligently created pockets that were asymmetrical and in the wrong location. There was a judgment for $1,000,000.

Comment: Postoperative asymmetry is a known risk of breast augmentation. Implants can move and form asymmetrical pockets without surgeon negligence. Complications from a secondary procedure are also known risks and may not be due to negligence. Severe deformity can sway a jury to give excessive compensation.

78.12
Discussion

Physicians should keep prevention of malpractice litigation in mind by keeping medical records that are more than adequate, especially including all informed consent discussions and their content. Physicians may have difficulty recalling discussions with patients unless that information is in writing. Patients have to understand that complications occur even in elective cases such as breast augmentation and that more than one procedure may be necessary. It is possible that the patient may not recall all the risks and complications discussed by the surgeon months or years previously and may think that some of the complications were not discussed [2]. It is also necessary for the patient to state that if the complication had been discussed, he or she would not have had the surgery.

Timely diagnosis and treatment of complications are essential to limit any damage. The surgeon must be prepared to discuss with the patient the cause of the complication, the treatment, the time it will take healing to occur, and further surgery that might be necessary.

For breast augmentation, chronic smokers either should be avoided as patients or the record must show reasonable efforts to have the patient stop smoking and that the patient complied. It should be explained to the patient that smoking, even in decreased amounts, will likely result in poor and delayed healing, possible tissue necrosis, and significantly increased scarring.

The surgeon should be aware that trials are unpredictable as to the results and that they depend quite a bit on the skilled attorney and the persuasive expert witness. Arbitration as an alternative to trial is less emotionally charged and shorter in time, but it is associated with more likelihood of payment to the plaintiff, but usually less an amount than would be given at trial.

Mediation is a method for the court to reduce the number of cases going to trial. In this instance the judge will have the attorneys argue both sides of the case in the absence of witnesses. The attorneys will try to wear each other down for a final settlement. In the meantime, the defendant and plaintiff sit outside the courtroom, and their attorneys bring them the offers for them to decide. This may go on for days.

References

1. Fragen R: Things I've learned and total submuscular breast implants. Presented at the American Society of Cosmetic Breast Surgery, 23rd ASCBS Annual Workshop, Newport Beach, CA, 4–7 May 2007

2. Shiffman MA: Cognitive dysfunction in the postoperative patient. Plast Reconstr Surg 2001;107(4):1079–1080

CHAPTER 79

Editor's Commentary

Melvin A. Shiffman

79.1
Introduction

A few commentaries are part of the privilege of being editor. This allows me to interject some of my own opinions on some perhaps controversial subjects. Forty-two years of experience with breast augmentation have taught me that complications are inevitable at some time or other and that we as surgeons should learn from our mistakes, misjudgments, and plain misfortunes.

79.2
Capsulectomy Versus Capsulotomy for the Treatment of Capsular Contraction

There are specific indications for capsulectomy for treating capsule contracture. These consist of patients with calcified [1] and thickened capsules and removal of ruptured gel implants intact without spillage. Performing a capsulectomy in a thin patient may result in palpable rippling or knuckling, especially with thicker-walled textured implants used for replacement [2]. Capsulectomy is more difficult than capsulotomy and causes more bleeding, which may result in a slightly higher incidence of recurrent capsular contracture (35%) [3].

When removing breast implants permanently, it may not be necessary to do capsulectomy because the capsules contract and dissipate gradually over a year with pericapsular vascular proliferation [3]. The capsule should not be left if calcified because it may become palpable after the implants are removed. However, if there is silicone spillage or excessive blood in the cavity while the capsule is still present, there may be tumor formation from siliconoma or hematoma [4, 5]. If the hematoma persists, calcification can occur. One alternative to capsulectomy is scoring the capsule anteriorly and posteriorly with electrocautery in criss-crossing patterns to stimulate fibrosis and attachment of the anterior capsule to the posterior capsule so that the space is obliterated.

There are very few complications with capsulotomy for treating capsular contracture except for a 30% incidence of recurrence [3, 6]. Closed compression capsulotomy should be avoided because this can cause a hematoma or rupture the prosthesis.

79.3
Retropectoral Versus Retromammary Breast Implantation

Placement of the prosthesis in a retropectoral position reduces the incidence of a grade II–IV capsule contracture requiring capsule release [7]. However, retropectoral placement of the implant involves more postoperative pain than with the retromammary position, and there can be distortion of the breast with contraction of the pectoralis major muscle.

The retropectoral implant tends to have less of the superior pole "drop-off" that makes the implant noticeable. Comparing retromammary and retropectoral implants in a variety of individuals, it is essentially impossible to tell by visualization which pocket the implant is in [8].

Retromammary placement of the prosthesis in a thin individual is likely to cause the implant to be more visible, with a cup-like appearance, and is objectionable to some patients.

In order for the patient to make an informed decision, all of this information should be explained to the patient prior to surgery.

79.4
Capsule Contracture After Breast Irradiation for Cancer

The treatment of early breast cancer is usually lumpectomy or quadrantectomy followed by irradiation and chemotherapy. There is a high incidence of capsule contracture in implant-augmented patients following irradiation [9–11]. This editor's experience has been a low incidence of capsule contracture in this situation if the patient manipulates the prosthesis firmly throughout the pocket during irradiation of the breast and for 12 months afterward.

79.5
Antibacterial Irrigation in Pocket Before Insertion of Prosthesis

It has always been my contention that antibacterial irrigation was essential when inserting the prosthesis into the breast pocket. In fact, the implants probably should also be soaked in the same solution. I used povidone (Betadine) for many years and then Ancef solution and had one patient with infection in over 1,000 cases. Burkhardt and Eades [12] found that povidone-iodine irrigation resulted in contracture in 4% of cases compared to 50% when only saline was used for irrigation. Subclinical infection in the pocket is a likely cause of the excessive capsule contracture when no antibacterial irrigation was used.

79.6
Textured Versus Smooth Implants

Hakelius and Ohlsen reported a study comparing smooth and textured silicone gel implants [13]. Twenty-five patients received a smooth implant on one side and a textured implant on the other side. On the textured implant side, 13% (17 patients) had grade II capsule contracture, and one patient had rippling. On the smooth side, 17 patients (68%) had the smooth implant changed to a textured implant because of firmness (six had rippling with the textured implant), and of the eight original breasts with smooth implants, four were grade I, three grade II, and one grade III.

This confirms the impression of most surgeons that textured silicone gel breast implants have less capsule contracture than smooth implants but more rippling. With smooth saline implants there is less rippling but more capsule contracture, except with the transumbilical approach (less bleeding).

79.7
Comparison of the Mentor Siltex Textured Implant and the McGhan BioCell Textured Implant

Both the Mentor Siltex implant and the McGhan Bio-Cell implant are generally effective in reducing capsular contracture [13–16]. However, the depth and width vary between the two implants [17]. Textured BioCell has better stability attributable to tissue adherence [18]. When the depth of the texture is over 100 μm there is more adherence, but that may not mean less capsule contracture. Further studies are needed to compare BioCell with Siltex as to the rate of capsule contracture.

79.8
Under or Over the Pectoralis Major Muscle: Capsule Contracture Rates

The general impression has been that placing the implant under the muscle results in a lower rate of capsule contracture than placing the implant over the muscle. Part of the reasoning was that the muscle action that massages the implant during body motion reduces the capsule contracture rate and that an implant's position under the muscle reduces the detection of capsule contracture that is present. However, there have been reports that the capsule contracture rate is the same whether the implant is under or over the muscle [19, 20].

79.9
Umbilical Approach to Breast Augmentation

Although there is not a large group of surgeons using the umbilical approach to augmentation, it is a procedure that leads to less capsule contracture, probably because there is less bleeding (the dissection is blunt, and an expander is used that expands the pocket but also compresses the vessels). The procedure requires training and experience. The inexperienced surgeon has more problems with an elevated implant, but this resolves with experience. There is a possibility of placing the implant in an incorrect pocket position, above or below the muscle, which may not be diagnosed during surgery even with an endoscope (the pectoralis minor muscle, with attachments to the 4th and 5th ribs, can appear to be the pectoralis major muscle). There is no standard of care requiring the use of an endoscope to perform the transumbilical approach because many surgeons, with experience, perform the procedure without using one.

79.10
Treatment of Implant Pocket Infection

If the breast develops erythema after implant augmentation, this can be a mastitis or infection. The conservative approach is to treat the problem by increasing the dose of the antibiotic or changing the antibiotic. If the inflamed area does not start to resolve within 72 h, then the surgeon should consider intravenous antibiotics or removal of the implant. If after 72 h there is no improvement, the implant should be removed, culture and sensitivity taken, and the pocket irrigated with saline and an antibiotic solution and then drained with either a Penrose or a suction catheter.

Replacement of the new implant should be delayed for at least 3 months after complete healing of the wound. Replacements any sooner than that have a high incidence of reinfection.

79.11
Autologous Fat Augmentation of the Breast

The use of autologous fat to augment the breast is not below the standard of care. The fat is not injected directly into the breast anymore but into the space under the pectoralis major muscle, in the muscle, and into the space above the muscle. Inadvertent injection of fat into the breast may still occur. Injection of fat into the breast itself has never been found to prevent or delay the diagnosis of cancer. If calcifications from fat necrosis cannot be identified as definitely benign, then a stereotactic needle biopsy will make a definitive diagnosis.

79.12
The Perfect Breast

"The breast that is symmetrical and perfect except for size will become the perfect breast after surgery." This is indeed rare. Most breast pairs are asymmetrical in some fashion, such as one breast being larger, one nipple–areolar complex being larger or higher, or the nipple–areolar complexes being too lateral or too medial. These problems sometimes need readjustments at the time of surgery, such as a larger implant on one side, periareolar reduction, or lateral or medial crescent mastopexy.

Many patients seem to expect perfection, and the limitations should be pointed out to them prior to surgery. The surgeon must know the limits of being able to correct small problems and know when "perfection is the enemy of good." The more surgeries performed to correct beast asymmetry, the more likely that there will be a major complication. Sometimes removal of both prostheses is the solution to the problem, such as with chronic recurrence of capsular contracture, and the patient should be advised that the prostheses need to be permanently removed. The surgeon should refuse to do more surgeries despite all the patient's protestations because litigation will otherwise result.

References

1. Riefkohl R: Augmentation mammoplasty. In: McCarthy JG (ed). Plastic Surgery. Philadelphia, WB Saunders 1990, pp 3879–3896

2. Collis N, Platt AJ, Batchelor AG: Pectoralis major "trap-door" flap for silicone breast implant medial knuckle deformities. Plast Reconstr Surg 2001;108(7):2133–2135

3. Hipps CJ, Raju DR: Straith RE: Influence of some operative and postoperative factors on capsular contracture around breast prostheses. Plast Reconstr Surg 1978;61(3):384–389

4. Friedman HI, Friedman AC, Carson K: The fate of the fibrous capsule after saline implant removal. Ann Plast Surg 2001;46(3):215–221

5. Sinclair DS, Spigos DG, Olsen J: Case 2: retained silicone and fibrous capsule in the right breast and retained fibrous capsule in the left breast after removal of implants. AJR Am J Roentgenol 2000;175(3):862–864

6. Little G, Baker JL: Results of closed compression capsulotomy for treatment of contracted breast implant capsules. Plast Reconstr Surg 1980;65(1):30–33

7. Biggs TM, Yarish RS: Augmentation mammaplasty: retropectoral versus retromammary implantation. Clin Plast Surg 1988;15(4):549–555

8. Morgan WR: How to do breast implant surgery. Presented at the American Society of Cosmetic Breast Surgery, Newport Beach, CA, 3–6 June 2005

9. Handel N, Lewinsky B, Jensen, JA, Silverstein MJ: Breast conservation therapy after breast augmentation: is it appropriate? Plast Reconstr Surg 1996;98(7):1216–1224

10. Mark RJ, Zimmerman RP, Grerif JM: Capsular contracture after lumpectomy and radiation therapy in patients who have undergone uncomplicated bilateral augmentation mammoplasty. Radiology 1996;200(3):621–625

11. Guenther JM, Tokita KM, Giuliano AE: Breast-conserving surgery and radiation after augmentation mammoplasty. Cancer 1994;73(10):2613–2618

12. Burkhardt BR, Eades E: The effect of Biocell texturing and povidone-iodine irrigation on capsular contracture around saline-inflatable breast implants. Plast Reconstr Surg 1995;96(6):1317–1325

13. Hakelius L, Ohlsen L: Tendency to capsular contracture around smooth and textured gel-filled silicone mammary implants: a 5-year follow-up. Plast Reconstr Surg 1997;100(6):1566–1569

14. Burkhardt BR, Demas CP: The effect of Siltex texturing and povidone-iodine irrigation on capsular contracture around saline inflatable breast implants. Plast Reconstr Surg 1994;93(1):123–128

15. Coleman DJ, Foo ITH, Sharpe DT: Textured or smooth implants for breast augmentation? A prospective controlled trial. Br J Plast Surg 1991;44(6):444–448

16. Hakelius L, Ohlsen L: A clinical comparison of the tendency to capsular contracture between smooth and textured gel-filled silicone mammary implants. Plast Reconstr Surg 1992;90(2):247–254

17. Danino AM, Basmacioglu P, Saito S, Rocher FBA, Blanchet-Bardon C, Revol M, Servant J-M: Comparison of the capsular response to the Biocell RTV and Mentor 1600 Siltex breast implant surface texturing: a scanning electron microscopic study. Plast Reconstr Surg 2001;108(7):2047–2052

18. Maxwell GP, Falcone PA: Eighty-four consecutive breast reconstructions using a textured silicone tissue expander. Plast Reconstr Surg 1992;89(6):1022–1034; discussion 1035–1036

19. Slade C: Subcutaneous mastectomy. Acute complications and long-term follow-up. Plast Reconstr Surg 1984;73(1):84–90

20. Baker J: Augmentation mammaplasty. Plast Reconstr Surg 1999;103(6):1763–1765

Subject Index